A Textbook of
Clinical Pharmacology
and Therapeutics

A Textbook of
Clinical Pharmacology and Therapeutics

FIFTH EDITION

JAMES M RITTER MA DPHIL FRCP FMedSci FBPHARMACOLS
Professor of Clinical Pharmacology at King's College London School of Medicine,
Guy's, King's and St Thomas' Hospitals, London, UK

LIONEL D LEWIS MA MB BCH MD FRCP
Professor of Medicine, Pharmacology and Toxicology at Dartmouth Medical School and
the Dartmouth-Hitchcock Medical Center, Lebanon, New Hampshire, USA

TIMOTHY GK MANT BSc FFPM FRCP
Senior Medical Advisor, Quintiles, Guy's Drug Research Unit, and Visiting Professor at
King's College London School of Medicine, Guy's, King's and St Thomas' Hospitals,
London, UK

ALBERT FERRO PHD FRCP FBPHARMACOLS
Reader in Clinical Pharmacology and Honorary Consultant Physician at King's College
London School of Medicine, Guy's, King's and St Thomas' Hospitals, London, UK

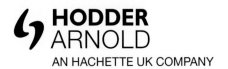
HODDER
ARNOLD
AN HACHETTE UK COMPANY

First published in Great Britain in 1981
Second edition 1986
Third edition 1995
Fourth edition 1999
This fifth edition published in Great Britain in 2008 by
Hodder Arnold, an imprint of Hodden Education, an Hachette UK Company,
338 Euston Road, London NW1 3BH

http://www.hoddereducation.com

©2008 James M Ritter, Lionel D Lewis, Timothy GK Mant and Albert Ferro

Whilst the advice and information in this book are believed to be true and accurate at the date of
going to press, neither the authors nor the publisher can accept any legal responsibility or liability
for any errors or omissions that may be made. In particular, (but without limiting the generality
of the preceding disclaimer) every effort has been made to check drug dosages; however it is
still possible that errors have been missed. Furthermore, dosage schedules are constantly being
revised and new side-effects recognized. For these reasons the reader is strongly urged to consult
the drug companies' printed instructions before administering any of the drugs recommended in
this book.

British Library Cataloguing in Publication Data
A catalogue record for this book is available from the British Library

Library of Congress Cataloging-in-Publication Data
A catalog record for this book is available from the Library of Congress

ISBN   978-0-340-90046-8

4 5 6 7 8 9 10

Commissioning Editor: Sara Purdy
Project Editor: Jane Tod
Production Controller: Andre Sim
Cover Design: Laura de Grasse
Indexer: John Sampson

Typeset in 9/12 pt palatino by Macmillan Publishing Solutions (www.macmillansolutions.com)
Printed and bound in India

What do you think about this book? Or any other Hodder Arnold title?
Please visit our website: www.hoddereducation.com

*This fifth edition is dedicated to the memory of Professors Howard Rogers and John Trounce,
two of the three authors of this textbook's first edition.*

COMPANION WEBSITE

The fifth edition of *A Textbook of Clinical Pharmacology and Therapeutics* is accompanied by an exciting new website featuring the images from the book for you to download. To visit the book's website, please go to www.hodderplus.com/clinicalpharmacology.

Your username is: student009
Your password is: pharma

CONTENTS

FOREWORD

John Trounce, who was the senior author of the first edition of this textbook, died on the 16 April 2007.

He considered a text in clinical pharmacology suitable for his undergraduate and postgraduate students to be an important part of the programme he developed in his department at Guy's Hospital Medical School, London. It is difficult to imagine today how much resistance from the medical and pharmacological establishments Trounce had to overcome in order to set up an academic department, a focussed course in the medical curriculum and a separate exam in final MB in clinical pharmacology. In other words, he helped to change a 'non-subject' into one of the most important areas of study for medical students. He was also aware of the need for a high quality textbook in clinical pharmacology that could also be used by nurses, pharmacists, pharmacology science students and doctors preparing for higher qualifications. (For example, it has been said that nobody knows more about acute pharmacology than an anaesthetist.)

The present edition of the textbook reflects the advances in therapeutics since the publication of the fourth edition. It is interesting to follow in all the editions of the book, for example, how the treatment of tumours has progressed. It was about the time of the first edition that Trounce set up the first oncology clinic at Guy's Hospital in which he investigated the value of combined radiation and chemotherapy and drug cocktails in the treatment of lymphomas. John Trounce was pleased to see his textbook (and his subject) in the expert hands of Professor Ritter and his colleagues.

Roy Spector
Professor Emeritus in Applied Pharmacology, University of London

PREFACE

Clinical pharmacology is the science of drug use in humans. Clinicians of all specialties prescribe drugs on a daily basis, and this is both one of the most useful but also one of the most dangerous activities of our professional lives. Understanding the principles of clinical pharmacology is the basis of safe and effective therapeutic practice, which is why this subject forms an increasingly important part of the medical curriculum.

This textbook is addressed primarily to medical students and junior doctors of all specialties, but also to other professionals who increasingly prescribe medicines (including pharmacists, nurses and some other allied professionals). Clinical pharmacology is a fast moving subject and the present edition has been completely revised and updated. It differs from the fourth edition in that it concentrates exclusively on aspects that students should know and understand, rather than including a lot of reference material. This has enabled us to keep its length down. Another feature has been to include many new illustrations to aid in grasping mechanisms and principles.

The first section deals with general principles including pharmacodynamics, pharmacokinetics and the various factors that modify drug disposition and drug interaction. We have kept algebraic formulations to a minimum. Drug metabolism is approached from a practical viewpoint, with discussion of the exciting new concept of personalized medicine. Adverse drug reactions and the use of drugs at the extremes of age and in pregnancy are covered, and the introduction of new drugs is discussed from the viewpoint of students who will see many new treatments introduced during their professional careers. Many patients use herbal or other alternative medicines and there is a new chapter on this important topic. There is a chapter on gene and cell-based therapies, which are just beginning to enter clinical practice. The remaining sections of the book deal comprehensively with major systems (nervous, musculoskeletal, cardiovascular, respiratory, alimentary, renal, endocrine, blood, skin and eye) and with multi-system issues including treatment of infections, malignancies, immune disease, addiction and poisoning.

JAMES M RITTER

LIONEL D LEWIS

TIMOTHY GK MANT

ALBERT FERRO

ACKNOWLEDGEMENTS

We would like to thank many colleagues who have helped us with advice and criticism in the revision and updating of this fifth edition. Their expertise in many specialist areas has enabled us to emphasize those factors most relevant. For their input into this edition and/or the previous edition we are, in particular, grateful to Professor Roy Spector, Professor Alan Richens, Dr Anne Dornhorst, Dr Michael Isaac, Dr Terry Gibson, Dr Paul Glue, Dr Mark Kinirons, Dr Jonathan Barker, Dr Patricia McElhatton, Dr Robin Stott, Mr David Calver, Dr Jas Gill, Dr Bev Holt, Dr Zahid Khan, Dr Beverley Hunt, Dr Piotr Bajorek, Miss Susanna Gilmour-White, Dr Mark Edwards, Dr Michael Marsh, Mrs Joanna Tempowski. We would also like to thank Dr Peter Lloyd and Dr John Beadle for their assistance with figures.

PART I

GENERAL PRINCIPLES

INTRODUCTION TO THERAPEUTICS

USE OF DRUGS

People consult a doctor to find out what (if anything) is wrong (the diagnosis), and what should be done about it (the treatment). If they are well, they may nevertheless want to know how future problems can be prevented. Depending on the diagnosis, treatment may consist of reassurance, surgery or other interventions. Drugs are very often either the primary therapy or an adjunct to another modality (e.g. the use of anaesthetics in patients undergoing surgery). Sometimes contact with the doctor is initiated because of a public health measure (e.g. through a screening programme). Again, drug treatment is sometimes needed. Consequently, doctors of nearly all specialties use drugs extensively, and need to understand the scientific basis on which therapeutic use is founded.

A century ago, physicians had only a handful of effective drugs (e.g. morphia, quinine, ether, aspirin and digitalis leaf) at their disposal. Thousands of potent drugs have since been introduced, and pharmaceutical chemists continue to discover new and better drugs. With advances in genetics, cellular and molecular science, it is likely that progress will accelerate and huge changes in therapeutics are inevitable. Medical students and doctors in training therefore need to learn something of the principles of therapeutics, in order to prepare themselves to adapt to such change. General principles are discussed in the first part of this book, while current approaches to treatment are dealt with in subsequent parts.

ADVERSE EFFECTS AND RISK/BENEFIT

Medicinal chemistry has contributed immeasurably to human health, but this has been achieved at a price, necessitating a new philosophy. A physician in Sir William Osler's day in the nineteenth century could safely adhere to the Hippocratic principle 'first do no harm', because the opportunities for doing good were so limited. The discovery of effective drugs has transformed this situation, at the expense of very real risks of doing harm. For example, cures of leukaemias, Hodgkin's disease and testicular carcinomas have been achieved through a preparedness to accept a degree of containable harm. Similar considerations apply in other disease areas.

All effective drugs have adverse effects, and therapeutic judgements based on risk/benefit ratio permeate all fields of medicine. Drugs are the physician's prime therapeutic tools, and just as a misplaced scalpel can spell disaster, so can a thoughtless prescription. Some of the more dramatic instances make for gruesome reading in the annual reports of the medical defence societies, but perhaps as important is the morbidity and expense caused by less dramatic but more common errors.

How are prescribing errors to be minimized? By combining a general knowledge of the pathogenesis of the disease to be treated and of the drugs that may be effective for that disease with specific knowledge about the particular patient. Dukes and Swartz, in their valuable work *Responsibility for drug-induced injury*, list eight basic duties of prescribers:

1. *restrictive use* – is drug therapy warranted?
2. *careful choice* of an appropriate drug and dose regimen with due regard to the likely risk/benefit ratio, available alternatives, and the patient's needs, susceptibilities and preferences;
3. *consultation and consent*;
4. *prescription and recording*;
5. *explanation*;
6. *supervision* (including monitoring);
7. *termination*, as appropriate;
8. *conformity* with the law relating to prescribing.

As a minimum, the following should be considered when deciding on a therapeutic plan:

1. age;
2. coexisting disease, especially renal and or hepatic impairment;
3. the possibility of pregnancy;
4. drug history;

5. the best that can reasonably be hoped for in this individual patient;
6. the patient's beliefs and goals.

DRUG HISTORY AND THERAPEUTIC PLAN

In the twenty-first century, a reliable drug history involves questioning the patient (and sometimes family, neighbours, other physicians, etc.). What prescription tablets, medicines, drops, contraceptives, creams, suppositories or pessaries are being taken? What over-the-counter remedies are being used including herbal or 'alternative' therapies? Does the patient use drugs socially or for 'life-style' purposes? Have they suffered from drug-induced allergies or other serious reactions? Have they been treated for anything similar in the past, and if so with what, and did it do the job or were there any problems? Has the patient experienced any problems with anaesthesia? Have there been any serious drug reactions among family members?

The prescriber must be both meticulous and humble, especially when dealing with an unfamiliar drug. Checking contraindications, special precautions and doses in a formulary such as the British National Formulary (BNF) (British Medical Association and Royal Pharmaceutical Society of Great Britain 2007) is the minimum requirement. The proposed plan is discussed with the patient, including alternatives, goals, possible adverse effects, their likelihood and measures to be taken if these arise. The patient must understand what is intended and be happy with the means proposed to achieve these ends. (This will not, of course, be possible in demented or delirious patients, where discussion will be with any available family members.) The risks of causing harm must be minimized. Much of the 'art' of medicine lies in the ability of the prescriber to agree to compromises that are acceptable to an individual patient, and underlies concordance (i.e. agreement between patient and prescriber) with a therapeutic plan.

Prescriptions must be written clearly and legibly, conforming to legal requirements. Electronic prescribing is currently being introduced in the UK, so these are changing. Generic names should generally be used (exceptions are mentioned later in the book), together with dose, frequency and duration of treatment, and paper prescriptions signed. It is prudent to print the prescriber's name, address and telephone number to facilitate communication from the pharmacist should a query arise. Appropriate follow up must be arranged.

FORMULARIES AND RESTRICTED LISTS

Historically, formularies listed the components of mixtures prescribed until around 1950. The perceived need for hospital formularies disappeared transiently when such mixtures were replaced by proprietary products prepared by the pharmaceutical industry. The BNF summarizes products licensed in the UK. Because of the bewildering array, including many alternatives, many hospital and primary care trusts have reintroduced formularies that are essentially restricted lists of the drugs stocked by the institution's pharmacy, from which local doctors are encouraged to prescribe. The objectives are to encourage rational prescribing, to simplify purchasing and storage of drugs, and to obtain the 'best buy' among alternative preparations. Such formularies have the advantage of encouraging consistency, and once a decision has been made with input from local consultant prescribers they are usually well accepted.

SCIENTIFIC BASIS OF USE OF DRUGS IN HUMANS

The scientific basis of drug action is provided by the discipline of pharmacology. Clinical pharmacology deals with the effects of drugs in humans. It entails the study of the interaction of drugs with their receptors, the transduction (second messenger) systems to which these are linked and the changes that they bring about in cells, organs and the whole organism. These processes (what the drug does to the body) are called 'pharmacodynamics'. The use of drugs in society is encompassed by pharmacoepidemiology and pharmacoeconomics – both highly politicized disciplines!

Man is a mammal and animal studies are essential, but their predictive value is limited. Modern methods of molecular and cell biology permit expression of human genes, including those that code for receptors and key signal transduction elements, in cells and in transgenic animals, and are revolutionizing these areas and hopefully improving the relevance of preclinical pharmacology and toxicology.

Important adverse effects sometimes but not always occur in other species. Consequently, when new drugs are used to treat human diseases, considerable uncertainties remain. Early-phase human studies are usually conducted in healthy volunteers, except when toxicity is inevitable (e.g. cytotoxic drugs used for cancer treatment, see Chapter 48).

Basic pharmacologists often use isolated preparations, where the concentration of drug in the organ bath is controlled precisely. Such preparations may be stable for minutes to hours. In therapeutics, drugs are administered to the whole organism by a route that is as convenient and safe as possible (usually by mouth), for days if not years. Consequently, the drug concentration in the vicinity of the receptors is usually unknown, and long-term effects involving alterations in receptor density or function, or the activation or modulation of homeostatic control mechanisms may be of overriding importance. The processes of absorption, distribution, metabolism and elimination (what the body does to the drug) determine the drug concentration–time relationships in plasma and at the receptors. These processes comprise 'pharmacokinetics'. There is considerable inter-individual variation due to both inherited and acquired factors, notably disease of the organs responsible for drug metabolism and excretion. Pharmacokinetic modelling is crucial in drug development to plan a rational therapeutic regime, and understanding pharmacokinetics is also important for prescribers individualizing therapy for a particular patient. Pharmacokinetic principles are described in Chapter 3 from the point of view of the prescriber. Genetic influences on pharmacodynamics and pharmacokinetics (pharmacogenetics) are discussed in Chapter 14 and effects of disease are addressed in Chapter 7, and the use of drugs in pregnancy and at extremes of age is discussed in Chapters 9–11.

There are no good animal models of many important human diseases. The only way to ensure that a drug with promising pharmacological actions is effective in treating or preventing disease is to perform a specific kind of human experiment, called a clinical trial. Prescribing doctors must understand the strengths and limitations of such trials, the principles of which are described in Chapter 15, if they are to evaluate the literature on drugs introduced during their professional lifetimes. Ignorance leaves the physician at the mercy of sources of information that are biased by commercial interests. Sources of unbiased drug information include Dollery's encyclopaedic *Therapeutic drugs*, 2nd edn (published by Churchill Livingstone in 1999), which is an invaluable source of reference. Publications such as the *Adverse Reaction Bulletin*, *Prescribers Journal* and the succinctly argued *Drug and Therapeutics Bulletin* provide up-to-date discussions of therapeutic issues of current importance.

Key points

- Drugs are prescribed by physicians of all specialties.
- This carries risks as well as benefits.
- Therapy is optimized by combining general knowledge of drugs with knowledge of an individual patient.
- Evidence of efficacy is based on clinical trials.
- Adverse drug effects may be seen in clinical trials, but the drug side effect profile becomes clearer only when widely prescribed.
- Rational prescribing is encouraged by local formularies.

Case history

A general practitioner reviews the medication of an 86-year-old woman with hypertension and multi-infarct dementia, who is living in a nursing home. Her family used to visit daily, but she no longer recognizes them, and needs help with dressing, washing and feeding. Drugs include bendroflumethiazide, atenolol, atorvastatin, aspirin, haloperidol, imipramine, lactulose and senna. On examination, she smells of urine and has several bruises on her head, but otherwise seems well cared for. She is calm, but looks pale and bewildered, and has a pulse of 48 beats/min regular, and blood pressure 162/96 mmHg lying and 122/76 mmHg standing, during which she becomes sweaty and distressed. Her rectum is loaded with hard stool. Imipramine was started three years previously. Urine culture showed only a light mixed growth. All of the medications were stopped and manual evacuation of faeces performed. Stool was negative for occult blood and the full blood count was normal. Two weeks later, the patient was brighter and more mobile. She remained incontinent of urine at night, but no longer during the day, her heart rate was 76 beats/min and her blood pressure was 208/108 mmHg lying and standing.
Comment
It is seldom helpful to give drugs in order to prevent something that has already happened (in this case multi-infarct dementia), and any benefit in preventing further ischaemic events has to be balanced against the harm done by the polypharmacy. In this case, drug-related problems probably include postural hypotension (due to imipramine, bendroflumethiazide and haloperidol), reduced mobility (due to haloperidol), constipation (due to imipramine and haloperidol), urinary incontinence (worsened by bendroflumethiazide and drugs causing constipation) and bradycardia (due to atenolol). Drug-induced torsades de pointes (a form of ventricular tachycardia, see Chapter 32) is another issue. Despite her pallor, the patient was not bleeding into the gastro-intestinal tract, but aspirin could have caused this.

FURTHER READING

Dukes MNG, Swartz B. *Responsibility for drug-induced injury.* Amsterdam: Elsevier, 1988.

Weatherall DJ. Scientific medicine and the art of healing. In: Warrell DA, Cox TM, Firth JD, Benz EJ (eds), *Oxford textbook of medicine*, 4th edn. Oxford: Oxford University Press, 2005.

CHAPTER 2

MECHANISMS OF DRUG ACTION (PHARMACODYNAMICS)

INTRODUCTION

Pharmacodynamics is the study of effects of drugs on biological processes. An example is shown in Figure 2.1, demonstrating and comparing the effects of a proton pump inhibitor and of a histamine H_2 receptor antagonist (both drugs used for the treatment of peptic ulceration and other disorders related to gastric hyperacidity) on gastric pH. Many mediators exert their effects as a result of high-affinity binding to specific receptors in plasma membranes or cell cytoplasm/nuclei, and many therapeutically important drugs exert their effects by combining with these receptors and either mimicking the effect of the natural mediator (in which case they are called 'agonists') or blocking it

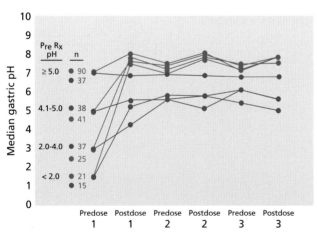

Figure 2.1: Effect of omeprazole and cimetidine on gastric pH in a group of critically ill patients. This was a study comparing the effect of immediate-release omeprazole with a loading dose of 40 mg, a second dose six to eight hours later, followed by 40 mg daily, with a continuous i.v. infusion of cimetidine. pH monitoring of the gastric aspirate was undertaken every two hours and immediately before and one hour after each dose. Red, omeprazole; blue, cimetidine. (Redrawn with permission from Horn JR, Hermes-DeSantis ER, Small, RE 'New Perspectives in the Management of Acid-Related Disorders: The Latest Advances in PPI Therapy'. *Medscape Today* http://www.medscape.com/viewarticle/503473_9 17 May 2005.)

(in which case they are termed 'antagonists'). Examples include oestrogens (used in contraception, Chapter 41) and anti-oestrogens (used in treating breast cancer, Chapter 48), alpha- and beta-adrenoceptor agonists and antagonists (Chapters 29 and 33) and opioids (Chapter 25).

Not all drugs work via receptors for endogenous mediators: many therapeutic drugs exert their effects by combining with an enzyme or transport protein and interfering with its function. Examples include inhibitors of angiotensin converting enzyme and serotonin reuptake. These sites of drug action are not 'receptors' in the sense of being sites of action of endogenous mediators.

Whether the site of action of a drug is a receptor or another macromolecule, binding is usually highly specific, with precise steric recognition between the small molecular ligand and the binding site on its macromolecular target. Binding is usually reversible. Occasionally, however, covalent bonds are formed with irreversible loss of function, e.g. aspirin binding to cyclo-oxygenase (Chapter 30).

Most drugs produce graded concentration-/dose-related effects which can be plotted as a dose–response curve. Such curves are often approximately hyperbolic (Figure 2.2a). If plotted semi-logarithmically this gives an S-shaped ('sigmoidal') shape (Figure 2.2b). This method of plotting dose–response curves facilitates quantitative analysis (see below) of full agonists (which produce graded responses up to a maximum value), antagonists (which produce no response on their own, but reduce the response to an agonist) and partial agonists (which produce some response, but to a lower maximum value than that of a full agonist, and antagonize full agonists) (Figure 2.3).

RECEPTORS AND SIGNAL TRANSDUCTION

Drugs are often potent (i.e. they produce effects at low concentration) and specific (i.e. small changes in structure lead to profound changes in potency). High potency is a consequence of high binding affinity for specific macromolecular receptors.

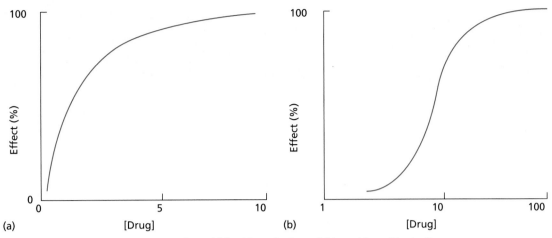

Figure 2.2: Concentration/dose–response curves plotted (a) arithmetically and (b) semi-logarithmically.

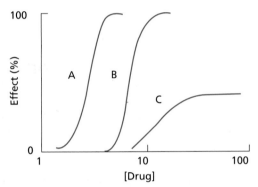

Figure 2.3: Concentration/dose–response curves of two full agonists (A, B) of different potency, and of a partial agonist (C).

Receptors were originally classified by reference to the relative potencies of agonists and antagonists on preparations containing different receptors. The order of potency of isoprenaline > adrenaline > noradrenaline on tissues rich in β-receptors, such as the heart, contrasts with the reverse order in α-receptor-mediated responses, such as vasoconstriction in resistance arteries supplying the skin. Quantitative potency data are best obtained from comparisons of different competitive antagonists, as explained below. Such data are supplemented, but not replaced, by radiolabelled ligand-binding studies. In this way, adrenoceptors were divided first into α and β, then subdivided into α_1/α_2 and β_1/β_2. Many other useful receptor classifications, including those of cholinoceptors, histamine receptors, serotonin receptors, benzodiazepine receptors, glutamate receptors and others have been proposed on a similar basis. Labelling with irreversible antagonists permitted receptor solubilization and purification. Oligonucleotide probes based on the deduced sequence were then used to extract the full-length DNA sequence coding different receptors. As receptors are cloned and expressed in cells in culture, the original functional classifications have been supported and extended. Different receptor subtypes are analogous to different forms of isoenzymes, and a rich variety has been uncovered – especially in the central nervous system – raising hopes for novel drugs targeting these.

Despite this complexity, it turns out that receptors fall into only four 'superfamilies' each linked to distinct types of signal transduction mechanism (i.e. the events that link receptor activation with cellular response) (Figure 2.4). Three families are located in the cell membrane, while the fourth is intracellular (e.g. steroid hormone receptors). They comprise:

- Fast (millisecond responses) neurotransmitters (e.g. nicotinic receptors), linked directly to a transmembrane ion channel.
- Slower neurotransmitters and hormones (e.g. muscarinic receptors) linked to an intracellular G-protein ('GPCR').
- Receptors linked to an enzyme on the inner membrane (e.g. insulin receptors) are slower still.
- Intranuclear receptors (e.g. gonadal and glucocorticosteroid hormones): ligands bind to their receptor in cytoplasm and the complex then migrates to the nucleus and binds to specific DNA sites, producing alterations in gene transcription and altered protein synthesis. Such effects occur over a time-course of minutes to hours.

AGONISTS

Agonists activate receptors for endogenous mediators – e.g. **salbutamol** is an agonist at β_2-adrenoceptors (Chapter 33). The consequent effect may be excitatory (e.g. increased heart rate) or inhibitory (e.g. relaxation of airway smooth muscle). Agonists at nicotinic acetylcholine receptors (e.g. **suxamethonium**, Chapter 24) exert an inhibitory effect (neuromuscular blockade) by causing long-lasting depolarization at the neuromuscular junction, and hence inactivation of the voltage-dependent sodium channels that initiate the action potential.

Endogenous ligands have sometimes been discovered long after the drugs that act on their receptors. Endorphins and enkephalins (endogenous ligands of morphine receptors) were discovered many years after morphine. Anandamide is a central transmitter that activates CB (cannabis) receptors (Chapter 53).

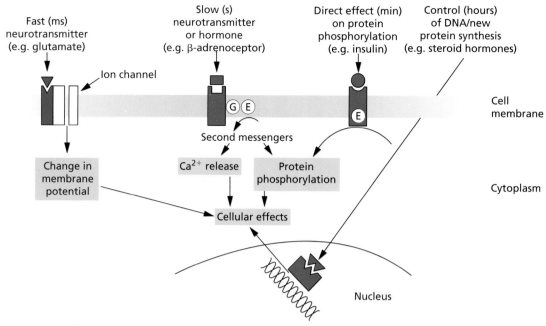

Figure 2.4: Receptors and signal transduction. G, G-protein; E, enzyme; Ca, calcium.

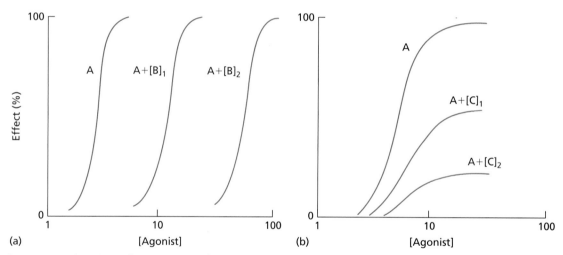

Figure 2.5: Drug antagonism. Control concentration/dose–response curves for an agonist A together with curves in the presence of (a) a competitive antagonist B and (b) a non-competitive antagonist C. Increasing concentrations of the competitive antagonist ($[B]_1$, $[B]_2$) cause a parallel shift to the right of the log dose–effect curve (a), while the non-competitive antagonist ($[C]_1$, $[C]_2$) flattens the curve and reduces its maximum (b).

ANTAGONISM

Competitive antagonists combine with the same receptor as an endogenous agonist (e.g. **ranitidine** at histamine H_2-receptors), but fail to activate it. When combined with the receptor, they prevent access of the endogenous mediator. The complex between competitive antagonist and receptor is reversible. Provided that the dose of agonist is increased sufficiently, a maximal effect can still be obtained, i.e. the antagonism is surmountable. If a dose (C) of agonist causes a defined effect when administered alone, then the dose (C′) needed to produce the same effect in the presence of antagonist is a multiple (C′/C)

known as the dose ratio (r). This results in the familiar parallel shift to the right of the log dose–response curve, since the addition of a constant length on a logarithmic scale corresponds to multiplication by a constant factor (Figure 2.5a). β-Adrenoceptor antagonists are examples of reversible competitive antagonists. By contrast, antagonists that do not combine with the same receptor (non-competitive antagonists) or drugs that combine irreversibly with their receptors, reduce the slope of the log dose–response curve and depress its maximum (Figure 2.5b). Physiological antagonism describes the situation where two drugs have opposing effects (e.g. adrenaline relaxes bronchial smooth muscle, whereas histamine contracts it).

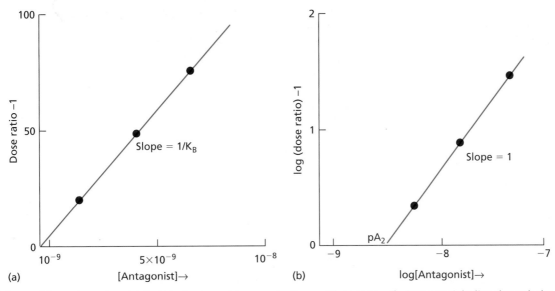

Figure 2.6: Competitive antagonism. (a) A plot of antagonist concentration vs. (dose ratio −1) gives a straight line through the origin. (b) A log–log plot (a Schildt plot) gives a straight line of unit slope. The potency of the antagonist (pA$_2$) is determined from the intercept of the Schildt plot.

The relationship between the concentration of a competitive antagonist [B], and the dose ratio (r) was worked out by Gaddum and by Schildt, and is:

$$r - 1 = [B]/K_B,$$

where K_B is the dissociation equilibrium constant of the reversible reaction of the antagonist with its receptor. K_B has units of concentration and is the concentration of antagonist needed to occupy half the receptors in the absence of agonist. The lower the value of K_B, the more potent is the drug. If several concentrations of a competitive antagonist are studied and the dose ratio is measured at each concentration, a plot of (r − 1) against [B] yields a straight line through the origin with a slope of $1/K_B$ (Figure 2.6a). Such measurements provided the means of classifying and subdividing receptors in terms of the relative potencies of different antagonists.

PARTIAL AGONISTS

Some drugs combine with receptors and activate them, but are incapable of eliciting a maximal response, no matter how high their concentration may be. These are known as partial agonists, and are said to have low efficacy. Several partial agonists are used in therapeutics, including **buprenorphine** (a partial agonist at morphine μ-receptors, Chapter 25) and **oxprenolol** (partial agonist at β-adrenoceptors).

Full agonists can elicit a maximal response when only a small proportion of the receptors is occupied (underlying the concept of 'spare' receptors), but this is not the case with partial agonists, where a substantial proportion of the receptors need to be occupied to cause a response. This has two clinical consequences. First, partial agonists antagonize the effect of a full agonist, because most of the receptors are occupied with low-efficacy partial agonist with which the full agonist must compete. Second, it is more difficult to reverse the effects of a partial agonist, such as **buprenorphine**, with a competitive antagonist such as **naloxone**, than it is to reverse the effects of a full agonist such as **morphine**. A larger fraction of the receptors is occupied by **buprenorphine** than by **morphine**, and a much higher concentration of **naloxone** is required to compete successfully and displace **buprenorphine** from the receptors.

SLOW PROCESSES

Prolonged exposure of receptors to agonists, as frequently occurs in therapeutic use, can cause down-regulation or desensitization. Desensitization is sometimes specific for a particular agonist (when it is referred to as 'homologous desensitization'), or there may be cross-desensitization to different agonists ('heterologous desensitization'). Membrane receptors may become internalized. Alternatively, G-protein-mediated linkage between receptors and effector enzymes (e.g. adenylyl cyclase) may be disrupted. Since G-proteins link several distinct receptors to the same effector molecule, this can give rise to heterologous desensitization. Desensitization is probably involved in the tolerance that occurs during prolonged administration of drugs, such as **morphine** or benzodiazepines (see Chapters 18 and 25).

Therapeutic effects sometimes depend on induction of tolerance. For example, analogues of gonadotrophin-releasing hormone (GnRH), such as **goserelin** or **buserelin**, are used to treat patients with metastatic prostate cancer (Chapter 48). Gonadotrophin-releasing hormone is released physiologically in a pulsatile manner. During continuous treatment with buserelin, there is initial stimulation of luteinizing hormone (LH) and follicle-stimulating hormone (FSH) release, followed by receptor desensitization and suppression of LH and FSH release. This results in regression of the hormone-sensitive tumour.

Conversely, reduced exposure of a cell or tissue to an agonist (e.g. by denervation) results in increased receptor numbers and supersensitivity. Prolonged use of antagonists may produce an analogous effect. One example of clinical importance is increased β-adrenoceptor numbers following prolonged use of beta-blockers. Abrupt drug withdrawal can lead to tachycardia and worsening angina in patients who are being treated for ischaemic heart disease.

NON-RECEPTOR MECHANISMS

In contrast to high-potency/high-selectivity drugs which combine with specific receptors, some drugs exert their effects via simple physical properties or chemical reactions due to their presence in some body compartment. Examples include antacids (which neutralize gastric acid), osmotic diuretics (which increase the osmolality of renal tubular fluid), and bulk and lubricating laxatives. These agents are of low potency and specificity, and hardly qualify as 'drugs' in the usual sense at all, although some of them are useful medicines. Oxygen is an example of a highly specific therapeutic agent that is used in high concentrations (Chapter 33). Metal chelating agents, used for example in the treatment of poisoning with ferrous sulphate, are examples of drugs that exert their effects through interaction with small molecular species rather than with macromolecules, yet which possess significant specificity.

General anaesthetics (Chapter 24) have low molar potencies determined by their oil/water partition coefficients, and low specificity.

Key points

- Most drugs are potent and specific; they combine with receptors for endogenous mediators or with high affinity sites on enzymes or other proteins, e.g. ion-transport mechanisms.
- There are four superfamilies of receptors; three are membrane bound:
  - directly linked to ion channel (e.g. nicotinic acetylcholine receptor);
  - linked via G-proteins to an enzyme, often adenylyl cyclase (e.g. β_2-receptors);
  - directly coupled to the catalytic domain of an enzyme (e.g. insulin)
- The fourth superfamily is intracellular, binds to DNA and controls gene transcription and protein synthesis (e.g. steroid receptors).
- Many drugs work by antagonizing agonists. Drug antagonism can be:
  - competitive;
  - non-competitive;
  - physiological.
- Partial agonists produce an effect that is less than the maximum effect of a full agonist. They antagonize full agonists.
- Tolerance can be important during chronic administration of drugs acting on receptors, e.g. central nervous system (CNS) active agents.

Case history

A young man is brought unconscious into the Accident and Emergency Department. He is unresponsive, hypoventilating, has needle tracks on his arms and pinpoint pupils. Naloxone is administered intravenously and within 30 seconds the patient is fully awake and breathing normally. He is extremely abusive and leaves hospital having attempted to assault the doctor.

Comment

The clinical picture is of opioid overdose, and this was confirmed by the response to naloxone, a competitive antagonist of opioids at μ-receptors (Chapter 25). It would have been wise to have restrained the patient before administering naloxone, which can precipitate withdrawal symptoms. He will probably become comatose again shortly after discharging himself, as naloxone has a much shorter elimination half-life than opioids such as morphine or diacetyl-morphine (heroin), so the agonist effect of the overdose will be reasserted as the concentration of the opiate antagonist falls.

FURTHER READING

Rang HP. The receptor concept: pharmacology's big idea. *British Journal of Pharmacology* 2006; 147 (Suppl. 1): 9–16.

Rang HP, Dale MM, Ritter JM, Flower RD. Chapter 2, How drugs act: general principles. Chapter 3, How drugs act: molecular aspects. In: *Rang and Dale's pharmacology*, 6th edn. London: Churchill Livingstone, 2007.

PHARMACOKINETICS

INTRODUCTION

Pharmacokinetics is the study of drug absorption, distribution, metabolism and excretion (ADME) – 'what the body does to the drug'. Understanding pharmacokinetic principles, combined with specific information regarding an individual drug and patient, underlies the individualized optimal use of the drug (e.g. choice of drug, route of administration, dose and dosing interval).

Pharmacokinetic modelling is based on drastically simplifying assumptions; but even so, it can be mathematically cumbersome, sadly rendering this important area unintelligible to many clinicians. In this chapter, we introduce the basic concepts by considering three clinical dosing situations:

- constant-rate intravenous infusion;
- bolus-dose injection;
- repeated dosing.

Bulk flow in the bloodstream is rapid, as is diffusion over short distances after drugs have penetrated phospholipid membranes, so the rate-limiting step in drug distribution is usually penetration of these membrane barriers. Permeability is determined mainly by the lipid solubility of the drug, polar water-soluble drugs being transferred slowly, whereas lipid-soluble, non-polar drugs diffuse rapidly across lipid-rich membranes. In addition, some drugs are actively transported by specific carriers.

The simplest pharmacokinetic model treats the body as a well-stirred single compartment in which an administered drug distributes instantaneously, and from which it is eliminated. Many drugs are eliminated at a rate proportional to their concentration – 'first-order' elimination. A single (one)-compartment model with first-order elimination often approximates the clinical situation surprisingly well once absorption and distribution have occurred. We start by considering this, and then describe some important deviations from it.

CONSTANT-RATE INFUSION

If a drug is administered intravenously via a constant-rate pump, and blood sampled from a distant vein for measurement of drug concentration, a plot of plasma concentration versus time can be constructed (Figure 3.1). The concentration rises from zero, rapidly at first and then more slowly until a plateau (representing steady state) is approached. At steady state, the rate of input of drug to the body equals the rate of elimination. The concentration at plateau is the steady-state concentration (C_{SS}). This depends on the rate of drug infusion and on its 'clearance'. The clearance is defined as the volume of fluid (usually plasma) from which the drug is totally eliminated (i.e. 'cleared') per unit time. At steady state,

administration rate = elimination rate

elimination rate = $C_{SS} \times$ clearance

so

clearance = administration rate$/C_{SS}$

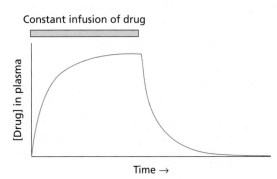

Constant infusion of drug

Figure 3.1: Plasma concentration of a drug during and after a constant intravenous infusion as indicated by the bar.

Clearance is the best measure of the efficiency with which a drug is eliminated from the body, whether by renal excretion, metabolism or a combination of both. The concept will be familiar from physiology, where clearances of substances with particular properties are used as measures of physiologically important processes, including glomerular filtration rate and renal or hepatic plasma flow. For therapeutic drugs, knowing the clearance in an individual patient enables the physician to adjust the maintenance dose to achieve a desired target steady-state concentration, since

required administration rate = desired $C_{SS} \times$ clearance

This is useful in drug development. It is also useful in clinical practice when therapy is guided by plasma drug concentrations. However, such situations are limited (Chapter 8). Furthermore, some chemical pathology laboratories report plasma concentrations of drugs in molar terms, whereas drug doses are usually expressed in units of mass. Consequently, one needs to know the molecular weight of the drug to calculate the rate of administration required to achieve a desired plasma concentration.

When drug infusion is stopped, the plasma concentration declines towards zero. The time taken for plasma concentration to halve is the half-life ($t_{1/2}$). A one-compartment model with first-order elimination predicts an exponential decline in concentration when the infusion is discontinued, as shown in Figure 3.1. After a second half-life has elapsed, the concentration will have halved again (i.e. a 75% drop in concentration to 25% of the original concentration), and so on. The increase in drug concentration when the infusion is started is also exponential, being the inverse of the decay curve. This has a very important clinical implication, namely that $t_{1/2}$ not only determines the time-course of disappearance when administration is stopped, but also predicts the time-course of its accumulation to steady state when administration is started.

Half-life is a very useful concept, as explained below. However, it is not a direct measure of drug elimination, since

differences in $t_{1/2}$ can be caused either by differences in the efficiency of elimination (i.e. the clearance) or differences in another important parameter, the apparent volume of distribution (V_d). Clearance and not $t_{1/2}$ must therefore be used when a measure of the efficiency with which a drug is eliminated is required.

SINGLE-BOLUS DOSE

The apparent volume of distribution (V_d) defines the relationship between the mass of a bolus dose of a drug and the plasma concentration that results. V_d is a multiplying factor relating the amount of drug in the body to the plasma concentration, C_p (i.e. the amount of drug in the body = $C_p \times V_d$). Consider a very simple physical analogy. By definition, concentration (c) is equal to mass (m) divided by volume (v):

$$c = \frac{m}{v}$$

Thus if a known mass (say 300 mg) of a substance is dissolved in a beaker containing an unknown volume (v) of water, v can be estimated by measuring the concentration of substance in a sample of solution. For instance, if the concentration is 0.1 mg/mL, we would calculate that $v = 3000$ mL ($v = m/c$). This is valid unless a fraction of the substance has become adsorbed onto the surface of the beaker, in which case the solution will be less concentrated than if all of the substance had been present dissolved in the water. If 90% of the substance is adsorbed in this way, then the concentration in solution will be 0.01 mg/mL, and the volume will be correspondingly overestimated, as 30 000 mL in this example. Based on the mass of substance dissolved and the measured concentration, we might say that it is 'as if' the substance were dissolved in 30 L of water, whereas the real volume of water in the beaker is only 3 L.

Now consider the parallel situation in which a known mass of a drug (say 300 mg) is injected intravenously into a human. Suppose that distribution within the body occurs instantaneously before any drug is eliminated, and that blood is sampled and the concentration of drug measured in the plasma is 0.1 mg/mL. We could infer that it is as if the drug has distributed in 3 L, and we would say that this is the apparent volume of distribution. If the measured plasma concentration was 0.01 mg/mL, we would say that the apparent volume of distribution was 30 L, and if the measured concentration was 0.001 mg/mL, the apparent volume of distribution would be 300 L.

What does V_d mean? From these examples it is obvious that it is not necessarily the real volume of a body compartment, since it may be greater than the volume of the whole body. At the lower end, V_d is limited by the plasma volume (approximately 3 L in an adult). This is the smallest volume in which a drug could distribute following intravenous injection, but there is no theoretical upper limit on V_d, with very large values occurring when very little of the injected dose remains in the plasma, most being taken up into fat or bound to tissues.

Key points

- Pharmacokinetics deals with how drugs are handled by the body, and includes drug absorption, distribution, metabolism and excretion.
- Clearance (*Cl*) is the volume of fluid (usually plasma) from which a drug is totally removed (by metabolism + excretion) per unit time.
- During constant i.v. infusion, the plasma drug concentration rises to a steady state (C_{SS}) determined by the administration rate (*A*) and clearance ($C_{SS} = A/Cl$).
- The rate at which C_{SS} is approached, as well as the rate of decline in plasma concentration when infusion is stopped are determined by the half-life ($t_{1/2}$).
- The volume of distribution (V_d) is an apparent volume that relates dose (*D*) to plasma concentration (*C*): it is 'as if' dose *D* mg was dissolved in V_d L to give a concentration of *C* mg/L.
- The loading dose is $C_p \times V_d$ where C_p is the desired plasma concentration.
- The maintenance dose = $C_{SS} \times Cl$, where C_{SS} is the steady-state concentration.

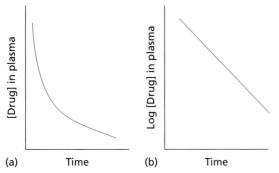

Figure 3.2: One-compartment model. Plasma concentration–time curve following a bolus dose of drug plotted (a) arithmetically and (b) semi-logarithmically. This drug fits a one-compartment model, i.e. its concentration falls exponentially with time.

In reality, processes of elimination begin as soon as the bolus dose (d) of drug is administered, the drug being cleared at a rate Cl_s (total systemic clearance). In practice, blood is sampled at intervals starting shortly after administration of the dose. Cl_s is determined from a plot of plasma concentration vs. time by measuring the area under the plasma concentration vs. time curve (AUC). (This is estimated mathematically using a method called the trapezoidal rule – important in drug development, but not in clinical practice.)

$$Cl_s = \frac{d}{\text{AUC}}$$

If the one-compartment, first-order elimination model holds, there is an exponential decline in plasma drug concentration, just as at the end of the constant rate infusion (Figure 3.2a). If the data are plotted on semi-logarithmic graph paper, with time on the abscissa, this yields a straight line with a negative slope (Figure 3.2b). Extrapolation back to zero time gives the concentration (c_0) that would have occurred at time zero, and this is used to calculate V_d:

$$V_d = \frac{d}{c_0}$$

Half-life can be read off the graph as the time between any point (c_1) and the point at which the concentration c_2 has decreased by 50%, i.e. $c_1/c_2 = 2$. The slope of the line is the elimination rate constant, k_{el}:

$$k_{el} = \frac{Cl_s}{V_d}$$

$t_{1/2}$ and k_{el} are related as follows:

$$t_{1/2} = \frac{l_n 2}{k_{el}} = \frac{0.693}{k_{el}}$$

V_d is related partly to characteristics of the drug (e.g. lipid solubility) and partly to patient characteristics (e.g. body size,

plasma protein concentration, body water and fat content). In general, highly lipid-soluble compounds that are able to penetrate cells and fatty tissues have a larger V_d than more polar water-soluble compounds.

V_d determines the peak plasma concentration after a bolus dose, so factors that influence V_d, such as body mass, need to be taken into account when deciding on dose (e.g. by expressing dose per kg body weight). Body composition varies from the usual adult values in infants or the elderly, and this also needs to be taken into account in dosing such patients (see Chapters 10 and 11).

V_d identifies the peak plasma concentration expected following a bolus dose. It is also useful to know V_d when considering dialysis as a means of accelerating drug elimination in poisoned patients (Chapter 54). Drugs with a large V_d (e.g. many tricyclic antidepressants) are not removed efficiently by haemodialysis because only a small fraction of the total drug in the body is present in plasma, which is the fluid compartment accessible to the artificial kidney.

If both V_d and $t_{1/2}$ are known, they can be used to estimate the systemic clearance of the drug using the expression:

$$Cl_s = 0.693 \times \frac{V_d}{t_{1/2}}$$

Note that clearance has units of volume/unit time (e.g. mL/min), V_d has units of volume (e.g. mL or L), $t_{1/2}$ has units of time (e.g. minutes) and 0.693 is a constant arising because $\ln -(0.5) = \ln 2 = 0.693$. This expression relates clearance to V_d and $t_{1/2}$, but unlike the steady-state situation referred to above during constant-rate infusion, or using the AUC method following a bolus, it applies only when a single-compartment model with first-order elimination kinetics is applicable.

> **Key points**
>
> - The 'one-compartment' model treats the body as a single, well-stirred compartment. Immediately following a bolus dose D, the plasma concentration rises to a peak (C_0) theoretically equal to D/V_d and then declines exponentially.
> - The rate constant of this process (k_{el}) is given by Cl/V_d. k_{el} is inversely related to $t_{1/2}$, which is given by $0.693/k_{el}$. Thus, $Cl = 0.693 \times V_d/t_{1/2}$.
> - Repeated bolus dosing gives rise to accumulation similar to that observed with constant-rate infusion, but with oscillations in plasma concentration rather than a smooth rise. The size of the oscillations is determined by the dose interval and by $t_{1/2}$. The steady state concentration is approached (87.5%) after three half-lives have elapsed.

REPEATED (MULTIPLE) DOSING

If repeated doses are administered at dosing intervals much greater than the drug's elimination half-life, little if any accumulation occurs (Figure 3.3a). Drugs are occasionally used in this way (e.g. **penicillin** to treat a mild infection), but a steady state concentration greater than some threshold value is often needed to produce a consistent effect throughout the dose interval. Figure 3.3b shows the plasma concentration–time curve when a bolus is administered repeatedly at an interval less than $t_{1/2}$. The mean concentration rises toward a plateau, as if the drug were being administered by constant-rate infusion. That is, after one half-life the mean concentration is 50% of the plateau (steady-state) concentration, after two half-lives it is 75%, after three half-lives it is 87.5%, and after four half-lives it is 93.75%. However, unlike the constant-rate infusion situation, the actual plasma concentration at any time swings above or below the mean level. Increasing the dosing frequency smoothes out the peaks and troughs between doses, while decreasing the frequency has the opposite effect. If the peaks are too high, toxicity may result, while if the troughs are too low there may be a loss of efficacy. If a drug is administered once every half-life, the peak plasma concentration (C_{max}) will be double the trough concentration (C_{min}). In practice, this amount of variation is tolerable in many therapeutic situations, so a dosing interval approximately equal to the half-life is often acceptable.

Knowing the half-life alerts the prescriber to the likely time-course over which a drug will accumulate to steady state. Drug clearance, especially renal clearance, declines with age (see Chapter 11). A further pitfall is that several drugs have active metabolites that are eliminated more slowly than

the parent drug. This is the case with several of the benzodiazepines (Chapter 18), which have active metabolites with half-lives of many days. Consequently, adverse effects (e.g. confusion) may appear only when the steady state is approached after several weeks of treatment. Such delayed effects may incorrectly be ascribed to cognitive decline associated with ageing, but resolve when the drug is stopped.

Knowing the half-life helps a prescriber to decide whether or not to initiate treatment with a loading dose. Consider **digoxin** (half-life approximately 40 hours). This is usually prescribed once daily, resulting in a less than two-fold variation in maximum and minimum plasma concentrations, and reaching >90% of the mean steady-state concentration in approximately one week (i.e. four half-lives). In many clinical situations, such a time-course is acceptable. In more urgent situations a more rapid response can be achieved by using a loading dose. The loading dose (LD) can be estimated by multiplying the desired concentration by the volume of distribution (LD = $C_p \times V_d$).

DEVIATIONS FROM THE ONE-COMPARTMENT MODEL WITH FIRST-ORDER ELIMINATION

TWO-COMPARTMENT MODEL

Following an intravenous bolus a biphasic decline in plasma concentration is often observed (Figure 3.4), rather than a simple exponential decline. The two-compartment model (Figure 3.5) is appropriate in this situation. This treats the body as a smaller central plus a larger peripheral compartment. Again, these compartments have no precise anatomical meaning, although the central compartment is assumed to consist of

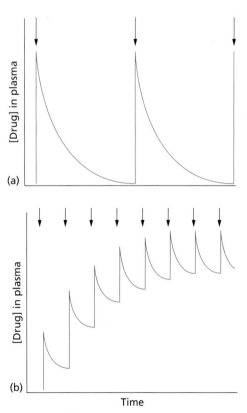

Figure 3.3: Repeated bolus dose injections (at arrows) at (a) intervals much greater than $t_{1/2}$ and (b) intervals less than $t_{1/2}$.

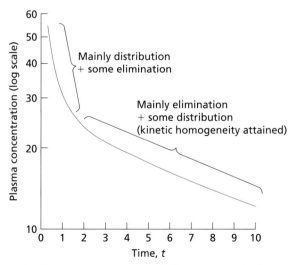

Figure 3.4: Two-compartment model. Plasma concentration–time curve (semi-logarithmic) following a bolus dose of a drug that fits a two-compartment model.

blood (from which samples are taken for analysis) plus the extracellular spaces of some well-perfused tissues. The peripheral compartment consists of less well-perfused tissues into which drug permeates more slowly.

The initial rapid fall is called the α phase, and mainly reflects distribution from the central to the peripheral compartment. The second, slower phase reflects drug elimination. It is called the β phase, and the corresponding $t_{1/2}$ is known as $t_{1/2\beta}$. This is the appropriate value for clinical use.

NON-LINEAR ('DOSE-DEPENDENT') PHARMACOKINETICS

Although many drugs are eliminated at a rate that is approximately proportional to their concentration ('first-order' kinetics), there are several therapeutically important exceptions. Consider a drug that is eliminated by conversion to an inactive metabolite by an enzyme. At high concentrations, the enzyme becomes saturated. The drug concentration and reaction velocity are related by the Michaelis–Menten equation (Figure 3.6). At low concentrations, the rate is linearly related

to concentration, whereas at saturating concentrations the rate is independent of concentration ('zero-order' kinetics). The same applies when a drug is eliminated by a saturable transport process. In clinical practice, drugs that exhibit non-linear kinetics are the exception rather than the rule. This is because most drugs are used therapeutically at doses that give rise to concentrations that are well below the Michaelis constant (K_m), and so operate on the lower, approximately linear, part of the Michaelis–Menten curve relating elimination velocity to plasma concentration.

Drugs that show non-linear kinetics in the therapeutic range include **heparin, phenytoin** and **ethanol**. Some drugs (e.g. barbiturates) show non-linearity in the part of the toxic range that is encountered clinically. Implications of non-linear pharmacokinetics include:

1. The decline in concentration vs. time following a bolus dose of such a drug is not exponential. Instead, elimination

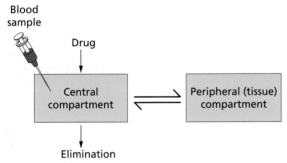

Figure 3.5: Schematic representation of a two-compartment model.

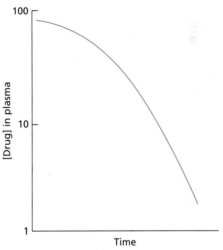

Figure 3.7: Non-linear kinetics: plasma concentration–time curve following administration of a bolus dose of a drug eliminated by Michaelis–Menten kinetics.

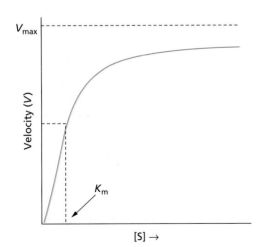

Figure 3.6: Michaelis–Menten relationship between the velocity (*V*) of an enzyme reaction and the substrate concentration ([S]). [S] at 50% V_{max} is equal to K_m, the Michaelis–Menten constant.

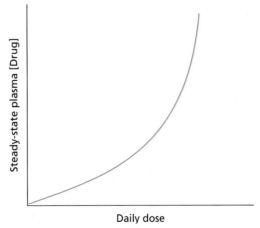

Figure 3.8: Non-linear kinetics: steady-state plasma concentration of a drug following repeated dosing as a function of dose.

begins slowly and accelerates as plasma concentration falls (Figure 3.7).

2. The time required to eliminate 50% of a dose increases with increasing dose, so half-life is not constant.

3. A modest increase in dose of such a drug disproportionately increases the amount of drug in the body once the drug-elimination process is saturated (Figure 3.8). This is very important clinically when using plasma concentrations of, for example, **phenytoin** as a guide to dosing.

Key points

- *Two-compartment model.* Following a bolus dose the plasma concentration falls bi-exponentially, instead of a single exponential as in the one-compartment model. The first (α) phase mainly represents distribution; the second (β) phase mainly represents elimination.
- *Non-linear ('dose-dependent') kinetics.* If the elimination process (e.g. drug-metabolizing enzyme) becomes saturated, the clearance rate falls. Consequently, increasing the dose causes a disproportionate increase in plasma concentration. Drugs which exhibit such properties (e.g. phenytoin) are often difficult to use in clinical practice.

Case history

A young man develops idiopathic epilepsy and treatment is started with phenytoin, 200 mg daily, given as a single dose last thing at night. After a week, the patient's serum phenytoin concentration is 25 μmol/L. (Therapeutic range is 40–80 μmol/L.) The dose is increased to 300 mg/day. One week later he is complaining of unsteadiness, there is nystagmus and the serum concentration is 125 μmol/L. The dose is reduced to 250 mg/day. The patient's symptoms slowly improve and the serum phenytoin concentration falls to 60 μmol/L (within the therapeutic range).
Comment
Phenytoin shows dose-dependent kinetics; the serum concentration at the lower dose was below the therapeutic range, so the dose was increased. Despite the apparently modest increase (to 150% of the original dose), the plasma concentration rose disproportionately, causing symptoms and signs of toxicity (see Chapter 22).

FURTHER READING

Rowland M, Tozer TN. Therapeutic regimens. In: *Clinical pharmacokinetics: concepts and applications*, 3rd edn. Baltimore, MD: Williams and Wilkins, 1995: 53–105.

Birkett DJ. *Pharmacokinetics made easy (revised)*, 2nd edn. Sydney: McGraw-Hill, 2002. (Lives up to the promise of its title!)

CHAPTER 4

DRUG ABSORPTION AND ROUTES OF ADMINISTRATION

INTRODUCTION

Drug absorption, and hence the routes by which a particular drug may usefully be administered, is determined by the rate and extent of penetration of biological phospholipid membranes. These are permeable to lipid-soluble drugs, whilst presenting a barrier to more water-soluble drugs. The most convenient route of drug administration is usually by mouth, and absorption processes in the gastro-intestinal tract are among the best understood.

BIOAVAILABILITY, BIOEQUIVALENCE AND GENERIC VS. PROPRIETARY PRESCRIBING

Drugs must enter the circulation if they are to exert a systemic effect. Unless administered intravenously, most drugs are absorbed incompletely (Figure 4.1). There are three reasons for this:

1. the drug is inactivated within the gut lumen by gastric acid, digestive enzymes or bacteria;
2. absorption is incomplete; and
3. presystemic ('first-pass') metabolism occurs in the gut wall and liver.

Together, these processes explain why the bioavailability of an orally administered drug is typically less than 100%. Bioavailability of a drug formulation can be measured experimentally (Figure 4.2) by measuring concentration vs. time curves following administration of the preparation via its intended route (e.g. orally) and of the same dose given intravenously (i.v.).

$$\text{Bioavailability} = \text{AUCoral}/\text{AUCi.v.} \times 100\%$$

Many factors in the manufacture of the drug formulation influence its disintegration, dispersion and dissolution in the gastro-intestinal tract. Pharmaceutical factors are therefore important in determining bioavailability. It is important to distinguish

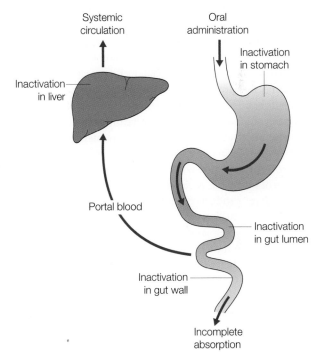

Figure 4.1: Drug bioavailability following oral administration may be incomplete for several reasons.

statistically significant from clinically important differences in this regard. The former are common, whereas the latter are not. However, differences in bioavailability did account for an epidemic of **phenytoin** intoxication in Australia in 1968–69. Affected patients were found to be taking one brand of **phenytoin**: the excipient had been changed from calcium sulphate to lactose, increasing **phenytoin** bioavailability and thereby precipitating toxicity. An apparently minor change in the manufacturing process of digoxin in the UK resulted in reduced potency due to poor bioavailability. Restoring the original manufacturing conditions restored potency but led to some confusion, with both toxicity and underdosing.

These examples raise the question of whether prescribing should be by generic name or by proprietary (brand) name. When a new preparation is marketed, it has a proprietary name

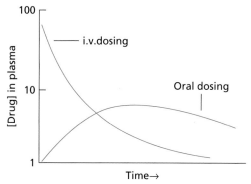

Figure 4.2: Oral vs. intravenous dosing: plasma concentration–time curves following administration of a drug i.v. or by mouth (oral).

supplied by the pharmaceutical company, and a non-proprietary (generic) name. It is usually available only from the company that introduced it until the patent expires. After this, other companies can manufacture and market the product, sometimes under its generic name. At this time, pharmacists usually shop around for the best buy. If a hospital doctor prescribes by proprietary name, the same drug produced by another company may be substituted. This saves considerable amounts of money. The attractions of generic prescribing in terms of minimizing costs are therefore obvious, but there are counterarguments, the strongest of which relates to the bioequivalence or otherwise of the proprietary product with its generic competitors. The formulation of a drug (i.e. excipients, etc.) differs between different manufacturers' products of the same drug, sometimes affecting bioavailability. This is a particular concern with slow-release or sustained-release preparations, or preparations to be administered by different routes. Drug regulatory bodies have strict criteria to assess whether such products can be licensed without the full dataset that would be required for a completely new product (i.e. one based on a new chemical entity).

It should be noted that the absolute bioavailability of two preparations may be the same (i.e. the same AUC), but that the kinetics may be very different (e.g. one may have a much higher peak plasma concentration than the other, but a shorter duration). The rate at which a drug enters the body determines the onset of its pharmacological action, and also influences the intensity and sometimes the duration of its action, and is important in addition to the completeness of absorption.

Prescribers need to be confident that different preparations (brand named or generic) are sufficiently similar for their substitution to be unlikely to lead to clinically important alterations in therapeutic outcome. Regulatory authorities have responded to this need by requiring companies who are seeking to introduce generic equivalents to present evidence that their product behaves similarly to the innovator product that is already marketed. If evidence is presented that a new generic product can be treated as therapeutically equivalent to the current 'market leader', this is accepted as 'bioequivalence'. This does not imply that all possible pharmacokinetic parameters are identical between the two products, but that any such differences are unlikely to be clinically important.

It is impossible to give a universal answer to the generic vs. proprietary issue. However, substitution of generic for brand-name products seldom causes obvious problems, and exceptions (e.g. different formulations of the calcium antagonist diltiazem, see Chapter 29) are easily flagged up in formularies.

Key points

- Drugs must cross phospholipid membranes to reach the systemic circulation, unless they are administered intravenously. This is determined by the lipid solubility of the drug and the area of membrane available for absorption, which is very large in the case of the ileum, because of the villi and microvilli. Sometimes polar drugs can be absorbed via specific transport processes (carriers).
- Even if absorption is complete, not all of the dose may reach the systemic circulation if the drug is metabolized by the epithelium of the intestine, or transported back into lumen of the intestine or metabolized in the liver, which can extract drug from the portal blood before it reaches the systemic circulation via the hepatic vein. This is called presystemic (or 'first-pass') metabolism.
- 'Bioavailability' describes the completeness of absorption into the systemic circulation. The amount of drug absorbed is determined by measuring the plasma concentration at intervals after dosing and integrating by estimating the area under the plasma concentration/time curve (AUC). This AUC is expressed as a percentage of the AUC when the drug is administered intravenously (100% absorption). Zero per cent bioavailability implies that no drug enters the systemic circulation, whereas 100% bioavailability means that all of the dose is absorbed into the systemic circulation. Bioavailability may vary not only between different drugs and different pharmaceutical formulations of the same drug, but also from one individual to another, depending on factors such as dose, whether the dose is taken on an empty stomach, and the presence of gastro-intestinal disease, or other drugs.
- The rate of absorption is also important (as well as the completeness), and is expressed as the time to peak plasma concentration (T_{max}). Sometimes it is desirable to formulate drugs in slow-release preparations to permit once daily dosing and/or to avoid transient adverse effects corresponding to peak plasma concentrations. Substitution of one such preparation for another may give rise to clinical problems unless the preparations are 'bioequivalent'. Regulatory authorities therefore require evidence of bioequivalence before licensing generic versions of existing products.
- Prodrugs are metabolized to pharmacologically active products. They provide an approach to improving absorption and distribution.

PRODRUGS

One approach to improving absorption or distribution to a relatively inaccessible tissue (e.g. brain) is to modify the drug molecule chemically to form a compound that is better absorbed and from which active drug is liberated after absorption. Such modified drugs are termed prodrugs (Figure 4.3). Examples are shown in Table 4.1.

ROUTES OF ADMINISTRATION

ORAL ROUTE

FOR LOCAL EFFECT

Oral drug administration may be used to produce local effects within the gastro-intestinal tract. Examples include antacids, and sulphasalazine, which delivers 5-amino salicylic acid (5-ASA) to the colon, thereby prolonging remission in patients with ulcerative colitis (Chapter 34). Mesalazine has a pH-dependent acrylic coat that degrades at alkaline pH as in the colon and distal part of the ileum. Olsalazine is a prodrug consisting of a dimer of two 5-ASA moieties joined by a bond that is cleaved by colonic bacteria.

FOR SYSTEMIC EFFECT

Oral administration of drugs is safer and more convenient for the patient than injection. There are two main mechanisms of drug absorption by the gut (Figure 4.4).

Passive diffusion

This is the most important mechanism. Non-polar lipid-soluble agents are well absorbed from the gut, mainly from the small intestine, because of the enormous absorptive surface area provided by villi and microvilli.

Active transport

This requires a specific carrier. Naturally occurring polar substances, including sugars, amino acids and vitamins, are absorbed by active or facilitated transport mechanisms. Drugs that are analogues of such molecules compete with them for transport via the carrier. Examples include L-dopa, methotrexate, 5-fluorouracil and lithium (which competes with sodium ions for absorption).

Other factors that influence absorption include:

1. *surgical interference with gastric function* – gastrectomy reduces absorption of several drugs;
2. *disease of the gastro-intestinal tract* (e.g. coeliac disease, cystic fibrosis) – the effects of such disease are unpredictable, but often surprisingly minor (see Chapter 7);
3. *the presence of food* – the timing of drug administration in relation to meal times can be important. Food and drink dilute the drug and can bind it, alter gastric emptying and increase mesenteric and portal blood flow;

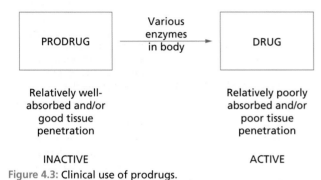

Figure 4.3: Clinical use of prodrugs.

Table 4.1: Prodrugs

Prodrug	Product
Enalapril	Enalaprilat
Benorylate	Aspirin and paracetamol
Levodopa	Dopamine
Minoxidil	Minoxidil sulphate
Carbimazole	Methimazole
Vanciclovir	Aciclovir

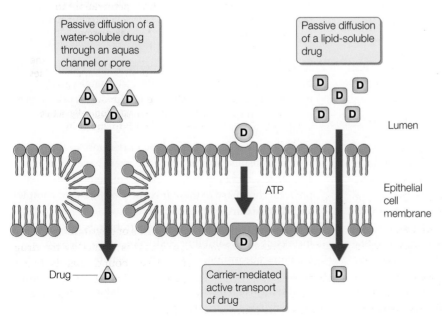

Figure 4.4: Modes of absorption of drugs from the gut.

4. *drug metabolism by intestinal flora* – this may affect drug absorption. Alteration of bowel flora (e.g. by concomitant use of antibiotics) can interrupt enterohepatic recycling and cause loss of efficacy of oral contraceptives (Chapter 13);
5. *drug metabolism by enzymes* (e.g. cytochrome P450 family 3A (CYP3A)) in the gastro-intestinal epithelium (Chapter 5);
6. *drug efflux* back into the gut lumen by drug transport proteins (e.g. P-glycoprotein (P-gp), ABCB1).

Prolonged action and sustained-release preparations

Some drugs with short elimination half-lives need to be administered frequently, at inconveniently short intervals, making adherence to the prescribed regimen difficult for the patient. A drug with similar actions, but a longer half-life, may need to be substituted. Alternatively, there are various pharmaceutical means of slowing absorption of a rapidly eliminated drug. The aim of such sustained-release preparations is to release a steady 'infusion' of drug into the gut lumen for absorption during transit through the small intestine. Reduced dosing frequency may improve compliance and, in the case of some drugs (e.g. **carbamazepine**), reduce adverse effects linked to high peak plasma concentrations. Absorption of such preparations is often incomplete, so it is especially important that bioavailability is established and substitution of one preparation for another may lead to clinical problems. Other limitations of slow-release preparations are:

1. Transit time through the small intestine is about six hours, so once daily dosing may lead to unacceptably low trough concentrations.
2. If the gut lumen is narrowed or intestinal transit is slow, as in the elderly, or due to other drugs (tricyclic antidepressants, opiates), there is a danger of high local drug concentrations causing mucosal damage. **Osmosin**™, an osmotically released formulation of **indometacin**, had to be withdrawn because it caused bleeding and ulceration of the small intestine.
3. Overdose with sustained-release preparations is difficult to treat because of delayed drug absorption.
4. Sustained-release tablets should not be divided.
5. Expense.

BUCCAL AND SUBLINGUAL ROUTE

Drugs are administered to be retained in the mouth for local disorders of the pharynx or buccal mucosa, such as aphthous ulcers (**hydrocortisone** lozenges or **carbenoxolone** granules).

Sublingual administration has distinct advantages over oral administration (i.e. the drug to be swallowed) for drugs with pronounced presystemic metabolism, providing direct and rapid access to the systemic circulation, bypassing the intestine and liver. **Glyceryl trinitrate**, **buprenorphine** and **fentanyl** are given sublingually for this reason. **Glyceryl trinitrate** is taken either as a sublingual tablet or as a spray. Sublingual administration provides short-term effects which can be terminated by

swallowing the tablet. Tablets for buccal absorption provide more sustained plasma concentrations, and are held in one spot between the lip and the gum until they have dissolved.

RECTAL ROUTE

Drugs may be given rectally for local effects (e.g. to treat proctitis). The following advantages have been claimed for the rectal route of administration of systemically active drugs:

1. Exposure to the acidity of the gastric juice and to digestive enzymes is avoided.
2. The portal circulation is partly bypassed, reducing presystemic (first pass) metabolism.
3. For patients who are unable to swallow or who are vomiting.

Rectal **diazepam** is useful for controlling status epilepticus in children. **Metronidazole** is well absorbed when administered rectally, and is less expensive than intravenous preparations. However, there are usually more reliable alternatives, and drugs that are given rectally can cause severe local irritation.

SKIN

Drugs are applied topically to treat skin disease (Chapter 51). Systemic absorption via the skin can cause undesirable effects, for example in the case of potent glucocorticoids, but the application of drugs to skin can also be used to achieve a systemic therapeutic effect (e.g. **fentanyl** patches for analgesia). The skin has evolved as an impermeable integument, so the problems of getting drugs through it are completely different from transport through an absorptive surface such as the gut. Factors affecting percutaneous drug absorption include:

1. *skin condition* – injury and disease;
2. *age* – infant skin is more permeable than adult skin;
3. *region* –plantar < forearm < scalp < scrotum < posterior auricular skin;
4. *hydration of the stratum corneum* – this is very important. Increased hydration increases permeability. Plastic-film occlusion (sometimes employed by dermatologists) increases hydration. Penetration of glucocorticosteroids is increased up to 100-fold, and systemic side effects are more common;
5. *vehicle* – little is known about the importance of the various substances which over the years have been empirically included in skin creams and ointments. The physical chemistry of these mixtures may be very complex and change during an application;
6. *physical properties of the drug* – penetration increases with increasing lipid solubility. Reduction of particle size enhances absorption, and solutions penetrate best of all;
7. *surface area to which the drug is applied* – this is especially important when treating infants who have a relatively large surface area to volume ratio.

Transdermal absorption is sufficiently reliable to enable systemically active drugs (e.g. **estradiol, nicotine, scopolamine**) to be administered by this route in the form of patches. Transdermal administration bypasses presystemic metabolism. Patches are more expensive than alternative preparations.

LUNGS

Drugs, notably steroids, β_2-adrenoceptor agonists and muscarinic receptor antagonists, are inhaled as aerosols or particles for their local effects on bronchioles. Nebulized antibiotics are also sometimes used in children with cystic fibrosis and recurrent *Pseudomonas* infections. Physical properties that limit systemic absorption are desirable. For example, **ipratropium** is a quaternary ammonium ion analogue of atropine which is highly polar, and is consequently poorly absorbed and has reduced atropine-like side effects. A large fraction of an 'inhaled' dose of **salbutamol** is in fact swallowed. However, the bioavailability of swallowed **salbutamol** is low due to inactivation in the gut wall, so systemic effects such as tremor are minimized in comparison to effects on the bronchioles.

The lungs are ideally suited for absorption from the gas phase, since the total respiratory surface area is about $60\,m^2$, through which only $60\,mL$ blood are percolating in the capillaries. This is exploited in the case of volatile anaesthetics, as discussed in Chapter 24. A nasal/inhaled preparation of insulin was introduced for type 2 diabetes (Chapter 37), but was not commercially successful.

NOSE

Glucocorticoids and sympathomimetic amines may be administered intranasally for their local effects on the nasal mucosa. Systemic absorption may result in undesirable effects, such as hypertension.

Nasal mucosal epithelium has remarkable absorptive properties, notably the capacity to absorb intact complex peptides that cannot be administered by mouth because they would be digested. This has opened up an area of therapeutics that was previously limited by the inconvenience of repeated injections. Drugs administered by this route include **desmopressin** (DDAVP, an analogue of antidiuretic hormone) for diabetes insipidus and **buserelin** (an analogue of gonadotrophin releasing hormone) for prostate cancer.

EYE, EAR AND VAGINA

Drugs are administered topically to these sites for their local effects (e.g. **gentamicin** or **ciprofloxacin** eyedrops for bacterial conjunctivitis, sodium bicarbonate eardrops for softening wax, and **nystatin** pessaries for *Candida* infections). Occasionally, they are absorbed in sufficient quantity to have undesirable systemic effects, such as worsening of bronchospasm in asthmatics caused by **timolol** eyedrops given for open-angle glaucoma. However, such absorption is not sufficiently reliable to make use of these routes for therapeutic ends.

INTRAMUSCULAR INJECTION

Many drugs are well absorbed when administered intramuscularly. The rate of absorption is increased when the solution is distributed throughout a large volume of muscle. Dispersion is enhanced by massage of the injection site. Transport away from the injection site is governed by muscle blood flow, and this varies from site to site (deltoid > vastus lateralis > gluteus maximus). Blood flow to muscle is increased by exercise and absorption rates are increased in all sites after exercise. Conversely, shock, heart failure or other conditions that decrease muscle blood flow reduce absorption.

The drug must be sufficiently water soluble to remain in solution at the injection site until absorption occurs. This is a problem for some drugs, including **phenytoin, diazepam** and **digoxin**, as crystallization and/or poor absorption occur when these are given by intramuscular injection, which should therefore be avoided. Slow absorption is useful in some circumstances where appreciable concentrations of drug are required for prolonged periods. Depot intramuscular injections are used to improve compliance in psychiatric patients (e.g. the decanoate ester of **fluphenazine** which is slowly hydrolysed to release active free drug).

Intramuscular injection has a number of disadvantages:

1. pain – distension with large volumes is painful, and injected volumes should usually be no greater than $5\,mL$;
2. sciatic nerve palsy following injection into the buttock – this is avoided by injecting into the upper outer gluteal quadrant;
3. sterile abscesses at the injection site (e.g. paraldehyde);
4. elevated serum creatine phosphokinase due to enzyme release from muscle can cause diagnostic confusion;
5. severe adverse reactions may be protracted because there is no way of stopping absorption of the drug;
6. for some drugs, intramuscular injection is less effective than the oral route;
7. haematoma formation.

SUBCUTANEOUS INJECTION

This is influenced by the same factors that affect intramuscular injections. Cutaneous blood flow is lower than in muscle so absorption is slower. Absorption is retarded by immobilization, reduction of blood flow by a tourniquet and local cooling.

Adrenaline incorporated into an injection (e.g. of local anaesthetic) reduces the absorption rate by causing vasoconstriction.

Sustained effects from subcutaneous injections are extremely important clinically, most notably in the treatment of insulin-dependent diabetics, different rates of absorption being achieved by different insulin preparations (see Chapter 37).

Sustained effects have also been obtained from subcutaneous injections by using oily suspensions or by implanting a pellet subcutaneously (e.g. **oestrogen** or **testosterone** for hormone replacement therapy).

INTRAVENOUS INJECTION

This has the following advantages:

1. rapid action (e.g. **morphine** for analgesia and **furosemide** in pulmonary oedema);
2. presystemic metabolism is avoided (e.g. **glyceryl trinitrate** infusion in patients with unstable angina);
3. intravenous injection is used for drugs that are not absorbed by mouth (e.g. aminoglycosides (**gentamicin**) and heparins). It is also used for drugs that are too painful or toxic to be given intramuscularly. Cytotoxic drugs must not be allowed to leak from the vein or considerable local damage and pain will result as many of them are severe vesicants (e.g. **vincristine, doxorubicin**);
4. intravenous infusion is easily controlled, enabling precise titration of drugs with short half-lives. This is essential for drugs such as **sodium nitroprusside** and **epoprostenol**.

The main drawbacks of intravenous administration are as follows:

1. Once injected, drugs cannot be recalled.
2. High concentrations result if the drug is given too rapidly – the right heart receives the highest concentration.
3. Embolism of foreign particles or air, sepsis or thrombosis.
4. Accidental extravascular injection or leakage of toxic drugs (e.g. **doxorubicin**) produce severe local tissue necrosis.
5. Inadvertent intra-arterial injection can cause arterial spasm and peripheral gangrene.

INTRATHECAL INJECTION

This route provides access to the central nervous system for drugs that are normally excluded by the blood–brain barrier. This inevitably involves very high risks of neurotoxicity, and this route should never be used without adequate training. (In the UK, junior doctors who have made mistakes of this kind have been held criminally, as well as professionally, negligent.) The possibility of causing death or permanent neurological disability is such that extra care must be taken in checking that both the drug and the dose are correct. Examples of drugs used in this way include **methotrexate** and local anaesthetics (e.g. **levobupivacaine**) or opiates, such as **morphine** and **fentanyl**. (More commonly anaesthetists use the extradural route to administer local anaesthetic drugs to produce regional analgesia without depressing respiration, e.g. in women during labour.) Aminoglycosides are sometimes administered by

neuro-surgeons via a cisternal reservoir to patients with Gram-negative infections of the brain. The antispasmodic **baclofen** is sometimes administered by this route.

Penicillin used to be administered intrathecally to patients with pneumococcal meningitis, because of the belief that it penetrated the blood–brain barrier inadequately. However, when the meninges are inflamed (as in meningitis), high-dose intravenous **penicillin** results in adequate concentrations in the cerebrospinal fluid. Intravenous **penicillin** should now always be used for meningitis, since **penicillin** is a predictable neurotoxin (it was formerly used to produce an animal model of seizures), and seizures, encephalopathy and death have been caused by injecting a dose intrathecally that would have been appropriate for intravenous administration.

Key points

- Oral – generally safe and convenient
- Buccal/sublingual – circumvents presystemic metabolism
- Rectal – useful in patients who are vomiting
- Transdermal – limited utility, avoids presystemic metabolism
- Lungs – volatile anaesthetics
- Nasal – useful absorption of some peptides (e.g. DDAVP; see Chapter 42)
- Intramuscular – useful in some urgent situations (e.g. behavioural emergencies)
- Subcutaneous – useful for insulin and heparin in particular
- Intravenous – useful in emergencies for most rapid and predictable action, but too rapid administration is potentially very dangerous, as a high concentration reaches the heart as a bolus
- Intrathecal – specialized use by anaesthetists

Case history

The health visitor is concerned about an eight-month-old girl who is failing to grow. The child's mother tells you that she has been well apart from a recurrent nappy rash, but on examination there are features of Cushing's syndrome. On further enquiry, the mother tells you that she has been applying **clobetasone**, which she had been prescribed herself for eczema, to the baby's napkin area. There is no biochemical evidence of endogenous over-production of glucocorticoids. The mother stops using the **clobetasone** cream on her daughter, on your advice. The features of Cushing's syndrome regress and growth returns to normal.
Comment
Clobetasone is an extremely potent steroid (see Chapter 50). It is prescribed for its top-ical effect, but can penetrate skin, especially of an infant. The amount prescribed that is appropriate for an adult would readily cover a large fraction of an infant's body surface area. If plastic pants are used around the nappy this may increase penetration through the skin (just like an occlusive dressing, which is often deliberately used to increase the potency of topical steroids; see Chapter 50), leading to excessive absorption and systemic effects as in this case.

FURTHER READING

Fix JA. Strategies for delivery of peptides utilizing absorption-enhancing agents. *Journal of Pharmaceutical Sciences* 1996; **85**: 1282–5.

Goldberg M, Gomez-Orellana I. Challenges for the oral delivery of macromolecules. *Nature Reviews Drug Discovery* 2003; **2**: 289–95.

Mahato RI, Narang AS, Thoma L, Miller DD. Emerging trends in oral delivery of peptide and protein drugs. *Critical Reviews in Therapeutic Drug Carrier Systems* 2003; **20**: 153–2.

Mathiovitz E, Jacobs JS, Jong NS et al. Biologically erodable microspheres as potential oral drug delivery systems. *Nature* 1997; **386**: 410–14.

Rowland M, Tozer TN. *Clinical pharmacokinetics: concepts and applications*, 3rd edn. Baltimore, MD: Williams and Wilkins, 1995: 11–50.

Skyler JS, Cefalu WT, Kourides I A et al. Efficacy of inhaled human insulin in type 1 diabetes mellitus: a randomized proof-of-concept study. *Lancet* 2001; **357**: 324–5.

Varde NK, Pack DW. Microspheres for controlled release drug delivery. *Expert Opinion on Biological Therapy* 2004; **4**: 35–51.

CHAPTER **5**

DRUG METABOLISM

INTRODUCTION

Drug metabolism is central to biochemical pharmacology. Knowledge of human drug metabolism has been advanced by the wide availability of human hepatic tissue, complemented by analytical studies of parent drugs and metabolites in plasma and urine.

The pharmacological activity of many drugs is reduced or abolished by enzymatic processes, and drug metabolism is one of the primary mechanisms by which drugs are inactivated. Examples include oxidation of **phenytoin** and of **ethanol**. However, not all metabolic processes result in inactivation, and drug activity is sometimes increased by metabolism, as in activation of prodrugs (e.g. hydrolysis of **enalapril**, Chapter 28, to its active metabolite **enalaprilat**). The formation of polar metabolites from a non-polar drug permits efficient urinary excretion (Chapter 6). However, some enzymatic conversions yield active compounds with a longer half-life than the parent drug, causing delayed effects of the long-lasting metabolite as it accumulates more slowly to its steady state (e.g. **diazepam** has a half-life of 20–50 hours, whereas its pharmacologically active metabolite **desmethyldiazepam** has a plasma half-life of approximately 100 hours, Chapter 18).

It is convenient to divide drug metabolism into two phases (phases I and II: Figure 5.1), which often, but not always, occur sequentially. Phase I reactions involve a metabolic modification of the drug (commonly oxidation, reduction or hydrolysis). Products of phase I reactions may be either pharmacologically active or inactive. Phase II reactions are synthetic conjugation reactions. Phase II metabolites have increased polarity compared to the parent drugs and are more readily excreted in the urine (or, less often, in the bile), and they are usually – but not always – pharmacologically inactive. Molecules or groups involved in phase II reactions include acetate, glucuronic acid, glutamine, glycine and sulphate, which may combine with reactive groups introduced during phase I metabolism ('functionalization'). For example, **phenytoin** is initially oxidized to 4-hydroxyphenytoin which is then glucuronidated to 4-hydroxyphenytoin-glucuronide, which is readily excreted via the kidney.

PHASE I METABOLISM

The liver is the most important site of drug metabolism. Hepatocyte endoplasmic reticulum is particularly important, but the cytosol and mitochondria are also involved.

ENDOPLASMIC RETICULUM

Hepatic smooth endoplasmic reticulum contains the cytochrome P450 (CYP450) enzyme superfamily (more than 50 different CYPs have been found in humans) that metabolize foreign substances – 'xenobiotics', i.e. drugs as well as pesticides, fertilizers and other chemicals ingested by humans. These metabolic reactions include oxidation, reduction and hydrolysis.

OXIDATION

Microsomal oxidation causes aromatic or aliphatic hydroxylation, deamination, dealkylation or *S*-oxidation. These reactions all involve reduced nicotinamide adenine dinucleotide phosphate (NADP), molecular oxygen, and one or more of a group of CYP450 haemoproteins which act as a terminal oxidase in the oxidation reaction (or can involve other mixed function oxidases, e.g. flavin-containing monooxygenases or epoxide hydrolases). CYP450s exist in several distinct isoenzyme families and subfamilies with different levels of amino acid homology. Each CYP subfamily has a different, albeit often overlapping, pattern of substrate specificities. The major drug metabolizing CYPs with important substrates, inhibitors and inducers are shown in Table 5.1.

CYP450 enzymes are also involved in the oxidative biosynthesis of mediators or other biochemically important intermediates. For example, synthase enzymes involved in the oxidation of arachidonic acid (Chapter 26) to prostaglandins and thromboxanes are CYP450 enzymes with distinct specificities.

REDUCTION

Reduction requires reduced NADP-cytochrome-c reductase or reduced NAD-cytochrome b5 reductase.

HYDROLYSIS

Pethidine (meperidine) is de-esterified to meperidinic acid by hepatic membrane-bound esterase activity.

NON-ENDOPLASMIC RETICULUM DRUG METABOLISM

OXIDATION

Oxidation of ethanol to acetaldehyde and of chloral to trichlorethanol is catalysed by a cytosolic enzyme (alcohol dehydrogenase) whose substrates also include vitamin A. Monoamine oxidase (MAO) is a membrane-bound mitochondrial enzyme that oxidatively deaminates primary amines to aldehydes (which are further oxidized to carboxylic acids) or ketones. Monoamine oxidase is found in liver, kidney, intestine and nervous tissue, and its substrates include catecholamines

(dopamine, noradrenaline and adrenaline), tyramine, phenylephrine and tryptophan derivatives (5-hydroxytryptamine and tryptamine). Oxidation of purines by xanthine oxidase (e.g. 6-mercaptopurine is inactivated to 6-thiouric acid) is non-microsomal.

REDUCTION

This includes, for example, enzymic reduction of double bonds, e.g. **methadone**, **naloxone**.

HYDROLYSIS

Esterases catalyse hydrolytic conversions of many drugs. Examples include the cleavage of suxamethonium by plasma cholinesterase, an enzyme that exhibits pharmacogenetic variation (Chapter 14), as well as hydrolysis of **aspirin** (acetylsalicylic acid) to **salicylate**, and the hydrolysis of **enalapril** to **enalaprilat**.

PHASE II METABOLISM (TRANSFERASE REACTIONS)

AMINO ACID REACTIONS

Glycine and glutamine are the amino acids chiefly involved in conjugation reactions in humans. Glycine forms conjugates with nicotinic acid and salicylate, whilst glutamine forms conjugates with p-aminosalicylate. Hepatocellular damage depletes the intracellular pool of these amino acids, thus restricting this pathway. Amino acid conjugation is reduced in neonates (Chapter 10).

ACETYLATION

Acetate derived from acetyl coenzyme A conjugates with several drugs, including **isoniazid**, **hydralazine** and **procainamide** (see Chapter 14 for pharmacogenetics of acetylation). Acetylating activity resides in the cytosol and occurs in leucocytes, gastrointestinal epithelium and the liver (in reticulo-endothelial rather than parenchymal cells).

GLUCURONIDATION

Conjugation reactions between glucuronic acid and carboxyl groups are involved in the metabolism of bilirubin, salicylates

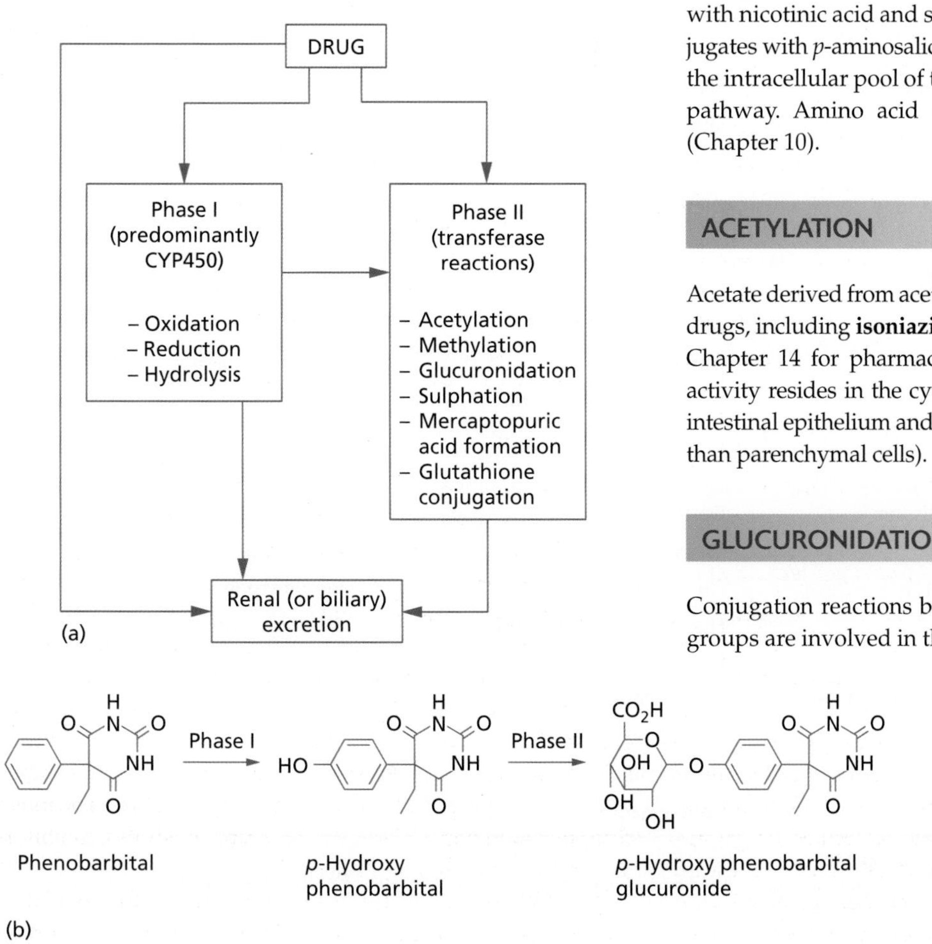

(a)

(b)

Phenobarbital

p-Hydroxy phenobarbital

p-Hydroxy phenobarbital glucuronide

Figure 5.1: (a) Phases I and II of drug metabolism. (b) A specific example of phases I and II of drug metabolism, in the case of phenobarbital.

Table 5.1: CYP450 isoenzymes most commonly involved in drug metabolism with representative drug substrates and their specific inhibitors and inducers

Enzyme	Substrate	Inhibitor	Inducer
CYP1A2	Caffeine	Amiodarone	Insulin
	Clozapine	Cimetidine	Cruciferous vegetables
	Theophylline	Fluoroquinolones	Nafcillin
	Warfarin (R)	Fluvoxamine	Omeprazole
CYP2C9[a]	Celecoxib		
	Losartan	Amiodarone	Barbiturates
	NSAIDs	Fluconazole	Rifampicin
	Sulphonylureas	Fluoxetine/Fluvoxamine	
	Phenytoin	Lansoprazole	
	Warfarin (S)	Sulfamethoxazole	
		Ticlopidine	
CYP2C19[a]	Diazepam	Fluoxetine	Carbamazepine
	Moclobamide	Ketoconazole	Prednisone
	Omeprazole		Rifampicin
	Pantoprazole		
	Proguanil		
CYP2D6[a]	Codeine (opioids)	Amiodarone	Dexamethasone
	Dextromethorphan	Celecoxib	Rifampicin
	Haloperidol	Cimetidine	
	Metoprolol	Ecstasy (MDMA)	
	Nortriptyline	Fluoxetine	
	Pravastatin	Quinidine	
	Propafenone		
CYP2E1	Chlormezanone	Diethyldithio-carbamate	Ethanol
	Paracetamol		Isoniazid
	Theophylline		
CYP3A4	Alprazolam	Amiodarone	Barbiturates
	Atorvastatin	Diltiazem	Carbamazepine
	Ciclosporin	Erythromycin (and other macrolides)	Efavirenz
			Glucocorticosteroids (and other steroids)
	Hydrocortisone	Gestodene	Nevirapine
	Lidocaine	Grapefruit juice	Phenytoin
	Lovastatin	Fluvoxamine	Pioglitazone
		Fluconazole/Itraconazole	St John's wort
	Midazolam	Ketoconazole	
	Nifedipine (many CCBs)	Nefazodone	
	Tamoxifen	Nelfinavir/Ritonavir	
	Tacrolimus	Verapamil	
	Vincristine	Voriconazole	

[a]Known genetic polymorphisms (Chapter 14).
Approximate percentage of clinically used drugs metabolized by each CYP isoenzyme: CYP3A4, 50%; CYP2D6, 20%; CYP2C, 20%; CYP1A2, 2%; CYP2E1, 2%; other CYPs, 6%.

and lorazepam. Some patients inherit a deficiency of glucuronide formation that presents clinically as a non-haemolytic jaundice due to excess unconjugated bilirubin (Crigler–Najjar syndrome). Drugs that are normally conjugated via this pathway aggravate jaundice in such patients. *O*-Glucuronides formed by reaction with a hydroxyl group result in an ether glucuronide. This occurs with drugs such as **paracetamol** and **morphine**.

METHYLATION

Methylation proceeds by a pathway involving *S*-adenosyl methionine as methyl donor to drugs with free amino, hydroxyl or thiol groups. Catechol *O*-methyltransferase is an example of such a methylating enzyme, and is of physiological as well as pharmacological importance. It is present in the cytosol, and catalyses the transfer of a methyl group to catecholamines, inactivating noradrenaline, dopamine and adrenaline. Phenylethanolamine *N*-methyltransferase is also important in catecholamine metabolism. It methylates the terminal – NH_2 residue of noradrenaline to form adrenaline in the adrenal medulla. It also acts on exogenous amines, including phenylethanolamine and phenylephrine. It is induced by corticosteroids, and its high activity in the adrenal medulla reflects the anatomical arrangement of the blood supply to the medulla which comes from the adrenal cortex and consequently contains very high concentrations of corticosteroids.

SULPHATION

Cytosolic sulphotransferase enzymes catalyse the sulphation of hydroxyl and amine groups by transferring the sulphuryl group from 3′-phosphoadenosine 5′-phosphosulphate (PAPS) to the xenobiotic. Under physiological conditions, sulphotransferases generate heparin and chondroitin sulphate. In addition, they produce ethereal sulphates from several oestrogens, androgens, from 3-hydroxycoumarin (a phase I metabolite of **warfarin**) and **paracetamol**. There are a number of sulphotransferases in the hepatocyte, with different specificities.

MERCAPTURIC ACID FORMATION

Mercapturic acid formation is via reaction with the cysteine residue in the tripeptide Cys-Glu-Gly, i.e. glutathione. It is very important in **paracetamol** overdose (Chapter 54), when the usual sulphation and glucuronidation pathways of **paracetamol** metabolism are overwhelmed, with resulting production of a highly toxic metabolite (*N*-acetyl-benzoquinone imine, NABQI). NABQI is normally detoxified by conjugation with reduced glutathione. The availability of glutathione is critical in determining the clinical outcome. Patients who have ingested large amounts of **paracetamol** are therefore treated

with thiol donors such as *N*-acetyl cysteine or methionine to increase the endogenous supply of reduced glutathione.

GLUTATHIONE CONJUGATES

Naphthalene and some sulphonamides also form conjugates with glutathione. One endogenous function of glutathione conjugation is formation of a sulphidopeptide leukotriene, leukotriene (LT) C4. This is formed by conjugation of glutathione with LTA4, analogous to a phase II reaction. LTA4 is an epoxide which is synthesized from arachidonic acid by a 'phase I'-type oxidation reaction catalysed by the 5′-lipoxygenase enzyme. LTC4, together with its dipeptide product LTD4, comprise the activity once known as 'slow-reacting substance of anaphylaxis' (SRS-A), and these leukotrienes play a role as bronchoconstrictor mediators in anaphylaxis and in asthma (see Chapters 12 and 33).

ENZYME INDUCTION

Enzyme induction (Figure 5.2, Table 5.1) is a process by which enzyme activity is enhanced, usually because of increased enzyme synthesis (or, less often, reduced enzyme degradation). The increase in enzyme synthesis is often caused by xenobiotics binding to nuclear receptors (e.g. pregnane X receptor, constitutive androstane receptor, aryl hydrocarbon receptor), which then act as positive transcription factors for certain CYP450s.

There is marked inter-individual variability in the degree of induction produced by a given agent, part of which is genetically determined. Exogenous inducing agents include not only drugs, but also halogenated insecticides (particularly dichloro-diphenyl-trichloroethane (DDT) and gamma-benzene hexachloride), herbicides, polycyclic aromatic hydrocarbons, dyes, food preservatives, nicotine, ethanol and hyperforin in St John's wort. A practical consequence of enzyme induction is that, when two or more drugs are given simultaneously, then if one drug is an inducing agent it can accelerate the metabolism of the other drug and may lead to therapeutic failure (Chapter 13).

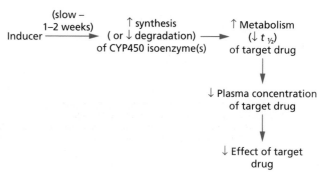

Figure 5.2: Enzyme induction.

TESTS FOR INDUCTION OF DRUG-METABOLIZING ENZYMES

The activity of hepatic drug-metabolizing enzymes can be assessed by measuring the clearance or metabolite ratios of probe drug substrates, e.g. **midazolam** for CYP3A4, **dextromethorphan** for CYP2D6, but this is seldom if ever indicated clinically. The ^{14}C-erythromycin breath test or the urinary molar ratio of 6-beta-hydroxycortisol/cortisol have also been used to assess CYP3A4 activity. It is unlikely that a single probe drug study will be definitive, since the mixed function oxidase (CYP450) system is so complex that at any one time the activity of some enzymes may be increased and that of others reduced. Induction of drug metabolism represents variable expression of a constant genetic constitution. It is important in drug elimination and also in several other biological processes, including adaptation to extra-uterine life. Neonates fail to form glucuronide conjugates because of immaturity of hepatic uridyl glucuronyl transferases with clinically important consequences, e.g. grey baby syndrome with **chloramphenicol** (Chapter 10).

ENZYME INHIBITION

Allopurinol, methotrexate, angiotensin converting enzyme inhibitors, non-steroidal anti-inflammatory drugs and many others, exert their therapeutic effects by enzyme inhibition (Figure 5.3). Quite apart from such direct actions, inhibition of drug-metabolizing enzymes by a concurrently administered drug (Table 5.1) can lead to drug accumulation and toxicity. For example, **cimetidine**, an antagonist at the histamine H_2-receptor, also inhibits drug metabolism via the CYP450 system and potentiates the actions of unrelated CYP450 metabolized drugs, such as **warfarin** and **theophylline** (see Chapters 13, 30 and 33). Other potent CYP3A4 inhibitors include the azoles (e.g. **fluconazole, voriconazole**) and HIV protease inhibitors (e.g. **ritonavir**).

The specificity of enzyme inhibition is sometimes incomplete. For example, **warfarin** and **phenytoin** compete with one another for metabolism, and co-administration results in elevation of plasma steady-state concentrations of both drugs. **Metronidazole** is a non-competitive inhibitor of microsomal enzymes and inhibits **phenytoin, warfarin** and **sulphonylurea** (e.g. **glyburide**) metabolism.

PRESYSTEMIC METABOLISM ('FIRST-PASS' EFFECT)

The metabolism of some drugs is markedly dependent on the route of administration. Following oral administration, drugs gain access to the systemic circulation via the portal vein, so the entire absorbed dose is exposed first to the intestinal mucosa and then to the liver, before gaining access to the rest of the body. A considerably smaller fraction of the absorbed dose goes through gut and liver in subsequent passes because of distribution to other tissues and drug elimination by other routes.

If a drug is subject to a high hepatic clearance (i.e. it is rapidly metabolized by the liver), a substantial fraction will be extracted from the portal blood and metabolized before it reaches the systemic circulation. This, in combination with intestinal mucosal metabolism, is known as presystemic or 'first-pass' metabolism (Figure 5.4).

The route of administration and presystemic metabolism markedly influence the pattern of drug metabolism. For example, when **salbutamol** is given to asthmatic subjects, the ratio of unchanged drug to metabolite in the urine is 2:1 after intravenous administration, but 1:2 after an oral dose. **Propranolol** undergoes substantial hepatic presystemic metabolism, and small doses given orally are completely metabolized before they reach the systematic circulation. After intravenous administration, the area under the plasma concentration–time curve is proportional to the dose administered and passes through the origin (Figure 5.5). After oral administration the relationship, although linear, does not pass through the origin and there is a threshold dose below which measurable concentrations of **propranolol** are not detectable in systemic venous plasma. The usual dose of drugs with substantial presystemic metabolism differs very markedly if the drug is given by the oral or by the systemic route (one must never estimate or guess the i.v. dose of a drug from its usual oral dose for this reason!) In patients with portocaval anastomoses bypassing the liver, hepatic presystemic metabolism is bypassed, so very small drug doses are needed compared to the usual oral dose.

Presystemic metabolism is not limited to the liver, since the gastro-intestinal mucosa contains many drug-metabolizing enzymes (e.g. CYP3A4, dopa-decarboxylase, catechol-O-methyl transferase (COMT)) which can metabolize drugs, e.g. **ciclosporin, felodipine, levodopa, salbutamol**, before they enter hepatic portal blood. Pronounced first-pass metabolism by either the gastro-intestinal mucosa (e.g. **felodipine, salbutamol, levodopa**) or liver (e.g. **felodipine, glyceryl trinitrate, morphine, naloxone, verapamil**) necessitates high oral doses by comparison with the intravenous route. Alternative routes of drug delivery (e.g. buccal, rectal, sublingual, transdermal) partly or completely bypass presystemic elimination (Chapter 4).

Drugs undergoing extensive presystemic metabolism usually exhibit pronounced inter-individual variability in drug disposition. This results in highly variable responses to therapy,

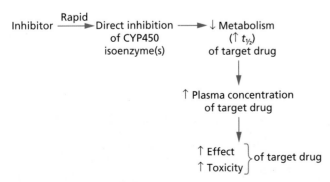

Figure 5.3: Enzyme inhibition.

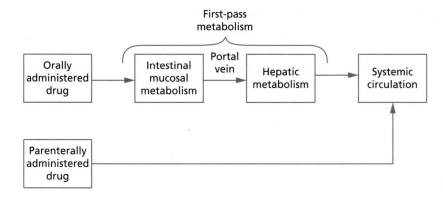

First-pass
metabolism

Figure 5.4: Presystemic ('first-pass') metabolism.

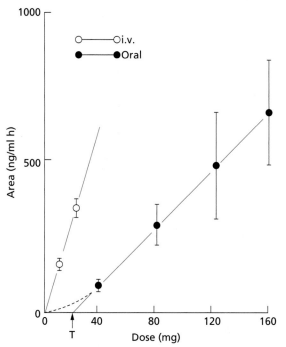

Figure 5.5: Area under blood concentration–time curve after oral
(●) and intravenous (○) administration of propranolol to humans
in various doses. T is the apparent threshold for propranolol
following oral administration. (Redrawn from Shand DG, Rangno
RE. *Pharmacology* 1972; **7**: 159, with permission of
S Karger AG, Basle.)

and is one of the major difficulties in their clinical use.
Variability in first-pass metabolism results from:

1. Genetic variations – for example, the bioavailability of
   hydralazine is about double in slow compared to fast
   acetylators. Presystemic hydroxylation of **metoprolol** and
   encainide also depends on genetic polymorphisms
   (CYP2D6, Chapter 14).
2. Induction or inhibition of drug-metabolizing enzymes.
3. Food increases liver blood flow and can increase the
   bioavailability of drugs, such as **propranolol**, **metoprolol**
   and **hydralazine**, by increasing hepatic blood flow and
   exceeding the threshold for complete hepatic extraction.
4. Drugs that increase liver blood flow have similar effects to
   food – for example, **hydralazine** increases **propranolol**
   bioavailability by approximately one-third, whereas drugs
   that reduce liver blood flow (e.g. β-adrenoceptor
   antagonists) reduce it.

5. Non-linear first-pass kinetics are common (e.g. **aspirin**,
   hydralazine, **propranolol**): increasing the dose
   disproportionately increases bioavailability.
6. Liver disease increases the bioavailability of some drugs
   with extensive first-pass extraction (e.g. **diltiazem**,
   ciclosporin, **morphine**).

METABOLISM OF DRUGS BY INTESTINAL ORGANISMS

This is important for drugs undergoing significant enterohepatic circulation. For example, in the case of **estradiol**, which is
excreted in bile as a glucuronide conjugate, bacteria-derived
enzymes cleave the glucuronide so that free drug is available
for reabsorption in the terminal ileum. A small proportion of
the dose (approximately 7%) is excreted in the faeces under
normal circumstances; this increases if gastro-intestinal disease or concurrent antibiotic therapy alter the intestinal flora.

Key points

- Drug metabolism involves two phases: phase I often
  followed sequentially by phase II.
- Phase I metabolism introduces a reactive group into a
  molecule, usually by oxidation, by a microsomal system
  present in the liver.
- The CYP450 enzymes are a superfamily of
  haemoproteins. They have distinct isoenzyme forms
  and are critical for phase I reactions.
- Products of phase I metabolism may be
  pharmacologically active, as well as being chemically
  reactive, and can be hepatotoxic.
- Phase II reactions involve conjugation (e.g. acetylation,
  glucuronidation, sulphation, methylation).
- Products of phase II metabolism are polar and can be
  efficiently excreted by the kidneys. Unlike the products
  of phase I metabolism, they are nearly always
  pharmacologically inactive.
- The CYP450 enzymes involved in phase I metabolism can
  be induced by several drugs and nutraceuticals (e.g.
  glucocorticosteroids, rifampicin, carbamazepine, St John's
  wort) or inhibited by drugs (e.g. cimetidine, azoles, HIV
  protease inhibitors, quinolones, metronidazole) and
  dietary constituents (e.g. grapefruit/grapefruit juice).
- Induction or inhibition of the CYP450 system are
  important causes of drug–drug interactions (see
  Chapter 13).

Case history

A 46-year-old woman is brought to the hospital Accident and Emergency Department by her sister, having swallowed an unknown number of paracetamol tablets washed down with vodka six hours previously, following an argument with her partner. She is an alcoholic and has been taking St John's wort for several weeks. Apart from signs of intoxication, examination was unremarkable. Plasma paracetamol concentration was 662 μmol/L (100 mg/L). Following discussion with the resident medical officer/ Poisons Information Service, it was decided to administer *N*-acetylcysteine.

Comment

In paracetamol overdose, the usual pathway of elimination is overwhelmed and a highly toxic product (*N*-acetyl benzo-quinone imine, known as NABQI) is formed by CYP1A2, 2E1 and CYP3A4 metabolism. A plasma paracetamol concentration of 100 mg/L six hours after ingestion would not usually require antidote treatment, but this woman is an alcoholic and is taking St John's wort and her hepatic drug-metabolizing enzymes (CYP1A2, CYP3A4 and probably others) will have been induced, so the paracetamol concentration threshold for antidote treatment is lowered (see Chapter 54). *N*-Acetylcysteine is the specific antidote, as it increases reduced glutathione which conjugates NABQI within hepatocytes.

FURTHER READING AND WEB MATERIAL

Boobis AR, Edwards RJ, Adams DA, Davies DS. Dissecting the function of P450. *British Journal of Clinical Pharmacology* 1996; **42**: 81–9.

Coon MJ. Cytochrome P450: nature's most versatile biological catalyst. *Annual Review of Pharmacology and Toxicology* 2005; **45**: 1–25.

Lin JH, Lu AY. Interindividual variability in inhibition and induction of cytochrome P450 enzymes. *Annual Review of Pharmacology and Toxicology* 2001; **41**: 535–67.

Nelson DR, Zeldin DC, Hoffman SM, Maltais LJ, Wain HM, Nebert DW. Comparison of cytochrome P450 (CYP) genes from the mouse and human genomes, including nomenclature recommendations for genes, pseudogenes and alternative-splice variants. *Pharmacogenetics* 2004; **14**: 1–18.

Website for CYP450 substrates, inhibitors and inducers: www.medicine.iupui.edu/flockhart/table, accessed April 2007.

RENAL EXCRETION OF DRUGS

INTRODUCTION

The kidneys are involved in the elimination of virtually every drug or drug metabolite (Figure 6.1). The contribution of renal excretion to total body clearance of any particular drug is determined by its lipid solubility (and hence its polarity). Elimination of non-polar drugs depends on metabolism (Chapter 5) to more polar metabolites, which are then excreted in the urine. Polar substances are eliminated efficiently by the kidneys, because they are not freely diffusible across the tubular membrane and so remain in the urine, even though there is a concentration gradient favouring reabsorption from tubular to interstitial fluid. Renal elimination is influenced by several processes that alter the drug concentration in tubular fluid. Depending on which of these predominates, the renal clearance of a drug may be either an important or a trivial component in its overall elimination.

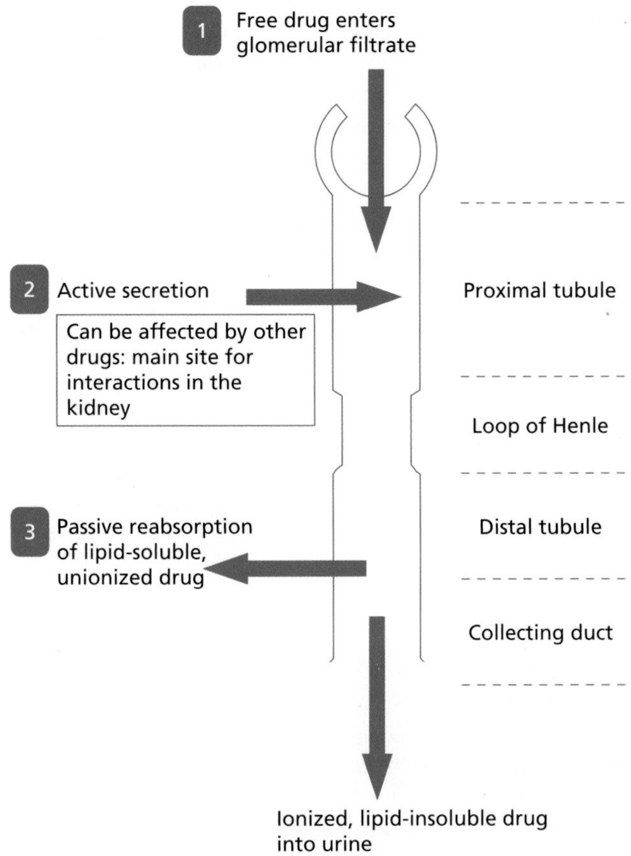

1 Free drug enters glomerular filtrate

2 Active secretion

Can be affected by other drugs: main site for interactions in the kidney

3 Passive reabsorption of lipid-soluble, unionized drug

Proximal tubule

Loop of Henle

Distal tubule

Collecting duct

Ionized, lipid-insoluble drug into urine

Figure 6.1: Urinary elimination of drugs and metabolites by glomerular filtration and/or tubular secretion and reabsorption.

GLOMERULAR FILTRATION

Glomerular filtrate contains concentrations of low-molecular-weight solutes similar to plasma. In contrast, molecules with a molecular weight of $\geq 66\,000$ (including plasma proteins and drug–protein complexes) do not pass through the glomerulus. Accordingly, only free drug passes into the filtrate. Renal impairment (Chapter 7) predictably reduces the elimination of drugs that depend on glomerular filtration for their clearance (e.g. **digoxin**). Drugs that are highly bound to albumin or α-1 acid glycoprotein in plasma are not efficiently filtered.

PROXIMAL TUBULAR SECRETION

There are independent mechanisms for active secretion of organic anions and organic cations (OAT and OCT) into the proximal tubule. These are relatively non-specific in their structural requirements, and share some of the characteristics of transport systems in the intestine. OAT excretes drugs, such as **probenecid** and **penicillin**. Para-aminohippuric acid (PAH) is excreted so efficiently that it is completely extracted from the renal plasma in a single pass through the kidney (i.e. during intravenous infusion of PAH its concentration in renal venous blood is zero). Clearance of PAH is therefore limited by the rate at which it is delivered to the kidney, i.e. renal plasma flow, so PAH clearance provides a non-invasive measure of renal plasma flow.

OCT contributes to the elimination of basic drugs (e.g. **cimetidine**, amphetamines).

Each mechanism is characterized by a maximal rate of transport for a given drug, so the process is theoretically saturable, although this maximum is rarely reached in practice. Because secretion of free drug occurs up a concentration gradient from peritubular fluid into the lumen, the equilibrium between unbound and bound drug in plasma can be disturbed, with bound drug dissociating from protein-binding sites. Tubular secretion can therefore eliminate drugs efficiently even if they are highly protein bound. Competition occurs between drugs transported via these systems. e.g. **probenecid** competitively inhibits the tubular secretion of **methotrexate**.

PASSIVE DISTAL TUBULAR REABSORPTION

The renal tubule behaves like a lipid barrier separating the high drug concentration in the tubular lumen and the lower concentration in the interstitial fluid and plasma. Reabsorption of drug down its concentration gradient occurs by passive diffusion. For highly lipid-soluble drugs, reabsorption is so effective that renal clearance is virtually zero. Conversely, polar substances, such as mannitol, are too water soluble to be absorbed, and are eliminated virtually without reabsorption.

Tubular reabsorption is influenced by urine flow rate. Diuresis increases the renal clearance of drugs that are passively reabsorbed, since the concentration gradient is reduced (Figure 6.2). Diuresis may be induced deliberately in order to increase drug elimination during treatment of overdose (Chapter 54).

Reabsorption of drugs that are weak acids (AH) or bases (B) depends upon the pH of the tubular fluid, because this determines the fraction of acid or base in the charged, polar form and the fraction in the uncharged lipid-soluble form. For acidic drugs, the more alkaline the urine, the greater the renal clearance, and vice versa for basic drugs, since:

$$AH \rightleftharpoons A^- + H^+$$

and

$$B + H^+ \rightleftharpoons BH^+.$$

Thus high pH favours A^-, the charged form of the weak acid which remains in the tubular fluid and is excreted in the urine, while low pH favours BH^+, the charged form of the base (Figure 6.3). This is utilized in treating overdose with **aspirin** (a weak acid) by alkalinization of the urine, thereby accelerating urinary elimination of salicylate (Chapter 54).

The extent to which urinary pH affects renal excretion of weak acids and bases depends quantitatively upon the pK_a of the drug. The critical range of pK_a values for pH-dependent excretion is about 3.0–6.5 for acids and 7.5–10.5 for bases.

Urinary pH may also influence the fraction of the total dose which is excreted unchanged. About 57% of a dose of amphetamine is excreted unchanged (i.e. as parent drug, rather than as a metabolite) in acid urine (pH 4.5–5.6), compared to about 7% in subjects with alkaline urine (pH 7.1–8.0). Administration of amphetamines with sodium bicarbonate has been used illicitly by athletes to enhance the pharmacological effects of the drug on performance, as well as to make its detection by urinary screening tests more difficult.

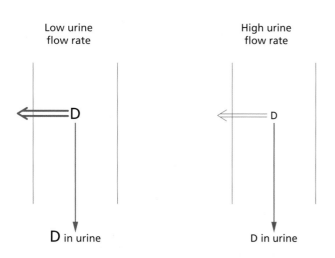

Figure 6.2: Effect of diuresis (urine flow rate) on renal clearance of a drug (D) passively reabsorbed in the distal tubule.

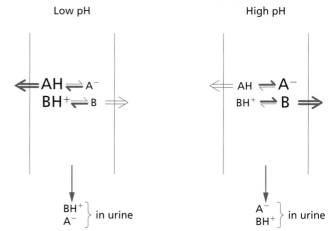

Figure 6.3: Effects of urine pH on renal clearance of a weak acid (AH) and a weak base (B).

ACTIVE TUBULAR REABSORPTION

This is of minor importance for most therapeutic drugs. Uric acid is reabsorbed by an active transport system which is inhibited by uricosuric drugs, such as **probenecid** and **sulfinpyrazone**. Lithium also undergoes active tubular reabsorption (hitching a ride on the proximal sodium ion transport mechanism).

Key points

- The kidney cannot excrete non-polar substances efficiently, since these diffuse back into blood as the urine is concentrated. Consequently, the kidney excretes polar drugs and/or the polar metabolites of non-polar compounds.
- Renal impairment reduces the elimination of drugs that depend on glomerular filtration, so the dose of drugs, such as digoxin, must be reduced, or the dose interval (e.g. between doses of aminoglycoside) must be increased, to avoid toxicity.
- There are specific secretory mechanisms for organic acids and organic bases in the proximal tubules which lead to the efficient clearance of weak acids, such as penicillin, and weak bases, such as cimetidine. Competition for these carriers can cause drug interactions, although less commonly than induction or inhibition of cytochrome P450.
- Passive reabsorption limits the efficiency with which the kidney eliminates drugs. Weak acids are best eliminated in an alkaline urine (which favours the charged form, A^-), whereas weak bases are best eliminated in an acid urine (which favours the charged form, BH^+).
- The urine may be deliberately alkalinized by infusing sodium bicarbonate intravenously in the management of overdose with weak acids such as aspirin (see Chapter 54, to increase tubular elimination of salicylate.
- Lithium ions are actively reabsorbed in the proximal tubule by the same system that normally reabsorbs sodium, so salt depletion (which causes increased proximal tubular sodium ion reabsorption) causes lithium toxicity unless the dose of lithium is reduced.

Case history

A house officer (HO) sees a 53-year-old woman in the Accident and Emergency Department with a six-hour history of fevers, chills, loin pain and dysuria. She looks very ill, with a temperature of 39.5°C, blood pressure of 80/60 mmHg and right loin tenderness. The white blood cell count is raised at 15 000/μL, and there are numerous white cells and rod-shaped organisms in the urine. Serum creatinine is normal at 90 μmol/L. The HO wants to start treatment with aminoglycoside antibiotic pending the availability of a bed on the intensive care unit. Despite the normal creatinine level, he is concerned that the dose may need to be adjusted and calls the resident medical officer for advice.
Comment
The HO is right to be concerned. The patient is hypotensive and will be perfusing her kidneys poorly. Serum creatinine may be normal in rapid onset acute renal failure. It is important to obtain an adequate peak concentration to combat her presumed Gram-negative septicaemia. It would therefore be appropriate to start treatment with the normal loading dose. This will achieve the usual peak concentration (since the volume of distribution will be similar to that in a healthy person). However, the subsequent and maintenance doses should not be given until urgent post-administration blood concentrations have been obtained – the dosing interval may be appropriately prolonged if renal failure does indeed supervene causing reduced aminoglycoside clearance.

FURTHER READING

Carmichael DJS. Chapter 19.2 Handling of drugs in kidney disease. In: AMA Davison, J Stewart Cameron, J-P Grunfeld, C Ponticelli, C Van Ypersele, E Ritz and C Winearls (eds). *Oxford textbook of clinical nephrology*, 3rd edn. Oxford: Oxford University Press, 2005: 2599–618.

Eraly SA, Bush KT, Sampogna RV, Bhatnagar V, Nigam SK. The molecular pharmacology of organic anion transporters: from DNA to FDA? *Molecular Pharmacology* 2004; **65**: 479–87.

Koepsell H. Polyspecific organic cation transporters: their functions and interactions with drugs. *Trends in Pharmacological Sciences* 2004; **25**: 375–81.

van Montfoort JE, Hagenbuch B, Groothuis GMM, Koepsell H, Meier PJ, Meijer DKF. Drug uptake systems in liver and kidney. *Current Drug Metabolism* 2003; **4**: 185–211.

CHAPTER 7

EFFECTS OF DISEASE ON DRUG DISPOSITION

INTRODUCTION

Several common disorders influence the way in which the body handles drugs and these must be considered before prescribing. Gastro-intestinal, cardiac, renal, liver and thyroid disorders all influence drug pharmacokinetics, and individualization of therapy is very important in such patients.

GASTRO-INTESTINAL DISEASE

Gastro-intestinal disease alters the absorption of orally administered drugs. This can cause therapeutic failure, so alternative routes of administration (Chapter 4) are sometimes needed.

GASTRIC EMPTYING

Gastric emptying is an important determinant of the rate and sometimes also the extent of drug absorption. Several pathological factors alter gastric emptying (Table 7.1). However, there is little detailed information about the effect of disease on drug absorption, in contrast to effects of drugs that slow gastric emptying (e.g. anti-muscarinic drugs) which delay C_{max}. Absorption of analgesics is delayed in migraine, and a more rapid absorption can be achieved by administering analgesics with **metoclopramide**, which increases gastric emptying.

SMALL INTESTINAL AND PANCREATIC DISEASE

The very large absorptive surface of the small intestine provides a substantial functional reserve, so even extensive involvement with, for example, coeliac disease may be present without causing a clinically important reduction in drug absorption. Crohn's disease typically affects the terminal ileum. Absorption of several antibiotics actually increases in Crohn's disease. Cystic fibrosis, because of its effects on

Table 7.1: Pathological factors influencing the rate of gastric emptying

Decreased rate	Increased rate
Trauma	Duodenal ulcer
Pain (including myocardial infarction, acute abdomen)	Gastroenterostomy
	Coeliac disease
Diabetic neuropathy	Drugs, e.g. metoclopramide
Labour	
Migraine	
Myxoedema	
Raised intracranial pressure	
Intestinal obstruction	
Gastric ulcer	
Anti-muscarinic drugs	

pancreatic secretions and bile flow, can impair the absorption of fat-soluble vitamins. Significant reductions in the absorption of **cefalexin** occur in cystic fibrosis, necessitating increased doses in such patients. Patients with small bowel resection may absorb lipophilic drugs poorly.

CARDIAC FAILURE

Cardiac failure affects pharmacokinetics in several ways and these are discussed below.

ABSORPTION

Absorption of some drugs (e.g. **furosemide**) is altered in cardiac failure because of mucosal oedema and reduced gastro-intestinal blood flow. Splanchnic vasoconstriction accompanies cardiac failure as an adaptive response redistributing blood to more vital organs.

DISTRIBUTION

Drug distribution is altered by cardiac failure. The apparent volume of distribution (V_d) of, for example, **quinidine** and **lidocaine** in patients with congestive cardiac failure is markedly reduced because of decreased tissue perfusion and altered partition between blood and tissue components. Usual doses can therefore result in elevated plasma concentrations, producing toxicity.

ELIMINATION

Elimination of several drugs is diminished in heart failure. Decreased hepatic perfusion accompanies reduced cardiac output. Drugs such as **lidocaine** with a high hepatic extraction ratio of >70% show perfusion-limited clearance, and steady-state levels are inversely related to cardiac output (Figure 7.1). During **lidocaine** infusion, the steady-state concentrations are almost 50% higher in patients with cardiac failure than in healthy volunteers. The potential for **lidocaine** toxicity in heart failure is further increased by the accumulation of its polar metabolites, which have cardiodepressant and pro-convulsant properties. This occurs because renal blood flow and glomerular filtration rate are reduced in heart failure.

Theophylline clearance is decreased and its half-life is doubled in patients with cardiac failure and pulmonary oedema, increasing the potential for accumulation and toxicity. The metabolic capacity of the liver is reduced in heart failure both by tissue hypoxia and by hepatocellular damage from hepatic congestion. Liver biopsy samples from patients with heart failure have reduced drug-metabolizing enzyme activity.

Heart failure reduces renal elimination of drugs because of reduced glomerular filtration, predisposing to toxicity from drugs that are primarily cleared by the kidneys, e.g. aminoglycosides and **digoxin**.

RENAL DISEASE

RENAL IMPAIRMENT

Renal excretion is a major route of elimination for many drugs (Chapter 6), and drugs and their metabolites that are excreted predominantly by the kidneys accumulate in renal failure. Renal disease also affects other pharmacokinetic processes (i.e. drug absorption, distribution and metabolism) in more subtle ways.

ABSORPTION

Gastric pH increases in chronic renal failure because urea is cleaved, yielding ammonia which buffers acid in the stomach. This reduces the absorption of ferrous iron and possibly also of other drugs. Nephrotic syndrome is associated with resistance to oral diuretics, and malabsorption of loop diuretics through the oedematous intestine may contribute to this.

DISTRIBUTION

Renal impairment causes accumulation of several acidic substances that compete with drugs for binding sites on albumin

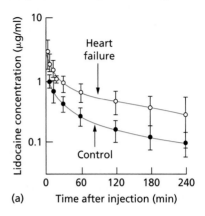

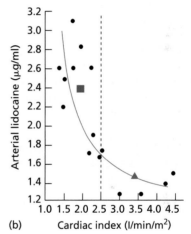

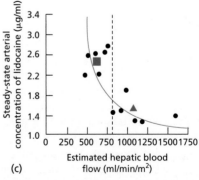

Figure 7.1: (a) Mean values (and standard deviations) of plasma lidocaine concentrations in seven heart failure patients and controls following a 50-mg intravenous bolus. (b) Relationship between arterial lidocaine level and cardiac index (dotted vertical line is lower limit of normal cardiac index, square is mean for low cardiac index patients, triangle is mean for patients with normal cardiac index). (c) Relationship of steady-state arterial lidocaine level following 50-mg bolus and infusion of 40 mg/kg/min (vertical line is lower limit of normal hepatic blood flow, square is mean for patients with low hepatic blood flow, triangle is mean for patients with normal flow). (Reproduced from: (a) Thompson PD et al. *American Heart Journal* 1971; **82**, 417; (b,c) Stenson RE et al. *Circulation* 1971; **43**: 205. With permission of the American Heart Association Inc.)

and other plasma proteins. This alters the pharmacokinetics of many drugs, but is seldom clinically important. **Phenytoin** is an exception, because therapy is guided by plasma concentration and routine analytical methods detect total (bound and free) drug. In renal impairment, **phenytoin** protein binding is reduced by competition with accumulated molecules normally cleared by the kidney and which bind to the same albumin drug-binding site as **phenytoin**. Thus, for any measured **phenytoin** concentration, free (active) drug is increased compared to a subject with normal renal function and the same measured total concentration. The therapeutic range therefore has to be adjusted to lower values in patients with renal impairment, as otherwise doses will be selected that cause toxicity.

Tissue binding of **digoxin** is reduced in patients with impaired renal function, resulting in a lower volume of distribution than in healthy subjects. A reduced loading dose of **digoxin** is therefore appropriate in such patients, although the effect of reduced glomerular filtration on **digoxin** clearance is even more important, necessitating a reduced maintenance dose, as described below.

The blood–brain barrier is more permeable to drugs in uraemia. This can result in increased access of drugs to the central nervous system, an effect that is believed to contribute to the increased incidence of confusion caused by **cimetidine**, **ranitidine** and **famotidine** in patients with renal failure.

METABOLISM

Metabolism of several drugs is reduced in renal failure. These include drugs that undergo phase I metabolism by CYP3A4. Drugs that are mainly metabolized by phase II drug metabolism are less affected, although conversion of **sulindac** to its active sulphide metabolite is impaired in renal failure, as is the hepatic conjugation of **metoclopramide** with glucuronide and sulphate.

RENAL EXCRETION

Glomerular filtration and tubular secretion of drugs usually fall in step with one another in patients with renal impairment. Drug excretion is directly related to glomerular filtration rate (GFR). Some estimate of GFR (eGFR) is therefore essential when deciding on an appropriate dose regimen. Serum creatinine concentration adjusted for age permits calculation of an estimate of GFR per $1.73\,m^2$ body surface area. This is now provided by most chemical pathology laboratories, and is useful in many situations. Alternatively, Figure 7.2 shows a nomogram given plasma creatinine, age, sex and body weight and is useful when a patient is markedly over- or underweight. The main limitation of such estimates is that they are misleading if GFR is changing rapidly as in acute renal failure. (Imagine that a patient with normal serum creatinine undergoes bilateral nephrectomy: an hour later, his serum creatinine would still be normal, but his GFR would be zero. Creatinine would rise gradually over the next few days as it continued to be produced in his body but was not cleared.) A normal creatinine level therefore does not mean that usual doses can be assumed to be safe in a patient who is acutely unwell.

eGFR is used to adjust the dose regimen in patients with some degree of chronic renal impairment for drugs with a low therapeutic index that are eliminated mainly by renal excretion. Dose adjustment must be considered for drugs for which there is >50% elimination by renal excretion. The British National Formulary tabulates drugs to be avoided or used with caution in patients with renal failure. Common examples are shown in Table 7.2.

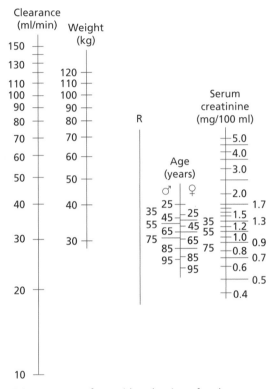

Figure 7.2: Nomogram for rapid evaluation of endogenous creatinine clearance – with a ruler joining weight to age. Keep ruler at crossing point on R, then move the right-hand side of the ruler to the appropriate serum creatinine value and read off clearance from the left-hand scale. To convert serum creatinine in μmol/L to mg/100 mL, as is used on this scale, simply divide by 88.4. (Reproduced with permission from Siersbaek-Nielson K et al. *Lancet* 1971; **1**: 1133. © The Lancet Ltd.)

Table 7.2: Examples of drugs to be used with particular caution or avoided in renal failure

Angiotensin-converting enzyme inhibitors[a]	Angiotensin receptor blockers[a]
Aldosterone antagonists	Aminoglycosides
Amphotericin	Atenolol
Ciprofloxacin	Cytotoxics
Digoxin	Lithium
Low molecular weight heparin	Metformin
NSAIDs	Methotrexate

[a]ACEI and ARB must be used with caution, but can slow progressive renal impairment (see Chapter 28).

Detailed recommendations on dosage reduction can be found in textbooks of nephrology. These are useful for getting treatment under way but, although precise, such recommendations are inevitably based only on the effects of reduced renal function on drug elimination in 'average' populations. Individual variation is substantial, and therapeutic monitoring of efficacy, toxicity and sometimes of drug concentrations is essential in patients with impaired renal function.

There are two ways of reducing the total dose to compensate for impaired renal function. Either each dose can be reduced, or the interval between each dose can be lengthened. The latter method is useful when a drug must achieve some threshold concentration to produce its desired effect, but does not need to remain at this level throughout the dose interval. This is the case with aminoglycoside antibiotics. Therapy with these drugs is appropriately monitored by measuring 'peak' concentrations (in blood sampled at a fixed brief interval after dosing, sufficient to permit at least partial tissue distribution), which indicate whether the dose is large enough to achieve a therapeutic plasma concentration, and 'trough' concentrations immediately before the next dose (see Chapter 8). If the peak concentration is satisfactory but the trough concentration is higher than desired (i.e. toxicity is present or imminent), the dose is not reduced but the interval between doses is extended. This type of therapeutic drug monitoring is modified to a single time point (after dosing and beyond the distribution phase) when extended interval dosing of aminoglycosides is used to treat patients (Chapter 43).

RENAL HAEMODYNAMICS

Patients with mild renal impairment depend on vasodilator prostaglandin biosynthesis to preserve renal blood flow and GFR. The same is true of patients with heart failure, nephrotic syndrome, cirrhosis or ascites. Such patients develop acute reversible renal impairment, often accompanied by salt and water retention and hypertension if treated with non-steroidal anti-inflammatory drugs (NSAIDs, see Chapter 26), because these inhibit cyclo-oxygenase and hence the synthesis of vasodilator prostaglandins, notably prostaglandin I_2 (prostacyclin) and prostaglandin E_2. **Sulindac** is a partial exception because it inhibits cyclo-oxygenase less in kidneys than in other tissues, although this specificity is incomplete and dose dependent.

Angiotensin converting enzyme inhibitors (e.g. **ramipril**) can also cause reversible renal failure due to altered renal haemodynamics. This occurs predictably in patients with bilateral renal artery stenosis (or with renal artery stenosis involving a single functioning kidney). The explanation is that in such patients GFR is preserved in the face of the fixed proximal obstruction by angiotensin-II-mediated efferent arteriolar vasoconstriction. Inhibition of angiotensin converting enzyme disables this homeostatic mechanism and precipitates renal failure.

NEPHROTIC SYNDROME

Plasma albumin in patients with nephrotic syndrome is low, resulting in increased fluctuations of free drug concentration following each dose. This could cause adverse effects, although in practice this is seldom clinically important. The high albumin concentration in tubular fluid contributes to the resistance to diuretics that accompanies nephrotic syndrome. This is because both loop diuretics and thiazides act on ion-transport processes in the luminal membranes of tubular cells (see Chapter 36). Protein binding of such diuretics within the tubular lumen therefore reduces the concentration of free (active) drug in tubular fluid in contact with the ion transporters on which they act.

PRESCRIBING FOR PATIENTS WITH RENAL DISEASE

1. Consider the possibility of renal impairment before drugs are prescribed and use available data to estimate GFR.
2. Check how drugs are eliminated before prescribing them. If renal elimination accounts for more than 50% of total elimination, then dose reduction will probably be necessary after the first dose, i.e. for maintenance doses.
3. Monitor therapeutic and adverse effects and, where appropriate, plasma drug concentrations.
4. If possible avoid potentially nephrotoxic drugs (e.g. aminoglycosides, NSAIDs); if such drugs are essential use them with great care.

Once a potential renal problem necessitating dose modification has been identified, there are a number of accepted reference sources that provide guidance for dose adjustment. These are useful approximations to get treatment under way, but their mathematical precision is illusory, and must not lull the inexperienced into a false sense of security – they do not permit a full 'course' of treatment to be prescribed safely. The patient must be monitored and treatment modified in the light of individual responses. The British National Formulary has a useful appendix which is concise, simple and accessible.

LIVER DISEASE

The liver is the main site of drug metabolism (Chapter 5). Liver disease has major but unpredictable effects on drug handling. Pharmacokinetic factors that are affected include absorption and distribution, as well as the metabolism of drugs.

Attempts to correlate changes in the pharmacokinetics of drugs with biochemical tests of liver function have been unsuccessful (in contrast to the use of plasma creatinine in chronic renal impairment described above). In chronic liver disease, serum albumin is the most useful index of hepatic drug-metabolizing activity, possibly because a low albumin level reflects depressed synthesis of hepatic proteins, including those involved in drug metabolism. Prothrombin time also shows a moderate correlation with drug clearance by the liver. However, in neither case has a continuous relationship been demonstrated, and such indices of hepatic function serve mainly to distinguish the severely affected from the milder cases. Clearances of indocyanine green, **antipyrine** and **lidocaine** have also been disappointing.

Currently, therefore, cautious empiricism coupled with an awareness of an increased likelihood of adverse drug effects and close clinical monitoring is the best way for a prescriber to approach a patient with liver disease. Drugs should be used only if necessary, and the risks weighed against potential benefit. If possible, drugs that are eliminated by routes other than the liver should be employed.

EFFECTS OF LIVER DISEASE ON DRUG ABSORPTION

Absorption of drugs is altered in liver disease because of portal hypertension, and because hypoalbuminaemia causes mucosal oedema. Portal/systemic anastomoses allow the passage of orally administered drug directly into the systemic circulation, bypassing hepatic presystemic metabolism and markedly increasing the bioavailability of drugs with high presystemic metabolism such as **propranolol, morphine, verapamil** and **ciclosporin**, which must therefore be started in low doses in such patients and titrated according to effect.

DISTRIBUTION OF DRUGS IN PATIENTS WITH LIVER DISEASE

Drug distribution is altered in liver disease. Reduced plasma albumin reduces plasma protein binding. This is also influenced by bilirubin and other endogenous substances that accumulate in liver disease and may displace drugs from binding sites. The free fraction of **tolbutamide** is increased by 115% in cirrhosis, and that of **phenytoin** is increased by up to 40%. It is particularly important to appreciate this when plasma concentrations of **phenytoin** are being used to monitor therapy, as unless the therapeutic range is adjusted downward, toxicity will be induced, as explained above in the section on drug distribution in renal disease.

Reduced plasma protein binding increases the apparent V_d if other factors remain unchanged. Increased V_d of several drugs (e.g. **theophylline**) is indeed observed in patients with liver disease. Disease-induced alterations in clearance and V_d often act in opposite directions with regard to their effect on $t_{1/2}$. Data on $t_{1/2}$ in isolation provide little information about the extent of changes in metabolism or drug distribution which result from liver disease.

DRUG METABOLISM IN LIVER DISEASE

CYP450-mediated phase I drug metabolism is generally reduced in patients with very severe liver disease, but drug metabolism is surprisingly little impaired in patients with moderate to severe disease. There is a poor correlation between microsomal enzyme activity from liver biopsy specimens in vitro and drug clearance measurements in vivo. Even in very severe disease, the metabolism of different drugs is not affected to the same extent. It is therefore hazardous to extrapolate from knowledge of the handling of one drug to effects on another in an individual patient with liver disease.

Prescribing for patients with liver disease

1. Weigh risks against hoped for benefit, and minimize non-essential drug use.
2. If possible, use drugs that are eliminated by routes other than the liver (i.e. in general, renally cleared drugs).
3. Monitor response, including adverse effects (and occasionally drug concentrations), and adjust therapy accordingly.
4. Avoid sedatives and analgesics if possible: they are common precipitants of hepatic coma.
5. Predictable hepatotoxins (e.g. cytotoxic drugs) should only be used for the strongest of indications, and then only with close clinical and biochemical monitoring.
6. Drugs that are known to cause idiosyncratic liver disease (e.g. **isoniazid**, **phenytoin**, **methyldopa**) are not necessarily contraindicated in stable chronic disease, as there is no evidence of increased susceptibility. Oral contraceptives are not advisable if there is active liver disease or a history of jaundice of pregnancy.
7. Constipation favours bacterial production of false neurotransmitter amines in the bowel: avoid drugs that cause constipation (e.g. **verapamil**, tricyclic antidepressants) if possible.
8. Drugs that inhibit catabolism of amines (e.g. monoamine oxidase inhibitors) also provoke coma and should be avoided.
9. Low plasma potassium provokes encephalopathy: avoid drugs that cause this if possible. Potassium-sparing drugs, such as **spironolactone**, are useful.
10. Avoid drugs that cause fluid overload or renal failure (e.g. NSAID) and beware those containing sodium (e.g. sodium-containing antacids and high-dose **carbenicillin**).
11. Avoid drugs that interfere with haemostasis (e.g. **aspirin**, anticoagulants and fibrinolytics) whenever possible, because of the increased risk of bleeding (especially in the presence of varices!).

THYROID DISEASE

Thyroid dysfunction affects drug disposition partly as a result of effects on drug metabolism and partly via changes in renal elimination. Existing data refer to only a few drugs, but it is prudent to anticipate the possibility of increased sensitivity of hypothyroid patients to many drugs when prescribing. Information is available for the following drugs.

DIGOXIN

Myxoedematous patients are extremely sensitive to **digoxin**, whereas unusually high doses are required in thyrotoxicosis. In general, hyperthyroid patients have lower plasma digoxin concentrations and hypothyroid patients have higher plasma concentrations than euthyroid patients on the same dose. There is no significant difference in half-life between these groups, and a difference in V_d has been postulated to explain the alteration of plasma concentration with thyroid activity. Changes in renal function, which occur with changes in thyroid status, complicate this interpretation. GFR is increased in thyrotoxicosis and decreased in myxoedema. These changes in renal function influence elimination, and the reduced plasma levels of **digoxin** correlate closely with the increased creatinine clearance in thyrotoxicosis. Other factors including enhanced biliary clearance, **digoxin** malabsorption due to intestinal hurry and increased hepatic metabolism, have all been postulated as factors contributing to the insensitivity of thyrotoxic patients to cardiac glycosides.

ANTICOAGULANTS

Oral anticoagulants produce an exaggerated prolongation of prothrombin time in hyperthyroid patients. This is due to increased metabolic breakdown of vitamin K-dependent clotting factors (Chapter 30), rather than to changes in drug pharmacokinetics.

GLUCOCORTICOIDS

Glucocorticoids are metabolized by hepatic mixed-function oxidases (CYP3A4) which are influenced by thyroid status. In hyperthyroidism, there is increased cortisol production and a reduced cortisol half-life, the converse being true in myxoedema.

THYROXINE

The normal half-life of **thyroxine** (six to seven days) is reduced to three to four days by hyperthyroidism and prolonged to nine to ten days by hypothyroidism. This is of considerable clinical importance when deciding on an appropriate interval at which to increase the dose of **thyroxine** in patients treated for myxoedema, especially if they have coincident ischaemic heart disease which would be exacerbated if an excessive steady-state **thyroxine** level were achieved.

ANTITHYROID DRUGS

The half-life of **propylthiouracil** and **methimazole** is prolonged in hypothyroidism and shortened in hyperthyroidism.

These values return to normal on attainment of the euthyroid state, probably because of altered hepatic metabolism.

OPIATES

Patients with hypothyroidism are exceptionally sensitive to opioid analgesics, which cause profound respiratory depression in this setting. This is probably due to reduced metabolism and increased sensitivity.

Key points

Disease profoundly influences the response to many drugs by altering pharmacokinetics and/or pharmacodynamics.

- Gastro-intestinal disease:
  (a) diseases that alter gastric emptying influence the response to oral drugs (e.g. migraine reduces gastric emptying, limiting the effectiveness of analgesics);
  (b) ileum/pancreas – relatively minor effects.
- Heart failure:
  (a) absorption of drugs (e.g. furosemide) is reduced as a result of splanchnic hypoperfusion;
  (b) elimination of drugs that are removed very efficiently by the liver (e.g. lidocaine) is reduced as a result of reduced hepatic blood flow, predisposing to toxicity;
  (c) tissue hypoperfusion increases the risk of lactic acidosis with metformin (cor pulmonale especially predisposes to this because of hypoxia).
- Renal disease:
  (a) chronic renal failure – as well as reduced excretion, drug absorption, distribution and metabolism may also be altered. Estimates of creatinine clearance or GFR based on serum creatinine concentration/ weight/age/sex/ ethnicity provide a useful index of the need for maintenance dose adjustment in chronic renal failure;
  (b) nephrotic syndrome leads to altered drug distribution because of altered binding to albumin and altered therapeutic range of concentrations for drugs that are extensively bound to albumin (e.g. some anticonvulsants). Albumin in tubular fluid binds diuretics and causes diuretic resistance. Glomerular filtration rate is preserved in nephrotic syndrome by compensatory increased prostaglandin synthesis, so NSAIDs (see Chapter 26) can precipitate renal failure.
- Liver disease – as well as effects on drug metabolism, absorption and distribution may also be altered because of portal systemic shunting, hypoalbuminaemia and ascites. There is no widely measured biochemical marker (analogous to serum creatinine in chronic renal failure) to guide dose adjustment in liver disease, and a cautious dose titration approach should be used.
- Thyroid disease:
  (a) hypothyroidism increases sensitivity to digoxin and opioids;
  (b) hyperthyroidism increases sensitivity to warfarin and reduces sensitivity to digoxin.

Case history

A 57-year-old alcoholic is admitted to hospital because of gross ascites and peripheral oedema. He looks chronically unwell, is jaundiced, and has spider naevi and gynaecomastia. His liver and spleen are not palpable in the presence of marked ascites. Serum chemistries reveal hypoalbuminuria (20 g/L), sodium 132 mmol/L, potassium 3.5 mmol/L, creatinine 105 μmol/L, and international normalized ratio (INR) is increased at 1.8. The patient is treated with furosemide and his fluid intake is restricted. Over the next five days he loses 10.5 kg, but you are called to see him because he has become confused and unwell. On examination, he is drowsy and has asterixis ('liver flap'). His blood pressure is 100/54 mmHg with a postural drop. His serum potassium is 2.6 mmol/L, creatinine has increased to 138 μmol/L and the urea concentration has increased disproportionately.

Comment

It is a mistake to try to eliminate ascites too rapidly in patients with cirrhosis. In this case, in addition to prerenal renal failure, the patient has developed profound hypokalaemia, which is commonly caused by furosemide in a patient with secondary hyperaldosteronism with a poor diet. The hypokalaemia has precipitated hepatic encephalopathy. It would have been better to have initiated treatment with spironolactone to inhibit his endogenous aldosterone. Low doses of furosemide could be added to this if increasing doses of spironolactone up to the maximum had not produced adequate fluid/weight loss. Great caution will be needed in starting such treatment now that the patient's renal function has deteriorated, and serum potassium levels must be monitored closely.

FURTHER READING

Carmichael DJS. Chapter 19.2 Handling of drugs in kidney disease. In: AMA Davison, J Stewart Cameron, J-P Grunfeld, C Ponticelli, C Van Ypersele, E Ritz and C Winearls (eds). *Oxford textbook of clinical nephrology*, 3rd edn. Oxford: Oxford University Press, 2005: 2599–618.

Rowland M, Tozer TN. Disease. In: *Clinical pharmacokinetics: concepts and applications*, 3rd edn. Baltimore: Williams and Wilkins, 1995: 248–66.

THERAPEUTIC DRUG MONITORING

INTRODUCTION

Drug response differs greatly between individuals. This variability results from two main sources:

1. variation in absorption, distribution, metabolism or elimination (pharmacokinetic);
2. variation at or beyond tissue receptors or other macromolecular drug targets (pharmacodynamic).

Monitoring of drug therapy by biological response encompasses both kinds of variability. There must be a continuous variable that is readily measured and is closely linked to the desired clinical outcome. Such responses are said to be good 'surrogate markers'. ('Surrogate' because what the prescriber really wants to achieve is to reduce the risk of a clinical event, such as a stroke, heart attack, pulmonary embolism, etc.) For example, antihypertensive drugs are monitored by their effect on blood pressure (Chapter 28), statins by their effect on serum cholesterol (Chapter 27), oral anticoagulants by their effect on the international normalized ratio (INR) (Chapter 30). Many other examples will be encountered in later chapters.

In some circumstances, however, there is no good continuous variable to monitor, especially for diseases with an unpredictable or fluctuating course. Measuring drug concentrations in plasma or serum identifies only pharmacokinetic variability, but can sometimes usefully guide dose adjustment, for example in treating an epileptic patient with an anticonvulsant drug. Measuring drug concentrations for use in this way is often referred to as 'therapeutic drug monitoring', and is the focus of this chapter.

ROLE OF DRUG MONITORING IN THERAPEUTICS

Measurement of drug concentrations is sometimes a useful complement to clinical monitoring to assist in selecting the best drug regimen for an individual patient. Accurate and convenient assays are necessary. Measurements of drug concentrations in plasma are most useful when:

1. There is a direct relationship between plasma concentration and pharmacological or toxic effect, i.e. a therapeutic range has been established. (Drugs that work via active metabolites, and drugs with irreversible actions, are unsuited to this approach. Tolerance also restricts the usefulness of plasma concentrations.)
2. Effect cannot readily be assessed quantitatively by clinical observation.
3. Inter-individual variability in plasma drug concentrations from the same dose is large (e.g. **phenytoin**).
4. There is a low therapeutic index (e.g. if the ratio of toxic concentration/effective concentration is <2).
5. Several drugs are being given concurrently and serious interactions are anticipated.
6. Replacement treatment (for example, of **thyroxine**) is to be optimized.
7. Apparent 'resistance' to the action of a drug needs an explanation, when non-compliance is suspected.

Another indication, distinct from therapeutic drug monitoring, for measuring drug concentrations in plasma is in clinical toxicology. Such measurements can guide management when specific intervention is contemplated in treating a poisoned patient (e.g. with **paracetamol** or **aspirin**).

PRACTICAL ASPECTS

Drug distribution and the location (tissue and cell) of the drug's target influence the relationship between plasma drug concentration and effect. A constant tissue to plasma drug concentration ratio only occurs during the terminal β-phase of elimination. Earlier in the dose interval, the plasma concentration does not reflect the concentration in the extracellular tissue space accurately. Figure 8.1 illustrates an extreme example of this in the case of digoxin. Measurements must be made when enough time has elapsed after a dose for distribution to

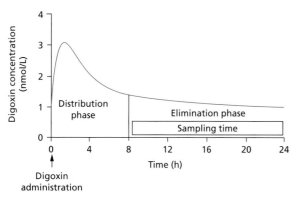

Figure 8.1: Serum concentration–time course following digoxin administration.

Table 8.1: Therapeutic range of several important drugs, for which therapeutic drug monitoring is often used.

Drug	Therapeutic range
Digoxin	0.8–2 mg/L (1–2.6 nmol/L)
Lithium	0.4–1.4 mmol/L[a]
Phenytoin	10–20 mg/L (40–80 μmol/L)
Theophylline	5–20 mg/L (28–110 μmol/L)
Ciclosporin	50–200 μg/L

[a]An upper limit of 1.6 mmol/L has also been advocated.

have occurred. Greater care is therefore required in the timing and labelling of specimens for drug concentration determination than is the case for 'routine' chemical pathology specimens. Usually during repeated dosing a sample is taken just before the next dose to assess the 'trough' concentration, and a sample may also be taken at some specified time after dosing (depending on the drug) to determine the 'peak' concentration.

Given this information, the laboratory should be able to produce useful information. Advice on the interpretation of this information is sometimes available from a local therapeutic drug-monitoring service, such as is provided by some clinical pharmacology and/or clinical pharmacy departments. In general, the cost of measuring drug concentrations is greater than for routine clinical chemical estimations, and to use expensive facilities to produce 'numbers' resulting from analysis of samples taken at random from patients described only by name or number is meaningless and misleading, as well as being a waste of money.

Analytical techniques of high specificity (often relying on high-performance liquid chromatography (HPLC), or HPLC-tandem mass spectroscopy or radioimmunoassay) avoid the pitfalls of less specific methods which may detect related compounds (e.g. drug metabolites). Even so, quality control monitoring of anticonvulsant analyses performed by laboratories both in the UK and in the USA have revealed that repeated analyses of a reference sample can produce some startlingly different results. The most important principle for the clinician is that plasma drug concentrations must always be interpreted in the context of the patient's clinical state.

There are few prospective studies of the impact of therapeutic drug-monitoring services on the quality of patient care. A retrospective survey conducted at the Massachusetts General Hospital showed that before the use of digoxin monitoring, 13.9% of all patients receiving **digoxin** showed evidence of toxicity, and that this figure fell to 5.9% following the introduction of monitoring.

DRUGS FOR WHICH THERAPEUTIC DRUG MONITORING IS USED

Table 8.1 lists those drugs which may be monitored therapeutically.

1. **Digoxin**: measuring the plasma concentration can help optimize therapy, especially for patients in sinus rhythm where there is no easy pharmacodynamic surrogate marker of efficacy, and is also useful in suspected toxicity or poor compliance.
2. **Lithium**: plasma concentrations are measured 12 hours after dosing.
3. Aminoglycoside antibiotics – for **gentamicin**, peak concentrations measured 30 minutes after dosing of 7–10 mg/L are usually effective against sensitive organisms, and trough levels, measured immediately before a dose, of 1–2 mg/L reduce the risk of toxicity; for **amikacin**, the desirable peak concentration is 4–12 mg/L, with a trough value of <4 mg/L. With extended interval aminoglycoside dosing (a single daily dose of 5–7 mg/kg), a single drug concentration determined at a time after the completion of the distribution phase is used to define further dosing intervals using validated nomograms.
4. **Phenytoin**: it is important to be aware of its non-linear pharmacokinetics (Chapters 3 and 22), and of the possible effects of concurrent renal or hepatic disease or of pregnancy on its distribution. Therapeutic drug monitoring is also widely used for some other anticonvulsants, such as **carbamazepine** and **sodium valproate**.
5. **Methotrexate**: plasma concentration is an important predictor of toxicity, and concentrations of >5 μmol/L 24 hours after a dose or 100 nmol/L 48 hours after dosing usually require folinic acid administration to prevent severe toxicity.
6. **Theophylline**: has a narrow therapeutic index (Figure 8.2) and many factors influence its clearance (Figure 8.3). Measurement of plasma **theophylline** concentration can help to minimize toxicity (e.g. cardiac dysrhythmias or seizures). A therapeutic range of 5–20 mg/L is quoted. (Plasma concentrations >15 mg/L are, however, associated with severe toxicity in neonates due to decreased protein binding and accumulation of caffeine, to which **theophylline** is methylated in neonates, but not in older children.)
7. The therapeutic ranges of plasma concentrations of several anti-dysrhythmic drugs (e.g. **lidocaine**) have been established with reasonable confidence. The therapeutic range of plasma **amiodarone** concentrations for ventricular dysrhythmias (1.0–2.5 mg/L) is higher than that needed

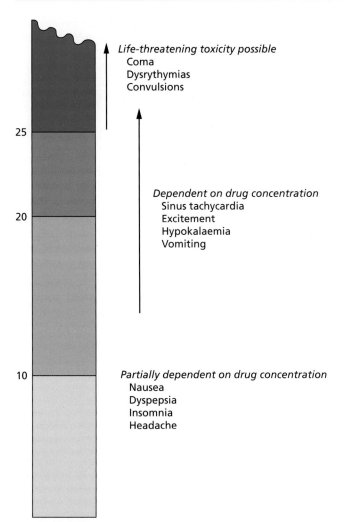

Figure 8.2: Theophylline plasma concentrations (mg/L). Note that there is a wide variation in the incidence and severity of adverse effects. (Adapted from Mant T, Henry J, Cochrane G. In: Henry J, Volans G (eds). *ABC of poisoning. Part 1: Drugs*. London: British Medical Journal.)

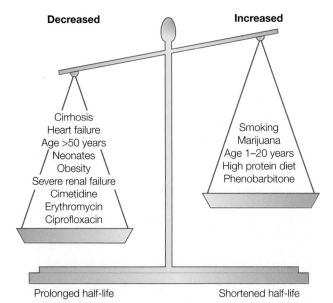

Figure 8.3: Theophylline clearance. (Adapted from Mant T, Henry J, Cochrane G. In: Henry J, Volans G (eds). *ABC of poisoning. Part 1: Drugs*. London: British Medical Journal.)

for atrial dysrhythmias (0.5–1.5 mg/L). The clinical utility of predicting toxicity by measuring a metabolite (desethyl amiodarone) is under evaluation.

8. Immunosuppressants: **Ciclosporin** compliance is a particular problem in children, and deterioration in renal function can reflect either graft rejection due to inadequate **ciclosporin** concentration or toxicity from excessive concentrations. **Sirolimus** use should be monitored, especially when used with **ciclosporin** or when there is hepatic impairment or during or after treatment with inducers or inhibitors of drug metabolism.

Key points

- Determining the plasma concentrations of drugs in order to adjust therapy is referred to as therapeutic drug monitoring. It has distinct but limited applications.
- Therapeutic drug monitoring permits dose individualization and is useful when there is a clear relationship between plasma concentration and pharmacodynamic effects.
- The timing of blood samples in relation to dosing is crucial. For aminoglycosides, samples are obtained for measurement of peak and trough concentrations. To guide chronic therapy (e.g. with anticonvulsants), sufficient time must elapse after starting treatment or changing dose for the steady state to have been achieved, before sampling.
- Drugs which may usefully be monitored in this way include digoxin, lithium, aminoglycosides, several anticonvulsants, methotrexate, theophylline, several anti-dysrhythmic drugs (including amiodarone) and ciclosporin.
- Individualization of dosage using therapeutic drug monitoring permits the effectiveness of these drugs to be maximized, while minimizing their potential toxicity.

Case history

A 35-year-old asthmatic is admitted to hospital at 6 a.m. because of a severe attack of asthma. She has been treated with salbutamol and beclometasone inhalers supplemented by a modified-release preparation of theophylline, 300 mg at night. She has clinical evidence of a severe attack and does not improve with nebulized salbutamol and oxygen. Treatment with intravenous aminophylline is considered.
Comment
Aminophylline is a soluble preparation of theophylline (80%) mixed with ethylenediamine (20%), which has a role in patients with life-threatening asthma. However, it is essential to have rapid access to an analytical service to measure plasma theophylline concentrations if this drug is to be used safely, especially in this situation where the concentration of theophylline resulting from the modified-release preparation that the patient took the night before admission must be determined before starting treatment. Theophylline toxicity (including seizures and potentially fatal cardiac dysrhythmias) can result if the dose is not individualized in relation to the plasma theophylline concentration.

FURTHER READING

Arns W, Cibrik DM, Walker RG et al. Therapeutic drug monitoring of mycophenolic acid in solid organ transplant patients treated with mycophenolate mofetil: Review of the literature. *Transplantation* 2006; **82**: 1004–12.

Aronson JK, Hardman M, Reynolds DJM. *ABC of monitoring drug therapy*. London: BMJ Publications, 1993.

Bartelink IH, Rademaker CMA, Schobben AFAM et al. Guidelines on paediatric dosing on the basis of developmental physiology and pharmacokinetic considerations. *Clinical Pharmacokinetics* 2006; **45**: 1077–97.

Fleming J, Chetty M. Therapeutic monitoring of valproate in psychiatry: How far have we progressed? *Clinical Neuropharmacology* 2006; **29**: 350–60.

Herxheimer A. Clinical pharmacology and therapeutics. In: Warrell DA (ed.). *Oxford textbook of medicine*, 4th edn. Oxford: Oxford University Press, 2006.

Johannessen SI, Tomson T. Pharmacokinetic variability of newer antiepileptic drugs – When is monitoring needed? *Clinical Pharmacokinetics* 2006; **45**: 1061–75.

Kaplan B. Mycophenolic acid trough level monitoring in solid organ transplant recipients treated with mycophenolate mofetil: association with clinical outcome. *Current Medical Research and Opinion* 2006; **22**: 2355–64.

Mitchell PB. Therapeutic drug monitoring of psychotropic medications. *British Journal of Clinical Pharmacology* 2000; **49**: 303–12.

Oellerich M, Armstrong VW. The role of therapeutic drug monitoring in individualizing immunosuppressive drug therapy: Recent developments. *Therapeutic Drug Monitoring* 2006; **28**: 720–25.

Stamp L, Roberts R, Kennedy M, Barclay M, O'Donnell J, Chapman P. The use of low dose methotrexate in rheumatoid arthritis – are we entering a new era of therapeutic drug monitoring and pharmacogenomics? *Biomedicine and Pharmacotherapy* 2006; **60**: 678–87.

DRUGS IN PREGNANCY

INTRODUCTION

The use of drugs in pregnancy is complicated by the potential for harmful effects on the growing fetus, altered maternal physiology and the paucity and difficulties of research in this field.

Key points

- There is potential for harmful effects on the growing fetus.
- Because of human variation, subtle effects to the fetus may be virtually impossible to identify.
- There is altered maternal physiology.
- There is notable paucity of and difficulties in research in this area.
- Assume all drugs are harmful until proven otherwise.

HARMFUL EFFECTS ON THE FETUS

Because experience with many drugs in pregnancy is severely limited, it should be assumed that all drugs are potentially harmful until sufficient data exist to indicate otherwise. 'Social' drugs (alcohol and cigarette smoking) are definitely damaging and their use must be discouraged.

In the placenta, maternal blood is separated from fetal blood by a cellular membrane (Figure 9.1). Most drugs with a molecular weight of less than 1000 can cross the placenta. This is usually by passive diffusion down the concentration gradient, but can involve active transport. The rate of diffusion depends first on the concentration of free drug (i.e. non-protein bound) on each side of the membrane, and second on the lipid solubility of the drug, which is determined in part by the degree of ionization. Diffusion occurs if the drug is in the unionized state. Placental function is also modified by changes in blood flow, and drugs which reduce placental blood flow can reduce birth weight. This may be the mechanism which causes the small reduction in birth weight following treatment

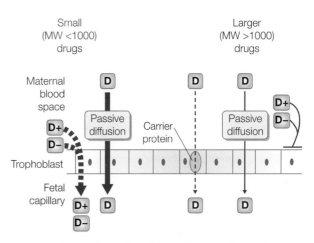

Figure 9.1: Placental transfer of drugs from mother to fetus.

of the mother with **atenolol** in pregnancy. Early in embryonic development, exogenous substances accumulate in the neuro-ectoderm. The fetal blood–brain barrier is not developed until the second half of pregnancy, and the susceptibility of the central nervous system (CNS) to developmental toxins may be partly related to this. The human placenta possesses multiple enzymes that are primarily involved with endogenous steroid metabolism, but which may also contribute to drug metabolism and clearance.

The stage of gestation influences the effects of drugs on the fetus. It is convenient to divide pregnancy into four stages, namely fertilization and implantation (<17 days), the organogenesis/embryonic stage (17–57 days), the fetogenic stage and delivery.

Key points

- A cellular membrane separates the maternal and fetal blood.
- Most drugs cross the placenta by passive diffusion.
- Placental function is modified by changes in blood flow.
- There are multiple placental enzymes, primarily involved with endogenous steroid metabolism, which may also contribute to drug metabolism.

FERTILIZATION AND IMPLANTATION

Animal studies suggest that interference with the fetus before 17 days gestation causes abortion, i.e. if pregnancy continues the fetus is unharmed.

ORGANOGENESIS/EMBRYONIC STAGE

At this stage, the fetus is differentiating to form major organs, and this is the critical period for teratogenesis. Teratogens cause deviations or abnormalities in the development of the embryo that are compatible with prenatal life and are observable post-natally. Drugs that interfere with this process can cause gross structural defects (e.g. **thalidomide** phocomelia).

Some drugs are confirmed teratogens (Table 9.1), but for many the evidence is inconclusive. **Thalidomide** was unusual in the way in which a very small dose of the drug given on only one or two occasions between the fourth and seventh weeks of pregnancy predictably produced serious malformations.

FETOGENIC STAGE

In this stage, the fetus undergoes further development and maturation. Even after organogenesis is almost complete, drugs can still have significant adverse effects on fetal growth and development.

- ACE inhibitors and angiotensin receptor blockers cause fetal and neonatal renal dysfunction.
- Drugs used to treat maternal hyperthyroidism can cause fetal and neonatal hypothyroidism.
- **Tetracycline** antibiotics inhibit growth of fetal bones and stain teeth.
- Aminoglycosides cause fetal VIIIth nerve damage.
- Opioids and **cocaine** taken regularly during pregnancy can lead to fetal drug dependency.
- **Warfarin** can cause fetal intracerebral bleeding.
- **Indometacin**, a potent inhibitor of prostaglandin synthesis, is used under specialist supervision to assist closure of patent ductus arteriosus in premature infants.
- Some hormones can cause inappropriate virilization or feminization.

Table 9.1: Some drugs that are teratogenic in humans.

Thalidomide	Androgens
Cytotoxic agents	Progestogens
Alcohol	Danazol
Warfarin	Diethylstilbestrol
Retinoids	Radioisotopes
Most anticonvulsants	Some live vaccines
Ribavarin	Lithium

- Anticonvulsants may possibly be associated with mental retardation.
- Cytotoxic drugs can cause intrauterine growth retardation and stillbirth.

DELIVERY

Some drugs given late in pregnancy or during delivery may cause particular problems. **Pethidine**, administered as an analgesic can cause fetal apnoea (which is reversed with **naloxone**, see Chapter 25). Anaesthetic agents given during Caesarean section may transiently depress neurological, respiratory and muscular functions. **Warfarin** given in late pregnancy causes a haemostasis defect in the baby, and predisposes to cerebral haemorrhage during delivery.

> **Key points**
>
> - Fertilization and implantation, <17 days.
> - Organogenesis/embryonic stage, 17–57 days.
> - Fetogenic stage.
> - Delivery.

THE MALE

Although it is generally considered that sperm cells damaged by drugs will not result in fertilization, the manufacturers of **griseofulvin**, an antifungal agent, advise men not to father children during or for six months after treatment. **Finasteride**, an anti-androgen used in the treatment of benign prostatic hyperplasia, is secreted in semen, and may be teratogenic to male fetuses.

RECOGNITION OF TERATOGENIC DRUGS

Major malformations that interfere with normal function occur in 2–3% of newborn babies, and a small but unknown fraction of these are due to drugs. Two principal problems face those who are trying to determine whether a drug is teratogenic when it is used to treat disease in humans:

1. Many drugs produce birth defects when given experimentally in large doses to pregnant animals. This does not necessarily mean that they are teratogenic in humans at therapeutic doses. Indeed, the metabolism and kinetics of drugs at high doses in other species is so different from that in humans as to limit seriously the relevance of such studies.
2. Fetal defects are common (2–3%). Consequently, if the incidence of drug-induced abnormalities is low, a very large number of cases has to be observed to define a significant increase above this background level. Effects on the fetus may take several years to become clinically manifest. For example, **diethylstilbestrol** was widely used in the late 1940s to prevent miscarriages and preterm births, despite little evidence of efficacy. In 1971, an association was reported between adenocarcinoma of the

vagina in girls in their late teens whose mothers had been given **diethylstilbestrol** during the pregnancy. Exposure to **stilbestrol** in utero has also been associated with a T-shaped uterus and other structural abnormalities of the genital tract, and increased rates of ectopic pregnancy and premature labour.

> ### Key points
>
> - The background incidence of serious congenital abnormality recognized at birth is 2–3%.
> - Environmental and genetic factors can influence a drug's effect.
> - Maternal disease can affect the fetus.
> - Studies of large doses in pregnant animals are of doubtful relevance.
> - Effects may be delayed (e.g. diethylstilbestrol).
> - Meticulous data collection is required for drugs administered during pregnancy and outcome, including long-term follow up. At present the Medicines and Healthcare products Regulatory Agency (MHRA) requests records of all drugs administered to a mother who bears an abnormal fetus. More complete (but with inherent practical difficulties) data collection by the MHRA, the National Teratology Information Services, the pharmaceutical industry and drug information agencies on all prescriptions during pregnancy with long-term follow up of offspring is required.

PHARMACOKINETICS IN PREGNANCY

Known differences in drug effects in pregnancy are usually explained by altered pharmacokinetics (Figure 9.2).

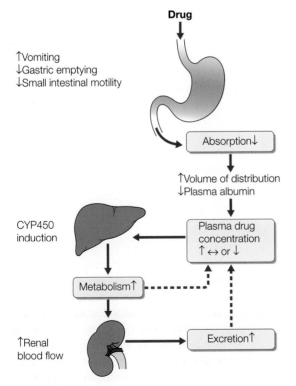

Figure 9.2: Pharmacokinetic changes in pregnancy.

ABSORPTION

Gastric emptying and small intestinal motility are reduced. This is of little consequence unless rapid drug action is required. Vomiting associated with pregnancy may make oral drug administration impractical.

DISTRIBUTION

During pregnancy, the blood volume increases by one-third, with expansion in plasma volume (from 2.5 to 4 L at term) being disproportionate to expansion in red cell mass, so that haematocrit falls. There is also an increase in body water due to a larger extravascular volume and changes in the uterus and breasts.

Oedema, which at least one-third of women experience during pregnancy, may add up to 8 L to the volume of extracellular water. For water-soluble drugs (which usually have a relatively small volume of distribution), this increases the apparent volume of distribution and, although clearance is unaltered, their half-life is prolonged. During pregnancy, the plasma protein concentration falls and there is increased competition for binding sites due to competition by endogenous ligands, such as increased hormone levels. These factors alter the total amount of bound drug and the apparent volume of distribution. However, the concentration of free drug usually remains unaltered, because a greater volume of distribution of free drug is accompanied by increased clearance of free drug. Thus, in practice, these changes are rarely of pharmacological significance. They may cause confusion in monitoring of plasma drug levels, since this usually measures total (rather than free) drug concentrations.

METABOLISM

Metabolism of drugs by the pregnant liver is increased, largely due to enzyme induction, perhaps by raised hormone levels. Liver blood flow does not change. This may lead to an increased rate of elimination of those drugs (e.g. **theophylline**), for which enzyme activity rather than liver blood flow is the main determinant of elimination rate.

RENAL EXCRETION

Excretion of drugs via the kidney increases because renal plasma flow almost doubles and the glomerular filtration rate increases by two-thirds during pregnancy. This has been documented for **digoxin**, **lithium**, **ampicillin**, **cefalexin** and **gentamicin**.

> ### Key points
>
> Known differences in drug effects can usually be explained by altered pharmacokinetics. Increased volume of distribution, hepatic metabolism and renal excretion all tend to reduce drug concentration. Decreased plasma albumin levels increase the ratio of free drug in plasma.

PRESCRIBING IN PREGNANCY

The prescription of drugs to a pregnant woman is a balance between possible adverse drug effects on the fetus and the risk to mother and fetus of leaving maternal disease inadequately treated. Effects on the human fetus cannot be reliably predicted from animal studies – hence one should prescribe drugs for which there is experience of safety over many years in preference to new or untried drugs. The smallest effective dose should be used. The fetus is most sensitive to adverse drug effects during the first trimester. It has been estimated that nearly half of all pregnancies in the UK are unplanned, and that most women do not present to a doctor until five to seven weeks after conception. Thus, sexually active women of childbearing potential should be assumed to be pregnant until it has been proved otherwise.

Delayed toxicity is a sinister problem (e.g. **diethylstilbestrol**) and if the teratogenic effect of **thalidomide** had not produced such an unusual congenital abnormality, namely phocomelia, its detection might have been delayed further. If drugs (or environmental toxins) have more subtle effects on the fetus (e.g. a minor reduction in intelligence) or cause an increased incidence of a common disease (e.g. atopy), these effects may never be detected. Many publications demand careful prospective controlled clinical trials, but the ethics and practicalities of such studies often make their demands unrealistic. A more rational approach is for drug regulatory bodies, the pharmaceutical industry and drug information agencies to collaborate closely and internationally to collate all information concerning drug use in pregnancy (whether inadvertent or planned) and associate these with outcome. This will require significant investment of time and money, as well as considerable encouragement to doctors and midwives to complete the endless forms.

Key points

Prescribing in pregnancy is a balance between the risk of adverse drug effects on the fetus and the risk of leaving maternal disease untreated. The effects on the human fetus are not reliably predicted by animal experiments. However, untreated maternal disease may cause morbidity and/or mortality to mother and/or fetus.
Therefore,

- minimize prescribing;
- use 'tried and tested' drugs whenever possible in preference to new agents;
- use the smallest effective dose;
- remember that the fetus is most sensitive in the first trimester;
- consider pregnancy in all women of childbearing potential;
- discuss the potential risks of taking or withholding therapy with the patient;
- seek guidance on the use of drugs in pregnancy in the British National Formulary, Drug Information Services, National Teratology Information Service (NTIS);
- warn the patient about the risks of smoking, alcohol, over-the-counter drugs and drugs of abuse.

Guidance on the use of drugs for a selection of conditions is summarized below. If in doubt, consult the British National Formulary, appendix 4 (which is appropriately conservative). Information for health professionals in the UK about the safety of drugs in pregnancy can also be obtained from the National Teratology Information Service (Tel. 0191 232 1525).

ANTIMICROBIAL DRUGS

Antimicrobial drugs are commonly prescribed during pregnancy. The safest antibiotics in pregnancy are the penicillins and cephalosporins. **Trimethoprim** is a theoretical teratogen as it is a folic acid antagonist. The aminoglycosides can cause ototoxicity. There is minimal experience in pregnancy with the fluoroquinolones (e.g. **ciprofloxacin**) and they should be avoided. **Erythromycin** is probably safe. **Metronidazole** is a teratogen in animals, but there is no evidence of teratogenicity in humans, and its benefit in serious anaerobic sepsis probably outweighs any risks. Unless there is a life-threatening infection in the mother, antiviral agents should be avoided in pregnancy. Falciparum malaria (Chapter 47) has an especially high mortality rate in late pregnancy. Fortunately, the standard regimens of intravenous and oral quinine are safe in pregnancy.

ANALGESICS

Opioids cross the placenta. This is particularly relevant in the management of labour when the use of opioids, such as **pethidine**, depresses the fetal respiratory centre and can inhibit the start of normal respiration. If the mother is dependent on opioids, the fetus can experience opioid withdrawal syndrome during and after delivery, which can be fatal. In neonates, the chief withdrawal symptoms are tremor, irritability, diarrhoea and vomiting. **Chlorpromazine** is commonly used to treat this withdrawal state. **Paracetamol** is preferred to aspirin when mild analgesia is required. In cases where a systemic anti-inflammatory action is required (e.g. in rheumatoid arthritis), **ibuprofen** is the drug of choice. Non-steroidal anti-inflammatory drugs can cause constriction of the ductus arteriosus. Occasionally, this may be used to therapeutic benefit.

ANAESTHESIA

Anaesthesia in pregnancy is a very specialist area and should only be undertaken by experienced anaesthetists. Local anaesthetics used for regional anaesthesia readily cross the placenta. However, when used in epidural anaesthesia, the drug remains largely confined to the epidural space. Pregnant women are at increased risk of aspiration. Although commonly used, **pethidine** frequently causes vomiting and may also lead to neonatal respiratory depression. **Metoclopramide** should be used in preference to **prochlorperazine** (which has an anti-analgesic effect when combined with **pethidine**), and **naloxone** (an opioid antagonist) must always be available. Respiratory depression in the newborn is not usually a problem with modern general anaesthetics currently in use in Caesarean section. Several studies have shown an increased incidence of spontaneous abortions in mothers who have had general anaesthesia during pregnancy, although a causal relationship is not proven, and in most circumstances failure to operate would have dramatically increased the risk to mother and fetus.

ANTI-EMETICS

Nausea and vomiting are common in early pregnancy, but are usually self-limiting, and ideally should be managed with reassurance and non-drug strategies, such as small frequent meals, avoiding large volumes of fluid and raising the head of the bed. If symptoms are prolonged or severe, drug treatment may be effective. An antihistamine, e.g. **promethazine** or **cyclizine** may be required. If ineffective, **prochlorperazine** is an alternative. **Metoclopramide** is considered to be safe and efficacious in labour and before anaesthesia in late pregnancy, but its routine use in early pregnancy cannot be recommended because of the lack of controlled data, and the significant incidence of dystonic reactions in young women.

DYSPEPSIA AND CONSTIPATION

The high incidence of dyspepsia due to gastro-oesophageal reflux in the second and third trimesters is probably related to the reduction in lower oesophageal sphincter pressure. Non-drug treatment (reassurance, small frequent meals and advice on posture) should be pursued in the first instance, particularly in the first trimester. Fortunately, most cases occur later in pregnancy when non-absorbable antacids, such as alginates, should be used. In late pregnancy, **metoclopromide** is particularly effective as it increases lower oesophageal sphincter pressure. H$_2$-receptor blockers should not be used for non-ulcer dyspepsia in this setting. Constipation should be managed with dietary advice. Stimulant laxatives may be uterotonic and should be avoided if possible.

PEPTIC ULCERATION

Antacids may relieve symptoms. **Cimetidine** and **ranitidine** have been widely prescribed in pregnancy without obvious damage to the fetus. There are inadequate safety data on the use of **omeprazole** or other proton pump inhibitors in pregnancy. **Sucralfate** has been recommended for use in pregnancy in the USA, and this is rational as it is not systemically absorbed. **Misoprostol**, a prostaglandin which stimulates the uterus, is contraindicated because it causes abortion.

ANTI-EPILEPTICS

Epilepsy in pregnancy can lead to fetal and maternal morbidity/mortality through convulsions, whilst all of the anticonvulsants used have been associated with teratogenic effects (e.g. **phenytoin** is associated with cleft palate and congenital heart disease). However, there is no doubt that the benefits of good seizure control outweigh the drug-induced teratogenic risk. Thorough explanation to the mother, ideally before a planned pregnancy, is essential, and it must be emphasized that the majority (>90%) of epileptic mothers have normal babies. (The usual risk of fetal malformation is 2–3% and in epileptic mothers it is up to 10%.) In view of the association of spina bifida with many anti-epileptics, e.g. **sodium valproate** and **carbamazepine** therapy, it is often recommended that the standard dose of folic acid should be increased to 5 mg daily. Both of these anti-epileptics can also cause hypospadias. As in non-pregnant epilepsy, single-drug therapy is preferable. Plasma concentration monitoring is particularly relevant for **phenytoin**, because the decrease in plasma protein binding and the increase in hepatic metabolism may cause considerable changes in the plasma concentration of free (active) drug. As always, the guide to the correct dose is freedom from fits and absence of toxicity. Owing to the changes in plasma protein binding, it is generally recommended that the therapeutic range is 5–15 mg/L, whereas in the non-pregnant state it is 10–20 mg/L. This is only a rough guide, as protein binding varies.

The routine injection of vitamin K recommended at birth counteracts the possible effect of some anti-epileptics on vitamin K-dependent clotting factors.

Magnesium sulphate is the treatment of choice for the prevention and control of eclamptic seizures.

Key points

- Epilepsy in pregnancy can lead to increased fetal and maternal morbidity/mortality.
- All anticonvulsants are teratogens.
- The benefits of good seizure control outweigh drug-induced teratogenic risk.
- Give a full explanation to the mother (preferably before pregnancy): most epileptic mothers (>90%) have normal babies.
- Advise an increase in the standard dose of folic acid up to 12 weeks.
- Make a referral to the neurologist and obstetrician.
- If epilepsy is well controlled, do not change therapy.
- Monitor plasma concentrations (levels tend to fall, and note that the bound:unbound ratio changes); the guide to the correct dose is freedom from fits and absence of toxicity.
- An early ultrasound scan at 12 weeks may detect gross neural tube defects.
- Detailed ultrasound scan and α-fetoprotein at 16–18 weeks should be considered.

ANTICOAGULATION

Warfarin has been associated with nasal hypoplasia and chondrodysplasia when given in the first trimester, and with CNS abnormalities after administration in later pregnancy, as well as a high incidence of haemorrhagic complications towards the end of pregnancy. Neonatal haemorrhage is difficult to prevent because of the immature enzymes in fetal liver and the low stores of vitamin K. It is not rcommended for use in pregnancy unless there are no other options. **Low molecular weight heparin (LMWH)**, which does not cross the placenta, is the anticoagulant of choice in pregnancy in preference to unfractionated heparin. **LMWH** has predictable pharmacokinetics and is safer – unlike unfractionated heparin there has never been a case of heparin-induced thrombocytopenia/thrombosis (HITT) associated with it in pregnancy. Moreover there has only been one case of osteoporotic fracture worldwide, whereas there is a 2% risk of osteoporotic fracture with nine months use of unfractionated heparin (see Chapter 30). **LMWH** is given twice daily in pregnancy due to the increased renal clearance of pregnancy. Women on long-term oral anticoagulants should be warned that these drugs are likely to affect the fetus in early pregnancy. Self-administered subcutaneous **LMWH** must be substituted for **warfarin** before six weeks' gestation. Subcutaneous **LMWH** can be continued throughout pregnancy and for the prothrombotic six weeks post partum. Patients with prosthetic heart valves present a special problem, and in these patients, despite the risks to the fetus, **warfarin** is often given up to 36 weeks. The prothrombin time/international normalized ratio (INR) should be monitored closely if **warfarin** is used.

> ### Key points
>
> - Pregnancy is associated with a hypercoagulable state.
> - **Warfarin** has been associated with nasal hypoplasia and chondrodysplasia in the first trimester, and with CNS abnormalities in late pregnancy, as well as haemorrhagic complications.
> - **Heparin** does not cross the placenta. Low molecular weight heparins (**LMWH**) are preferable as they have better and more predictable pharmacokinetics, are safer with no evidence of heparin-induced thrombocytopenia and thrombosis (HITT) and osteoporotic fracture is very rare.
> - Refer to the guidelines of the Royal College of Obstetricians for thromboprophylaxis and management of established venous thromboembolism in pregnancy.

CARDIOVASCULAR DRUGS

Hypertension in pregnancy (see Chapter 28) can normally be managed with either **methyldopa** which has the most extensive safety record in pregnancy, or **labetalol**. Parenteral **hydralazine** is useful for lowering blood pressure in preeclampsia. Diuretics should not be started to treat hypertension in pregnancy, although some American authorities continue thiazide diuretics in women with essential hypertension, who are already stabilized on these drugs. Modified-release preparations of **nifedipine** are also used for hypertension in pregnancy, but angiotensin-converting enzyme inhibitors and angitensin II receptor antagonists must be avoided.

HORMONES

Progestogens, particularly synthetic ones, can masculinize the female fetus. There is no evidence that this occurs with the small amount of **progestogen** (or oestrogen) present in the oral contraceptive – the risk applies to large doses. Corticosteroids do not appear to give rise to any serious problems when given via inhalation or in short courses. Transient suppression of the fetal hypothalamic–pituitary–adrenal axis has been reported. Rarely, cleft palate and congenital cataract have been linked with steroids in pregnancy, but the benefit of treatment usually outweighs any such risk. **Iodine** and antithyroid drugs cross the placenta and can cause hypothyroidism and goitre.

TRANQUILLIZERS AND ANTIDEPRESSANTS

Benzodiazepines accumulate in the tissues and are slowly eliminated by the neonate, resulting in prolonged hypotonia ('floppy baby'), subnormal temperatures (hypothermia), periodic cessation of respiration and poor sucking. There is no evidence that the phenothiazines, tricyclic antidepressants or **fluoxetine** are teratogenic. **Lithium** can cause fetal goitre and possible cardiovascular abnormalities.

NON-THERAPEUTIC DRUGS

Excessive **ethanol** consumption is associated with spontaneous abortion, craniofacial abnormalities, mental retardation, congenital heart disease and impaired growth. Even moderate alcohol intake may adversely affect the baby – the risk of having an abnormal child is about 10% in mothers drinking 30–60 mL ethanol per day, rising to 40% in chronic alcoholics. Fetal alcohol syndrome describes the distinct pattern of abnormal morphogenesis and central nervous system dysfunction in children whose mothers were chronic alcoholics, and this syndrome is a leading cause of mental retardation. After birth, the characteristic craniofacial malformations diminish, but microcephaly and to a lesser degree short stature persist. Cigarette smoking is associated with spontaneous abortion, premature delivery, small babies, increased perinatal mortality and a higher incidence of sudden infant death syndrome (cot death). **Cocaine** causes vasoconstriction of placental vessels. There is a high incidence of low birth weight, congenital abnormalities and, in particular, delayed neurological and behavioural development.

Case history

A 20-year-old female medical student attended her GP requesting a course of Septrin® (co-trimoxazole) for cystitis. She tells her GP that her last menstrual bleed was about six weeks earlier. She did not think she was at risk of pregnancy as her periods had been irregular since stopping the oral contraceptive one year previously due to fears about thrombosis, and her boyfriend used a condom. Physical examination, which did not include a vaginal examination, was normal. Urinalysis was 1+ positive for blood and a trace of protein.

Question

Why should the GP not prescribe co-trimoxazole for this patient?

Answer

Until proven otherwise, it should be assumed that this woman is pregnant. Co-trimoxazole (a combination of sulfamethoxazole and trimethoprim) has been superseded by trimethoprim alone as a useful drug in lower urinary tract infection (UTI). The sulfamethoxazole does not add significant antibacterial advantage in lower UTI, but does have sulphonamide-associated side effects, including the rare but life-threatening Stevens–Johnson syndrome. Both sulfamethoxazole and trimethoprim inhibit folate synthesis and are theoretical teratogens. If pregnancy is confirmed (urinary frequency is an early symptom of pregnancy in some women, due to a progesterone effect) and if the patient has a lower UTI confirmed by pyuria and bacteria on microscopy whilst awaiting culture and sensitivity results, amoxicillin is the treatment of choice. Alternatives include an oral cephalosporin or nitrofurantoin. Note that lower urinary tract infection in pregnancy can rapidly progress to acute pyelonephritis.

FURTHER READING

Anon. Antiepileptics, pregnancy and the child. *Drugs and Therapeutics Bulletin* 2005; **43** no 2.

Koren G. *Medication, safety in pregnancy and breastfeeding: the evidence-based A–Z clinicians pocket guide*. Maidenhead: McGraw-Hill, 2006.

Rubin PC. *Prescribing in pregnancy*, 3rd edn. London: Blackwell, BMJ Books, 2000.

McElhatton PR. General principles of drug use in pregnancy. *Pharmaceutical Journal* 2003; 270: 305–7.

FURTHER INFORMATION FOR HEALTH PROFESSIONALS

National Teratology Information Service
Regional Drug and Therapeutics Centre
Wolfson Unit
Clarement Place
Newcastle upon Tyne
NE1 4LP
Tel. 0191 232 1525

CHAPTER 10

DRUGS IN INFANTS AND CHILDREN

INTRODUCTION

Children cannot be regarded as miniature adults in terms of drug response, due to differences in body constitution, drug absorption and elimination, and sensitivity to adverse reactions. Informed consent is problematic and commercial interest has been limited by the small size of the market, so clinical trials in children have lagged behind those in adults. Regulatory agencies in the USA and Europe now recognize this problem and are attempting to address it, for example, by introducing exclusivity legislation designed to attract commercial interest. Traditionally, paediatricians have used drugs 'off-label' (i.e. for unlicensed indications), often gaining experience in age groups close to those for which a product is licensed and then extending this to younger children. That this empirical approach has worked (at least to some extent) is testament to the biological fact that while not just 'miniature adults' children do share the same drug targets (e.g. receptors, enzymes), cellular transduction mechanisms and physiological processes with their parents. Drug responses are thus usually qualitatively similar in children and adults, although there are important exceptions, including some central nervous system (CNS) responses and immunological responses to **ciclosporin**. Furthermore, some adverse effects occur only during certain stages of development, for example, retrolental fibroplasia induced by excess oxygen in the premature neonate and staining of teeth by **tetracycline** which occurs only in developing enamel. The processes of drug elimination are, however, immature at birth so quantitative differences (e.g. in dose) are important. Establishing optimal doses for drugs prescribed for children is thus an extremely important clinical challenge. Current regimes have been arrived at empirically, but guidelines are evolving for paediatric dosing in clinical trials and in future greater use may be made of pharmacokinetic/pharmacodynamic modelling in children, so hopefully this Cinderella of therapeutics will soon be making her (belated) entry to the ball.

PHARMACOKINETICS

ABSORPTION

Gastro-intestinal absorption is slower in infancy, but absorption from intramuscular injection is faster. The rate of gastric emptying is very variable during the neonatal period and may be delayed by disease, such as respiratory distress syndrome and congenital heart disease. To ensure that adequate blood concentrations reach the systemic circulation in the sick neonate, it is common practice to use intravenous preparations. In older and less severely ill children, oral liquid preparations are commonly used, resulting in less accurate dosing and a more rapid rate of absorption. This is important for drugs with adverse effects that occur predictably at high plasma concentration, and which show lack of efficacy if trough concentration is low (e.g. **carbamazepine** and **theophylline**). Infant skin is thin and percutaneous absorption can cause systemic toxicity if topical preparations (e.g. of potent corticosteroids) are applied too extensively.

DISTRIBUTION

Body fat content is relatively low in children, whereas water content is greater, leading to a lower volume of distribution of fat-soluble drugs (e.g. **diazepam**) in infants. Plasma protein binding of drugs is reduced in neonates due to a lower plasma albumin concentration and altered binding properties. The risk of kernicterus caused by displacement of bilirubin from albumin by sulphonamides (see Chapter 12) is well recognized. The blood–brain barrier is more permeable in neonates and young children, leading to an increased risk of CNS adverse effects.

METABOLISM

At birth, the hepatic microsomal enzyme system (see Chapter 5) is relatively immature (particularly in the preterm infant), but after the first four weeks it matures rapidly. **Chloramphenicol** can produce 'grey baby syndrome' in neonates due to high plasma levels secondary to inefficient elimination. Conversely, hepatic drug metabolism can be increased once enzyme activity has matured in older infants and children, because the ratio of the weight of the liver to body weight is up to 50% higher than in adults. Drugs administered to the mother can induce neonatal enzyme activity (e.g. barbiturates). **Phenobarbitone** metabolism is faster in children than in adults because of greater induction of hepatic enzyme activity.

Key points

Prevalence of chronic illness in children requiring drug therapy:

- one in eight children have asthma;
- one in 250 children have epilepsy;
- one in 750 children have diabetes mellitus.

Key points

At birth, renal and hepatic function are less efficient than in adulthood. Drug effects may be prolonged and accumulation may occur. These factors are exaggerated in the premature infant.

EXCRETION

All renal mechanisms (filtration, secretion and reabsorption) are reduced in neonates, and renal excretion of drugs is relatively reduced in the newborn. Glomerular filtration rate (GFR) increases rapidly during the first four weeks of life, with consequent changes in the rate of drug elimination (Table 10.1).

Table 10.1: Changes in rate of drug elimination with development

Stage of development	Plasma half-life of gentamicin
Premature infant	
<48 hours old	18 hours
5–22 days old	6 hours
Normal infant	
1–4 weeks old	3 hours
Adult	2 hours

PHARMACODYNAMICS

Documented evidence of differences in receptor sensitivity in children is lacking, and the apparently paradoxical effects of some drugs (e.g. hyperkinesia with **phenobarbitone**, sedation of hyperactive children with **amphetamine**) are as yet unexplained. Augmented responses to **warfarin** in prepubertal patients occur at similar plasma concentrations as in adults, implying a pharmacodynamic mechanism. **Ciclosporin** added in vitro to cultured monocytes (hence there is no opportunity for a pharmacokinetic effect) has greater effects in cells isolated from infants, providing another example of an age-related pharmacodynamic difference.

BREAST-FEEDING

Breast-feeding can lead to toxicity in the infant if the drug enters the milk in pharmacological quantities. The milk concentration of some drugs (e.g. iodides) may exceed the maternal plasma concentration, but the total dose delivered to the baby is usually very small. However, drugs in breast milk may cause hypersensitivity reactions even in very low doses. Virtually all drugs that reach the maternal systemic circulation will enter breast milk, especially lipid-soluble unionized low-molecular-weight drugs. Milk is weakly acidic, so drugs that are weak bases are concentrated in breast milk by trapping of the charged form of the drug (compare with renal elimination; see Chapter 6). However, the resulting dose administered to the fetus in breast milk is seldom clinically appreciable, although some drugs are contraindicated (Table 10.2), and breast-feeding should cease during treatment if there is no safer alternative. Appendix 5 of the British National Formulary provides very helpful practical advice.

Table 10.2: Some drugs to be avoided during breast-feeding

Amiodarone
Aspirin
Benzodiazepines
Chloramphenicol
Ciclosporin
Ciprofloxacin
Cocaine
Combined oral contraceptives
Cytotoxics
Ergotamine
Octreotide
Stimulant laxatives
Sulphonylureas
Thiazide diuretics
Vitamin A/retinoid analogues (e.g. etretinate)

The infant should be monitored if β-adrenoceptor antagonists, **carbimazole**, corticosteroids or **lithium** are prescribed to the mother. β-Adrenoceptor antagonists rarely cause significant bradycardia in the suckling infant. **Carbimazole** should be prescribed at its lowest effective dose to reduce the risk of hypothyroidism in the neonate/infant. In high doses, corticosteroids can affect the infant's adrenal function and **lithium** may cause intoxication. There is a theoretical risk of Reye's syndrome if **aspirin** is prescribed to the breast-feeding mother. **Warfarin** is not contraindicated during breast-feeding. **Bromocriptine** suppresses lactation and large doses of diuretics may do likewise. **Metronidazole** gives milk an unpleasant taste.

PRACTICAL ASPECTS OF PRESCRIBING

COMPLIANCE AND ROUTE OF ADMINISTRATION

Sick neonates will usually require intravenous drug administration. Accurate dosage and attention to fluid balance are essential. Sophisticated syringe pumps with awareness of 'dead space' associated with the apparatus are necessary.

Children under the age of five years may have difficulty in swallowing even small tablets, and hence oral preparations which taste pleasant are often necessary to improve compliance. Liquid preparations are given by means of a graduated syringe. However, chronic use of sucrose-containing elixirs encourages tooth cavities and gingivitis. Moreover, the dyes and colourings used may induce hypersensitivity.

Pressurized aerosols (e.g. **salbutamol** inhaler, see Chapter 33) are usually only practicable in children over the age of ten years, as co-ordinated deep inspiration is required unless a device such as a spacer is used. Spacers can be combined with a face mask from early infancy. Likewise, nebulizers may be used to enhance local therapeutic effect and reduce systemic toxicity.

Only in unusual circumstances, i.e. extensive areas of application (especially to inflamed or broken skin), or in infants, does systemic absorption of drugs (e.g. steroids, **neomycin**) become significant following topical application to the skin.

Intramuscular injection should only be used when absolutely necessary. Intravenous therapy is less painful, but skill is required to cannulate infants' veins (and a confident colleague to keep the target still!). Children find intravenous infusions uncomfortable and restrictive. Rectal administration (see Chapter 4) is a convenient alternative (e.g. **metronidazole** to treat anaerobic infections). Rectal **diazepam** is particularly valuable in the treatment of status epilepticus when intravenous access is often difficult. Rectal **diazepam** may also be administered by parents. Rectal administration should also be considered if the child is vomiting.

Paramount to ensuring compliance is full communication with the child's parents and teachers. This should include information not only on how to administer the drug, but also on why it is being prescribed, for how long the treatment should continue and whether any adverse effects are likely.

Case history

A two-year-old epileptic child is seen in the Accident and Emergency Department. He has been fitting for at least 15 minutes. The casualty officer is unable to cannulate a vein to administer intravenous diazepam. The more experienced medical staff are dealing with emergencies elsewhere in the hospital.
Question
Name two drugs, and their route of administration, with which the casualty officer may terminate the convulsions.
Answer
Rectal diazepam solution.
Rectal or intramuscular paraldehyde.

DOSAGE

Even after adjustment of dose according to surface area, calculation of the correct dose must consider the relatively large volume of distribution of polar drugs in the first four months of life, the immature microsomal enzymes and reduced renal function. The British National Formulary and specialist paediatric textbooks and formularies provide appropriate guidelines and must be consulted by physicians who are not familiar with prescribing to infants and children.

ADVERSE EFFECTS

With a few notable exceptions, drugs in children generally have a similar adverse effect profile to those in adults. Of particular significance is the potential of chronic corticosteroid use, including high-dose inhaled corticosteroids, to inhibit growth. **Aspirin** is avoided in children under 16 years (except in specific indications, such as Kawasaki syndrome) due to an association with Reye's syndrome, a rare but often fatal illness of unknown aetiology consisting of hepatic necrosis and encephalopathy, often in the aftermath of a viral illness. Tetracyclines are deposited in growing bone and teeth, causing staining and occasionally dental hypoplasia, and should not be given to children. Fluoroquinolone antibacterial drugs may damage growing cartilage. Dystonias with **metoclopramide** occur more frequently in children and young adults than in older adults. **Valproate** hepatotoxicity is increased in young children with learning difficulties receiving multiple anticonvulsants. Some adverse effects cause lifelong effects as a result of toxicity occurring at a sensitive point in development (a 'critical window') during fetal or neonatal life ('programming') as with **thalidomide**/phocomelia or hypothyroid drugs/congenital hypothyroidism

RESEARCH

Research in paediatric clinical pharmacology is limited. Not only is there concern about the potential for adverse effects of new drugs on those who are growing and developing mentally, but there are also considerable ethical problems encountered in research involving individuals who are too young to give informed consent. New drugs are often given to children for the first time only when no alternative is available or when unacceptable side effects have been encountered in a particular individual with established drugs. Pharmaceutical companies seldom seek to license their products for use in children. When drugs are prescribed to children that are not licensed for use in this age group, it is important to make careful records of both efficacy and possible adverse effects. Prescribers take sole responsibility for prescribing unlicensed preparations (e.g. formulated to appeal to children) or for prescribing licensed preparations outside the licensed age range. Parents should be informed and their consent obtained.

Case history

A 14-year-old boy with a history of exercise-induced asthma, for which he uses salbutamol as necessary (on average two puffs twice daily and before exercise) is seen by his GP because of malaise and nocturnal cough. On examination, he has a mild fever (38°C), bilateral swollen cervical lymph nodes and bilateral wheeze. Ampicillin is prescribed for a respiratory tract infection. The next day the boy develops a widespread maculopapular rash.
Question 1
What is the cause of the rash?
Question 2
What is the likely cause of the nocturnal cough and how may this be treated?
Answer 1
Ampicillin rash in infectious mononucleosis (glandular fever).
Answer 2
Poorly controlled asthma. Regular inhaled glucocorticosteroid or cromoglicate.

FURTHER READING

Baber N, Pritchard D. Dose estimation in children. *British Journal of Clinical Pharmacology* 2003; **56**: 489–93.

British National Formulary for Children 2007. www.bnfc.org

Kearns GL, Abdel-Rahmen SM. Developmental pharmacology – drug disposition, action and therapy in infants and children. *New England Journal of Medicine* 2003; **349**: 1157–67.

Paediatric Special Issue. *British Journal of Clinical Pharmacology* 2005; **59** (6).

Paediatric formulary, 7th edn. London: Guy's, St Thomas', King's College and Lewisham Hospitals, revised 2005.

DRUGS IN THE ELDERLY

INTRODUCTION

The proportion of elderly people in the population is increasing steadily in economically developed countries. The elderly are subject to a variety of complaints, many of which are chronic and incapacitating, and so they receive a great deal of drug treatment. There is a growing evidence base for the use of drugs in elderly patients, with important implications for prescribing of many important classes of drugs, including statins, β-adrenoceptor antagonists, thrombolytics, ACE inhibitors, angiotensin receptor blockers, vitamin D and bisphosphonates (see reviews by Mangoni and Jackson, 2006). Adverse drug reactions and drug interactions become more common with increasing age. In one study, 11.8% of patients aged 41–50 years experienced adverse reactions to drugs, but this increased to 25% in patients over 80 years of age. There are several reasons for this.

1. Elderly people take more drugs. In one survey in general practice, 87% of patients over 75 years of age were on regular drug therapy, with 34% taking three to four different drugs daily. The most commonly prescribed drugs were diuretics (34% of patients), analgesics (27%), tranquillizers and antidepressants (24%), hypnotics (22%) and digoxin (20%). All of these are associated with a high incidence of important adverse effects.
2. Drug elimination becomes less efficient with increasing age, leading to drug accumulation during chronic dosing.
3. Homeostatic mechanisms become less effective with advancing age, so individuals are less able to compensate for adverse effects, such as unsteadiness or postural hypotension.
4. The central nervous system becomes more sensitive to the actions of sedative drugs.
5. Increasing age produces changes in the immune response that can cause an increased liability to allergic reactions.
6. Impaired cognition combined with relatively complex dose regimens may lead to inadvertent overdose.

PHARMACOKINETIC CHANGES

ABSORPTION

Absorption of carbohydrates and of several nutrients, including iron, calcium and thiamine, is reduced in elderly people. Lipid-soluble drugs are absorbed by simple diffusion down the concentration gradient (Chapter 3), and this is not impaired by age. Intestinal blood flow is reduced by up to 50% in the elderly. However, age per se does not affect drug absorption to a large extent (Figure 11.1).

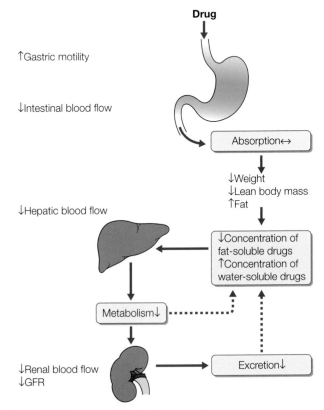

Figure 11.1: Pharmacokinetic changes with age.

DISTRIBUTION

Ageing is associated with loss of lean body mass, and with an increased ratio of fat to muscle and body water. This enlarges the volume of distribution of fat-soluble drugs, such as **diazepam** and **lidocaine**, whereas the distribution of polar drugs such as **digoxin** is reduced compared to younger adults. Changes in plasma proteins also occur with ageing, especially if associated with chronic disease and malnutrition, with a fall in albumin and a rise in gamma-globulin concentrations.

HEPATIC METABOLISM

There is a decrease in the hepatic clearance of some but not all drugs with advancing age. A prolonged plasma half-life (Figure 11.2), can be the result either of reduced clearance or of increased apparent volume of distribution. Ageing reduces metabolism of some drugs (e.g. benzodiazepines) as evidenced by reduced hepatic clearance. The reduced clearance of benzodiazepines has important clinical consequences, as does the long half-life of several active metabolites (Chapter 18). Slow accumulation may lead to adverse effects whose onset may occur days or weeks after initiating therapy. Consequently, confusion or memory impairment may be falsely attributed to ageing rather than to adverse drug effects.

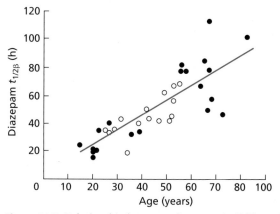

Figure 11.2: Relationship between diazepam half-life and age in 33 normal individuals. Non-smokers, o; smokers, •. (Redrawn with permission from Klotz U et al. *Journal of Clinical Investigation* 1975; **55**: 347.)

Table 11.1: Examples of drugs requiring dose adjustment in the elderly

Aminoglycosides (e.g. gentamicin)

Atenolol

Cimetidine

Diazepam

Digoxin

Non-steroidal anti-inflammatory drugs

Oral hypoglycaemic agents

Warfarin

RENAL EXCRETION

The most important cause of drug accumulation in the elderly is declining renal function. Many healthy elderly individuals have a glomerular filtration rate (GFR) <50 mL/min. Although glomerular filtration rate declines with age, this is not necessarily reflected by serum creatinine, which can remain within the range defined as 'normal' for a younger adult population despite a marked decline in renal function. This is related to the lower endogenous production of creatinine in the elderly secondary to their reduced muscle mass. Under-recognition of renal impairment in the elderly is lessened by the routine reporting by many laboratories of an estimated GFR (eGFR) based on age, sex and serum creatinine concentration and reported in units normalized to $1.73\,m^2$ body surface area $(mL/min/1.73\,m^2)$. When estimating doses of nephrotoxic drugs, it is important to remember that the drug elimination depends on the absolute GFR (in mL/min) rather than that normalized to an ideal body surface area (in $mL/min/1.73\,m^2$), and to estimate this if necessary using a nomogram (see Chapter 7) that incorporates height and weight, as well as age, sex and creatinine.

Examples of drugs which may require reduced dosage in the elderly secondary to reduced renal excretion and/or hepatic clearance are listed in Table 11.1.

The principal age-related changes in pharmacokinetics are summarized in Figure 11.1.

> **Key points**
>
> Pharmacokinetic changes in the elderly include:
>
> - Absorption of iron, calcium and thiamine is reduced.
> - There is an increased volume of distribution of fat-soluble drugs (e.g. diazepam).
> - There is a decreased volume of distribution of polar drugs (e.g. digoxin).
> - There is reduced hepatic clearance of long half-life benzodiazepines.
> - Declining renal function is the most important cause of drug accumulation.

PHARMACODYNAMIC CHANGES

Evidence that the elderly are intrinsically more sensitive to drugs than the young is scarce. However, the sensitivity of the elderly to benzodiazepines as measured by psychometric tests is increased, and their effects last longer than in the young. It is common clinical experience that benzodiazepines given to the elderly at hypnotic doses used for the young can produce prolonged daytime confusion even after single doses. The incidence of confusion associated with **cimetidine** is increased in the elderly. Other drugs may expose physiological defects that are a normal concomitant of ageing. Postural hypotension can occur in healthy elderly people, and the incidence of postural hypotension from drugs such as phenothiazines, β-adrenoceptor antagonists, tricyclic antidepressants and diuretics is increased in elderly patients. The QT interval is longer in the elderly, which may predispose to drug-induced ventricular tachy-dysrhythmias. Clotting factor synthesis by the liver is reduced in the elderly, and old people often require lower **warfarin** doses for effective anticoagulation than younger adults.

Key points

Pharmacodynamic changes in the elderly include:

- increased sensitivity to central nervous system (CNS) effects (e.g. benzodiazepines, cimetidine);
- increased incidence of postural hypotension (e.g. phenothiazines, beta-blockers, tricyclic antidepressants, diuretics);
- reduced clotting factor synthesis, reduced warfarin for anticoagulation;
- increased toxicity from NSAIDs;
- increased incidence of allergic reactions to drugs.

COMPLIANCE IN THE ELDERLY

Incomplete compliance is extremely common in elderly people. This is commonly due to a failure of memory or to not understanding how the drug should be taken. In addition, many patients store previously prescribed drugs in the medicine cupboard which they take from time to time. It is therefore essential that the drug regimen is kept as simple as possible and explained carefully. There is scope for improved methods of packaging to reduce over- or under-dosage. Multiple drug regimens are confusing and increase the risk of adverse interactions (see Chapter 13).

EFFECT OF DRUGS ON SOME MAJOR ORGAN SYSTEMS IN THE ELDERLY

CENTRAL NERVOUS SYSTEM

Cerebral function in old people is easily disturbed, resulting in disorientation and confusion. Drugs are one of the factors that contribute to this state; sedatives and hypnotics can easily precipitate a loss of awareness and clouding of consciousness.

NIGHT SEDATION

The elderly do not sleep as well as the young. They sleep for a shorter time, their sleep is more likely to be broken and they are more easily aroused. This is quite normal, and old people should not have the expectations of the young as far as sleep is concerned. Before hypnotics are commenced, other possible factors should be considered and treated if possible. These include:

1. pain, which may be due to such causes as arthritis;
2. constipation – the discomfort of a loaded rectum;
3. urinary frequency;
4. depression;
5. anxiety;
6. left ventricular failure;
7. dementia;
8. nocturnal xanthine alkaloids, e.g. caffeine in tea, **theophylline**.

A little more exercise may help, and 'catnapping' in the day reduced to a minimum and regularized (as in Mediterranen cultures).

The prescription of hypnotics (see Chapter 18) should be minimized and restricted to short-term use.

ANTIDEPRESSANTS

Although depression is common in old age and may indeed need drug treatment, this is not without risk. Tricyclic antidepressants (see Chapter 20) can cause constipation, urinary retention and glaucoma (due to their muscarinic blocking action which is less marked in the case of **lofepramine** than other drugs of this class), and also drowsiness, confusion, postural hypotension and cardiac dysrhythmias. Tricyclic antidepressants can produce worthwhile remissions of depression but should be started at very low dosage.

Selective 5-hydroxytryptamine reuptake inhibitors (e.g. **fluoxetine**) are as effective as the tricyclics and have a distinct side-effect profile (see chapter 20). They are generally well tolerated by the elderly, although hyponatraemia has been reported more frequently than with other antidepressants.

ANTI-PARKINSONIAN DRUGS

The anticholinergic group of anti-parkinsonian drugs (e.g. **trihexyphenidyl, orphenadrine**) commonly cause side effects in the elderly. Urinary retention is common in men. Glaucoma may be precipitated or aggravated and confusion may occur with quite small doses. **Levodopa** combined with a peripheral dopa decarboxylase inhibitor such as **carbidopa** can be effective, but it is particularly important to start with a small dose, which can be increased gradually as needed. In patients with dementia, the use of antimuscarinics, **levodopa** or **amantidine** may produce adverse cerebral stimulation and/or hallucinations, leading to decompensation of cerebral functioning, with excitement and inability to cope.

CARDIOVASCULAR SYSTEM

HYPERTENSION

There is excellent evidence that treating hypertension in the elderly reduces both morbidity and mortality. The agents used (starting with a C or D drug) are described in Chapter 28. It is important to start with a low dose and monitor carefully. Some adverse effects (e.g. hyponatraemia from diuretics) are much more common in the elderly, who are also much more likely to suffer severe consequences, such as falls/fractures from common effects like postural hypotension. Alpha-blockers in particular should be used as little as possible. **Methyldopa** might be expected to be problematic in this age group but was in fact surprisingly well tolerated when used as add-on therapy in a trial by the European Working Party on Hypertension in the Elderly (EWPHE).

DIGOXIN

Digoxin toxicity is common in the elderly because of decreased renal elimination and reduced apparent volume of distribution. Confusion, nausea and vomiting, altered vision and an acute abdominal syndrome resembling mesenteric artery obstruction are all more common features of **digoxin** toxicity in the elderly than in the young. Hypokalaemia due to decreased potassium intake (potassium-rich foods are often expensive), faulty homeostatic mechanisms resulting in increased renal loss and the concomitant use of diuretics is more common in the elderly, and is a contributory factor in some patients. **Digoxin** is sometimes prescribed when there is no indication for it (e.g. for an irregular pulse which is due to multiple ectopic beats rather than atrial fibrillation). At other times, the indications for initiation of treatment are correct but the situation is never reviewed. In one series of geriatric patients on **digoxin**, the drug was withdrawn in 78% of cases without detrimental effects.

DIURETICS

Diuretics are more likely to cause adverse effects (e.g. postural hypotension, glucose intolerance and electrolyte disturbances) in elderly patients. Too vigorous a diuresis may result in urinary retention in an old man with an enlarged prostate, and necessitate bladder catheterization with its attendant risks. Brisk diuresis in patients with mental impairment or reduced mobility can result in incontinence. For many patients, a thiazide diuretic, such as **bendroflumethiazide**, is adequate. Loop diuretics, such as **furosemide**, should be used in acute heart failure or in the lowest effective dose for maintenance treatment of chronic heart failure. Clinically important hypokalaemia is uncommon with low doses of diuretics, but plasma potassium should be checked after starting treatment. If clinically important hypokalaemia develops, a thiazide plus potassium-retaining diuretic (**amiloride** or **triamterene**) can be considered, but there is a risk of hyperkalaemia due to renal impairment, especially if an ACE inhibitor and/or angiotensin receptor antagonist and aldosterone antagonist are given together with the diuretic for hypertension or heart failure. Thiazide-induced gout and glucose intolerance are important side effects.

ISCHAEMIC HEART DISEASE

This is covered in Chapter 29.

ANGIOTENSIN CONVERTING ENZYME INHIBITORS (ACEI) AND ANGIOTENSIN RECEPTOR BLOCKERS (ARB)

These drugs plays an important part in the treatment of chronic heart failure, as well as hypertension (see Chapters 28 and 31), and are effective and usually well tolerated in the elderly. However, hypotension, hyperkalaemia and renal failure are more common in this age group. The possibility of atheromatous renal artery stenosis should be borne in mind and serum creatinine levels checked before and after starting treatment. Potassium-retaining diuretics should be co-administered only with extreme caution, because of the reduced GFR and plasma potassium levels monitored. Despite differences in their pharmacology, ACEI and ARB appear similar in efficacy, but ARB do not cause the dry cough that is common with ACEI. The question of whether co-administration of ACEI with ARB has much to add remains controversial; in elderly patients with reduced GFR, the safety of such combined therapy is an important consideration.

ORAL HYPOGLYCAEMIC AGENTS

Diabetes is common in the elderly and many patients are treated with oral hypoglycaemic drugs (see Chapter 37). It is best for elderly patients to be managed with diet if at all possible. In obese elderly diabetics who remain symptomatic on diet, **metformin** should be considered, but coexisting renal, heart or lung disease may preclude its use. Short-acting sulphonylureas (e.g. **gliclazide**) are preferred to longer-acting drugs because of the risk of hypoglycaemia: **chlorpropamide** (half-life 36 hours) can cause prolonged hypoglycaemia and is specifically contraindicated in this age group, **glibenclamide** should also be avoided. **Insulin** may be needed, but impaired visual and cognitive skills must be considered on an individual basis, and the potential need for dose reduction with advancing age and progressive renal impairment taken into account.

ANTIBIOTICS

The decline in renal function must be borne in mind when an antibiotic that is renally excreted is prescribed, especially if it is nephrotoxic (e.g. an aminoglycoside or **tetracycline**). Appendix 3 of the British National Formulary is an invaluable practical guide. Over-prescription of antibiotics is a threat to all age groups, but especially in the elderly. Broad-spectrum drugs including cephalosporins and other beta-lactams, and fluoroquinones are common precursors of *Clostridium difficile* infection which has a high mortality rate in the elderly. **Amoxicillin** is the most common cause of drug rash in the elderly. Flucloxacillin induced cholestatic jaundice and hepatitis is more common in the elderly.

Case history

An 80-year-old retired publican was referred with 'congestive cardiac failure and acute retention of urine'. His wife said his symptoms of ankle swelling and breathlessness had gradually increased over a period of six months despite the GP doubling the water tablet (co-amilozide) which he was taking for high blood pressure. Over the previous week he had become mildly confused and restless at night, for which the GP had prescribed chlorpromazine. His other medication included ketoprofen for osteoarthritis and frequent magnesium trisilicate mixture for indigestion. He had been getting up nearly ten times most nights for a year to pass urine. During the day, he frequently passed small amounts of urine. Over the previous 24 hours, he had been unable to pass urine. His wife thought most of his problems were due to the fact that he drank two pints of beer each day since his retirement seven years previously.

On physical examination he was clinically anaemic, but not cyanosed. Findings were consistent with congestive cardiac failure. His bladder was palpable up to his umbilicus. Rectal examination revealed an enlarged, symmetrical prostate and black tarry faeces. Fundoscopy revealed a grade II hypertensive retinopathy.

Initial laboratory results revealed that the patient had acute on chronic renal failure, dangerously high potassium levels (7.6 mmol/L) and anaemia (Hb 7.4 g/dL). Emergency treatment included calcium chloride, dextrose and insulin, urinary catheterization, furosemide and haemodialysis. Gastroscopy revealed a bleeding gastric ulcer. The patient was discharged two weeks later, when he was symptomatically well. His discharge medication consisted of regular doxazosin and ranitidine, and paracetamol as required.

Question

Describe how each of this patient's drugs prescribed before admission may have contributed to his clinical condition.

Answer

Co-amilozide – hyperkalaemia: amiloride, exacerbation of prostatic symptoms: thiazide

Chlorpromazine – urinary retention

Ketoprofen – gastric ulcer, antagonism of thiazide diuretic, salt retention, possibly interstitial nephritis

Magnesium trisilicate mixture – additional sodium load (6 mmol Na$^+$/10 mL).

Comment

Iatrogenic disease due to multiple drug therapy is common in the elderly. The use of amiloride in renal impairment leads to hyperkalaemia. This patient's confusion and restlessness were most probably related to his renal failure. Chlorpromazine may mask some of the symptoms/signs and delay treatment of the reversible organic disease. The analgesic of choice in osteoarthritis is paracetamol, due to its much better tolerance than NSAID. The sodium content of some antacids can adversely affect cardiac and renal failure.

NON-STEROIDAL ANTI-INFLAMMATORY DRUGS

The elderly are particularly susceptible to non-steroidal anti-inflammatory drug (NSAID)-induced peptic ulceration, gastro-intestinal irritation and fluid retention. An NSAID is frequently prescribed inappropriately for osteoarthritis before physical and functional interventions and oral **paracetamol** have been adequately utilized. If an NSAID is required as adjunctive therapy, the lowest effective dose should be used. **Ibuprofen** is probably the NSAID of choice in terms of minimizing gastro-intestinal side effects. A proton pump inhibitor should be considered as prophylaxis against upper gastro-intestinal complications in those most at risk.

PRACTICAL ASPECTS OF PRESCRIBING FOR THE ELDERLY

Improper prescription of drugs is a common cause of morbidity in elderly people. Common-sense rules for prescribing do not apply only to the elderly, but are especially important in this vulnerable group.

1. Take a full drug history (see Chapter 1), which should include any adverse reactions and use of over-the-counter drugs.
2. Know the pharmacological action of the drug employed.
3. Use the lowest effective dose.
4. Use the fewest possible number of drugs the patient needs.
5. Consider the potential for drug interactions and co-morbidity on drug response.
6. Drugs should seldom be used to treat symptoms without first discovering the cause of the symptoms (i.e. first diagnosis, then treatment).
7. Drugs should not be withheld because of old age, but it should be remembered that there is no cure for old age either.
8. A drug should not be continued if it is no longer necessary.
9. Do not use a drug if the symptoms it causes are worse than those it is intended to relieve.
10. It is seldom sensible to treat the side effects of one drug by prescribing another.

In the elderly, it is often important to pay attention to matters such as the formulation of the drug to be used – many old people tolerate elixirs and liquid medicines better than tablets or capsules. Supervision of drug taking may be necessary, as an elderly person with a serious physical or mental disability cannot be expected to comply with any but the simplest drug regimen. Containers require especially clear labelling, and should be easy to open – child-proof containers are often also grandparent-proof!

RESEARCH

Despite their disproportionate consumption of medicines, the elderly are often under-represented in clinical trials. This may result in the data being extrapolated to an elderly population inappropriately, or the exclusion of elderly patients from new treatments from which they might benefit. It is essential that, both during a drug's development and after it has been licensed, subgroup analysis of elderly populations is carefully examined both for efficacy and for predisposition to adverse effects.

Case history

A previously mentally alert and well-orientated 90-year-old woman became acutely confused two nights after hospital admission for bronchial asthma which, on the basis of peak flow and blood gases, had responded well to inhaled salbutamol and oral prednisolone. Her other medication was cimetidine (for dyspepsia), digoxin (for an isolated episode of atrial fibrillation two years earlier) and nitrazepam (for night sedation).

Question

Which drugs may be related to the acute confusion?

Answer

Prednisolone, cimetidine, digoxin and nitrazepam.

Comment

If an H$_2$-antagonist is necessary, ranitidine is preferred in the elderly. It is likely that the patient no longer requires digoxin (which accumulates in the elderly). Benzodiazepines should not be used for sedation in elderly (or young) asthmatics. They may also accumulate in the elderly. The elderly tend to be more sensitive to adverse drug effects on the central nervous system (CNS).

FURTHER READING

Dhesi JK, Allain TJ, Mangoni AA, Jackson SHD. The implications of a growing evidence base for drug use in elderly patients. Part 4. Vitamin D and bisphosphonates for fractures and osteoporosis. *British Journal of Clinical Pharmacology* 2006; **61**: 520–8.

Hanratty CG, McGlinchey P, Johnston GD, Passmore AP. Differential pharmacokinetics of digoxin in elderly patients. *Drugs and Aging* 2000; **17**: 353–62.

Mangoni AA, Jackson SHD. The implications of a growing evidence base for drug use in elderly patients. Part 1. Statins for primary and secondary cardiovascular prevention. *British Journal of Clinical Pharmacology* 2006; **61**: 494–501.

Mangoni AA, Jackson SHD. The implications of a growing evidence base for drug use in elderly patients. Part 2. ACE inhibitors and angiotensin receptor blockers in heart failure and high cardiovascular risk patients. *British Journal of Clinical Pharmacology* 2006; **61**: 502–12.

Mangoni AA, Jackson SHD. The implications of a growing evidence base for drug use in elderly patients. Part 3. β-adrenoceptor blockers in heart failure and thrombolytics in acute myocardial infarction. *British Journal of Clinical Pharmacology* 2006; **61**: 513–20.

Sproule BA, Hardy BG, Shulman KI. Differential pharmacokinetics in elderly patients. *Drugs and Aging* 2000; **16**: 165–77.

ADVERSE DRUG REACTIONS

INTRODUCTION

Adverse drug reactions are unwanted effects caused by normal therapeutic doses. Drugs are great mimics of disease, and adverse drug reactions present with diverse clinical signs and symptoms. The classification proposed by Rawlins and Thompson (1977) divides reactions into type A and type B (Table 12.1).

Type A reactions, which constitute approximately 80% of adverse drug reactions, are usually a consequence of the drug's primary pharmacological effect (e.g. bleeding from **warfarin**) or a low therapeutic index (e.g. nausea from **digoxin**), and they are therefore predictable. They are dose-related and usually mild, although they may be serious or even fatal (e.g. intracranial bleeding from **warfarin**). Such reactions are usually due to inappropriate dosage, especially when drug elimination is impaired. The term 'side effects' is often applied to minor type A reactions.

Type B ('idiosyncratic') reactions are not predictable from the drug's main pharmacological action, are not dose-related and are severe, with a considerable mortality. The underlying pathophysiology of type B reactions is poorly if at all understood, and often has a genetic or immunological basis. Type B reactions occur infrequently (1:1000–1:10 000 treated subjects being typical).

Table 12.1: Some examples of type A and type B reactions.

Drug	Type A	Type B
Chlorpromazine	Sedation	Cholestatic jaundice
Naproxen	Gastro-intestinal haemorrhage	Agranulocytosis
Phenytoin	Ataxia	Hepatitis, lymphadenopathy
Thiazides	Hypokalaemia	Thrombocytopenia
Quinine	Tinnitus	Thrombocytopenia
Warfarin	Bleeding	Breast necrosis

Adverse drug reactions due to specific drug–drug interactions are considered in Chapter 13. Three further minor categories of adverse drug reaction have been proposed:

1. *type C* – continuous reactions due to long-term drug use (e.g. neuroleptic-related tardive dyskinesia or analgesic nephropathy);
2. *type D* – delayed reactions (e.g. alkylating agents leading to carcinogenesis, or retinoid-associated teratogenesis);
3. *type E* end-of-use reactions, such as adrenocortical insufficiency following withdrawal of glucocorticosteroids, or withdrawal syndromes following discontinuation of treatment with benzodiazepines or β-adrenoceptor antagonists.

In the UK there are between 30 000 and 40 000 medicinal products available directly or on prescription. Surveys suggest that approximately 80% of adults take some kind of medication during any two-week period. Exposure to drugs in the population is thus substantial, and the incidence of adverse reactions must be viewed in this context. Type A reactions are reported to be responsible for 2–3% of consultations in general practice. In a recent prospective analysis of 18 820 hospital admissions by Pirmohamed et al. (2004), 1225 were related to an adverse drug reaction (prevalence 6.8%), with the adverse drug reaction leading directly to admission in 80% of cases. Median bed stay was eight days, accounting for 4% of hospital bed capacity. The projected annual cost to the NHS is £466 million. Overall fatality was 0.15%. Most reactions were either definitely or probably avoidable. Adverse drug reactions are most frequent and severe in the elderly, in neonates, women, patients with hepatic or renal impairment, and individuals with a history of previous adverse drug reactions. Such reactions often occur early in therapy (during the first one to ten days). Drugs most commonly implicated include low-dose **aspirin** (antiplatelet agents), diuretics, **warfarin** and NSAIDs. A systematic review by Howard et al. (2006) of preventable adverse drug reactions which caused hospitalization, implicated the same major drug classes.

Factors involved in the aetiology of adverse drug reactions can be classified as shown in Table 12.2.

IDENTIFICATION OF THE DRUG AT FAULT

It is often difficult to decide whether a clinical event is drug related, and even when this is probable, it may be difficult to determine which drug is responsible, as patients are often taking multiple drugs. One or more of several possible approaches may be appropriate.

1. A careful drug history is essential. The following considerations should be made to assess causality of the effect to the drug: did the clinical event and the time-course of its development fit with the duration of suspected drug treatment and known adverse drug effects? Did the adverse effect reverse upon drug withdrawal and, upon rechallenge with the drug, reappear? Were other possible causes reasonably excluded? A patient's drug history may not always be conclusive because, although allergy to a drug implies previous exposure, the antigen may have occurred in foods (e.g. antibiotics are often fed to livestock and drug residues remain in the flesh), in drug mixtures or in some casual manner.

2. Provocation testing. This involves giving a very small amount of the suspected drug and seeing whether a reaction ensues, e.g. skin testing, where a drug is applied as a patch, or is pricked or scratched into the skin or injected intradermally. Unfortunately, prick and scratch testing is less useful for assessing the systemic reaction to drugs than it is for the more usual atopic antigens (e.g. pollens), and both false-positive and false-negative results can occur. Patch testing is safe, and is useful for the diagnosis of contact sensitivity, but does not reflect systemic reactions and may itself cause allergy. Provocation tests should only be undertaken under expert guidance, after obtaining informed consent, and with resuscitation facilities available.

3. Serological testing and lymphocytes testing. Serological testing is rarely helpful, circulating antibodies to the drug do not mean that they are necessarily the cause of the symptoms. The demonstration of transformation occurring when the patient's lymphocytes are exposed to a drug ex vivo suggests that the patient's T-lymphocytes are sensitized to the drug. In this type of reaction, the hapten itself will often provoke lymphocyte transformation, as well as the conjugate.

4. The best approach in patients on multiple drug therapy is to stop all potentially causal drugs and reintroduce them one by one until the drug at fault is discovered. This should only be done if the reaction is not serious, or if the drug is essential and no chemically unrelated alternative is available. All drug allergies should be recorded in the case notes and the patient informed of the risks involved in taking the drug again.

Table 12.2: Factors involved in adverse drug reactions.

Intrinsic	Extrinsic
Patient factors	
Age – neonatal, infant and elderly	Environment – sun
Sex – hormonal environment	Xenobiotics (e.g. drugs, herbicides)
Genetic abnormalities (e.g. enzyme or receptor polymorphisms)	Malnutrition
Previous adverse drug reactions, allergy, atopy	
Presence of organ dysfunction – disease	
Personality and habits – adherence (compliance), alcoholic, drug addict, nicotine	
Prescriber factors	
Incorrect drug or drug combination	
Incorrect route of administration	
Incorrect dose	
Incorrect duration of therapy	
Drug factors	
Drug–drug interactions (see Chapter 13)	
Pharmaceutical – batch problems, shelf-life, incorrect dispensing	

> ### Key points
>
> - *Type A reaction* – an extension of the pharmacology of the drug, dose related, and accounts for most adverse reactions (e.g. β-adrenoreceptor antagonist-induced bradycardia or AV block).
> - *Type B reaction* – idiosyncratic reaction to the drug, not dose related, rare but severe (e.g. chloramphenicol-induced aplastic anaemia).
> - Other types of drug reaction (much rarer):
>   - *type C reaction* – continuous reactions due to long-term use: analgesic nephropathy;
>   - *type D reaction* – delayed reactions of carcinogenesis or teratogenesis;
>   - *type E reaction* – drug withdrawal reactions (e.g. benzodiazepines).

ADVERSE DRUG REACTION MONITORING/ SURVEILLANCE (PHARMACOVIGILANCE)

The evaluation of drug safety is complex, and there are many methods for monitoring adverse drug reactions. Each of these has its own advantages and shortcomings, and no single system can offer the 100% accuracy that current public opinion expects. The ideal method would identify adverse drug reactions with a high degree of sensitivity and specificity and respond rapidly. It would detect rare but severe adverse drug reactions, but would not be overwhelmed by common ones, the incidence of which it would quantify together with predisposing factors. Continued surveillance is mandatory after a new drug has been marketed, as it is inevitable that the preliminary testing of medicines in humans during drug development, although excluding many ill effects, cannot identify uncommon adverse effects. A variety of early detection systems have been introduced to identify adverse drug reactions as swiftly as possible.

PHASE I/II/III TRIALS

Early (phase I/II) trials (Chapter 15) are important for assessing the tolerability and dose–response relationship of new therapeutic agents. However, these studies are, by design, very insensitive at detecting adverse reactions because they are performed on relatively few subjects (perhaps 200–300). This is illustrated by the failure to detect the serious toxicity of several drugs (e.g. **benoxaprofen**, **cerivastatin**, **felbamate**, **dexfenfluramine** and **fenfluramine**, **rofecoxib**, **temofloxacin**, **troglitazone**) before marketing. However, phase III clinical trials can establish the incidence of common adverse reactions and relate this to therapeutic benefit. Analysis of the reasons given for dropping out of phase III trials is particularly valuable in establishing whether common events, such as headache, constipation, lethargy or male sexual dysfunction are truly drug related. The Medical Research Council Mild Hypertension Study unexpectedly identified impotence as more commonly associated with thiazide diuretics than with placebo or β-adrenoceptor antagonist therapy. Table 12.3 illustrates how difficult it is to detect adverse drug reactions with 95% confidence, even when there is no background incidence and the diagnostic accuracy is 100%. This 'easiest-case' scenario approximates to the actual situation with **thalidomide** teratogenicity: spontaneous phocomelia is almost unknown, and the condition is almost unmistakable. It is sobering to consider that an estimated 10 000 malformed babies were born world-wide before **thalidomide** was withdrawn. Regulatory authorities may act after three or more documented events.

The problem of adverse drug reaction recognition is much greater if the reaction resembles spontaneous disease in the population, such that physicians are unlikely to attribute the reaction to drug exposure: the numbers of patients that must then be exposed to enable such reactions to be detected are greater than those quoted in Table 12.3, probably by several orders of magnitude.

YELLOW CARD SCHEME AND POST-MARKETING (PHASE IV) SURVEILLANCE

Untoward effects that have not been detected in clinical trials become apparent when the drug is used on a wider scale. Case

Table 12.3: Numbers of subjects that would need to be exposed in order to detect adverse drug reactions

Expected frequency of the adverse effect	Approximate number of patients required to be exposed	
	For one event	For three events
1 in 100	300	650
1 in 1000	3000	6500
1 in 10 000	30 000	65 000

reports, which may stimulate further reports, remain the most sensitive means of detecting rare but serious and unusual adverse effects. In the UK, a Register of Adverse Reactions was started in 1964. Currently, the Medicines and Healthcare products Regulatory Agency (MHRA) operates a system of spontaneous reporting on prepaid yellow postcards. Doctors, dentists, pharmacists, nurse practitioners and (most recently) patients are encouraged to report adverse events whether actually or potentially causally drug-related. Analogous schemes are employed in other countries. The yellow card scheme consists of three stages:

1. data collection;
2. analysis;
3. feedback.

Such surveillance methods are useful, but under-reporting is a major limitation. Probably fewer than 10% of appropriate adverse reactions are reported. This may be due partly to confusion about what events to report, partly to difficulty in recognizing the possible relationship of a drug to an adverse event – especially when the patient has been taking several drugs, and partly to ignorance or laziness on the part of potential reporters. A further problem is that, as explained above, if a drug increases the incidence of a common disorder (e.g. ischaemic heart disease), the change in incidence must be very large to be detectable. This is compounded when there is a delay between starting the drug and occurrence of the event (e.g. cardiovascular thrombotic events including myocardial infarction following initiation of **rofecoxib** therapy). Doctors are inefficient at detecting such adverse reactions to drugs, and those reactions that are reported are in general the obvious or previously described and well-known ones. Initiatives are in progress to attempt to improve this situation by involvement of trained clinical pharmacologists and pharmacists in and outside hospitals.

The Committee on Safety of Medicines (CSM), now part of MHRA, introduced a system of high vigilance for newly marketed drugs. For its first two years on the general market, any newly marketed drug has a black triangle on its data sheet and against its entry in the British National Formulary. This conveys to prescribers that any unexpected event should be reported by the yellow card system. The pharmaceutical company is also responsible for obtaining accurate reports on all patients treated up to an agreed number. This scheme was successful in the case of **benoxaprofen**, an anti-inflammatory analgesic. Following its release, there were spontaneous reports to the CSM of photosensitivity and onycholysis. Further reports appeared in the elderly, in whom its half-life is prolonged, of cholestatic jaundice and hepatorenal failure, which was fatal in eight cases. **Benoxaprofen** was subsequently taken off the market when 3500 adverse drug reaction reports were received with 61 fatalities. The yellow card/black triangle scheme was also instrumental in the early identification of urticaria and cough as adverse effects of angiotensin-converting enzyme inhibitors. Although potentially the population under study by this system consists of all the patients using a drug, in fact under-reporting yields a population that is not uniformly sampled. Such data can be unrepresentative and difficult to work with statistically, contributing to the paucity of accurate incidence data for adverse drug reactions.

Systems such as the yellow card scheme (e.g. FDA MedWatch in the USA) are relatively inexpensive and easy to manage, and facilitate ongoing monitoring of all drugs, all consumers and all types of adverse reaction. Reports from the drug regulatory bodies of 22 countries are collated by the World Health Organization (WHO) Unit of Drug Evaluation and Monitoring in Geneva. Rapid access to reports from other countries should be of great value in detecting rare adverse reactions, although the same reservations apply to this register as apply to national systems. In addition, this database could reveal geographical differences in the pattern of untoward drug effects.

CASE–CONTROL STUDIES

A very large number of patients have to be monitored to detect a rare type B adverse effect. An alternative approach is to identify patients with a disorder which it is postulated could be caused by an adverse reaction to a drug, and to compare the frequency of exposure to possible aetiological agents with a control group. A prior suspicion (hypothesis) must exist to prompt the setting up of such a study – examples are the possible connection between irradiation or environmental pollution and certain malignancies, especially where they are observed in clusters. Artefacts can occur as a result of unrecognized bias from faulty selection of patients and controls, and the approach remains controversial among epidemiologists, public health physicians and statisticians. Despite this, there is really no practicable alternative for investigating a biologically plausible hypothesis relating to a disease which is so uncommon that it is unlikely to be represented even in large trial or cohort populations. This methodology has had notable successes: the association of **stilboestrol** with vaginal adenocarcinoma, **gatifloxacin** with hypo- and hyperglycaemia, and **salmeterol** or **fenoterol** use with increased fatality in asthmatics.

INTENSIVE MONITORING

Several hospital-based intensive monitoring programmes are currently in progress. The Aberdeen–Dundee system abstracts data from some 70 000 hospital admissions each year, storing these on a computer file before analysis. The Boston Collaborative Drug Surveillance Program (BCDSP), involving selected hospitals in several countries, is even more comprehensive. In the BCDSP, all patients admitted to specially designated general wards are included in the analysis. Specially trained personnel obtain the following information from hospital patients and records:

1. background information (i.e. age, weight, height, etc.);
2. medical history;
3. drug exposure;
4. side effects;
5. outcome of treatment and changes in laboratory tests during hospital admission.

A unique feature of comprehensive drug-monitoring systems lies in their potential to follow up and investigate adverse reactions suggested by less sophisticated detection systems, or by isolated case reports in medical journals. Furthermore, the frequency of side effects can be determined more cheaply than by a specially mounted trial to investigate a simple adverse effect. Thus, for example, the risk of developing a rash with **ampicillin** was found to be around 7% both by clinical trial and by the BCDSP, which can quantify such associations almost automatically from data on its files. New adverse reactions or drug interactions are sought by multiple correlation analysis. Thus, when an unexpected relationship arises, such as the 20% incidence of gastro-intestinal bleeding in severely ill patients treated with **ethacrynic acid** compared to 4.3% among similar patients treated with other diuretics, this cannot be attributed to bias arising from awareness of the hypothesis during data collection, since the data were collected before the hypothesis was proposed. Conversely, there is a possibility of chance associations arising from multiple comparisons ('type I' statistical error), and such associations must be reviewed critically before accepting a causal relationship. It is possible to identify predisposing risk factors. In the association between **ethacrynic acid** and gastro-intestinal bleeding, these were female sex, a high blood urea concentration, previous heparin administration and intravenous administration of the drug. An important aspect of this type of approach is that lack of clinically important associations can also be investigated. Thus, no significant association between **aspirin** and renal disease was found, whereas long-term **aspirin** consumption is associated with a decreased incidence of myocardial infarction, an association which has been shown to be of therapeutic importance in randomized clinical trials (Chapter 29). There are plans to extend intensive drug monitoring to cover other areas of medical practice.

However, in terms of new but uncommon adverse reactions, the numbers of patients undergoing intensive monitoring while taking a particular drug will inevitably be too small for the effect to be detectable. Such monitoring can therefore only provide information about relatively common, early reactions to drugs used under hospital conditions. Patients are not in hospital long enough for detection of delayed effects, which are among the reactions least likely to be recognized as such even by an astute clinician.

MONITORING FROM NATIONAL STATISTICS

A great deal of information is available from death certificates, hospital discharge diagnoses and similar records. From these data, it may be possible to detect a change in disease trends and relate this to drug therapy. Perhaps the best-known example of this is the increased death rate in young asthmatics noted in the mid-1960s, which was associated with overuse of bronchodilator inhalers containing non-specific β-adrenoceptor agonists (e.g. **adrenaline** and/or **isoprenaline**). Although relatively inexpensive, the shortcomings of this method are obvious, particularly in diseases with an appreciable mortality, since large numbers of patients must suffer before the change is detectable. Data interpretation is particularly difficult when hospital discharges are used as a source of information, since discharge diagnosis is often provisional or incomplete, and may be revised during follow up.

Key points

- Rare (and often severe) adverse drug events may not be detected in early drug development but only defined in the first few years post marketing (phase IV of drug development).
- Be aware of and participate in the MHRA yellow card system for reporting suspected adverse drug reactions.
- Use of any recently marketed drug, which is identified with a black triangle on its data sheet or in the British National Formulary, indicates the need to be particularly suspicious about adverse drug reactions and to report any suspected adverse drug reaction via the yellow card system.
- Constant vigilance by physicians for drug-induced disease, particularly for new drugs, but also for more established agents, is needed.

FEEDBACK

There is no point in collecting vast amounts of data on adverse reactions unless they are analysed and conclusions reported back to prescribing doctors. In addition to articles in the medical journals and media, the *Current Problems in Pharmacovigilance* series deals with important and recently identified adverse drug reactions. If an acute and serious problem is recognized, doctors will usually receive notification from the MHRA/Commission on Human Medicines, and often from the pharmaceutical company marketing the product.

ALLERGIC ADVERSE DRUG REACTIONS

Immune mechanisms are involved in a number of adverse effects caused by drugs (see below and Chapter 50). The development of allergy implies previous exposure to the drug or to some closely related substance. Most drugs are of low molecular weight (300–500 Da) and thus are not antigenic.

However, they can combine with high molecular weight entities, usually proteins, to form an antigenic hapten conjugate.

The factors that determine the development of allergy to a drug are not fully understood. Some drugs (e.g. **penicillin**) are more likely to cause allergic reactions than others, and type I (immediate anaphylactic) reactions are more common in patients with a history of atopy. A correlation between allergic reactions involving immunoglobulin E (IgE) and human leukocyte antigen (HLA) serotypes has been reported, so genetic factors may also be important. There is some evidence that drug allergies are more common in older people, in women and in those with a previous history of drug reaction. However, this may merely represent increased frequencies of drug exposure in these patient groups.

TYPES OF ALLERGY

Drugs cause a variety of allergic responses (Figure 12.1) and sometimes a single drug can be responsible for more than one type of allergic response.

TYPE I REACTIONS

Type I reactions are due to the production of reaginic (IgE) antibodies to an antigen (e.g. penicillins and cephalosporins). The antigen binds to surface bound IgE on mast cells causing degranulation and release of histamine, eicosanoids and cytokines. It commonly occurs in response to a foreign serum or **penicillin**, but may also occur with **streptomycin** and some local anaesthetics. With **penicillin**, it is believed that the penicilloyl moiety of the **penicillin** molecule is responsible for the production of antibodies. Treatment of anaphylactic shock is detailed in Chapter 50.

TYPE II REACTIONS

These are due to antibodies of class IgG and IgM which, on contact with antibodies on the surface of cells, bind complement, causing cell lysis (e.g. **penicillin**, cephalosporins, **methyldopa** or **quinine**) causing, for example, Coombs' positive haemolytic anaemia.

TYPE III IMMUNE COMPLEX ARTHUS REACTIONS

Circulating immune complexes can produce several clinical allergic states, including serum sickness and immune complex glomerulonephritis, and a syndrome resembling systemic lupus erythematosus. The onset of serum sickness is delayed for several days until features develop such as fever, urticaria, arthropathy, lymphadenopathy, proteinuria and eosinophilia. Recovery takes a few days. Examples of causative agents include serum, **penicillin**, **sulfamethoxazole/trimethoprim**, **streptomycin** and **propylthiouracil**. **Amiodarone** lung and **hydralazine**-induced systemic lupus syndrome are also possibly mediated by immune complex-related mechanisms, although these reactions are less well understood.

TYPE IV DELAYED HYPERSENSITIVITY REACTIONS

Type IV reactions are delayed hypersensitivity reactions, the classical example of which is contact dermatitis (e.g. to topical

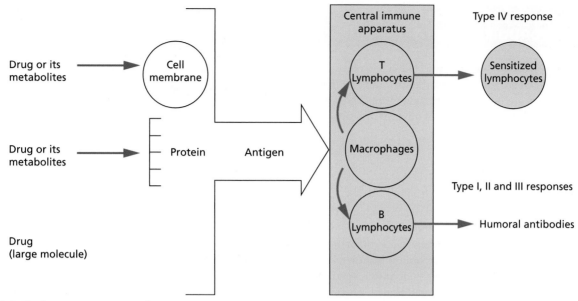

Figure 12.1: The immune response to drugs.

antibiotics, such as **penicillin** or **neomycin**). The mechanism here is that the drug applied to the skin forms an antigenic conjugate with dermal proteins, stimulating formation of sensitized T-lymphocytes in the regional lymph nodes, with a resultant rash if the drug is applied again. Drug photosensitivity is due to a photochemical combination between the drug (e.g. **amiodarone**, **chlorpromazine**, **ciprofloxacin**, tetracyclines) and dermal protein. Delayed sensitivity can also result from the systemic administration of drugs.

Key points

How to attempt to define the drug causing the adverse drug reaction:

- Attempt to define the likely causality of the effect to the drug, thinking through the following: Did the reaction and its time-course fit with the duration of suspected drug treatment and known adverse drug effects? Did the adverse effect disappear on drug withdrawal and, if rechallenged with the drug, reappear? Were other possible causes excluded?
- Provocation testing with skin testing – intradermal tests are neither very sensitive nor specific.
- Test the patient's serum for anti-drug antibodies, or test the reaction of the patient's lymphocytes in vitro to the drug and/or drug metabolite if appropriate.
- Consider stopping all drugs and reintroducing essential ones sequentially.
- Carefully document and highlight the adverse drug reaction and the most likely culprit in the case notes.

PREVENTION OF ALLERGIC DRUG REACTIONS

Although it is probably not possible to avoid all allergic drug reactions, the following measures can decrease their incidence:

1. Taking a detailed drug history (prescription and over-the-counter drugs, drugs of abuse, nutritional and vitamin supplements and alternative remedies) is essential. A history of atopy, although not excluding the use of drugs, should make one wary.
2. Drugs given orally are less likely to cause severe allergic reactions than those given by injection.
3. Desensitization (hyposensitization) should only be used when continued use of the drug is essential. It involves giving a very small dose of the drug and increasing the dose at regular intervals, sometimes under cover of a glucocorticosteroid and β_2-adrenoceptor agonist. An antihistamine may be added if a drug reaction occurs, and equipment for resuscitation and therapy of anaphylactic shock must be close at hand. It is often successful, although the mechanism by which it is achieved is not fully understood.
4. Prophylactic skin testing is not usually practicable, and a negative test does not exclude the possibility of an allergic reaction.

Key points

Classification of immune-mediated adverse drug reactions:

- *Type I* – urticaria or anaphylaxis due to the production of IgE against drug bound to mast cells, leading to massive release of mast cell mediators locally or systemically (e.g. ampicillin skin allergy or anaphylaxis).
- *Type II* – IgG and IgM antibodies to drug which, on contact with antibodies on the cell surface, cause cell lysis by complement fixation (e.g. penicillin, haemolytic anaemia; quinidine, thrombocytopenia).
- *Type III* – circulating immune complexes produced by drug and antibody to drug deposit in organs, causing drug fever, urticaria, rash, lymphadenopathy, glomerulonephritis, often with eosinophilia (e.g. co-trimoxazole, β-lactams).
- *Type IV* – delayed-type hypersensitivity due to drug forming an antigenic conjugate with dermal proteins and sensitized T cells reacting to drug, causing a rash (e.g. topical antibiotics).

EXAMPLES OF ALLERGIC AND OTHER ADVERSE DRUG REACTIONS

Adverse drug reactions can be manifested in any one or multiple organ systems, and in extraordinarily diverse forms. Specific instances are dealt with throughout this book. Some examples to illustrate the diversity of adverse drug reactions are given here.

RASHES

These are one of the most common manifestations of drug reactions. A number of immune and non-immune mechanisms may be involved which produce many different types of rash ranging from a mild maculopapular rash to a severe erythema multiforme major (Stevens Johnson syndrome; Figures 12.2 and 12.3). Commonly implicated drugs/drug classes include beta-lactams, sulphonamides and other antimicrobial agents; anti-seizure medications (e.g. **phenytoin**, **carbamazepine**); NSAIDs. Some drugs may give rise to direct tissue toxicity (e.g. DMPS, used as chelating therapy in patients with heavy metal poisoning; Figure 12.4, see Chapter 54).

LYMPHADENOPATHY

Lymph-node enlargement can result from taking drugs (e.g. **phenytoin**). The mechanism is unknown, but allergic factors

may be involved. The reaction may be confused with a lymphoma, and the drug history is important in patients with lymphadenopathy of unknown cause.

BLOOD DYSCRASIAS

Thrombocytopenia, anaemia (aplastic, iron deficiency, macrocytic, haemolytic) and agranulocytosis can all be caused by drugs.

Thrombocytopenia can occur with many drugs, and in many but not all instances the mechanism is direct suppression of the megakaryocytes rather than immune processes. Drugs that cause thrombocytopenia include:

- heparin;
- gold salts;
- cytotoxic agents (e.g. azathioprine/6-mercaptopurine);
- quinidine;
- sulphonamides;
- thiazides.

Haemolytic anaemia can be caused by a number of drugs, and sometimes immune mechanisms are responsible. Glucose-6-phosphate dehydrogenase deficiency (Chapter 14)

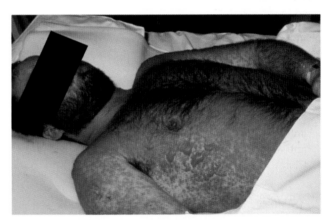

Figure 12.3: Stevens Johnson syndrome following commencement of penicillin therapy (see Chapter 43).

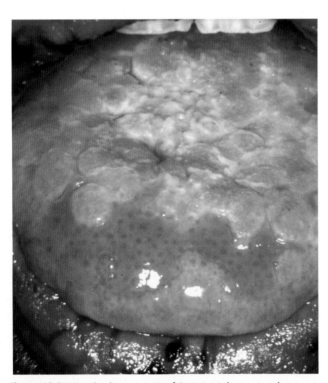

Figure 12.2: Mouth ulcer as part of Stevens Johnson syndrome as a reaction to phenytoin therapy (see Chapter 22).

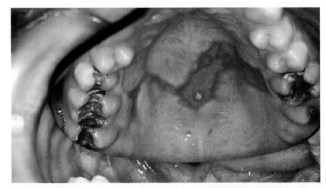

Figure 12.4: Mouth ulcer following DMPS treatment (see Chapter 54).

predisposes to non-immune haemolysis (e.g. **primaquine**). Immune mechanisms include the following:

1. Combination of the drug with the red-cell membrane, with the conjugate acting as an antigen. This has been shown to occur with **penicillin**-induced haemolysis, and may also occur with **chlorpromazine** and sulphonamides.
2. Alteration of the red-cell membrane by the drug so that it becomes autoimmunogenic. This may happen with **methyldopa**, and a direct positive Coombs' test develops in about 20% of patients who have been treated with this drug for more than one year. Frank haemolysis occurs in only a small proportion of cases. Similar changes can take place with **levodopa**, **mefenamic acid** and beta-lactam antibiotics.
3. Non-specific binding of plasma protein to red cells, and thus causing haemolysis. This is believed to occur with cephalosporins.

Aplastic anaemia as an isolated entity is not common, but may occur either in isolation or as part of a general depression of bone marrow activity (pancytopenia). Examples include **chloramphenicol** and (commonly and predictably) cytotoxic drugs.

Agranulocytosis can be caused by many drugs. Several different mechanisms are implicated, and it is not known whether allergy plays a part. The drugs most frequently implicated include the following:

- most cytotoxic drugs (Chapter 48);
- antithyroid drugs (**methimazole, carbimazole, propylthiouracil**; Chapter 38);
- sulphonamides and sulphonylureas (e.g. **tolbutamide, glipizide**; Chapter 37);
- antidepressants (especially **mianserin**; Chapter 20) and antipsychotics (e.g. phenothiazines, **clozapine**; Chapter 20);
- anti-epileptic drugs (e.g. **carbamazepine, felbamate**; Chapter 22).

SYSTEMIC LUPUS ERYTHEMATOSUS

Several drugs (including **procainamide, isoniazid, hydralazine, chlorpromazine** and anticonvulsants) produce a syndrome that resembles systemic lupus together with a positive antinuclear factor test. The development of this is closely related to dose, and in the case of **hydralazine** it also depends on the rate of acetylation, which is genetically controlled (Chapter 14). There is some evidence that the drugs act as haptens, combining with DNA and forming antigens. Symptoms usually disappear when the drug is stopped, but recovery may be slow.

VASCULITIS

Both acute and chronic vasculitis can result from taking drugs, and may have an allergic basis. Acute vasculitis with purpura and renal involvement occurs with penicillins, sulphonamides and **penicillamine**. A more chronic form can occur with **phenytoin**.

RENAL DYSFUNCTION

All clinical manifestations of renal disease can be caused by drugs, and common culprits are non-steroidal anti-inflammatory drugs and angiotensin-converting enzyme inhibitors (which cause functional and usually reversible renal failure in susceptible patients; Chapters 26 and 28). Nephrotic syndrome results from several drugs (e.g. **penicillamine**, high-dose **captopril, gold salts**) which cause various immune-mediated glomerular injuries. Interstitial nephritis can be caused by several drugs, including non-steroidal anti-inflammatory drugs and penicillins, especially **meticillin**. **Cisplatin**, aminoglycosides, **amphotericin**, radiocontrast media and **vancomycin** cause direct tubular toxicity. Many drugs cause electrolyte or acid-base disturbances via their predictable direct or indirect effects on renal electrolyte excretion (e.g. hypokalaemia and hypomagnesaemia from loop diuretics, hyperkalaemia from potassium-sparing diuretics, converting enzyme inhibitors and angiotensin II receptor antagonists, proximal renal tubular acidosis from carbonic anhydrase inhibitors), and some cause unpredictable toxic effects on acid-base balance (e.g. distal renal tubular acidosis from **amphotericin**). Obstructive uropathy can be caused by uric acid crystals consequent upon initiation of chemotherapy in patients with haematological malignancy, and – rarely – poorly soluble drugs, such as sulphonamides, **methotrexate** or **indinavir**, can cause crystalluria.

OTHER REACTIONS

Fever is a common manifestation of drug allergy, and should be remembered in patients with fever of unknown cause.

Liver damage (hepatitis with or without obstructive features) as a side effect of drugs is important. It may be insidious, leading slowly to end-stage cirrhosis (e.g. during chronic treatment with **methotrexate**) or acute and fulminant (as in some cases of **isoniazid, halothane** or **phenytoin** hepatitis). **Chlorpromazine** or **erythromycin** may cause liver involvement characterized by raised alkaline phosphatase and bilirubin ('obstructive' pattern). Gallstones (and mechanical obstruction) can be caused by fibrates and other lipid-lowering drugs (Chapter 27), and by **octreotide**, a somatostatin analogue used to treat a variety of enteropancreatic tumours, including carcinoid syndrome and VIPomas (vasoactive intestinal polypeptide) (see Chapter 42). Immune mechanisms are implicated in some forms of hepatic injury by drugs, but are seldom solely responsible.

Case history

A 73-year-old man develops severe shoulder pain and is diagnosed as having a frozen shoulder, for which he is prescribed physiotherapy and given naproxen, 250 mg three times a day, by his family practitioner. The practitioner knows him well and checks that he has normal renal function for his age. When he attends for review about two weeks later, he is complaining of tiredness and reduced urine frequency. Over the past few days he noted painful but non-swollen joints and a maculopapular rash on his trunk and limbs. He is afebrile and apart from the rash there are no other abnormal physical signs. Laboratory studies show a normal full blood count; an absolute eosinophil count raised at 490/mm³. His serum creatinine was 110 μmol/L at baseline and is now 350 μmol/L with a urea of 22.5 mmol/L; electrolytes and liver function tests are normal. Urinalysis shows 2+ protein, urine microscopy contains 100 leukocytes/hpf with 24% eosinophils.

Question 1

If this is an adverse drug reaction, what type of reaction is it and what is the diagnosis?

Question 2

What is the best management plan and should this patient ever receive naproxen again?

Answer 1

The patient has developed an acute interstitial nephritis, probably secondary to the recent introduction of naproxen treatment. This is a well-recognized syndrome, with the clinical features that the patient displays in this case. It can be associated with many NSAIDs (both non selective NSAIDs and COX-2 inhibitors), particularly in the elderly. This is a type B adverse drug reaction whose pathophysiology is probably a combination of type III and type IV hypersensitivity reactions.

Answer 2

Discontinuation of the offending agent is vital and this is sometimes sufficient to produce a return to baseline values of renal function and the disappearance of systemic symptoms of fever and the rash. Recovery may possibly be accelerated and further renal toxicity minimized by a short course (five to seven days) of high-dose oral corticosteroids, while monitoring renal function. The offending agent should not be used again in this patient unless the benefits of using it vastly outweigh the risks associated with its use in a serious illness.

FURTHER READING AND WEB MATERIAL

Davies DM, Ferner RE de Glanville H. *Textbook of adverse drug reactions*, 5th edn. Oxford: Oxford Medical Publications, 1998.

Dukes MNG, Aronson JA: 2000: *Meylers's side-effects of drugs*, vol. 14. Amsterdam: Elsevier (see also companion volumes *Side-effects of drugs annuals*, 2003, published annually since 1977).

FDA Medwatch website. www.fda.gov/medwatch

Gruchalla RS, Pirmohamed M. Antibiotic allergy. *New England Journal of Medicine* 2006; **354**: 601–609 (practical clinical approach).

Howard RL, Avery AJ, Slavenburg S et al. Which drugs cause preventable admissions to hospital? A systematic review. *British Journal of Clinical Pharmacology* 2006; **63**: 136–47.

MHRA and the Committee on Safety of Medicines and the Medicine Control Agency. *Current problems in pharmacovigilance*. London: Committee on Safety of Medicines and the Medicine Control Agency. (Students are advised to monitor this publication for ongoing and future adverse reactions.)

MHRA Current problems in pharmacovigilance website. www.mhra.gov.uk/home/idcplg?IdcService=SS_GET_PAGE&nodeId=368.

Pirmohamed M, James S, Meakin S et al. Adverse drug reactions as cause of admission to hospital: prospective analysis of 18.820 patients. *British Medical Journal* 2004; **329**: 15–19.

Rawlins MD, Thompson JW. *Pathogenesis of adverse drug reactions*, 2nd edn. Oxford: Oxford University Press, 1977.

DRUG INTERACTIONS

INTRODUCTION

Drug interaction is the modification of the action of one drug by another. There are three kinds of mechanism:

1. pharmaceutical;
2. pharmacodynamic;
3. pharmacokinetic.

Pharmaceutical interactions occur by chemical reaction or physical interaction when drugs are mixed. Pharmacodynamic interactions occur when different drugs each infuence the same physiological function (e.g. drugs that influence state of alertness or blood pressure); the result of adding a second such drug during treatment with another may be to increase the effect of the first (e.g. alcohol increases sleepiness caused by benzodiazepines). Conversely, for drugs with opposing actions, the result may be to reduce the effect of the first (e.g. **indometacin** increases blood pressure in hypertensive patients treated with an antihypertensive drug such as **losartan**). Pharmacokinetic interactions occur when one drug affects the pharmocokinetics of another (e.g. by reducing its elimin-ation from the body or by inhibiting its metabolism). These mechanisms are discussed more fully below in the section on adverse interactions grouped by mechanism. A drug interaction can result from one or a combination of these mechanisms.

Drug interaction is important because, whereas judicious use of more than one drug at a time can greatly benefit patients, adverse interactions are not uncommon, and may be catastrophic, yet are often avoidable. Multiple drug use ('polypharmacy') is extremely common, so the potential for drug interaction is enormous. One study showed that on average 14 drugs were prescribed to medical in-patients per admission (one patient received 36 different drugs). The problem is likely to get worse, for several reasons.

1. Many drugs are not curative, but rather ameliorate chronic conditions (e.g. arthritis). The populations of western countries are ageing, and elderly individuals not uncommonly have several co-morbid conditions.
2. It is all too easy to enter an iatrogenic spiral in which a drug results in an adverse effect that is countered by the introduction of another drug, and so on. Prescribers should heed the moral of the nursery rhyme about the old lady who swallowed a fly! Hospital admission provides an opportunity to review all medications that any patient is receiving, to ensure that the overall regimen is rational.

Out-patients also often receive several prescribed drugs, plus proprietary over-the-counter medicines, 'alternative' remedies

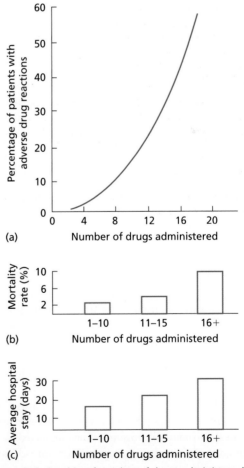

Figure 13.1: Relationship of number of drugs administered to (a) adverse drug reactions, (b) mortality rate and (c) average duration of hospital stay. (Redrawn by permission of the British Medical Journal from Smith JW et al. *Annals of Internal Medicine* 1966; **65**: 631.)

(see Chapter 17) and 'lifestyle' drugs taken for social reasons. The greater the number of drugs taken, the more likely things are to go wrong (Figure 13.1).

Drug interactions can be useful, of no consequence, or harmful.

USEFUL INTERACTIONS

INCREASED EFFECT

Drugs can be used in combination to enhance their effectiveness. Disease is often caused by complex processes, and drugs that influence different components of the disease mechanism may have additive effects (e.g. an antiplatelet drug with a fibrinolytic in treating myocardial infarction, Chapter 29). Other examples include the use of a β_2 agonist with a glucocorticoid in the treatment of asthma (to cause bronchodilation and suppress inflammation, respectively; Chapter 33).

Combinations of antimicrobial drugs are used to prevent the selection of drug-resistant organisms. Tuberculosis is the best example of a disease whose successful treatment requires this approach (Chapter 44). Drug resistance via synthesis of a microbial enzyme that degrades antibiotic (e.g. penicillinase-producing staphylococci) can be countered by using a combination of the antibiotic with an inhibitor of the enzyme: **co-amoxiclav** is a combination of **clavulanic acid**, an inhibitor of penicillinase, with **amoxicillin**.

Increased efficacy can result from pharmacokinetic interaction. **Imipenem** (Chapter 43) is partly inactivated by a dipeptidase in the kidney. This is overcome by administering **imipenem** in combination with **cilastin**, a specific renal dipeptidase inhibitor. Another example is the use of the combination of **ritonavir** and **saquinavir** in antiretroviral therapy (Chapter 46). **Saquinavir** increases the systemic bioavailability of **ritonavir** by inhibiting its degradation by gastro-intestinal CYP3A and inhibits its faecal elimination by blocking the P-glycoprotein that pumps it back into the intestinal lumen.

Some combinations of drugs have a more than additive effect ('synergy'). Several antibacterial combinations are synergistic, including **sulfamethoxazole** with **trimethoprim** (**co-trimoxazole**), used in the treatment of *Pneumocystis carinii* (Chapter 46). Several drugs used in cancer chemotherapy are also synergistic, e.g. **cisplatin** plus **paclitaxel** (Chapter 48).

Therapeutic effects of drugs are often limited by the activation of a physiological control loop, particularly in the case of cardiovascular drugs. The use of a low dose of a second drug that interrupts this negative feedback may therefore enhance effectiveness substantially. Examples include the combination of an angiotensin converting enzyme inhibitor (to block the renin-angiotensin system) with a diuretic (the effect of which is limited by activation of the renin-angiotensin system) in treating hypertension (Chapter 28).

MINIMIZE SIDE EFFECTS

There are many situations (e.g. hypertension) where low doses of two drugs may be better tolerated, as well as more effective, than larger doses of a single agent. Sometimes drugs with similar therapeutic effects have opposing undesirable metabolic effects, which can to some extent cancel out when the drugs are used together. The combination of a loop diuretic (e.g. **furosemide**) with a potassium-sparing diuretic (e.g. **spironolactone**) provides an example.

Predictable adverse effects can sometimes be averted by the use of drug combinations. **Isoniazid** neuropathy is caused by pyridoxine deficiency, and is prevented by the prophylactic use of this vitamin. The combination of a peripheral dopa decarboxylase inhibitor (e.g. **carbidopa**) with levodopa permits an equivalent therapeutic effect to be achieved with a lower dose of levodopa than is needed when it is used as a single agent, while reducing dose-related peripheral side effects of nausea and vomiting (Chapter 21).

BLOCK ACUTELY AN UNWANTED (TOXIC) EFFECT

Drugs can be used to block an undesired or toxic effect, as for example when an anaesthetist uses a cholinesterase inhibitor to reverse neuromuscular blockade, or when antidotes such as **naloxone** are used to treat opioid overdose (Chapter 54). Uses of vitamin K or of fresh plasma to reverse the effect of **warfarin** (Chapter 30) are other important examples.

TRIVIAL INTERACTIONS

Many interactions are based on in vitro experiments, the results of which cannot be extrapolated uncritically to the clinical situation. Many such potential interactions are of no practical consequence. This is especially true of drugs with shallow dose–response curves and of interactions that depend on competition for tissue binding to sites that are not directly involved in drug action but which influence drug distribution (e.g. to albumin in blood).

SHALLOW DOSE–RESPONSE CURVES

Interactions are only likely to be clinically important when there is a steep dose–response curve and a narrow therapeutic window between minimum effective dose and minimum toxic dose of one or both interacting drugs (Figure 13.2). This is often not the case. For example, **penicillin**, when used in most clinical situations, is so non-toxic that the usual dose is more than adequate for therapeutic efficacy, yet far below that which would cause dose-related toxicity. Consequently, a second drug that interacts with **penicillin** is unlikely to cause either toxicity or loss of efficacy.

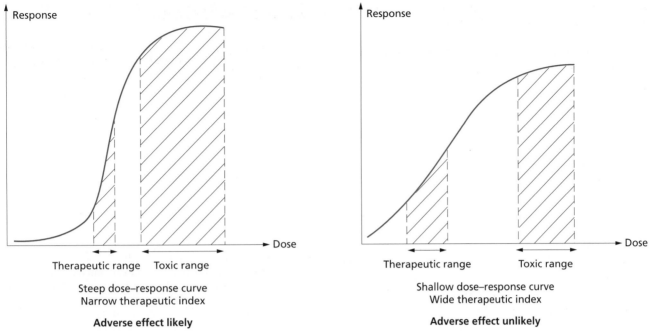

Figure 13.2: Drug dose–response curves illustrating likelihood of adverse effect if an interaction increases its blood level.

PLASMA AND TISSUE BINDING SITE INTERACTIONS

One large group of potential drug interactions that are seldom clinically important consists of drugs that displace one another from binding sites on plasma albumin or α-1 acid glycoprotein (AAG) or within tissues. This is a common occurrence and can readily be demonstrated in plasma or solutions of albumin/AAG in vitro. However, the simple expectation that the displacing drug will increase the effects of the displaced drug by increasing its free (unbound) concentration is seldom evident in clinical practice. This is because drug clearance (renal or metabolic) also depends directly on the concentration of free drug. Consider a patient receiving a regular maintenance dose of a drug. When a second displacing drug is commenced, the free concentration of the first drug rises only transiently before increased renal or hepatic elimination reduces total (bound plus free) drug, and restores the free concentration to that which prevailed before the second drug was started. Consequently, any increased effect of the displaced drug is transient, and is seldom important in practice. It must, however, be taken into account if therapy is being guided by measurements of plasma drug concentrations, as most such determinations are of total (bound plus free) rather than just free concentration (Chapter 8).

An exception, where a transient increase in free concentration of a circulating substance (albeit not a drug) can have devastating consequences, is provided by bilirubin in premature babies whose ability to metabolize bile pigments is limited. Unconjugated bilirubin is bound by plasma albumin, and injudicious treatment with drugs, such as sulphonamides, that displace it from these binding sites permits diffusion of free bilirubin across the immature blood–brain barrier, consequent staining of and damage to basal ganglia ('kernicterus') and subsequent choreoathetosis in the child.

Instances where clinically important consequences do occur on introducing a drug that displaces another from tissue binding sites are in fact often due to additional actions of the second drug on elimination of the first. For instance, **quinidine** displaces **digoxin** from tissue binding sites, and can cause **digoxin** toxicity, but only because it simultaneously reduces the renal clearance of **digoxin** by a separate mechanism. **Phenylbutazone** (an NSAID currently reserved for ankylosing spondylitis unresponsive to other drugs, Chapter 26) displaces **warfarin** from binding sites on albumin, and causes excessive anticoagulation, but only because it also inhibits the metabolism of the active isomer of **warfarin** (S-warfarin), causing this to accumulate at the expense of the inactive isomer. **Indometacin** (another NSAID) also displaces **warfarin** from binding sites on albumin, but does not inhibit its metabolism and does not further prolong prothrombin time in patients treated with **warfarin**, although it can cause bleeding by causing peptic ulceration and interfering with platelet function.

HARMFUL INTERACTIONS

It is impossible to memorize reliably the many clinically important drug interactions, and prescribers should use suitable references (e.g. the British National Formulary) to check for potentially harmful interactions. There are certain drugs with steep dose–response curves and serious dose-related toxicities for which drug interactions are especially liable to cause harm (Figure 13.2), and where special caution is required with concurrent therapy. These include:

- warfarin and other anticoagulants;
- anticonvulsants;
- cytotoxic drugs;
- drugs for HIV/AIDS;
- immunosuppressants;
- digoxin and other anti-dysrhythmic drugs;
- oral hypoglycaemic agents;
- xanthine alkaloids (e.g. theophylline);
- monoamine oxidase inhibitors.

The frequency and consequences of an adverse interaction when two drugs are used together are seldom known precisely. Every individual has a peculiar set of characteristics that determine their response to therapy.

RISK OF ADVERSE DRUG INTERACTIONS

In the Boston Collaborative Drug Surveillance Program, 234 of 3600 (about 7%) adverse drug reactions in acute-care hospitals were identified as being due to drug interactions. In a smaller study in a chronic-care setting, the prevalence of adverse interactions was much higher (22%), probably because of the more frequent use of multiple drugs in elderly patients with multiple pathologies. The same problems exist for the detection of adverse drug interactions as for adverse drug reactions (Chapter 12). The frequency of such interactions will be underestimated by attribution of poor therapeutic outcome to an underlying disease. For example, graft rejection following renal transplantation is not uncommon. Historically, it took several years for nephrologists to appreciate that epileptic patients suffered much greater rejection rates than did non-epileptic subjects. These adverse events proved to be due to an interaction between anticonvulsant medication and immunosuppressant cortico-steroid therapy, which was rendered ineffective because of increased drug metabolism. In future, a better understanding of the potential mechanisms of such interactions should lead to their prediction and prevention by study in early-phase drug evaluation.

SEVERITY OF ADVERSE DRUG INTERACTIONS

Adverse drug interactions are diverse, including unwanted pregnancy (from failure of the contraceptive pill due to concomitant medication), hypertensive stroke (from hypertensive crisis in patients on monoamine oxidase inhibitors), gastrointestinal or cerebral haemorrhage (in patients receiving **warfarin**), cardiac arrhythmias (e.g. secondary to interactions leading to electrolyte disturbance or prolongation of the QTc) and blood dyscrasias (e.g. from interactions between **allopurinol** and **azathioprine**). Adverse interactions can be severe. In one study, nine of 27 fatal drug reactions were caused by drug interactions.

Key points

- Drug interactions may be clinically useful, trivial or adverse.
- Useful interactions include those that enable efficacy to be maximized, such as the addition of an angiotensin converting enzyme inhibitor to a thiazide diuretic in a patient with hypertension inadequately controlled on diuretic alone (see Chapter 28). They may also enable toxic effects to be minimized, as in the use of pyridoxine to prevent neuropathy in malnourished patients treated with isoniazid for tuberculosis, and may prevent the emergence of resistant organisms (e.g. multi-drug regimens for treating tuberculosis, see Chapter 44).
- Many interactions that occur in vitro (e.g. competition for albumin) are unimportant in vivo because displacement of drug from binding sites leads to increased elimination by metabolism or excretion and hence to a new steady state where the total concentration of displaced drug in plasma is reduced, but the concentration of active, free (unbound) drug is the same as before the interacting drug was introduced. Interactions involving drugs with a wide safety margin (e.g. penicillin) are also seldom clinically important.
- Adverse drug interactions are not uncommon, and can have profound consequences, including death from hyperkalaemia and other causes of cardiac dysrhythmia, unwanted pregnancy, transplanted organ rejection, etc.

ADVERSE INTERACTIONS GROUPED BY MECHANISM

PHARMACEUTICAL INTERACTIONS

Inactivation can occur when drugs (e.g. **heparin** with **gentamicin**) are mixed. Examples are listed in Table 13.1. Drugs may also interact in the lumen of the gut (e.g. **tetracycline** with iron, and **colestyramine** with **digoxin**).

PHARMACODYNAMIC INTERACTIONS

These are common. Most have a simple mechanism consisting of summation or opposition of the effects of drugs with, respectively, similar or opposing actions. Since this type of interaction depends broadly on the effect of a drug, rather than on its specific chemical structure, such interactions are non-specific. Drowsiness caused by an H_1-blocking antihistamine and by alcohol provides an example. It occurs to a greater or lesser degree with all H_1-blockers irrespective of the chemical structure of the particular drug used. Patients must be warned of the dangers of consuming alcohol concurrently when such antihistamines are prescribed, especially if they drive or operate machinery. Non-steroidal anti-inflammatory agents and antihypertensive drugs provide another clinically important example. Antihypertensive drugs are rendered less effective by concurrent use of non-steroidal anti-inflammatory drugs, irrespective of the chemical group to which they belong, because of inhibition of biosynthesis of vasodilator prostaglandins in the kidney (Chapter 26).

Table 13.1: Interactions outside the body

Mixture	Result
Thiopentone and suxamethonium	Precipitation
Diazepam and infusion fluids	Precipitation
Phenytoin and infusion fluids	Precipitation
Heparin and hydrocortisone	Inactivation of heparin
Gentamicin and hydrocortisone	Inactivation of gentamicin
Penicillin and hydrocortisone	Inactivation of penicillin

Drugs with negative inotropic effects can precipitate heart failure, especially when used in combination. Thus, beta-blockers and **verapamil** may precipitate heart failure if used sequentially intravenously in patients with supraventricular tachycardia.

Warfarin interferes with haemostasis by inhibiting the coagulation cascade, whereas **aspirin** influences haemostasis by inhibiting platelet function. **Aspirin** also predisposes to gastric bleeding by direct irritation and by inhibition of prostaglandin E_2 biosynthesis in the gastric mucosa. There is therefore the potential for serious adverse interaction between them.

Important interactions can occur between drugs acting at a common receptor. These interactions are generally useful when used deliberately, for example, the use of naloxone to reverse opiate intoxication.

One potentially important type of pharmacodynamic drug interaction involves the interruption of physiological control loops. This was mentioned above as a desirable means of increasing efficacy. However, in some situations such control mechanisms are vital. The use of β-blocking drugs in patients with insulin-requiring diabetes is such a case, as these patients may depend on sensations initiated by activation of β-receptors to warn them of insulin-induced hypoglycaemia.

Alterations in fluid and electrolyte balance represent an important source of pharmacodynamic drug interactions (see Table 13.2). Combined use of diuretics with actions at different parts of the nephron (e.g. **metolazone** and **furosemide**) is valuable in the treatment of resistant oedema, but without close monitoring of plasma urea levels, such combinations readily cause excessive intravascular fluid depletion and pre-renal renal failure (Chapter 36). Thiazide and loop diuretics commonly cause mild hypokalaemia, which is usually of no consequence. However, the binding of **digoxin** to plasma membrane Na^+/K^+ adenosine triphosphatase (Na^+/K^+ ATPase), and hence its toxicity, is increased when the extracellular potassium concentration is low. Concurrent use of such diuretics therefore increases the risk of digoxin toxicity. β_2-Agonists, such as **salbutamol**, also reduce the plasma potassium concentration, especially when used intravenously. Conversely, potassium-sparing diuretics may cause hyperkalaemia if combined with potassium supplements and/or angiotensin converting enzyme inhibitors (which reduce circulating aldosterone), especially in patients with renal impairment. Hyperkalaemia is one of the most common causes of fatal adverse drug reactions.

Table 13.2: Interactions secondary to drug-induced alterations of fluid and electrolyte balance

Primary drug	Interacting drug effect	Result of interaction
Digoxin	Diuretic-induced hypokalaemia	Digoxin toxicity
Lidocaine	Diuretic-induced hypokalaemia	Antagonism of anti-dysrhythmic effects
Diuretics	NSAID-induced salt and water retention	Antagonism of diuretic effects
Lithium	Diuretic-induced reduction in lithium clearance	Raised plasma lithium
Angiotensin converting enzyme inhibitor	Potassium chloride and/or potassium-retaining diuretic-induced hyperkalaemia	Hyperkalaemia

NSAID, non-steroidal anti-inflammatory drug.

PHARMACOKINETIC INTERACTIONS
Absorption

In addition to direct interaction within the gut lumen (see above), drugs that influence gastric emptying (e.g. **metoclopramide**, **propantheline**) can alter the rate or completeness of absorption of a second drug, particularly if this has low bioavailability. Drugs can interfere with the enterohepatic recirculation of other drugs. Failure of oral contraception can result from concurrent use of antibiotics, due to this mechanism. Many different antibiotics have been implicated. **Phenytoin** reduces the effectiveness of **ciclosporin** partly by reducing its absorption.

Distribution

As explained above, interactions that involve only mutual competition for inert protein- or tissue-binding sites seldom, if ever, give rise to clinically important effects. Examples of complex interactions where competition for binding sites occurs in conjunction with reduced clearance are mentioned below.

Metabolism

Decreased efficacy can result from enzyme induction by a second agent (Table 13.3). Historically, barbiturates were clinically the most important enzyme inducers, but with the decline in their use, other anticonvulsants, notably **carbamazepine** and the antituberculous drug **rifampicin**, are now the most common cause of such interactions. These necessitate special care in concurrent therapy with **warfarin**, **phenytoin**, oral contraceptives, glucocorticoids or immunosuppressants (e.g. **ciclosporin**, **sirolimus**).

Table 13.3: Interactions due to enzyme induction

Primary drug	Inducing agent	Effect of interaction
Warfarin	Barbiturates Ethanol Rifampicin	Decreased anticoagulation
Oral contraceptives	Rifampicin	Pregnancy
Prednisolone/ ciclosporin	Anticonvulsants	Reduced immunosuppression (graft rejection)
Theophylline	Smoking	Decreased plasma theophylline

Table 13.4: Interactions due to CYP450 or other enzyme inhibition

Primary drug	Inhibiting drug	Effect of interaction
Phenytoin	Isoniazid Cimetidine Chloramphenicol	Phenytoin intoxication
Warfarin	Allopurinol Metronidazole Phenylbutazone Co-trimoxazole	Haemorrhage
Azathioprine, 6-MP	Allopurinol	Bone-marrow suppression
Theophylline	Cimetidine Erythromycin	Theophylline toxicity
Cisapride	Erythromycin Ketoconazole	Ventricular tachycardia

6-MP, 6-mercaptopurine.

Withdrawal of an inducing agent during continued administration of a second drug can result in a slow decline in enzyme activity, with emergence of delayed toxicity from the second drug due to what is no longer an appropriate dose. For example, a patient receiving **warfarin** may be admitted to hospital for an intercurrent event and receive treatment with an enzyme inducer. During the hospital stay, the dose of **warfarin** therefore has to be increased in order to maintain measurements of international normalized ratio (INR) within the therapeutic range. The intercurrent problem is resolved, the inducing drug discontinued and the patient discharged while taking the larger dose of **warfarin**. If the INR is not checked frequently, bleeding may result from an excessive effect of **warfarin** days or weeks after discharge from hospital, as the effect of the enzyme inducer gradually wears off.

Inhibition of drug metabolism also produces adverse effects (Table 13.4). The time-course is often more rapid than for enzyme induction, since it depends merely on the attainment of a sufficiently high concentration of the inhibiting drug at the metabolic site. Xanthine oxidase is responsible for inactivation of **6-mercaptopurine**, itself a metabolite of **azathioprine**. **Allopurinol** markedly potentiates these drugs by inhibiting xanthine oxidase. Xanthine alkaloids (e.g. **theophylline**) are not inactivated by xanthine oxidase, but rather by a form of CYP450. **Theophylline** has serious (sometimes fatal) dose-related toxicities, and clinically important interactions occur with inhibitors of the CYP450 system, notably several antibiotics, including **ciprofloxacin** and **clarithromycin**. Severe exacerbations in asthmatic patients are often precipitated by chest infections, so an awareness of these interactions before commencing antibiotic treatment is essential.

Hepatic CYP450 inhibition also accounts for clinically important interactions with **phenytoin** (e.g. **isoniazid**) and with **warfarin** (e.g. sulphonamides). Non-selective monoamine oxidase inhibitors (e.g. **phenelzine**) potentiate the action of indirectly acting amines such as tyramine, which is present in a wide variety of fermented products (most famously soft cheeses: 'cheese reaction').

Clinically important impairment of drug metabolism may also result indirectly from haemodynamic effects rather than enzyme inhibition. **Lidocaine** is metabolized in the liver and the hepatic extraction ratio is high. Consequently, any drug that reduces hepatic blood flow (e.g. a negative inotrope) will reduce hepatic clearance of **lidocaine** and cause it to accumulate. This accounts for the increased **lidocaine** concentration and toxicity that is caused by β-blocking drugs.

Excretion

Many drugs share a common transport mechanism in the proximal tubules (Chapter 6) and reduce one another's excretion by competition (Table 13.5). **Probenecid** reduces **penicillin** elimination in this way. **Aspirin** and non-steroidal anti-inflammatory drugs inhibit secretion of **methotrexate** into urine, as well as displacing it from protein-binding sites, and can cause **methotrexate** toxicity. Many diuretics reduce sodium absorption in the loop of Henle or the distal tubule (Chapter 36). This leads indirectly to increased proximal tubular reabsorption of monovalent cations. Increased proximal tubular reabsorption of **lithium** in patients treated with lithium salts can cause lithium accumulation and toxicity. **Digoxin** excretion is reduced by **spironolactone**, **verapamil** and **amiodarone**, all of which can precipitate **digoxin** toxicity as a consequence, although several of these interactions are complex in mechanism, involving displacement from tissue binding sites, in addition to reduced **digoxin** elimination.

Changes in urinary pH alter the excretion of drugs that are weak acids or bases, and administration of systemic alkalinizing or acidifying agents influences reabsorption of such drugs

Table 13.5: Competitive interactions for renal tubular transport

Primary drug	Competing drug	Effect of interaction
Penicillin	Probenecid	Increased penicillin blood level
Methotrexate	Salicylates	Bone marrow suppression
	Sulphonamides	
Salicylate	Probenecid	Salicylate toxicity
Indometacin	Probenecid	Indometacin toxicity
Digoxin	Spironolactone	Increased plasma digoxin
	Amiodarone	
	Verapamil	

from urine (e.g. the excretion of **salicylate** is increased in an alkaline urine). Such effects are used in the management of overdose (Chapter 54).

Key points

- There are three main types of adverse interaction:
  – pharmaceutical;
  – pharmacodynamic;
  – pharmacokinetic.
- Pharmaceutical interactions are due to in vitro incompatibilities, and they occur outside the body (e.g. when drugs are mixed in a bag of intravenous solution, or in the port of an intravenous cannula).
- Pharmacodynamic interactions between drugs with a similar effect (e.g. drugs that cause drowsiness) are common. In principle, they should be easy to anticipate, but they can cause serious problems (e.g. if a driver fails to account for the interaction between an antihistamine and ethanol).
- Pharmacokinetic interactions are much more difficult to anticipate. They occur when one drug influences the way in which another is handled by the body:
  (a) *absorption* (e.g. broad-spectrum antibiotics interfere with enterohepatic recirculation of oestrogens and can cause failure of oral contraception);
  (b) *distribution* – competition for binding sites seldom causes problems on its own but, if combined with an effect on elimination (e.g. amiodarone/digoxin or NSAID/methotrexate), serious toxicity may ensue;
  (c) *metabolism* – many serious interactions stem from enzyme induction or inhibition. Important inducing agents include ethanol, rifampicin, rifabutin, many of the older anticonvulsants, St John's wort, nevirapine and pioglitazone. Common inhibitors include many antibacterial drugs (e.g. isoniazid, macrolides, co-trimoxazole and metronidazole), the azole antifungals, cimetidine, allopurinol, HIV protease inhibitors;
  (d) *excretion* (e.g. diuretics lead to increased reabsorption of lithium, reducing its clearance and predisposing to lithium accumulation and toxicity).

Case history

A 64-year-old Indian male was admitted to hospital with miliary tuberculosis. In the past he had had a mitral valve replaced, and he had been on warfarin ever since. Treatment was commenced with isoniazid, rifampicin and pyrazinamide, and the INR was closely monitored in anticipation of increased warfarin requirements. He was discharged after several weeks with the INR in the therapeutic range on a much increased dose of warfarin. Rifampicin was subsequently discontinued. Two weeks later the patient was again admitted, this time drowsy and complaining of headache after mildly bumping his head on a locker. His pupils were unequal and the INR was 7.0. Fresh frozen plasma was administered and neurosurgical advice was obtained.
Comment
This patient's warfarin requirement increased during treatment with rifampicin because of enzyme induction, and the dose of warfarin was increased to maintain anticoagulation. When rifampicin was stopped, enzyme induction gradually receded, but the dose of warfarin was not readjusted. Consequently, the patient became over-anticoagulated and developed a subdural haematoma in response to mild trauma. Replacment of clotting factors (present in fresh frozen plasma) is the quickest way to reverse the effect of warfarin overdose (Chapter 30).

FURTHER READING

There is a very useful website for CYP450 substrates with inhibitors and inducers: http://medicine.iupui.edu/flockhart/

British Medical Association and Royal Pharmaceutical Society of Great Britain. *British National Formulary* 54. London: Medical Association and Royal Pharmaceutical Society of Great Britian, 2007. (Appendix 1 provides an up-to-date and succinct alphabetical list of interacting drugs, highlighting interactions that are potentially hazardous.)

Brown HS, Ito K, Galetin A et al. Prediction of in vivo drug–drug interactions from in vitro data: impact of incorporating parallel pathways of drug elimination and inhibitor absorption rate constant. *British Journal of Clinical Pharmacology* 2005; **60**: 508–18.

Constable S, Ham A, Pirmohamed M. Herbal medicines and acute medical emergency admissions to hospital. *British Journal of Clinical Pharmacology* 2007; **63**: 247–8.

De Bruin ML, Langendijk PNJ, Koopmans RP et al. In-hospital cardiac arrest is associated with use of non-antiarrhythmic QTc-prolonging drugs. *British Journal of Clinical Pharmacology* 2007; **63**: 216–23.

Fugh-Berman A, Ernst E. Herb–drug interactions: Review and assessment of report reliability. *British Journal of Clinical Pharmacology* 2001; **52**: 587–95.

Hurle AD, Navarro AS, Sanchez MJG. Therapeutic drug monitoring of itraconazole and the relevance of pharmacokinetic interactions. *Clinical Microbiology and Infection* 2006; **12** (Suppl. 7): 97–106.

Jackson SHD, Mangoni AA, Batty GM. Optimization of drug prescribing. *British Journal of Clinical Pharmacology* 2004; **57**: 231–6.

Karalleidde L, Henry J. *Handbook of drug interactions*. London: Edward Arnold, 1998.

Mertens-Talcott SU, Zadezensky I, De Castro WV et al. Grapefruit–drug interactions: Can interactions with drugs be avoided? *Journal of Clinical Pharmacology* 2006; **46**: 1390–1416.

Neuvonen PJ, Niemi M, Backman JT. Drug interactions with lipid-lowering drugs: mechanisms and clinical relevance. *Clinical Pharmacology and Therapeutics* 2006; **80**: 565–81.

Perucca E. Clinically relevant drug interactions with antiepileptic drugs. *British Journal of Clinical Pharmacology* 2006; **61**: 246–55.

Stockley I. *Drug interactions*, 2nd edn. Oxford: Blackwell Scientific Publications, 1991.

Westphal JF. 2000 Macrolide-induced clinically relevant drug interactions with cytochrome P-450A (CYP) 3A4: an update focused on clarithromycin, azithromycin and dirithromycin. *British Journal of Clinical Pharmacology* 2000; **50**: 285–95.

Whitten DL, Myers SP, Hawrelak JA et al. The effect of St John's wort extracts on CYP3A: a systematic review of prospective clinical trials. *British Journal of Clinical Pharmacology* 2006; **62**: 512–26.

CHAPTER 14

PHARMACOGENETICS

INTRODUCTION: 'PERSONALIZED MEDICINE'

Variability in drug response between individuals is due to genetic and environmental effects on drug absorption, distribution, metabolism or excretion (pharmacokinetics) and on target protein (receptor) or downstream protein signalling (pharmacodynamics). Several idiosyncratic adverse drug reactions (ADRs) have been explained in terms of genetically determined variation in the activity of enzymes involved in metabolism, or of other proteins (e.g. variants of haemoglobin and haemolysis). The study of variation in drug responses under hereditary control is known as pharmacogenetics. Mutation results in a change in the nucleotide sequence of DNA. Single nucleotide polymorphisms (SNPs) are very common. They may change the function or level of expression of the corresponding protein. (Not all single nucleotide variations change the coded protein because the genetic code is 'redundant' – i.e. more than one triplet of nucleotides codes for each amino acid – so a change in one nucleotide does not always change the amino acid coded by the triplet, leaving the structure of the coded protein unaltered.) Balanced polymorphisms, when a substantial fraction of a population differs from the remainder in such a way over many generations, results when heterozygotes experience some selective advantage. Tables 14.1 and 14.2 detail examples of genetic influences on drug metabolism and response. It is hoped that by defining an individual's DNA sequence from a blood sample, physicians will be able to select a drug that will be effective without adverse effects. This much-hyped 'personalized medicine' has one widely used clinical application currently, that of genotyping the enzyme thiopurine methyl-transferase (which inactivates **6-mercaptopurine (6-MP)**) to guide dosing **6-MP** in children with acute lymphocytic leukaemia, but could revolutionize therapeutics in the future.

Throughout this chapter, italics are used for the gene and plain text for the protein product of the gene.

GENETIC INFLUENCES ON DRUG METABOLISM

Abnormal sensitivity to a drug may be the result of a genetic variation of the enzymes involved in its metabolism.

Inheritance may be autosomal recessive and such disorders are rare, although they are important because they may have severe consequences. However, there are also dominant patterns of inheritance that lead to much more common variations within the population. Balanced polymorphisms of drug metabolizing enzymes are common. Different ethnic populations often have a different prevalence of the various enzyme polymorphisms.

PHASE I DRUG METABOLISM

CYP2D6

The *CYP2D6* gene is found on chromosome 22 and over 50 polymorphic variants have been defined in humans. The function of this enzyme (e.g. 4-hydroxylation of **debrisoquine**, an adrenergic neurone-blocking drug previously used to treat hypertension but no longer used clinically) is deficient in about 7–10% of the UK population (Table 14.1). Hydroxylation polymorphisms in *CYP2D6* explain an increased susceptibility to several ADRs:

- **nortriptyline** – headache and confusion (in poor metabolizers);
- **codeine** – weak (or non-existent) analgesia in poor metabolizers (poor metabolizers convert little of it to **morphine**);
- **phenformin** – excessive incidence of lactic acidosis (in poor metabolizers).

Several drugs (including other opioids, e.g. **pethidine, morphine** and **dextromethorphan**; beta-blockers, e.g. **metoprolol, propranolol**; SSRIs, e.g. **fluoxetine**; antipsychotics, e.g. **haloperidol**) are metabolized by CYP2D6. The many genotypic variants yield four main phenotypes of CYP2D6 – poor metabolizers (PM) (7–10% of a Caucasian population), intermediate (IM) and extensive metabolizers (EM) (85–90% of Caucasians) and ultra-rapid metabolizers (UM) (1–2% of Caucasians, but up to 30% in Egyptians) due to possession of multiple copies of the *CYP2D6* gene. UM patients require higher doses of CYP2D6 drug substrates for efficacy.

Table 14.1: Variations in drug metabolism/pharmacodynamics due to genetic polymorphisms

Pharmacogenetic variation	Mechanism	Inheritance	Occurrence	Drugs involved
Phase I drug metabolism:				
Defective CYP2D6	Functionally defective	Autosomal recessive	7–10% Caucasians, 1% Saudi Arabians, 30% Chinese	Originally defined by reduced CYP2D6 debrisoquine hydroxylation; Beta blockers: metoprolol; TCAs: nortriptyline; SSRIs: fluoxetine; Opioids: morphine; Anti-dysrhythmics: encainide
Ultra-rapid metabolism:				
CYP2D6	Duplication 2D6		1–2% Caucasians, 30% Egyptians	Rapid metabolism of 2D6 drug substrates above
Phase II drug metabolism:				
Rapid-acetylator status	Increased hepatic N-acetyltransferase	Autosomal dominant	45% Caucasians	Isoniazid; hydralazine; some sulphonamides; phenelzine; dapsone; procainamide
Impaired glucuronidation	Reduced activity UGT1A1		7–10% Caucasians	Irinotecan (CPT-11)
Abnormal pharmacodynamic responses:				
Malignant hyperthermia with muscular rigidity	Polymorphism in ryanodine receptors (RyR1)	Autosomal dominant	1:20 000 of population	Some anaesthetics, especially inhalational, e.g. isoflurane, suxamethonium
Other:				
Suxamethonium sensitivity	Several types of abnormal plasma pseudocholinesterase	Autosomal recessive	Most common form 1:2500	Suxamethonium
Ethanol sensitivity	Relatively low rate of ethanol metabolism by aldehyde dehydrogenase	Usual in some ethnic groups	Orientals	Ethanol

CYP2C9 POLYMORPHISM (TOLBUTAMIDE POLYMORPHISM)

The *CYP2C9* gene is found on chromosome 10 and six polymorphic variants have been defined. Pharmacogenetic variation was first described after the finding of a nine-fold range between individuals in the rate of oxidation of a sulphonylurea drug, **tolbutamide**. *CYP2C9* polymorphisms cause reduced enzyme activity, with 1–3% of Caucasians being poor (slow) metabolizers. Drugs metabolized by CYP2C9 are eliminated slowly in poor metabolizers, who are therefore susceptible to dose-related ADRs. Such drugs include **S-warfarin**, **losartan** and **celecoxib**, as well as the sulphonylureas.

CYP2C19 POLYMORPHISM

CYP2C19 is found on chromosome 10 and four polymorphic variants have been defined. These polymorphisms produce reduced enzyme activity and 3–5% of Caucasians and 15–20% of Asians have genotypes which yield a poor (slow) metabolizer phenotype. Such patients require lower doses of drugs metabolized by the CYP2C19 enzyme. These include proton pump inhibitors (**omeprazole**, **lansoprazole**, **pantoprazole**) and some anticonvulsants, e.g. **phenytoin**, **phenobarbitone**.

PHASE II DRUG METABOLISM

ACETYLATOR STATUS (N-ACETYLTRANSFERASE-2)

Administration of identical doses (per kilogram body weight) of **isoniazid** (INH), an antituberculous drug, results in great variation in blood concentrations. A distribution histogram of such concentrations shows two distinct groups (i.e. a 'bimodal' distribution; Figure 14.1). INH is metabolized in the liver by

Table 14.2: Variations in drug response due to disease caused by genetic mutations

Pharmacogenetic variation	Mechanism	Inheritance	Occurrence	Drugs involved
G6PD deficiency, favism, drug-induced haemolytic anaemia	80 distinct forms of G6PD	X-linked incomplete codominant	10 000 000 affected world-wide	Many – including 8-aminoquinolines, antimicrobials and minor analgesics (see text)
Methaemoglobinaemia: drug-induced haemolysis	Methaemoglobin reductase deficiency	Autosomal recessive (heterozygotes show some response)	1:100 are heterozygotes	Same drugs as for G6PD deficiency
Acute intermittent porphyria: exacerbation induced by drugs	Increased activity of D-amino levulinic synthetase secondary to defective porphyrin synthesis	Autosomal dominant	Acute intermittent type 15:1 000 000 in Sweden; Porphyria cutanea tarda 1:100 in Afrikaaners	Barbiturates, cloral, chloroquine, ethanol, sulphonamides, phenytoin, griseofulvin and many others

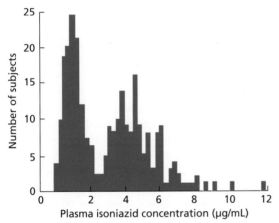

Figure 14.1: Plasma isoniazid concentrations in 483 subjects six hours after oral isoniazid (9.8 mg/kg). Acetylator polymorphism produces a bimodal distribution into fast and slow acetylators. (Redrawn from Evans DAP et al. *British Medical Journal* 1960; **2**: 485, by permission of the editor.)

acetylation. Individuals who acetylate the drug more rapidly because of a greater hepatic enzyme activity demonstrate lower concentrations of INH in their blood following a standard dose than do slow acetylators. Acetylator status may be measured using **dapsone** by measuring the ratio of monoacetyldapsone to **dapsone** in plasma following a test dose.

Slow and rapid acetylator status are inherited in a simple Mendelian manner. Heterozygotes, as well as homozygotes, are rapid acetylators because rapid metabolism is autosomal dominant. Around 55–60% of Europeans are slow acetylators and 40–45% are rapid acetylators. The rapid acetylator phenotype is most common in Eskimos and Japanese (95%) and rarest among some Mediterranean Jews (20%).

INH toxicity, in the form of peripheral neuropathy, most commonly occurs in slow acetylators, whilst slower response and higher risk of relapse of infection are more frequent in rapid acetylators, particularly when the drug is not given daily, but twice weekly. In addition, slow acetylators are more likely to show **phenytoin** toxicity when this drug is given with INH, because the latter inhibits hepatic microsomal hydroxylation of **phenytoin**. Isoniazid hepatitis may be more common among rapid acetylators, but the data are conflicting.

Acetylator status affects other drugs (e.g. **procainamide**, **hydralazine**) that are inactivated by acetylation. Approximately 40% of patients treated with **procainamide** for six months or longer develop antinuclear antibodies. Slow acetylators are more likely to develop such antibodies than rapid acetylators (Figure 14.2) and more slow acetylators develop **procainamide**-induced lupus erythematosus. Similarly, lower doses of **hydralazine** are needed to control hypertension in slow acetylators (Figure 14.3) and these individuals are more susceptible to **hydralazine**-induced systemic lupus erythematosus (SLE).

SULPHATION

Sulphation by sulfotransferase (SULT) enzymes shows polymorphic variation. SULT enzymes metabolize oestrogens, progesterones and catecholamines. The polymorphic forms have reduced activity and contribute to the considerable variability in metabolism of these compounds.

SUXAMETHONIUM SENSITIVITY

The usual response to a single intravenous dose of **suxamethonium** is muscular paralysis for three to six minutes. The effect is brief because **suxamethonium** is rapidly hydrolysed by plasma pseudocholinesterase. Occasional individuals show a much more prolonged response and may remain

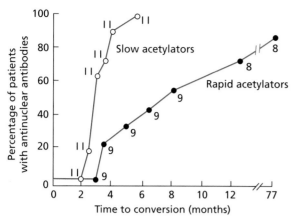

Figure 14.2: Development of procainamide-induced antinuclear antibody in slow acetylators (○) and rapid acetylators (●) with time. Number of patients shown at each point. (Redrawn with permission from Woosley RL et al. *New England Journal of Medicine* 1978; **298**: 1157.)

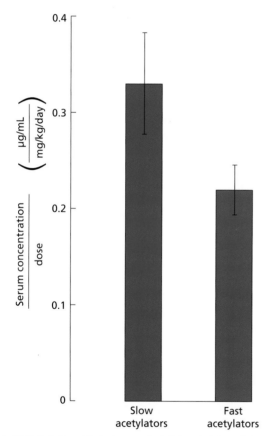

Figure 14.3: Relationship between acetylator status and dose-normalized serum hydralazine concentration (i.e. serum concentration corrected for variable daily dose). Serum concentrations were measured one to two hours after oral hydralazine doses of 25–100 mg in 24 slow and 11 fast acetylators. (Redrawn with permission from Koch-Weser J. *Medical Clinics of North America* 1974; **58**: 1027.)

paralysed and require artificial ventilation for two hours or longer. This results from the presence of an aberrant form of plasma cholinesterase. The most common variant which causes **suxamethonium** sensitivity occurs at a frequency of around one in 2500 and is inherited as an autosomal recessive.

Heterozygotes are unaffected carriers and represent about 4% of the population.

GENETIC INFLUENCES ON DRUG DISPOSITION

Several genotypic variants occur in the drug transporter proteins known as ATP binding cassette proteins (ABC proteins). The best known is P-glycoprotein now renamed ABCB1. This has several polymorphisms leading to altered protein expression/activity. Effects of drug transporter polymorphisms on drug disposition depend on the individual drug and the genetic variant, and are still incompletely understood.

GENETIC INFLUENCES ON DRUG ACTION

RECEPTOR/DRUG TARGET POLYMORPHISMS

There are many polymorphic variants in receptors, e.g. oestrogen receptors, β-adrenoceptors, dopamine D_2 receptors and opioid μ receptors. Such variants produce altered receptor expression/activity. One of the best studied is the β_2-adrenoceptor polymorphism. SNPs resulting in an Arg-to-Gly amino acid change at codon 16 yield a reduced response to **salbutamol** with increased desensitization.

Variants in platelet glycoprotein IIb/IIIa receptors modify the effects of **eptifibatide**. Genetic variation in serotonin transporters influences the effects of antidepressants, such as **fluoxetine** and **clomiprimine**. There is a polymorphism of the angiotensin-converting enzyme (ACE) gene which involves a deletion in a flanking region of DNA that controls the activity of the gene; suggestions that the double-deletion genotype may be a risk factor for various disorders are controversial.

WARFARIN SUSCEPTIBILITY

Warfarin inhibits the vitamin K epoxide complex 1 (VKORC1) (Chapter 30). Sensitivity to **warfarin** has been associated with the genetically determined combination of reduced metabolism of the S-warfarin stereoisomer by CYP2C9 *2/*3 and *3/*3 polymorphic variants and reduced activity (low amounts) of VKORC1. This explains approximately 40% of the variability in **warfarin** dosing requirement. **Warfarin** resistance (requirement for very high doses of **warfarin**) has been noted in a few pedigrees and may be related to poorly defined variants in *CYP2C9* combined with *VKORC1*.

FAMILIAL HYPERCHOLESTEROLAEMIA

Familial hypercholesterolaemia (FH) is an autosomal disease in which the ability to synthesize receptors for low-density lipoprotein (LDL) is impaired. LDL receptors are needed for hepatic uptake of LDL and individuals with FH consequently have very high circulating concentrations of LDL, and suffer from atheromatous disease at a young age. Homozygotes completely lack the ability to synthesize LDL receptors and may suffer from coronary artery disease in childhood, whereas the much more common heterozygotes have intermediate numbers of receptors between homozygotes and healthy individuals, and commonly suffer from coronary disease in young adulthood. β-Hydroxy-β-methylglutaryl coenzyme A (HMG CoA) reductase inhibitors (otherwise known as statins, an important class of drug for lowering circulating cholesterol levels) function largely by indirectly increasing the number of hepatic LDL receptors. Such drugs are especially valuable for treating heterozygotes with FH, because they restore hepatic LDL receptors towards normal in such individuals by increasing their synthesis. In contrast, they are relatively ineffective in homozygotes because such individuals entirely lack the genetic material needed for LDL-receptor synthesis.

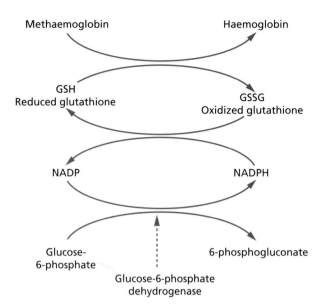

Figure 14.4: Physiological role of glucose-6-phosphate dehydrogenase.

INHERITED DISEASES THAT PREDISPOSE TO DRUG TOXICITY

GLUCOSE-6-PHOSPHATE DEHYDROGENASE DEFICIENCY

Glucose-6-phosphatase dehydrogenase (G6PD) catalyses the formation of reduced nicotinamide adenine dinucleotide phosphate (NADPH), which maintains glutathione in its reduced form (Figure 14.4). The gene for G6PD is located on the X-chromosome, so deficiency of this enzyme is inherited in a sex-linked manner. G6PD deficiency is common, especially in Mediterranean peoples, those of African or Indian descent and in East Asia. Reduced enzyme activity results in methaemoglobinaemia and haemolysis when red cells are exposed to oxidizing agents (e.g. as a result of ingestion of broad beans (*Vicia faba*), naphthalene or one of several drugs). There are over 80 distinct variants of G6PD, but not all of them produce haemolysis. The lower the activity of the enzyme, the more severe is the clinical disease. The following drugs can produce haemolysis in such patients:

1. analgesics – **aspirin**;
2. antimalarials – **primaquine, quinacrine, quinine**;
3. antibacterials – sulphonamides, sulphones, **nitrofurantoin**, fluoroquinolones: **ciprofloxacin**
4. miscellaneous – **quinidine, probenecid**.

Patients with G6PD deficiency treated with an 8-aminoquinoline (e.g. **primaquine**) should spend at least the first few days in hospital under supervision. If acute severe haemolysis occurs, **primaquine** may have to be withdrawn and blood transfusion may be needed. **Hydrocortisone** is given intravenously and the urine is alkalinized to reduce the likelihood of deposition of acid haematin in the renal tubules. The high incidence of this condition in some areas is attributed to a balanced polymorphism. It is postulated that the selective advantage conferred on heterozygotes is due to a protective effect of partial enzyme deficiency against falciparum malaria.

METHAEMOGLOBINAEMIA

Several xenobiotics oxidize haemoglobin to methaemoglobin, including nitrates, nitrites, chlorates, sulphonamides, sulphones, nitrobenzenes, nitrotoluenes, anilines and topical local anesthetics. In certain haemoglobin variants (e.g. HbM, HbH), the oxidized (methaemoglobin) form is not readily converted back into reduced, functional haemoglobin. Exposure to the above substances causes methaemoglobinaemia in individuals with these haemoglobin variants. Similarly, nitrites, chlorates, **dapsone** and **primaquine** can cause cyanosis in patients with a deficiency of NADH-methaemoglobin reductase.

MALIGNANT HYPERTHERMIA

This is a rare but potentially fatal complication of general anaesthesia (Chapter 24). The causative agent is usually an inhalational anaesthetic (e.g. **halothane, isoflurane**) and/or **suxamethonium**. Sufferers exhibit a rapid rise in temperature, muscular rigidity, tachycardia, increased respiratory rate, sweating, cyanosis and metabolic acidosis. There are several forms, one of the more common ones (characterized by **halothane**-induced rigidity) being inherited as a Mendelian dominant. The underlying abnormality is a variant in the ryanodine R1 receptor (Ry1R) responsible for controlling intracellular calcium flux from the sarcolemma. The prevalence is approximately 1:20 000. Individuals can be genotyped for Ry1R or undergo muscle biopsy to assess their predisposition to this condition. Muscle from affected individuals is abnormally sensitive to **caffeine** in vitro, responding with a strong contraction to low concentrations. (Pharmacological doses of **caffeine** release calcium from intracellular stores and cause contraction even in normal muscle at sufficiently high concentration.) Affected muscle responds similarly to **halothane** or **suxamethonium**.

ACUTE PORPHYRIAS

This group of diseases includes acute intermittent porphyria, variegate porphyria and hereditary coproporphyria. In each of these varieties, acute illness is precipitated by drugs because of inherited enzyme deficiencies in the pathway of haem biosynthesis (Figure 14.5). Drugs do not precipitate acute attacks in porphyria cutanea tarda, a non-acute porphyria, although this condition is aggravated by alcohol, oestrogens, iron and polychlorinated aromatic compounds.

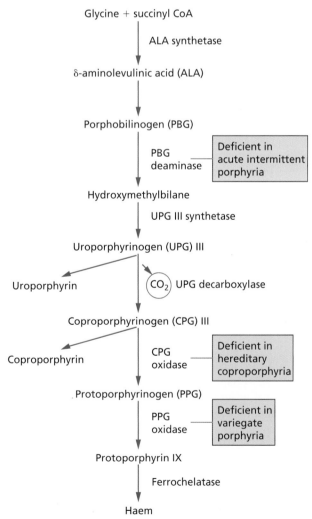

Figure 14.5: Porphyrin metabolism, showing sites of enzyme deficiency.

Drug-induced exacerbations of acute porphyria (neurological, psychiatric, cardiovascular and gastro-intestinal disturbances that are occasionally fatal) are accompanied by increased urinary excretion of 5-aminolevulinic acid (ALA) and porphobilinogen. An extraordinarily wide array of drugs can cause such exacerbations. Most of the drugs that have been incriminated are enzyme inducers that raise hepatic ALA synthetase levels. These drugs include **phenytoin**, sulphonyl-ureas, **ethanol**, **griseofulvin**, sulphonamides, sex hormones, **methyldopa**, **imipramine**, **theophylline**, **rifampicin** and **pyrazinamide**. Often a single dose of one drug of this type can precipitate an acute episode, but in some patients repeated doses are necessary to provoke a reaction.

Specialist advice is essential. A very useful list of drugs that are unsafe to use in patients with porphyrias is included in the British National Formulary.

GILBERT'S DISEASE

This is a benign chronic form of primarily unconjugated hyperbilirubinaemia caused by an inherited reduced activity/lack of the hepatic conjugating enzyme uridine phosphoglucuronyl transferase (UGT1A1). Oestrogens impair bilirubin uptake and aggravate jaundice in patients with this condition, as does protracted fasting. The active metabolite of **irinotecan** is glucuronidated by UGT1A1, so **irinotecan** toxicity is increased in Gilbert's disease.

Case history

A 26-year-old Caucasian woman has a three-month history of intermittent bloody diarrhoea and is diagnosed with ulcerative colitis. She is initially started on oral prednisolone 30 mg/day and sulfasalazine 1 g four times a day with little improvement in her colitic symptoms. Her gastroenterologist, despite attempting to control her disease with increasing doses of her initial therapy, reverts to starting low-dose azathioprine at 25 mg three times a day and stopping her sulfasalazine. Two weeks later, on review, her symptoms of colitis have improved, but she has ulcers on her oropharynx with a sore mouth. Her Hb is 9.8 g/dL and absolute neutrophil count is 250/mm³ and platelet count 85 000.

Question
What is the most likely cause of this clinical situation?

Answer
The patient has haematopoietic toxicity due to azathioprine (a prodrug of 6-MP). 6-MP is inactivated by the enzyme thiopurine methyltransferase (TPMT). In Caucasians 0.3% (one in 300) of patients are genetically deficient in this enzyme because of polymorphisms in the gene (*3/*4 is most common) and 11% of Caucasians who have a heterozygous genotype have low levels of the enzyme. Patients with absent or low TPMT expression are at a higher risk of bone marrow suppression. In this patient, the azathioprine should be stopped and her TPMT genotype defined. Once her bone marrow has recovered (with or without haematopoietic growth factors), she could be restarted on very low doses (e.g 6.25–12 mg azathioprine daily).

Key points

- Genetic differences contribute substantially to individual (pharmacokinetic and pharmacodynamic) variability (20–50%) in drug response.
- Mendelian traits that influence drug metabolism include:
  - (a) deficient thiopurine methyltransferase (TPMT) which inactivates 6-MP (excess haematopoietic suppression);
  - (b) deficient CYP2D6 activity which hydroxylates several drug classes, including opioids, β-blockers, tricyclic antidepressants and SSRIs;
  - (c) deficient CYP2C9 activity which hydroxylates several drugs including sulphonylureas, S-warfarin, losartan;
  - (d) acetylator status (NAT-2), a polymorphism that affects acetylation of drugs, including isoniazid, hydralazine and dapsone;
  - (e) pseudocholinesterase deficiency; this leads to prolonged apnoea after suxamethonium, which is normally inactivated by this enzyme.
- Several inherited diseases predispose to drug toxicity:
  - (a) glucose-6-phosphate dehydrogenase deficiency predisposes to haemolysis following many drugs, including primaquine;
  - (b) malignant hyperthermia is a Mendelian dominant affecting the ryanodine receptor in striated muscle, leading to potentially fatal attacks of hyperthermia and muscle spasm after treatment with suxamethonium and/or inhalational anaesthetics;
  - (c) acute porphyrias, attacks of which are particularly triggered by enzyme-inducing agents, as well as drugs, e.g. sulphonamides, rifampicin and anti-seizure medications.

FURTHER READING

Evans DA, McLeod HL, Pritchard S, Tariq M, Mobarek A. Inter-ethnic variability in human drug responses. *Drug Metabolism and Disposition* 2001; **29**: 606–10.

Evans WE, McLeod HL. Drug therapy: pharmacogenomics – drug disposition, drug targets, and side effects. *New England Journal of Medicine* 2003; **348**: 538–49.

Wang L, Weinshilboum R. Thiopurine S-methyltransferase pharmaco-genetics: insights, challenges and future directions. *Oncogene* 2006; **25**: 1629–38.

Weinshilboum R. Inheritance and drug response. *New England Journal of Medicine* 2003; **348**: 529–37.

Weinshilboum R, Wang L. Pharmacogenomics: bench to bedside. *Nature Reviews. Drug Discovery* 2004; **3**: 739–48.

Wilkinson GR. Drug therapy: drug metabolism and variability among patients in drug response. *New England Journal of Medicine* 2005; **352**: 2211–21.

CHAPTER 15

INTRODUCTION OF NEW DRUGS AND CLINICAL TRIALS

HISTORY

Many years before Christ, humans discovered that certain plants influence the course of disease. Primitive tribes used extracts containing active drugs such as **opium**, **ephedrine**, **cascara**, **cocaine**, **ipecacuanha** and **digitalis**. These were probably often combined with strong psychosomatic therapies and the fact that potentially beneficial agents survived the era of magic and superstition says a great deal about the powers of observation of those early 'researchers'.

Many useless and sometimes deleterious treatments also persisted through the centuries, but the desperate situation of the sick and their faith in medicine delayed recognition of the harmful effects of drugs. Any deterioration following drug administration was usually attributed to disease progression, rather than to adverse drug effects. There were notable exceptions to this faith in medicine and some physicians had a short life expectancy as a consequence!

Over the last 100 years, there has been an almost exponential growth in the number of drugs introduced into medicine. Properly controlled clinical trials, which are the cornerstone of new drug development and for which the well-organized vaccine trials of the Medical Research Council (MRC) must take much credit, only became widespread after the Second World War. Some conditions did not require clinical trials (e.g. the early use of **penicillin** in conditions with a predictable natural history and high fatality rate). (Florey is credited with the remark that 'if you make a real discovery, you don't need to call in the statisticians'.) Ethical considerations relating to the use of a 'non-treatment' group in early trials were sometimes rendered irrelevant by logistic factors such as the lack of availability of drugs.

It was not until the 1960s that the appalling potential of drug-induced disease was realized world-wide. **Thalidomide** was first marketed in West Germany in 1956 as a sedative/hypnotic, as well as a treatment for morning sickness. The drug was successfully launched in various countries, including the UK in 1958, and was generally accepted as a safe and effective compound, and indeed its advertising slogan was 'the safe hypnotic'. However, in 1961, it became clear that its use in early pregnancy was causally related to rare congenital abnormality, phocomelia, in which the long bones fail to develop. At least 600 such babies were born in England and more than 10 000 afflicted babies were born world-wide. The **thalidomide** tragedy stunned the medical profession, the pharmaceutical industry and the general public. In 1963, the Minister of Health of the UK established a Committee on the Safety of Drugs, since it was clear that some control over the introduction and marketing of drugs was necessary. These attempts at regulation culminated in the Medicines Act (1968).

UK REGULATORY SYSTEM

The UK comes under European Community (EC) legislation regarding the control of human medicines, which is based upon safety, quality and efficacy. The UK Medicines and Healthcare products Regulation Agency (MHRA) or the European Agency for the Evaluation of Medicinal Products (EMEA) must approve any new medicine before it can be marketed in the UK. All UK clinical trials involving a medicinal product must be approved by the MHRA. The MHRA is assisted by expert advisory groups through the Commission on Human Medicines (CHM) to assess new medicines during their development and licensing. The MHRA is also responsible for the quality and safety monitoring of medicines after licensing. Product labels, patient leaflets, prescribing information and advertising are subject to review by the MHRA. In the UK, there is also extensive 'self-regulation' of the pharmaceutical industry through the Association of the British Pharmaceutical Industry (ABPI). The National Institute for Health and Clinical Excellence (NICE) is independent of the MHRA.

THE PROCESS OF DRUG DEVELOPMENT

Drug development is a highly regulated process which should be performed under internationally recognized codes

- Discovery
- Screening
- Preclinical testing

| Early (exploratory) development |

- Phase I (usually healthy volunteers) Proof of principle
- Phase IIa Proof of concept
- -
- Phase IIb
- Phase III (1000–5000 patients)
- * Registration
- Phase IV

| Late (confirmatory) development |

Cost is approximately £500 million, 60% of which is spent in clinical trials. Time from discovery to registration approximately 10–13 years

Figure 15.1: Stages of drug development.

of practice, namely Good Manufacturing Practice (GMP), Good Laboratory Practice (GLP) and Good Clinical Practice (GCP). Good Clinical Practice is an international ethical and scientific quality standard for designing, conducting, recording and reporting trials that involve the participation of human subjects. The stages of drug development are outlined in Figure 15.1.

DRUG DISCOVERY, DESIGN AND SYNTHESIS

Whilst random screening and serendipity remain important in the discovery of new drugs, new knowledge of the role of receptors, enzymes, ion channels and carrier molecules in both normal physiological processes and disease now permits a more focused approach to drug design. Using advances in combinatorial chemistry, biotechnology, genomics, high output screening and computer-aided drug design, new drugs can now be identified more rationally.

PRECLINICAL STUDIES

New chemical entities are tested in animals to investigate their pharmacology, toxicology, pharmacokinetics and potential efficacy in order to select drugs of potential value in humans. Although there is considerable controversy concerning the value of some studies performed in animals, human drug development has an excellent safety record, and there is understandable reluctance on the part of the regulatory authorities to reduce requirements. At present, the European guidelines require that the effects of the drug should be assessed in two mammalian species (one non-rodent) after two weeks of dosing before a single dose is administered to a human. In addition, safety pharmacology and mutagenicity tests will have been assessed. Additional and longer duration studies are conducted before product licence approval. The timing, specific tests and duration of studies may relate to the proposed human usage in both the clinical trials and eventual indications.

CLINICAL TRIALS

Physicians read clinical papers, review articles and pharmaceutical advertisements describing clinical trial results. Despite peer review, the incompetent or unscrupulous author can conceal deficiencies in design and possibly publish misleading data. The major medical journals are well refereed, although supplements to many medical journals are less rigorously reviewed for scientific value. An understanding of the essential elements of clinical trial design enables a more informed interpretation of published data.

Assessment of a new treatment by clinical impression is not adequate. Diseases may resolve or relapse spontaneously, coincidental factors may confound interpretation, and the power of placebo and enthusiastic investigators are a major influence on subjective response. In order to minimize these factors and eliminate bias, any new treatment should be rigorously assessed by carefully designed, controlled clinical trials.

All physicians involved in clinical trials must follow the guidelines of the Declaration of Helsinki and subsequent amendments.

OBJECTIVES

The first step in clinical trial design is to determine the questions to be addressed. Primary and achievable objectives must be defined. The question may be straightforward. For example, does treatment A prolong survival in comparison with treatment B following diagnosis of small-cell carcinoma of the lung? Survival is a clear and objective end-point. Less easily measured end-points such as quality of life must also be assessed as objectively as possible. Prespecified subgroups of patients may be identified and differences in response determined. For example, treatment A may be found to be most effective in those patients with limited disease at diagnosis, whereas treatment B may be most effective in those with widespread disease at diagnosis. Any physician conducting a clinical trial must not forget that the ultimate objective of all studies is to benefit patients. The patients' welfare must be of paramount importance.

RANDOMIZATION

Patients who agree to enter such a study must be randomized so that there is an equal likelihood of receiving treatment A or B. If treatment is not truly randomized, then bias will occur. For example, the investigator might consider treatment B to be less well tolerated and thus decide to treat particularly frail patients with treatment A. Multicentre studies are often necessary in order to recruit adequate numbers of patients, and it is essential to ensure that the treatments are fairly compared. If treatment A is confined to one centre/hospital and treatment B to another, many factors may affect the outcome of the study due to differences between the centres, such as interval between diagnosis and treatment, individual differences in determining entry criteria, facilities for treatment of complications, differing attitude to pain control, ease of transport, etc.

INCLUSION AND EXCLUSION CRITERIA

For any study, inclusion and exclusion criteria must be defined. It is essential to maximize safety and minimize confounding factors, whilst also ensuring that the criteria are not so strict that the findings will be applicable only to an unrepresentative subset of the patient population encountered in usual practice. The definition of a healthy elderly subject is problematic. Over the age of 65 years, it is 'normal' (in the sense that it is common) to have a reduced creatinine clearance, to be on some concomitant medication and to have a history of allergy. If these are exclusion criteria, a trial will address a 'superfit' elderly population and not a normal population.

DOUBLE-BLIND DESIGN

A 'double-blind' design is often desirable to eliminate psychological factors such as enthusiasm for the 'new' remedy. This is not always possible. For example, if in the comparison of treatment A and treatment B described above, treatment A consists of regular intravenous infusions whilst treatment B consists of oral medication, the 'blind' is broken. As 'survival' duration is 'hard' objective data, this should not be influenced markedly, whereas softer end-points, such as the state of well-being, are more easily confounded. In trials where these are especially important, it may be appropriate to use more elaborate strategies to permit blinding, such as the use of a 'double dummy' where there is a placebo for both dosage forms. In this case patients are randomized to active tablets plus placebo infusion or to active infusion plus placebo tablets.

WITHDRAWALS

The number of patients who are withdrawn from each treatment and the reason for withdrawal (subjective, objective or logistic) must be taken into account. For example, if in an antihypertensive study comparing two treatments administered for three months only the data from those who completed three months of therapy with treatment X or Y are analysed, this may suggest that both treatments were equally effective. However, if 50% of the patients on treatment X withdrew after one week because of lack of efficacy, that conclusion is erroneous. Again, if patients are withdrawn after randomization but before dosing, this can lead to unrecognized bias if more patients in one group die before treatment is started than in the other group, leading to one group containing a higher proportion of fitter 'survivors'. Conversely, if patients are withdrawn after randomization but before dosing, adverse events cannot be attributed to the drug. Hence both an 'intention-to-treat' analysis and a 'treatment-received' analysis should be presented.

PLACEBO

If a placebo control is ethical and practical, this simplifies interpretation of trial data and enables efficacy to be determined more easily (and with much smaller numbers of subjects) than if an effective active comparator is current standard treatment (and hence ethically essential). It is well recognized that placebo treatment can have marked effects (e.g. lowering of blood pressure). This is partly due to patient familiarization with study procedures, whose effect can be minimized by a placebo 'run-in' phase.

TRIAL DESIGN

There is no one perfect design for comparing treatments. Studies should be prospective, randomized, double-blind and placebo-controlled whenever possible. Parallel-group studies are those in which patients are randomized to receive different treatments. Although tempting, the use of historical data as a control is often misleading and should only be employed in exceptional circumstances. Usually one of the treatments is the standard, established treatment of choice, i.e. the control, whilst the other is an alternative – often a new treatment which is a potential advance. In chronic stable diseases, a crossover design in which each subject acts as his or her own control can be employed. Intra-individual variability in response is usually much less than inter-individual variability. The treatment sequence must be evenly balanced to avoid order effects and there must be adequate 'washout' to prevent a carry-over effect from the first treatment. This design is theoretically more 'economical' in subject numbers, but is often not applicable in practice.

STATISTICS

It is important to discuss the design and sample size of any clinical trial with a statistician at the planning phase.

Research papers often quote P values as a measure of whether or not an observed difference is 'significant'. Conventionally, the null hypothesis is often rejected if $P < 0.05$ (i.e. a difference of the magnitude observed would be expected to occur by chance in less than one in 20 trials – so-called type I error, see Figure 15.2). This is of limited value, as a clinically important difference may be missed if the sample size is too small (type II error, see Figure 15.2). To place reliance on a negative result, the statistical power of the study should be at least >0.8 and preferably >0.9 (i.e. a true difference of the magnitude pre-specified would be missed in 20% or 10% of such trials, respectively). It is possible to calculate the number of patients required to establish a given difference between treatments at a specified level of statistical confidence. For a continuous variable, one needs an estimate of the mean and standard deviation which one would expect in the control group. This is usually available from historical data, but a pilot study may be necessary. The degree of uncertainty surrounding observed

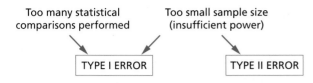

Figure 15.2: Different types of statistical error.

differences should be reported as confidence intervals (usually 95% confidence intervals). Such intervals will diminish as the sample size is increased. Confidence intervals reflect the effects of sampling variability on the precision of a procedure, and it is important to quote them when a 'non-significant' result is obtained, and when comparing different estimates of effectiveness (e.g. drug A in one trial may have performed twice as well as placebo, whereas drug B in another trial may have performed only 1.5 times as well as placebo; whether drug A is probably superior to drug B will be apparent from inspection of the two sets of confidence intervals).

If many parameters are analysed, some apparently 'significant' differences will be identified by chance. For example, if 100 parameters are analysed in a comparison of two treatments, one would expect to see a 'significant' difference in approximately five of those parameters. It is therefore very important to prespecify the primary trial end-point and secondary end-points that will be analysed. Statistical corrections can be applied to allow for the number of comparisons made. One must also consider the clinical importance of any statistically significant result. For example, a drug may cause a statistically significant decrease in blood pressure in a study, but if it is only 0.2 mmHg it is not of any clinical relevance.

CLINICAL DRUG DEVELOPMENT

For most new drugs, the development process – following a satisfactory preclinical safety evaluation – proceeds through four distinct phases. These are summarized below. Figure 15.3 illustrates the overall decision-making process for determining whether or not a new therapy will be clinically useful.

PHASE I

The initial studies of drugs in humans usually involve healthy male volunteers unless toxicity is predictable (e.g. cytotoxic agents, murine monoclonal antibodies). The first dose to be administered to humans is usually a fraction of the dose that produced any effect in the most sensitive animal species tested. Subjective adverse events, clinical signs, haematology, biochemistry, urinalysis and electrocardiography are used to assess tolerability. Depending on the preclinical data, further, more specific evaluations may be appropriate. The studies are placebo controlled to reduce the influence of environment and normal variability. If the dose is well tolerated, a higher dose will be administered either to a different subject in a parallel design, or to the same group in an incremented crossover design.

This process is repeated until some predefined end-point such as a particular plasma concentration, a pharmacodynamic effect or maximum tolerated dose is reached. Data from the single-dose study will determine appropriate doses and dose intervals for subsequent multiple-dose studies. If the drug is administered by mouth, a food interaction study should be conducted before multiple-dose studies.

The multiple-dose study provides further opportunity for pharmacodynamic assessments, which may demonstrate a desired pharmacological effect and are often crucial for the selection of doses for phase II. Having established the dose range that is well tolerated by healthy subjects, and in some cases identified doses that produce the desired pharmacological effect, the phase II studies are initiated.

Key points

Phase I studies:

- initial exposure of humans to investigational drug;
- assessment of tolerance, pharmacokinetics and pharmacodynamics in healthy subjects or patients;
- usually healthy male volunteers;
- usually single site;
- 40–100 subjects in total.

PHASE II

Phase II studies are usually conducted in a small number of patients by specialists in the appropriate area to explore efficacy, tolerance and the dose–response relationship. If it is ethical and practicable, a double-blind design is used, employing either a placebo control or a standard reference drug therapy as control. These are the first studies in the target population, and it is possible that drug effects, including adverse drug reactions and pharmacokinetics, may be different to those observed in the healthy subjects. If the exploratory phase II studies are promising, larger phase III studies are instigated, using a dosage regimen defined on the basis of the phase II studies.

Key points

Phase II studies:

- initial assessment of tolerance in 'target' population;
- initial assessment of efficacy;
- identification of doses for phase III studies;
- well controlled with a narrowly defined patient population;
- 100–300 patients in total;
- usually double-blind, randomized and controlled.

PHASE III

Phase III is the phase of large-scale formal clinical trials in which the efficacy and tolerability of the new drug is established.

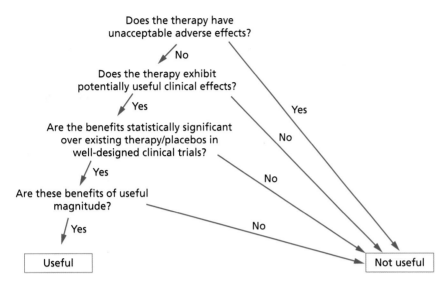

Figure 15.3: Flow chart for deciding usefulness of a new therapy.

Patient groups who respond more or less well may be identified, patient exposure (both numbers and duration of therapy) is increased, and less common type B (see Chapter 12) adverse reactions may be identified. During this period, the manufacturers will be setting up plant for large-scale manufacture and undertaking further pharmaceutical studies on drug formulation, bioavailability and stability. The medical advisers to the company, in association with their pharmacological, pharmaceutical and legal colleagues, will begin to collate the large amount of data necessary to make formal application to the MHRA or EMEA for a product licence. Marketing approval may be general or granted subject to certain limitations which may include restriction to hospital practice only, restriction in indications for use, or a requirement to monitor some particular action or organ function in a specified number of patients. Doctors are reminded (by means of a black triangle symbol beside its entry in the British National Formulary) that this is a recently introduced drug, and that any suspected adverse reaction should be reported to the MHRA or Commission on Human Medicines.

> **Key points**
>
> Phase III studies:
>
> - confirmation of effective doses;
> - expanded tolerability profile;
> - collection of data on a more varied patient population with indication;
> - data on overall benefit/risk;
> - can be placebo or more usually active controls;
> - multicentre;
> - commonly 1000–5000 patients in total;
> - usually double-blind.

PHASE IV

Phase IV studies are prospective trials performed after marketing approval (the granting of a product licence). These may assess the drug's clinical effectiveness in a wider population and may also help in the detection of previously unrecognized adverse events (see Chapter 12).

> **Key points**
>
> Phase IV studies:
>
> - performed after marketing approval and related to the approved indications;
> - exposure of drug to a wider population;
> - different formulations, dosages, duration of treatment, drug interactions and other drug comparisons are studied;
> - detection and definition of previously unknown or inadequately quantified adverse events and related risk factors.

POSTMARKETING SURVEILLANCE

The MHRA closely monitors newly licensed drugs for adverse events through the yellow card reporting system (see Chapter 12). Direct reporting by patients of adverse events was introduced in 2004. SAMM (Safety Assessment of Marketed Medicines) studies may be initiated which can involve many thousands of patients.

GENERIC DRUGS

Once the patent life of a drug has expired, anyone may manufacture and sell their version of that drug. The generic drug producer does not have to perform any of the research and development process other than to demonstrate that their version of the drug is 'bioequivalent' to the standard formulation. The convention accepted for such 'bioequivalence' is generous, and the issue is the subject of current debate by biostatisticians. In practice, the essential point is that clinically untoward consequences should not ensue if one preparation is substituted for the other.

ETHICS COMMITTEES

Protocols for all clinical trials must be reviewed and approved by a properly constituted independent ethics committee. Research Ethics Committees are coordinated by NRES (National Research Ethics Services) working on behalf of the Department of Health in the UK.

NRES maintains a UK-wide system of ethical review that protects the safety, dignity and well-being of research participants whilst facilitating and promoting research within the NHS.

Interestingly, studies have shown that patients taking part in clinical trials often have better health outcomes than those not involved in a trial.

GLOBALIZATION

In order to facilitate world-wide drug development and encourage good standards of practice, a series of international conferences on harmonization of requirements for registration of pharmaceuticals for human use have been conducted. International Conferences on Harmonisation (ICH) are leading to a globally accepted system of drug development, hopefully without stifling research with excessive bureaucracy and without any lowering of standards. The goal is to facilitate the early introduction of valuable new therapies, while at the same time maximizing patient protection.

Case history

Rather than a clinical case history, consider a chapter in the history of drug regulation which is instructive in illustrating the value of toxicity testing. Triparanol is a drug that lowers the concentration of cholesterol in plasma. It was marketed in the USA in 1959. In 1962, the Food and Drug Administration (FDA) received a tip-off and undertook an unannounced inspection. This revealed that toxicology data demonstrating cataract formation in rats and dogs had been falsified. Triparanol was withdrawn, but some of the patients who had been taking it for a year or longer also developed cataracts.

FURTHER READING

Collier J (ed.). *Drug and therapeutics bulletin; from trial outcomes to clinical practice*. London: Which? Ltd, 1996.

Griffin JP, O'Grady J (eds). *The textbook of pharmaceutical medicine*, 5th edn. London: BMJ Books, 2005.

Wilkins MR (ed.). *Experimental therapeutics. Section 1: Drug discovery and development*. London: Martin Dunitz, 2003.

CHAPTER 16

CELL-BASED AND RECOMBINANT DNA THERAPIES

The term 'biotechnology' encompasses the application of advances in our knowledge of cell and molecular biology since the discovery of DNA to the diagnosis and treatment of disease. Recent progress in molecular genetics, cell biology and the human genome has assisted the discovery of the mechanisms and potential therapies of disease. The identification of a nucleotide sequence that has a particular function (e.g. production of a protein), coupled with our ability to insert that human nucleotide sequence into a bacterial or yeast chromosome and to extract from those organisms large quantities of human proteins, has presented a whole array of new opportunities in medicine. (Human gene sequences have also been inserted into mice to develop murine models of human disease.) In 1982, the first recombinant pharmaceutical product, human recombinant insulin, was marketed. Since then, more than 100 medicines derived via biotechnology have been licensed for use in patients, whilst hundreds more are currently undergoing clinical trials. Successes include hormones, coagulation factors, enzymes and monoclonal antibodies, extending the range of useful therapeutic agents from low molecular weight chemical entities to macromolecules. Once discovered, some biotechnology products are manufactured by chemical synthesis rather than by biological processes. Examples of recombinant products are listed in Table 16.1. In parallel with these advances, the human genome project is establishing associations between specific genes and specific diseases. Detailed medical histories and genetic information are being collected and collated from large population samples. This will identify not only who is at risk of a potential disease and may thus benefit from prophylactic therapy, but also who may be at risk of particular side effects of certain drugs. This carries potentially momentous implications for selecting the right drug for the individual patient – a 'holy grail' known as personalized medicine. Achieving this grail is not imminent. It is not just the physical presence but, more importantly, the expression of a gene that is relevant. Often a complex interaction between many genes and the environment gives rise to disease. Despite these complexities, the human genome project linked with products of recombinant DNA technology, including gene therapy, offers unprecedented opportunities for the treatment of disease.

Most recombinant proteins are not orally bioavailable, due to the efficiency of the human digestive system. However, the ability to use bacteria to modify proteins systematically may aid the identification of orally bioavailable peptides. Nucleic acids for gene therapy (see below) are also inactive when administered by mouth. Drug delivery for such molecules is very specialized and at present consists mainly of incorporating the gene in a virus which acts as a vector, delivering the DNA into the host cell for incorporation into the host genome and subsequent transcription and translation by the cellular machinery of the host cell.

Human proteins from transgenic animals and bacteria are used to treat diseases that are caused by the absence or impaired function of particular proteins. Before gene cloning permitted the synthesis of these human proteins in large quantities, their only source was human tissues or body fluids, carrying an inherent risk of viral (e.g. hepatitis B and C and HIV) or prion infections. An example in which protein replacement is life-saving is the treatment of Gaucher's disease, a lysosomal storage disease, which is caused by an inborn error of metabolism inherited as an autosomal recessive trait, which results in a deficiency of glucocerebrosidase, which in turn results in the accumulation of glucosylceramide in the lysosomes of the reticulo-endothelial system, particularly the liver, bone marrow and spleen. This may result in hepatosplenomegaly, anaemia and pathological fractures. Originally, a modified form of the protein, namely alglucerase, had to be extracted from human placental tissue. The deficient enzyme is now produced by recombinant technology.

The production of recombinant factor VIII for the treatment of haemophilia has eliminated the risk of blood-borne viral infection. Likewise, the use of human recombinant growth hormone has eliminated the risk of Creutzfeldt–Jakob disease that was associated with human growth hormone extracted from bulked cadaver-derived human pituitaries.

Recombinant technology is used to provide deficient proteins (Table 16.1) and can also be used to introduce modifications of human molecules. In the human insulin analogue, **lispro insulin**, produced using recombinant technology, the order of just two amino acids is reversed in one chain of the insulin molecule, resulting in a shorter duration of action than

Table 16.1: Recombinant proteins/enzymes licensed in the UK (examples)

Protein/enzyme	Indication
Recombinant coagulation factors VIII and VIIa	Haemophilia
Imiglucerase	Gaucher's disease
Interferon alfa	Hepatitis B and C, certain lymphomas and solid tumours
Interferon beta	Multiple sclerosis
Epoetin alfa and beta (recombinant human erythropoietin)	Anaemia of chronic renal failure. To increase yield of autologous blood, e.g. during cancer chemotherapy
Drotrecogin alfa (activated) (recombinant activated protein C which reduces microvascular dysfunction)	Severe sepsis

Table 16.2: Hormones/hormone antagonists (examples)

	Mode of action	Indication
Somatropin	Synthetic human growth hormone (hGH)	Growth hormone deficiency
Pegvisomant	Genetically modified hGH that blocks hGH receptors	Acromegaly
Follitropin alfa and beta	Recombinant human follicle stimulating hormone	Infertility
Insulin aspart, glulisine and lispro	Recombinant human insulin analogues, faster onset of action	Diabetes (helps glucose control in some patients/ situations)

soluble insulin, a real advance for some patients (see Chapter 37). Other 'designer' insulins have longer actions or other kinetic features that are advantageous in specific circumstances.

In addition to producing recombinant human hormones (see Table 16.2) and other recombinant proteins (e.g. hirudin, the anticoagulant protein of the leech), recombinant monoclonal antibodies for treating human diseases have been produced originally in immortalized clones of mouse plasma cells. Not surprisingly, the original murine antibodies induced antibody responses in humans which in turn caused disease or neutralizing antibodies, rendering the monoclonal antibodies ineffective if used repeatedly (Table 16.3). Immunoglobulins have been gradually humanized to reduce the risk of an immune response on repeated treatments.

In cancer therapy, monoclonal antibodies have been developed against a tumour-associated antigen, e.g. **trastuzumab** against the HER2 protein (over-expressed in certain breast cancers in particular). Most facilitate the body's immune system in destroying the cancer cells or reduce the blood supply to the tumour. **Abciximab** (see Chapter 30) inhibits platelet aggregation by blocking the glycoprotein receptor that is a key convergence point in different pathways of platelet aggregation. It is used as an adjunct to **heparin** and **aspirin** for the prevention of ischaemic complications in high-risk patients undergoing percutaneous coronary intervention. It is a murine monoclonal antibody and can only be used in an individual patient once. Most recently developed monoclonal antibodies have been fully humanized. In comparison to most conventional 'small molecule' drugs, the antibodies' activities are very specific and toxicity is usually directly related to the targeted effect either through excessive effect or a 'downstream' consequence of the effect. The effects are usually very species-specific, so extrapolation from animal studies is more difficult. The initial doses in humans should be a fraction of the minimum anticipated biological effect level (MABEL, see Figure 16.1) taking into account concentration, receptor occupancy, relative potency, likely dose–response curve, and effects of excessive pharmacology rather than just the 'no observable adverse effect level' (NOAEL) which is the mainstay of first dose calculation for conventional small molecule drugs.

Recombinant techniques have also been of value in the development of vaccines, thereby avoiding the use of intact virus. Suspensions of hepatitis B surface antigen prepared from yeast cells by recombinant DNA techniques are already widely used to prevent hepatitis B infection in high-risk groups in the UK. In comparison to traditional egg-based and cell-based vaccines, DNA vaccines using plasmid DNA coding for specific epitopes of influenza virus may be developed, manufactured and distributed much more rapidly and effectively. With the current likelihood of an influenza pandemic caused by a new strain of virus predicted by the World Health Organization (WHO), the ability to produce such DNA vaccines may save millions of lives.

Table 16.3: Licensed monoclonal antibodies (examples)

Monoclonal antibody	Mode of action	Indication
Abciximab	Inhibits glycoprotein IIb/IIIa, platelet aggregation	Angioplasty
Omalizumab	Anti-IgE	Prophylaxis of severe allergic asthma
Infliximab, Adalimumab	Anti-TNFα	Rheumatoid arthritis, psoriatic arthritis
Basiliximab, Daclizumab	Bind to IL-2Rα receptor on T cells, prevent T-cell proliferation, causing immunosuppression	Prophylaxis of acute rejection in allogenic renal transplantation
Bevacizumab (Avastin®)	Inhibits vascular endothelial growth factor (VEGF), hence inhibits angiogenesis	Metastatic colorectal cancer
Pegaptanib and ranibizumab	Inhibit VEGF	Neovascular age-related macular degeneration

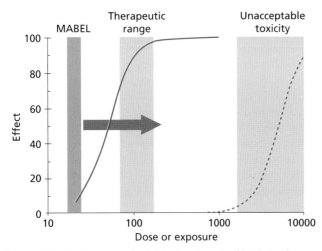

Figure 16.1: Explanation of minimum anticipated biological effect level (MABEL) (kindly provided by P Lloyd, Novartis, Basel, Switzerland). Unbroken line, desired effect; dashed line, undesired effect.

Table 16.4: Prevalence of some genetic disorders which result from a defect in a single gene

Disorder	Estimated prevalence
Familial hypercholesterolaemia	1 in 500
Polycystic kidney disease	1 in 1250
Cystic fibrosis	1 in 2000
Huntington's chorea	1 in 2500
Hereditary spherocytosis	1 in 5000
Duchenne muscular dystrophy	1 in 7000
Haemophilia	1 in 10 000
Phenylketonuria	1 in 12 000

GENE THERAPY

The increasing potential to exploit advances in genetics and biotechnology raises the possibility of prevention by gene therapy both of some relatively common diseases which are currently reliant on symptomatic drug therapy, and of genetic disorders for which there is currently no satisfactory treatment, let alone cure.

Gene therapy is the deliberate insertion of genes into human cells for therapeutic purposes. Potentially, gene therapy may involve the deliberate modification of the genetic material of either somatic or germ-line cells. Germ-line genotherapy by the introduction of a normal gene and/or deletion of the abnormal gene in germ cells (sperm, egg or zygote) has the potential to correct the genetic defect in many devastating inherited diseases and to be subsequently transmitted in Mendelian fashion from one generation to the next.

The prevalence figures for inherited diseases in which a single gene is the major factor are listed in Table 16.4. However, germ-line gene therapy is prohibited at present because of the unknown possible consequences and hazards, not only to the individual but also to future generations. Thus, currently, gene therapy only involves the introduction of genes into human somatic cells. Whereas gene therapy research was initially mainly directed at single-gene disorders, most of the research currently in progress is on malignant disease. Gene therapy trials in cancer usually involve destruction of tumour cells by the insertion of a gene that causes protein expression that induces an immune response against those cells, or by the introduction of 'suicide genes' into tumour cells.

Cystic fibrosis (CF) is the most common life-shortening autosomal-recessive disease in Europeans. It is caused by a mutation in the cystic fibrosis transmembrane conductance regulator (CFTR) gene. Over 600 different CF mutations have been recognized, although one mutation (F508) is present on over 70% of CF chromosomes. Phase I studies using adenoviral or liposomal vectors to deliver the normal CFTR gene to the airway epithelium have shown that gene transfer is feasible, but with current methods is only transient in duration and benefit. Adenoviral vectors are more efficient than liposomes but themselves cause serious inflammatory reactions.

A dramatic example of the potential benefit and danger of gene therapy has been seen in the treatment of severe combined immunodeficiency (SCID) secondary to adenosine deaminase deficiency by reinfusing genetically corrected autologous T cells into affected children. Whilst the gene therapy was effective in the immunological reconstitution of the patients, allowing a normal life including socializing with other children rather than living in an isolation 'bubble', T-cell leukaemia has developed in some patients. This probably reflects problems with the retrovirus vector.

A success in gene therapy has occurred with recipients of allogenic bone marrow transplants with recurrent malignancies. T cells from the original bone marrow donor can mediate regression of the malignancy, but can then potentially damage normal host tissues. A suicide gene was introduced into the donor T cells, rendering them susceptible to **ganciclovir** before they were infused into the patients, so that they could be eliminated after the tumours had regressed and so avoid future damage to normal tissues.

From the above, it will be appreciated that a major problem in gene therapy is introducing the gene into human cells. In some applications, 'gene-gun' injection of 'naked' (i.e. not incorporated in a vector) plasmid DNA may be sufficient. Minute metal (e.g. gold) particles coated with DNA are 'shot' into tissues using gas pressure (Figure 16.2). Some DNA is recognized as foreign by a minority of cells, and this may be sufficient to induce an immune response. This method underpins DNA vaccines. The other major problem is that for most diseases it is not enough simply to replace a defective protein, it is also necessary to control the expression of the inserted gene. It is for reasons such as these that gene therapy has been slower in finding clinical applications than had been hoped, but the long-term prospects remain bright.

Despite the inherent problems of gene therapy and societal concerns as to how information from the genotyping of individuals will be used, the development of gene therapy has dramatic potential – not only for the replacement of defective genes in disabling diseases such as cystic fibrosis, Duchenne muscular dystrophy and Friedreich's ataxia, but also for the treatment of malignant disease, and for prevention of cardiovascular disease and other diseases for which there is a genetic predisposition or critical protein target.

Another gene-modulating therapy that is currently being evaluated is the role of anti-sense oligonucleotides. These are nucleotides (approximately 20mers in length) whose sequence is complementary to part of the mRNA of the gene of interest. When the anti-sense enters cells it binds to the complementary sequence, forming a short piece of double-stranded DNA that is then degraded by RNase enzymes, thus inhibiting gene expression. Examples of such agents in development or near approval include **fomiversen**, which binds to cytomegalovirus (CMV) RNA (used intraocularly for CMV infection) and anti-Bcl-2, used to enhance apoptosis in lymphoma cells.

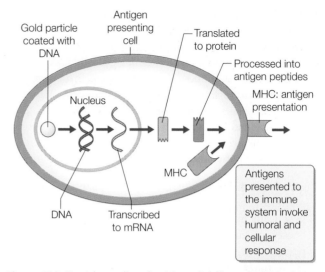

Figure 16.2: Particle-mediated epidermal delivery (PMED) of DNA into an antigen presenting cell (APC). The DNA elutes from the gold particle and enters the nucleus where it is transcribed into mRNA. The mRNA is then translated using the cellular synthetic pathways to produce the encoded protein of interest. This intracellular foreign protein is then processed by proteasomes into small antigenic peptides that are presented on the cell surface by the major histocompatibility complex (MHC).

HUMAN STEM CELL THERAPY

The discovery of stem cells' ability to replace damaged cells has led to much interest in cell-based therapies. Stem cells retain the potential to differentiate, for example into cardiac muscle cells or pancreatic insulin-producing cells, under particular physiological conditions.

In the UK, stem cell therapy is already established in the treatment of certain leukaemias and has also been used successfully in skin grafting, certain immune system and corneal disorders. Autologous and allogenic haemopoietic stem cells collected from bone marrow or via leukophoresis from peripheral blood following granulocyte colony-stimulating factor (G-CSF) stimulation (see Chapter 49) have been used for some years in the management of certain leukaemias. Allogenic stem cell transplantation is associated with graft-versus-host disease, hence concomitant immunosuppressant treatment with prophylactic anti-infective treatment including anti-T-cell antibodies is required. Graft-versus-host disease and opportunistic infections remain the principal complications.

Non-myeloblastic allogenic stem cell transplantation is being increasingly used, particularly in the elderly. This has an additional benefit from a graft-versus-tumour effect as immunosuppression is less severe.

Although there has been much publicity over the potential of stem cell regenerative and reparative effects in chronic central nervous system disorders, such as Parkinson's disease, Alzheimer's disease, motor neurone disease and multiple sclerosis, to date there is no convincing evidence of benefit for these conditions. There is ongoing ethical debate over the use of embryonic stem cells, which have more therapeutic potential than adult stem cells for research and possible therapy.

The Gene Therapy Advisory Committee (GTAC) is the national research ethics committee for gene therapy clinical research. GTAC's definition of gene therapy is as follows: 'The deliberate introduction of genetic material into human somatic cells for therapeutic, prophylactic or diagnostic purposes.' This definition, and hence the remit of GTAC, encompasses techniques for delivering synthetic or recombinant nucleic acids into humans:

- genetically modified biological vectors, such as viruses or plasmids;
- genetically modified stem cells;
- oncolytic viruses;
- nucleic acids associated with delivery vehicles;
- naked nucleic acids;
- antisense techniques (for example, gene silencing, gene correction or gene modification);
- genetic vaccines;
- DNA or RNA technologies, such as RNA interference;
- xenotransplantation of animal cells, but not solid organs.

FURTHER READING

Anon. Understanding monoclonal antibodies. *Drugs and Therapeutics Bulletin* 2007; **45**.

Anson DS. The use of retroviral vectors for gene therapy – what are the risks? A review of retroviral pathogenesis and its relevance to retroviral vector-mediated gene delivery. *Genetic Vaccines and Therapy* 2004; **2**: 9.

Check E. A tragic setback. *Nature* 2002; **420**: 116–18.

Guttmacher AE, Collins FS. Genomic medicine a primer. *New England Journal of Medicine* 2002; **347**: 1512–20.

Marshall E. Gene therapy death prompts review of adenovirus vector. *Science* 1999; **286**: 2244–5.

Nathwani AC, Davidoff AM, Linch DC. A review of gene therapy for haematological disorders. *British Journal of Haematology* 2005; **128**: 3–17.

Rang HP, Dale MM, Ritter JM, Flower RJ. Chapter 55 Biopharmaceuticals and gene therapy. In: *Pharmacology*, 6th edn. Oxford: Elsevier, 2007.

Safer medicines. A report from the Academy. London: The Academy of Medical Sciences, 2005.

Walsh G. Second-generation biopharmaceuticals. *European Journal of Pharmaceutics and Biopharmaceutics* 2004; **58**: 185–96.

CHAPTER 17

ALTERNATIVE MEDICINES: HERBALS AND NUTRACEUTICALS

INTRODUCTION

'Alternative' therapies (i.e. alternative to licensed products of proven quality, safety and efficacy) span a huge range from frank charlatanry (e.g. products based on unscientific postulates, composed of diluent or of snake oil), through physical therapies such as massage and aroma therapies which certainly please ('placebo' means 'I will please') and do a great deal less harm than some conventional therapies (e.g. surgery, chemotherapy), through to herbal medications with undoubted pharmacological activity and the potential to cause desired or adverse effects, albeit less predictably than the licensed products that have been derived from them in the past and will no doubt be so derived in the future. Medicine takes an empirical, evidence-based view of therapeutics and, if supported by sufficiently convincing evidence, alternative therapies can enter the mainstream of licensed products. Overall, efforts to test homeopathic products have been negative (Ernst, 2002) and it has been argued that no more resource should be wasted on testing products on the lunatic fringe, even when they come with royal endorsement and (disgracefully) public funding. Here we focus on herbal and nutraceutical products that may cause pharmacological effects.

Herbal remedies include dietary supplements (any product other than tobacco intended for ingestion as a supplement to the diet, including vitamins, minerals, anti-oxidants – Chapter 35 – and herbal products), phytomedicines (the use of plants or plants components to achieve a therapeutic effect/outcome) and botanical medicines (botanical supplements used as medicine). The recent increase in the use of herbal remedies by normal healthy humans, as well as patients, is likely to be multifactorial and related to: (1) patient dissatisfaction with conventional medicine; (2) patient desire to take more control of their medical treatment; and (3) philosophical/cultural bias. In the USA, approximately one-third of the population used some form of complementary or alternative medicine (the majority consuming herbal products) in the past 12 months. At a clinical therapeutic level, it is disconcerting that 15–20 million Americans regularly take herbal remedies, while concomitantly receiving modern prescription drugs, implying a significant risk for herb–drug interactions. In Scotland, some 12% of general practitioners and 60% of general practices prescribe homeopathic medicines! Herbal remedies are particularly used by certain groups of patients, notably HIV and cancer patients. The stereotypical user is a well-educated, career professional, white female. From a therapeutic perspective, many concerns arise from the easy and widespread availability, lack of manufacturing or regulatory oversight, potential adulteration and contamination of these herbal products. Furthermore, there is often little or no rigorous clinical trial evidence for efficacy and only anecdotes about toxicity. Many patients who are highly attuned to potential harms of conventional drugs (such as **digoxin**, a high quality drug derived historically from extracts of dried foxglove of variable quality and potency) fail to recognize that current herbals have as great or greater potential toxicities, often putting their faith in the 'naturalness' of the herbal product as an assurance of safety. This chapter briefly reviews the most commonly used herbals (on the basis of sales, Table 17.1) from a therapeutic perspective and addresses some of the recently identified problems caused by these agents.

GARLIC

Garlic has been used as a culinary spice and medicinal herb for thousands of years. One active compound in garlic is allicin, and this is produced along with many additional sulphur compounds by the action of the enzyme allinase when fresh garlic is crushed or chewed. Initial clinical trials suggested the potential of garlic to lower serum cholesterol and triglyceride, but a recent trial has shown limited to no benefit. Garlic has been advocated to treat many conditions, ranging from many cardiovascular diseases, e.g. atherosclerosis including peripheral vascular disease, hypertension, lipid disorders and sickle

Table 17.1: Most commonly used herbal products based on dollar sales

Product	Plant	Intended condition to be used for	Annual sales in USA ($ millions)
Garlic	*Allium sativum*	Hyperlipidaemia–hypercholesterolaemia	34.5
Ginkgo	*Ginkgo biloba*	Dementia and claudication	33.0
Echinacea	*Echinacea purpurea*	Prevention of common cold	32.5
Soy	*Glycine max*	Symptoms of menopause	28.0
Saw palmetto	*Serenoa repens*	Prostatic hypertrophy	23.0
Ginseng	*Panax ginseng*	Fatigue	22.0
St John's wort	*Hypericum perforatum*	Depression (mild)	15.0
Black cohosh	*Actaea racemosa*	Menopausal symptoms	12.3
Cranberry	*Vaccinia macrocarpon*	Cystitis and UTI	12.0
Valerian	*Valeriana officinalis*	Stress and sleeplessness	8.0
Milk thistle	*Silybum marianum*	Hepatitis and cirrhosis	7.5
Evening primrose	*Oenothera biennis*	Premenstrual symptoms	6.0
Bilberry	*Vaccinia myrtillus*	Diabetic retinopathy	3.5
Grape seed	*Vitis vinifera*	Allergic rhinitis	3

UTI: urinary tract infection

cell anaemia. Garlic can alter blood coagulability by decreasing platelet aggregation and increasing fibrinolysis.

Adverse effects

The adverse effects of garlic use involve gastro-intestinal symptoms including halitosis, dyspepsia, flatulence and heartburn. Other reported adverse effects include headache, haematoma and contact dermatitis.

Drug interactions

Garlic inhibits many drug-metabolizing (CYP450) enzymes in vitro, but induces CYP450s when administered chronically in vivo (reminiscent of many anticonvulsant drugs – Chapter 22 – as well as ethanol). Clinical studies using probe-drug cocktails have shown that garlic has no significant effect on the activity of CYP1A2 (**caffeine**), CYP2D6 (**debrisoquine, dextromethorphan**) and CYP3A4 (**alprazolam, midazolam**). Clinical studies suggest that garlic significantly decreases the bioavailability of **saquinavir** and **ritonavir**. These HIV protease inhibitors are not only metabolized by CYP3A4, but are also substrates for P-glycoprotein. The clinical importance of these interactions is uncertain, but potentially appreciable.

GINSENG

There are several types of ginseng (Siberian, Asian, American and Japanese), the most common type used in herbal preparations being the Asian variety (*Panax ginseng*). In humans, ginseng has been suggested to be a sedative-hypnotic, an aphrodisiac, an antidepressant and a diuretic, and therapeutic

benefits have been claimed for many indications (see below). Its pharmacologic properties include actions as a phytoestrogen, suggesting that its use, as with soy supplementation, could be disadvantageous in women with oestrogen-sensitive cancers (e.g. breast or endometrium). The active component of ginseng, ginsenoside, inhibits cAMP phosphodiesterase and monamine oxidase. These properties may partly explain purported central nervous system (CNS) stimulant actions of ginseng (though not sedative/hypnotic effects), potential modulation of the immune system and increase of glycogen storage. However, possible efficacy of ginseng in improving physical or psychomotor performance, cognitive function, immune function, diabetes mellitus and herpes simplex type 2 infections is not established beyond reasonable doubt.

Adverse effects

The adverse effects of ginseng are primarily CNS effects – agitation, irritability, insomnia and headache. Others noted include hypertension and mastalgia.

Drug interactions

In vitro evidence suggests that ginseng extracts inhibit CYP3A4 in human hepatocytes. These in vitro data are consistent with study data during an 18-day course of ginseng where it significantly increased the peak plasma concentration of **nifedipine**, a CYP3A4 substrate, in healthy volunteers. As with other herbs (e.g. echinacea), substantial variability in **ginsenoside** content has been reported among commercially available ginseng preparations, indicating that clinically significant effects on the pharmacokinetics of drugs that are metabolized by CYP3A4 could be highly variable between batches.

A case report has suggested a possible interaction between ginseng consumption and **warfarin**, but animal studies do not support this.

GINKGO BILOBA

Originating from Chinese medicine, ginkgo (derived from the nuts of *Ginkgo biloba* – a beautiful and threatened tree rather than the western culinary stereotype of a 'herb') is used for a variety of ailments and has multiple purported actions, including antihypoxic, antioxidant, antiplatelet, free radical-scavenging and microcirculatory properties. It has been used in patients with asthma, brain trauma, cochlear deafness, depression, retinitis, impotence, myocardial reperfusion and vertigo. The evidence for efficacy in many of these conditions is unconvincing. A recent clinical trial, in which a leading ginkgo extract did not improve cognitive function, may have contributed to a decline of ginkgo from the top-selling position it had held among such products since 1995. One of the principal components of ginkgo, ginkgolide B, is a moderately potent antagonist of platelet-activating factor. 'Anti-stress' effects claimed for ginkgo products are postulated to be due to monamine oxidase inhibition by ginkgolides.

Adverse effects

Serious or fatal side effects of gingko include spontaneous bleeding, fatal intracerebral bleeding, seizures and anaphylactic shock. Less serious side effects are nausea, vomiting, flatulence, diarrhoea, headaches and pruritus.

Drug interactions

In vitro data suggest ginkgo can inhibit hepatic drug metabolizing enzymes. Long-term administration of ginkgo to volunteers (for up to 28 days) had no effect on the pharmacokinetics of **midazolam**, a marker of CYP3A4 activity. In another study, however, ginkgo increased the plasma concentrations of the CYP3A4 substrate **nifedipine** by 53%, confirming the potential for enzyme inhibition observed in vitro. The discrepant findings for effects of ginkgo on CYP3A4 observed in this trial and in the phenotyping studies is possibly related to the highly variable phytochemical composition of commercially available ginkgo extracts. The potential importance of the change in CYP2C19 activity noted previously in a cocktail screening approach, was verified by the observation that ginkgo significantly reduced the metabolism of **omeprazole**, a CYP2C19 substrate, in Chinese patients. Collectively, these clinical data indicate that ginkgo may interfere with the pharmacokinetics of drugs metabolized by CYP2C19 or CYP3A4. If it does inhibit MAO at therapeutic doses, adverse interactions with tyramine-containing foods and possibly with selective serotonin reuptake inhibitors (SSRI) (Chapter 20) are to be anticipated.

ECHINACEA

Echinacea is one of the most commonly used alternative medicines, representing 10% of the herbal market. There are nine species of the genus *Echinacea*, a member of the sunflower family, found in North America. The most common and widespread of these are *Echinacea angustifolia*, *E. purpurea* and *E. pallida*, each of which has a long history of medicinal use. The majority of pharmacologic studies since 1939 have been conducted on *E. purpurea* preparations made from the fresh pressed juice of the flowering plant. Many chemical compounds have been identified from *Echinacea* species and it is currently not possible to attribute the pharmacological effects to any specific substance. Constituents that have been identified include volatile oil, caffeic acid derivatives, polysaccharides, polyines, polyenes, isobutylamides and flavonoids of the quercetin and kaempferol type. Many studies of echinacea have pointed to effects on the immune system. Proposed mechanisms of action include increased circulating granulocytes, enhanced phagocytosis, inhibition of virus proliferation, cytokine activation, increased T-lymphocyte production and an increase in the CD4/CD8 T-cell ratio. Echinacea is currently most widely used in attempts to prevent the common cold and influenza symptoms, but is also used for *Candida* infections, chronic respiratory infections, prostatitis and rheumatoid arthritis. Well-controlled studies have shown little, if any, benefit. One recent placebo-controlled study of echinacea in the treatment of the common cold actually suggested echinacea did not prevent people catching a 'cold' and if they did get symptoms they lasted slightly longer in patients taking echinacea.

Adverse effects

Adverse effects of echinacea use involve rashes, including erythema multiforme, arthralgias, allergic reactions, gastrointestinal disturbances including dysgeusia, dyspepsia and diarrhoea.

Drug interactions

Some flavonoids present in echinacea extracts can either inhibit or activate human CYPs and drug transporters, depending on their structures, concentrations and assay conditions. **Midazolam**, a substrate for CYP3A4 and CYP3A5, was cleared 42% faster during an eight-day echinacea treatment in 12 volunteers and there was a 23% reduction in **midazolam** area under the curve (AUC). The oral bioavailability of **midazolam** in this study was significantly increased from 24 to 36% in the presence of echinacea, indicating that the hepatic and intestinal availabilities were altered in opposite directions. These data suggest that echinacea is likely to interact with other oral drugs that are substrates for CYP3A4 and that the interaction will depend on the relative extraction of drugs at the hepatic and intestinal sites and the route of administration. Echinacea from retail stores often does not contain the labelled species (a similar situation affects other herbal preparations). The high variability observed in concentration of constituents of the herb has implications for echinacea's ability to modulate drug absorption and disposition.

SOY

The use of soy (*Glycine max*) and soy-derived products for the treatment of menopause in women is growing with the fear of possible side effects of traditional hormone replacement therapy. The principal constituents of soy, the isoflavones genistein and daidzein, are structurally similar to 17α-oestradiol and produce weak oestrogenic effects (i.e. they are phytoestrogens). It is prudent to discourage soy-derived products in patients with oestrogen-dependent tumours (e.g. breast cancer or endometrial cancer) because experimental data indicate that soy can stimulate the growth of these tumours in mice. Furthermore, as genistein can negate the inhibitory effect of **tamoxifen** on breast cancer growth, women taking this agent should especially avoid soy. Acute vasodilatation caused by 17β-oestradiol is mediated by nitric oxide, and genistein (which is selective for the oestrogen receptor ER_β, as well as having quite distinct effects attributable to tyrosine kinase inhibition) is as potent as 17β-oestradiol in this regard, raising the possibility of beneficial vascular effects.

Adverse reactions

Adverse reactions in soy use include allergic reactions (pruritus, rash, anaphylaxis) and gastro-intestinal disturbances (nausea, dyspepsia, diarrhoea).

Drug interactions

Isoflavones, such as genistein and daidzein, also inhibit oxidative and conjugative metabolism in vitro and in vivo. In 20 healthy volunteers, a 14-day course of soy extract (50 mg twice a day) did not alter the ratio of the amounts of 6β-hydroxycortisol and cortisol excreted in the urine, suggesting that soy is not an inducer of CYP3A4 in humans. However, genistein interacts with transporters such as P-glycoprotein (MDR-1, ABCB1), MRP1 (ABCC1) and MRP2 (ABCC2). Given that these transporters are involved in the intestinal absorption and biliary secretion of many drugs, it is reasonable to suspect that soy may alter drug absorption and/or disposition of such agents in humans.

SAW PALMETTO

Saw palmetto (*Serenoa repens*) is derived from a tree native to southeastern North America, particularly Florida. The main constituents of saw palmetto include carbohydrates, fixed oils, steroids, flavonoids, resin, tannin and volatile oil. Saw palmetto is used in men with the hope of 'toning and strengthening the reproductive system, and specifically for symptoms of prostate enlargement'. It has oestrogenic activity and reduces plasma testosterone concentration. In women, the principal use of saw palmetto is to (hopefully) reduce ovarian enlargement and to increase the size of small breasts. Although no drug interactions with, or medical contraindications to, the use of saw palmetto have been reported, it would be prudent to avoid concomitant use with other hormonal therapies, especially oestrogens, and in patients with oestrogen-dependent cancers.

Adverse effects

The adverse effects of saw palmetto involve gastro-intestinal intolerance, nausea and diarrhoea, hepatitis and cholestasis, gynaecomastia and impotence.

ST JOHN'S WORT

St John's wort (*Hypericum perforatum*, Figure 17.1), a perennial plant native to Europe, North America and western Asia, is one of the most extensively studied herbal products and many of its uses are based on observations noted in early Greek and Roman medicine. Currently, St John's wort is still widely used for the treatment of mild to moderate depression and other nervous conditions. Reported cases and trials have shown varying results of therapy with St John's wort for depressive and mood disorders. A meta-analysis of trials in 1757 patients concluded that treatment of depression with St John's wort was comparable to standard, prescription antidepressants and superior to placebo. More recently, a randomized, double-blind, placebo-controlled trial evaluating the safety and efficacy of St John's wort in the treatment of patients with major depressive disorders revealed that St John's wort was no more effective than placebo.

St John's wort extract is a very complex mixture of over 20 constituent compounds. These include catechin-type tannins and condensed-type proanthocyanidins, flavonoids (mostly hyperoside, rutin, quercetin and kaempferol), biflavonoids (e.g. biapigenin), phloroglutinol derivatives like hyperforin, phenolic acids, volatile oils and naphthodianthrones,

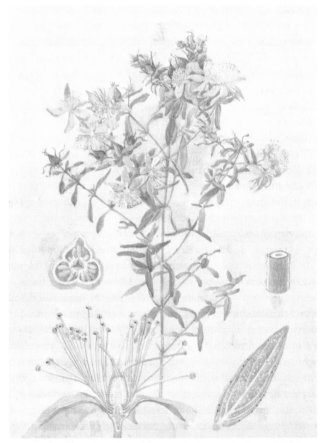

Figure 17.1: Drawing of perforate St John's wort (*Hypericum perforatum*). (© Natural History Museum, London. Reproduced with permission.)

including hypericin and pseudohypericin. With regard to the putative antidepressant effects of St John's wort, the pharmacological activities of hypericin and hyperforin, which inhibit synaptic 5HT and catecholamine reuptake, could contribute.

Adverse effects

Adverse CNS effects include headaches, drowsiness, restlessness, serotonin syndrome (Chapter 20) if used with SSRIs or TCAs, skin photosensitivity. Gastro-intestinal disturbances involve abdominal pain or discomfort, and xerostomia. Drug interactions with therapeutic failure of concomitant drugs, e.g. HIV protease inhibitors, **ciclosporin**, warfarin, **theophylline**, antidepressants, oral contraceptives and anti-cancer agents, such as **irinotecan**.

Drug interactions

Many clinical trials are now reporting significant pharmacokinetic interactions with long-term treatment with St John's wort and drugs from a variety of therapeutic classes. These studies followed a number of case reports of serious interactions between St John's wort and **digoxin**, **theophylline**, **ciclosporin**, oral contraceptives, **phenprocoumon**, **warfarin** and **sertraline**, thought to be secondary to enzyme induction. The mechanism for most of the interactions observed in subsequent clinical trials remains unclear, although for some agents, induction of CYP3A4 (e.g. **indinavir**, **midazolam**, **simvastatin**), P-glycoprotein-ABCB1 (e.g. **digoxin**, **fexofenadine**), or both (e.g. **ciclosporin**) may explain their increased clearance. St John's wort produced significantly greater increases in CYP3A4 expression in women compared to men, unexplained by differences in body mass index. More recently, it was shown that St John's wort enhanced the activity of transcription factors, including the pregnane X receptor to transcribe the *CYP3A4* and *P-gp* (*ABCB1*) genes. Other drug metabolism enzymes induced by St John's wort include CYP1A2, CYP2C9 and 2C19 and possibly UGT1A1 (Chapter 13). It should be noted that studies of St John's wort on CYP activity in vitro suggest acute inhibition, followed by induction in the long term.

GLUCOSAMINE

Glucosamine is available as a non-prescription dietary supplement and in many products is obtained from shellfish. It is one of several naturally occurring 6-carbon amino sugars found in the body. Amino sugars are essential building blocks for mucopolysaccharides, mucoproteins and mucolipids. Some commercial products contain glucosamine in combination with chondroitin. The precise mechanism of action of glucosamine is unknown. In vitro data suggest glucosamine can stimulate cartilage cells to synthesize glycosaminoglycans and proteoglycans. It is more likely that the cell produces smaller, soluble subunits; assembly of these smaller, soluble subunits outside of the cell into a soluble form of collagen has been proposed. Solubilized collagen, or tropocollagen, is a precursor

of mature collagen fibres. Chondroitin inhibits the enzymes that degrade cartilage.

Several clinical studies have documented the efficacy of glucosamine in the treatment of patients with osteoarthritis: data from double-blind studies showed glucosamine was superior to placebo and to **ibuprofen** in patients with osteoarthritis of the knee. Although there is a scientific basis for administering glucosamine in combination with chrondroitin, there is currently no evidence that the combination is more effective than glucosamine alone for osteoarthritis. A randomized, placebo-controlled, double-blind study evaluated the effects of glucosamine on disease progression and supported the use of glucosamine long term (three years) for slowing progression of knee osteoarthritis.

Adverse effects

The adverse effects associated with glucosamine involve gastro-intestinal disturbances, including dyspepsia, nausea, constipation and diarrhoea, skin rashes and allergic reactions in patients with known shellfish allergy.

Drug interactions

No drug interactions have been defined with the use of glucosamine.

MISCELLANEOUS HERBS RECENTLY FOUND TO BE TOXIC OR MERITING THEIR WITHDRAWAL FROM THE MARKET

Warnings about the toxicity of herbal products such as kava kava (hepatotoxicity), aristocholic acid (nephrotoxicity) and phen phen (pulmonary hypertension) have recently been communicated to prescribers and the public. PC-SPES, which was used by many prostate cancer patients because of anecdotal and uncontrolled studies of evidence of activity in prostate cancer, was withdrawn from sale by its suppliers after the FDA found it contained **alprazolam** and phytoestrogens.

Key points

- Herbal and nutraceutical products are widely available over the counter in many shops and are not regulated.
- The most commonly used products are garlic, ginkgo biloba, echinacea, soy, saw palmetto, ginseng and St John's wort.
- The efficacy of such products in many cases is not supported by rigorous clinical trials.
- Patients believe herbals are safe and are unaware of documented or potential toxicities.
- Many patients take herbal products in conjunction with prescription medications, unknowingly risking herb–drug interactions.
- When a patient develops an unusual reaction to his or her drug therapy (either therapeutic failure or toxicity) a careful history concerning the use of herbal products should be obtained.

Case history

A 45-year-old Caucasian female undergoes a successful liver transplant for primary biliary cirrhosis. Following the successful operation, her immunosuppressive regimen consists of tacrolimus, mycophenolic acid and relatively low doses of prednisolone, which are being further reduced. During the first six months, she remains well and her trough tacrolimus concentrations remain between 5 and 15 μg/L. This is therapeutic. When seen in follow up at approximately nine months post transplant, she is not quite feeling herself generally. Her only other symptoms noted on systematic enquiry are that she has not been sleeping well recently and has been anxious about driving her car. This was because four weeks ago she was involved in a head to head collision in a road traffic accident, but neither she nor the other driver were injured. Current clinical examination revealed some mild subcostal tenderness, without guarding and an otherwise normal clinical examination. Her liver function tests show an increased AST and ALT (five-fold the upper limit of normal) and a mildly elevated conjugated bilirubin. Thorough clinical and laboratory investigation revealed no infectious cause. A liver biopsy is compatible with hepatic rejection and a random tacrolimus concentration is 2 μg/L. She is adamant that she is adhering to her medication regimen.

Question 1

Could these problems all be attributed to her liver dysfunction? Is this a possible drug–drug interaction, if so which CYP450 enzyme system is involved?

Question 2

What else might she be taking in addition to her immunosuppressive regimen that could lead to this clinical situation?

Answer 1

The patient's hepatic dysfunction is most likely due to a late rejection episode. However, if her hepatic dysfunction were severe enough to compromise hepatic drug metabolism this would be accompanied by evidence of hepatic biosynthetic dysfunction and drugs metabolized by the liver would accumulate to toxic concentrations, rather than be subtherapeutic. An alternative drug interaction with an inducer of hepatic drug metabolism could explain the clinical picture, but whereas high-dose corticosteroids would cause a 15–30% induction of hepatic CYP3A4 enzymes, the enzymes involved in metabolism of tacrolimus, she is on a relatively low dose of prednisolone.

Answer 2

It is possible, but should be clarified with the patient, that she has been taking St John's wort for anxiety and insomnia. The current public view of St John's wort is that it is a harmless, herbal therapy that can be used to help patients with anxiety, insomnia and depression. Some of its chemical constituents act as GABA and 5-HT receptor agonists. In addition, one of the constituents of St John's wort (hyperforin) has been shown to be a potent inducer of several CYP450 enzymes, including 3A4, and the drug efflux transporter protein P-gp (ABCB1). The induction of CYP3A4/ABCB1 by St John's wort constituents occurs over eight to ten days. In the case of the magnitude of the induction caused by CYP3A and P-gp, St Johns wort is similar to that caused by rifampicin, and induction of both proteins is mediated via the pregnane X nuclear receptor. St John's wort could be the likely cause of this patient's subtherapeutic tacrolimus concentrations (a 3A4/ABCB1 substrate) and could thus have led over time to this rejection episode. Carefully enquiring about this possibility with the patient would be mandatory in this case. Apart from rifampicin, other drugs that induce 3A4 (but which the patient has not been prescribed) include phenobarbitone, carbamazepine, other rifamycins, pioglitazone, nevirapine (see Chapter 13).

FURTHER READING AND WEB MATERIAL

Ernst E. A systematic review of systematic reviews of homeopathy. *British Journal of Clinical Pharmacology* 2002; **54**: 577–82.

Goggs R, Vaughan-Thomas A, Clegg PD et al. Nutraceutical therapies for degenerative joint diseases: a critical review. *Critical Reviews in Food Science and Nutrition* 2005; **45**: 145–64.

Linde K, Berner M, Egger M, Mulrow C. St John's wort for depression: meta-analysis of randomised controlled trials. *British Journal of Psychiatry* 2005; **186**: 99–107.

Linde K, Barrett B, Wolkart K et al. Echinacea for preventing and treating the common cold. *Cochrane Database of Systematic Reviews* 2006; CD000530.

Reginster JY, Bruyere O, Fraikin G, Henrotin Y. Current concepts in the therapeutic management of osteoarthritis with glucosamine. *Bulletin (Hospital for Joint Diseases (New York))* 2005; **63**: 31–6.

Ross S, Simpson CR, McLay JS. Homoeopathic and herbal prescribing in general practice in Scotland. *British Journal of Clinical Pharmacology* 2006; **62**: 646–51.

Sparreboom A, Cox MC, Acahrya MR, Figg WD. Herbal remedies in the USA: Potential adverse reactions with anti-cancer agents. *Journal of Clinical Oncology* 2004; **20**: 2489–503.

Walker HA, Dean TS, Sanders TAB et al. The phytoestrogen genistein produces acute nitric oxide-dependent dilation of human forearm vasculature with similar potency to 17 beta-estradiol. *Circulation* 2001; **103**: 258–62.

Xie HG, Kim RB. St John's wort-associated drug interactions: short-term inhibition and long-term induction? *Clinical Pharmacology and Therapeutics* 2005; **78**: 19–24.

Useful websites: www.nccam.nih.gov and www.fda.gov

PART II

THE NERVOUS SYSTEM

HYPNOTICS AND ANXIOLYTICS

INTRODUCTION

Hypnotics induce sleep and anxiolytics reduce anxiety. There is considerable overlap between them. Thus, drugs that induce sleep also reduce anxiety, and as most anxiolytic drugs are sedative, will assist sleep when given at night. Neither hypnotics nor anxiolytics are suitable for the long-term management of insomnia or anxiety, due to tolerance and dependence. In this chapter, we discuss the management – both non-pharmacological and pharmacological – of sleep difficulties and of anxiety, and this is summarized in Figure 18.1.

SLEEP DIFFICULTIES AND INSOMNIA

Insomnia is common. Although no general optimal sleep duration can be defined, sleep requirements decline in old age. The average adult requires seven to eight hours, but some function well on as little as four hours, while others perceive more than nine hours to be necessary. Dissatisfaction with sleep reportedly occurs in 35% of adults and is most frequent in women aged over 65 years. Insomnia may include complaints such as difficulty in falling or staying asleep, and waking unrefreshed. Hypnotics are widely prescribed despite their ineffectiveness in chronic insomnia, as well as the problems associated with their long-term use. Persistent insomnia is a risk factor for or precursor of mood disorders, and may be associated with an increased incidence of daytime sleepiness predisposing to road traffic accidents, social and work-related problems. Insomnia lasting only a few days is commonly the result of acute stress, acute medical illness or jet lag. Insomnia lasting longer than three weeks is 'chronic'.

SLEEP

Although we spend about one-third of our lives asleep, the function of sleep is not known. Sleep consists of two alternating states, namely rapid eye movement (REM) sleep and non-REM sleep. During REM sleep, dreaming occurs. This is accompanied by maintenance of synaptic connections and increased cerebral blood flow. Non-REM sleep includes sleep of different depths, and in the deepest form the electroencephalogram (EEG) shows a slow wave pattern, growth hormone is secreted and protein synthesis occurs.

Drugs produce states that superficially resemble physiological sleep, but lack the normal mixture of REM and non-REM phases. Hypnotics usually suppress REM sleep, and when discontinued, there is an excess of REM (rebound) which is associated with troubled dreams punctuated by repeated wakenings. During this withdrawal state, falling from wakefulness to non-REM sleep is also inhibited by feelings of tension and anxiety. The result is that both patient and doctor are tempted to restart medication to suppress the withdrawal phenomena, resulting in a vicious cycle.

GENERAL PRINCIPLES OF MANAGEMENT OF INSOMNIA

It is important to exclude causes of insomnia that require treating in their own right. These include:

- pain (e.g. due to arthritis or dyspepsia);
- dyspnoea (e.g. as a result of left ventricular failure, bronchospasm or cough);
- frequency of micturition;
- full bladder and/or loaded colon in the elderly;
- drugs (see Table 18.1);

Table 18.1: Drugs that may cause sleep disturbances

Caffeine
Nicotine
Alcohol withdrawal
Benzodiazepine withdrawal
Amphetamines
Certain antidepressants (e.g. imipramine)
Ecstasy
Drugs that can cause nightmares (e.g. cimetidine, corticosteroids, digoxin and propranolol)

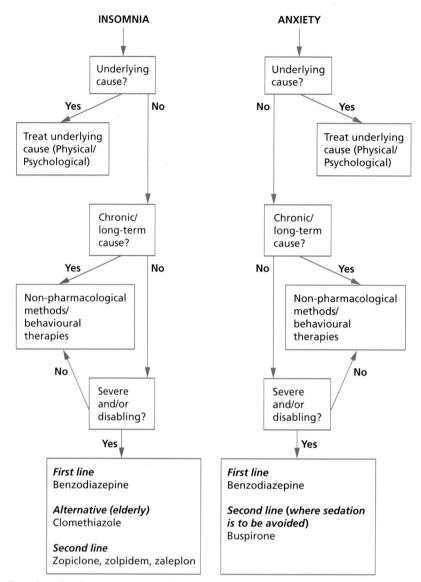

Figure 18.1: Decision tree/flow chart for the management of insomnia and anxiety.

- depression;
- anxiety.

Much chronic insomnia is due to dependence on hypnotic drugs. In addition, external factors such as noise, snoring partner and an uncomfortable bed may be relevant.

Drug therapy is inappropriate in individuals who need little sleep. Shortened sleep time is common in the elderly, and patients with dementia often have a very disturbed sleep pattern.

- Hypnotics should be considered if insomnia is severe and causing intolerable distress. They should be used for short periods (two to four weeks at most) and, if possible, taken intermittently. On withdrawal the dose and frequency of use should be tailed off gradually.
- Benzodiazepines are currently the hypnotics of choice, but may fail in the elderly, and alternatives such as **clomethiazole** can be helpful. There is currently no evidence of superiority for the newer 'non-benzodiazepine' hypnotics that act nonetheless on benzodiazepine receptors (see below).

- Prescribing more than one hypnotic at a time is not recommended, and there is no pharmacological rationale for doing this.
- Drugs of other types may be needed when insomnia complicates psychiatric illness. Sleep disturbances accompanying depressive illness usually respond to sedative antidepressives, such as **amitriptyline**. Antipsychotics, such as **chlorpromazine**, may help to settle patients suffering from dementia who have nocturnal restlessness.
- Hypnotics should not be routinely given to hospital patients or in any other situation, except where specifically indicated and for short-term use only.
- Whenever possible, non-pharmacological methods such as relaxation techniques, meditation, cognitive therapy, controlled breathing or mantras should be used. Some people experience sleepiness after a warm bath and/or sexual activity. A milk-based drink before bed can promote sleep, but may cause nocturia and, in the long run, weight gain. Caffeine-containing beverages should be avoided,

and daytime sleeping should be discouraged. Increased daytime exercise improves sleep at night.

- Alcohol should be avoided because it causes rebound restlessness and sleep disturbance after the initial sedation has worn off. Tolerance and dependence develop rapidly. It also causes dehydration (*gueule de bois*) and other unpleasant manifestations of hangover.

SPECIAL PROBLEMS AND SPECIAL GROUPS

JET LAG

Jet lag consists of fatigue, sleep disturbances, headache and difficulty in concentrating. It is due to mismatching of the body clock (circadian dysrhythmia) against a new time environment with its own time cues (*Zeitgebers*). Resetting the internal clock is hastened by conforming to the new time regime. Thus, one should rest in a dark room at night, even if not tired, and eat, work and socialize during the day. Sufferers should not allow themselves to sleep during the day (easier said than done!). Taking hypnotics at night can make things worse if sleepiness is experienced the next day. However, short-acting benzodiazepines may be effective if taken before going to bed for two or three nights.

Melatonin is of uncertain usefulness but may help sleep patterns, and improves daytime well-being if taken in the evening. It is not generally available in the UK, although it is in several other countries including the USA.

NIGHT WORK

Night work causes more serious sleep difficulties than jet lag because hypnotics cannot be used for long periods. Moreover, drug-induced sleep during the day precludes family and other non-work activities. A better strategy is to allow the subject to have a short, non-drug-induced sleep during the night shift. This improves efficiency towards the end of the night shift and reduces sleep needs during the day.

CHILDREN

The use of hypnotics in children is not recommended, except in unusual situations (e.g. on the night before an anticipated unpleasant procedure in hospital). Hypnotics are sometimes used for night terrors. Children are, however, prone to experience paradoxical excitement with these drugs. **Promethazine**, an antihistamine which is available without a prescription, is often used, but is of doubtful benefit.

ELDERLY

Anxiety and insomnia are prevalent in the elderly, for a variety of psychological and physical reasons. As a rule, elderly patients are more sensitive to the action of central nervous system (CNS) depressant drugs than younger patients, and the pharmacokinetics of these drugs are also altered such that their action is more prolonged with increasing age. Hypnotics increase the risk of falls and nocturnal confusion. Even short-acting drugs can lead to ataxia and hangover the next morning. In the treatment of insomnia, when short-term treatment with drugs is considered necessary, short-acting hypnotics should be used in preference to long-acting drugs but with

explanation from the outset that these will not be continued long term. (Short-acting benzodiazepines have the greatest abuse potential.) Insomnia occurring in the context of documented psychiatric disorders or dementia may be better treated with low doses of antipsychotic drugs.

Case history

A 42-year-old man with chronic depression presents to his general practitioner with a long history of difficulty in sleeping at night, associated with early morning waking. His general practitioner had made the diagnosis of depression and referred him some years previously for cognitive behavioural therapy, but this had not resulted in significant improvement of his symptoms. His difficulty in sleeping is now interfering with his life quite significantly, so that he feels tired most of the day and is having difficulty holding down his job as an insurance clerk. The GP decides that he would benefit from taking **temazepam** at night; he prescribes him this, but says that he will only give it for a maximum of a month, as he does not want his patient to become addicted.
Question 1
Is this the correct management?
Question 2
What would be a suitable alternative treatment?
Answer 1
No. Although the benzodiazepine might help in the short term, it does not provide the patient with a long-term solution, and does not tackle the root cause of his insomnia.
Answer 2
A more appropriate treatment would be with a regular dose of a sedating antidepressant drug, for example **amitriptyline** at night.

ANXIETY

Anxiety is fear and is usually a normal reaction. Pathological anxiety is fear that is sufficiently severe as to be disabling. Such a reaction may be a response to a threatening situation (e.g. having to make a speech) or to a non-threatening event (e.g. leaving one's front door and going into the street). Episodes of paroxysmal severe anxiety associated with severe autonomic symptoms (e.g. chest pain, dyspnoea and palpitations) are termed panic attacks and often accompany a generalized anxiety disorder.

GENERAL PRINCIPLES AND MANAGEMENT OF ANXIETY

- Distinguish anxiety as a functional disturbance from a manifestation of organic brain disease or somatic illness (e.g. systemic lupus erythematosus).
- Assess the severity of any accompanying depression, which may need treatment in itself.
- Most patients are best treated with cognitive therapy, relaxation techniques and simple psychotherapy and without drugs.
- Some patients are improved by taking regular exercise.
- In severely anxious patients who are given anxiolytic drugs, these are only administered for a short period (up to two to four weeks) because of the risk of dependence.

- Desensitization can be useful when severe anxiety develops in well-recognized situations (e.g. agoraphobia, arachnophobia, etc.). Anxiolytic drugs are sometimes given intermittently and with a flexible-dose scheme in such situations.
- Benzodiazepines are the anxiolytics normally used where pharmacological therapy is indicated. **Buspirone** is as effective as and less hypnotic than the benzodiazepines, but has slower onset.
- β-Blockers are sometimes useful in patients with prominent symptoms, such as palpitations or tremor.
- Tricyclic antidepressants may be effective in anxiety and in preventing panic attacks.
- Monoamine oxidase inhibitors (used only by specialists) can be useful for treating anxiety with depression, phobic anxiety, recurrent panic attacks and obsessive-compulsive disorders.
- Individual panic attacks are usually terminated by benzodiazepines, which may have to be supplemented with short-term treatment with phenothiazines (e.g. **chlorpromazine**).
- If hyperventilation is the principal 'trigger', advice on controlled breathing exercises can be curative.

DRUGS USED TO TREAT SLEEP DISTURBANCES AND ANXIETY

The distinction between hypnotics and anxiolytics is rather arbitrary, and the same classes of drugs are used for both purposes. Compounds with a short half-life tend to be used as hypnotics, because they cause less 'hangover' effects; longer half-life drugs tend to be used as anxiolytics, since a longer duration of action is generally desirable in this setting. Benzodiazepines are used for the short-term alleviation of anxiety, but should not be used long term, where antidepressants (Chapter 20) are usually the treatment of choice.

BENZODIAZEPINES

These drugs are anxiolytic, anticonvulsant muscle relaxants that induce sleepiness; they remain drugs of choice for the pharmacological treatment of insomnia and anxiety. **Clonazepam** is believed to be more anticonvulsant than other members of the group at equi-sedating doses. Benzodiazepines bind to specific binding sites in the $GABA_A$ receptor–chloride channel complex in the brain, and facilitate the opening of the channel in the presence of GABA; this increases hyperpolarization-induced neuronal inhibition.

Examples

- **Diazepam** – used as an anxiolytic, because of its long half-life.
- **Temazepam** – used as a hypnotic, because of its short half-life.
- **Lorazepam** – potent short half-life benzodiazepine. Should generally be avoided for more than very

short-term use, as it causes intense withdrawal phenomena and dependence.
- **Diazepam** or **midazolam** i.v. before procedures such as endoscopy, cardioversion and operations under local anaesthesia. Early short-lived high peak blood levels are accompanied by anterograde amnesia.

Cautions

- respiratory failure;
- breast-feeding;
- previous addiction.

Adverse effects

- drowsiness;
- confusion;
- paradoxical disinhibition and aggression.

Adverse effects of intravenous diazepam include:

1. Cardiovascular and respiratory depression (uncommon). Patients with chronic lung disease, and those who have been previously given other central depressant drugs are at risk.
2. Local pain following i.v. injection. An emulsion of **diazepam** in **intralipid** is less irritating to the vein. Intra-arterial benzodiazepine can cause arterial spasm and gangrene.

Drug dependence, tolerance and withdrawal

Benzodiazepine dependence is usually caused by large doses taken for prolonged periods, but withdrawal states have arisen even after limited drug exposure. Pharmacological evidence of tolerance may develop within three to 14 days. The full withdrawal picture can manifest within hours of the last dose for the shorter-acting drugs, or may develop over up to three weeks with the longer-duration benzodiazepines. Withdrawal syndrome includes a cluster of features including frank anxiety and panic attacks. Perceptual distortions (e.g. feelings of being surrounded by cotton wool), visual and auditory hallucinations, paranoia, feelings of unreality, depersonalization, paraesthesiae, sweating, headaches, blurring of vision, dyspepsia and influenza-like symptoms can occur. Depression and agoraphobia are also common. The syndrome may persist for weeks. Withdrawal from benzodiazepines in patients who have become dependent should be gradual. If this proves difficult, then an equivalent dose of a long-acting benzodiazepine should be given as a single night-time dose instead of shorter-acting drugs. The dose should then be reduced in small fortnightly steps. Psychological support is important.

Drug interactions

Pharmacodynamic interactions with other centrally acting drugs are common, whereas pharmacokinetic interactions are not. Pharmacodynamic interactions include potentiation of the sedative actions of alcohol, histamine (H_1) antagonists and other hypnotics.

FLUMAZENIL

Flumazenil is a benzodiazepine antagonist. It can be used to reverse benzodiazepine sedation. It is short acting, so sedation may return. It can cause nausea, flushing, anxiety and fits, so is not routinely used in benzodiazepine overdose which seldom causes severe adverse outcome.

OTHERS

- Barbiturates are little used and dangerous in overdose.
- **Clomethiazole** – causes conjunctival, nasal and gastric irritation. Useful as a hypnotic in the elderly because its short action reduces the risk of severe hangover, ataxia and confusion the next day. It is effective in acute withdrawal syndrome in alcoholics, but its use should be carefully supervised and treatment limited to a maximum of nine days. It can be given intravenously to terminate status epilepticus. It can also be used as a sedative during surgery under local anaesthesia.
- **Zopiclone**, **zolpidem** and **zaleplon** – are non-benzodiazepine hypnotics which enhance GABA activity by binding to the GABA–chloride channel complex at the benzodiazepine-binding site. Although they lack structural features of benzodiazepines, they also act by potentiating GABA. Their addictive properties are probably similar to benzodiazepines.
- **Buspirone** – is a $5HT_{1A}$ receptor partial agonist. Its use has not been associated with addiction or abuse, but may be a less potent anxiolytic than the benzodiazepines. Its therapeutic effects take much longer to develop (two to three weeks). It has mild antidepressant properties.
- **Cloral** and derivatives – formerly often used in paediatric practice. Cloral shares properties with alcohol and volatile anaesthetics. Cloral derivatives have no advantages over benzodiazepines, and are more likely to cause rashes and gastric irritation.
- Sedative antihistamines, e.g. **promethazine**, are of doubtful benefit, and may be associated with prolonged drowsiness, psychomotor impairment and antimuscarinic effects.

BENZODIAZEPINES VS. NEWER DRUGS

Since the advent of the newer non-benzodiazepine hypnotics (**zopiclone**, **zolpidem** and **zaleplon**), there has been much discussion and a considerable amount of confusion, as to which type of drug should be preferred. The National Institute for Health and Clinical Excellence (NICE) has given guidance based on evidence and experience. In essence,

1. When hypnotic drug therapy is appropriate for severe insomnia, hypnotics should be prescribed for short periods only.
2. There is no compelling evidence to distinguish between **zaleplon**, **zolpidem**, **zopiclone** or the shorter-acting benzodiazepine hypnotics. It is reasonable to prescribe the drug whose cost is lowest, other things being equal. (At present, this means that benzodiazepines are preferred.)
3. Switching from one hypnotic to another should only be done if a patient experiences an idiosyncratic adverse effect.
4. Patients who have not benefited from one of these hypnotic drugs should not be prescribed any of the others.

Case history

A 67-year-old widow attended the Accident and Emergency Department complaining of left-sided chest pain, palpitations, breathlessness and dizziness. Relevant past medical history included generalized anxiety disorder following the death of her husband three years earlier. She had been prescribed lorazepam, but had stopped it three weeks previously because she had read in a magazine that it was addictive. When her anxiety symptoms returned she attended her GP, who prescribed buspirone, which she had started the day before admission.

Examination revealed no abnormality other than a regular tachycardia of 110 beats/minute, dilated pupils and sweating hands. Routine investigations, including ECG and chest x-ray, were unremarkable.

Question 1
Assuming a panic attack is the diagnosis, what is a potential precipitant?
Question 2
Give two potential reasons for the tachycardia.
Answer 1
Benzodiazepine withdrawal.
Answer 2
1. Buspirone (note that buspirone, although anxiolytic, is not helpful in benzodiazepine withdrawal and may also cause tachycardia).
2. Anxiety.
3. Benzodiazepine withdrawal.

FURTHER READING

Fricchione G. Clinical practice. Generalized anxiety disorder. *New England Journal of Medicine* 2004; **351**: 675–82.

National Institute for Clinical Excellence. 2004: Guidance on the use of zaleplon, zolpidem and zopiclone for the short-term management of insomnia. www.nice.org.uk/TA077guidance, 2004.

Sateia MJ, Nowell PD. Insomnia. *Lancet* 2004; **364**: 1959–73.

Stevens JC, Pollack MH. Benzodiazepines in clinical practice: consideration of their long-term use and alternative agents. *Journal of Clinical Psychiatry* 2005; **66** (Suppl. 2), 21–7.

CHAPTER 19

SCHIZOPHRENIA AND BEHAVIOURAL EMERGENCIES

SCHIZOPHRENIA

INTRODUCTION

Schizophrenia is a devastating disease that affects approximately 1% of the population. The onset is often in adolescence or young adulthood and the disease is usually characterized by recurrent acute episodes which may develop into chronic disease. The introduction of antipsychotic drugs such as **chlorpromazine** revolutionized the treatment of schizophrenia so that the majority of patients, once the acute symptoms are relieved, can now be cared for in the community. Previously, they would commonly be sentenced to a lifetime in institutional care.

PATHOPHYSIOLOGY

The aetiology of schizophrenia, for which there is a genetic predisposition, is unknown, although several precipitating factors are recognized (Figure 19.1). Neurodevelopmental delay has been implicated and it has been postulated that the disease is triggered by some life experience in individuals predisposed by an abnormal (biochemical/anatomical) mesolimbic system.

There is heterogeneity in clinical features, course of disease and response to therapy. The concept of an underlying neurochemical disorder is advanced by the dopamine theory of schizophrenia, summarized in Box 19.1. The majority of antipsychotics block dopamine receptors in the forebrain. 5-Hydroxytryptamine is also implicated, as indicated in Box 19.2. Glutamine hypoactivity, GABA hypoactivity and α-adrenergic hyperactivity are also potential neurochemical targets.

About 30% of patients with schizophrenia respond inadequately to conventional dopamine D_2 receptor antagonists. A high proportion of such refractory patients respond to clozapine, an 'atypical' antipsychotic drug which binds only transiently to D_2 receptors, but acts on other receptors, especially muscarinic, 5-hydroxytryptamine receptors ($5HT_2$) and D_1, and displays an especially high affinity for D_4 receptors. The D_4 receptor is localized to cortical regions and may be overexpressed in schizophrenia. Regional dopamine differences may be involved, such as low mesocortical activity with high mesolimbic activity. Magnetic resonance imaging (MRI) studies indicate enlargement of ventricles and loss of brain tissue, whilst functional MRI and positron emission tomography (PET) suggest hyperactivity in some cerebral areas, consistent with loss of inhibitory neurone function.

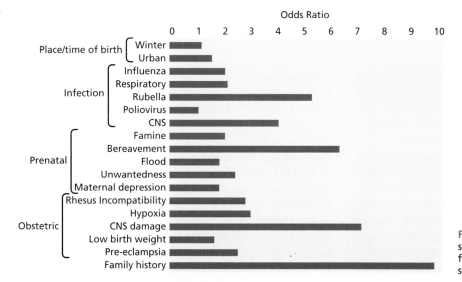

Figure 19.1: Predispositions to schizophrenia. Redrawn with permission from Sullivan PF. The genetics of schizophrenia. *PLoS Medicine* 2005; **2**: e212.

Box 19.1: Dopamine theory of schizophrenia

- There is excess dopamine activity in the mesolimbic system in schizophrenia.
- Antipsychotic potency is often proportional to D_2-blocking potency.
- Amphetamine (which increases dopamine release) can produce acute psychosis that is indistinguishable from acute schizophrenia (positive symptoms).
- D_2 agonists (bromocriptine and apomorphine) aggravate schizophrenia in schizophrenic patients.
- There is an increase in D_2 and D_4 receptors on PET in schizophrenic patients.
- L-Dopa can cause hallucinations and acute psychotic reactions and paranoia, but does not cause all the features of these conditions.
- There is no definite increase in brain dopamine in vivo and post mortem.
- Dopamine receptor blockade does not fully alleviate symptoms.

Box 19.2: 5-Hydroxytryptamine and schizophrenia

- LSD acts on 5HT receptors, causing hallucinations and dramatic psychological effects which may mimic some features of schizophrenia.
- 5HT has a modulatory effect on dopamine pathways.
- Many effective antipsychotic drugs have dopamine and $5HT_2$ receptor-blocking properties.
- $5HT_2$ receptor blockade is not essential for drug efficacy.

Figure 19.2 shows a summary of putative pathways for the development of schizophrenia.

GENERAL PRINCIPLES OF MANAGEMENT

ACUTE TREATMENT

The main principles are:

- Prompt drug treatment should be instigated, usually as an in-patient.
- Oral 'atypical antipsychotics' should be administered, e.g. **risperidone** or **olanzapine**.
- If the patient is very disturbed/aggressive, add benzodiazepine, e.g. **lorazepam**.

- Chlorpromazine may be preferred if sedation is advantageous, e.g. in very agitated patients.
- Antimuscarinic drugs, e.g. **procyclidine**, should be used if acute dystonia or Parkinsonian symptoms develop.
- Psychosocial support/treatment should be offered.
- Behaviour usually improves quickly, but hallucinations, delusions and affective disturbance may take weeks or months to improve.
- Once first-rank symptoms have been relieved, the patient can usually return home and resume work on low-dose antipsychotic treatment.
- Conventional drugs, e.g. **chlorpromazine** or **haloperidol**, are as effective in treatment of acute positive symptoms as atypical antipsychotic drugs and are less expensive, but adverse effects may be troublesome.

MAINTENANCE TREATMENT

- Only 10–15% of patients remain in permanent remission after stopping drug therapy following a first schizophrenic episode.
- The decision to attempt drug withdrawal should be taken with regard to the individual patient, their views, adverse drug effects, social support, relatives and carers.
- Cognitive behavioural therapy is a treatment option.
- Most patients require lifelong drug therapy, so the correct diagnosis is essential (e.g. beware drug-induced psychosis, as amphetamines in particular can produce acute schizophreniform states). All antipsychotic drugs have adverse effects. Continuing psychosocial support is critical.
- Oral or intramuscular depot therapy (Box 19.3), e.g. **olanzapine** (oral) or **flupentixol** (i.m.) should be considered. The latter ensures compliance.

Box 19.3: Intramuscular depot treatment

- Esters of the active drug are formulated in oil.
- There is slow absorption into the systemic circulation.
- It takes several months to reach steady state.
- After an acute episode, reduce the oral dose gradually and overlap with depot treatment.
- Give a test dose in case the patient is allergic to the oil vehicle or very sensitive to extrapyramidal effects.
- Rotate the injection site, e.g. flupentixol is given once every two to four weeks (ester of active drug formulated in an oil) or risperidone once every two weeks.

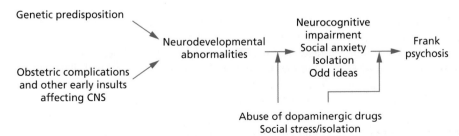

Figure 19.2: Pathways for development of schizophrenia.

DRUGS USED IN TREATMENT

CONVENTIONAL ANTIPSYCHOTIC DRUGS

The principal action of the conventional antipsychotic drugs (see Table 19.1), such as **chlorpromazine** (a phenothiazine) and **haloperidol** (a butyrophenone), is an antagonism of D_2 receptors in the forebrain. The effect on D_1 receptors is variable. Blockade of the D_2 receptors induces extrapyramidal effects. Repeated adminstration causes an increase in D_2-receptor sensitivity due to an increase in abundance of these receptors. This appears to underlie the tardive dyskinesias that are caused by prolonged use of the conventional antipsychotic drugs.

The choice of drug is largely determined by the demands of the clinical situation, in particular the degree of sedation needed and the patient's susceptibility to extrapyramidal toxicity and hypotension.

Uses

These include the following:

1. schizophrenia – antipsychotic drugs are more effective against first-rank (positive) symptoms (hallucinations, thought disorder, delusions, feelings of external control) than against negative symptoms (apathy and withdrawal);
2. other excited psychotic states, including mania and delirium;
3. anti-emetic and anti-hiccough;
4. premedication and in neuroleptanalgesia;
5. terminal illness, including potentiating desired actions of opioids while reducing nausea and vomiting;
6. severe agitation and panic;
7. aggressive and violent behaviour;
8. movement and mental disorders in Huntington's disease.

Adverse effects

1. The most common adverse effects are dose-dependent extensions of pharmacological actions:
   - extrapyramidal symptoms (related to tight binding to, and receptor occupancy of, D_2 receptors) – parkinsonism including tremor, acute dystonias, e.g. torticollis, fixed upward gaze, tongue protrusion; akathisia (uncontrollable restlessness with feelings of anxiety and agitation) and tardive dyskinesia. Tardive dyskinesia consists of persistent, repetitive, dystonic athetoid or choreiform movements of voluntary muscles. Usually the face and mouth are involved, causing repetitive sucking, chewing and lip smacking. The tongue may be injured. The movements are usually mild, but can be severe and incapacitating. This effect follows months or years of antipsychotic treatment;
   - anticholinergic – dry mouth, nasal stuffiness, constipation, urinary retention, blurred vision;
   - postural hypotension due to α-adrenergic blockade. Gradual build up of the dose improves tolerability;
   - sedation (which may be desirable in agitated patients), drowsiness and confusion. Tolerance usually develops after several weeks on a maintenance dose. Emotional flattening is common, but it may be difficult to distinguish this feature from schizophrenia. Depression may develop, particularly following treatment of hypomania, and is again difficult to distinguish confidently from the natural history of the disease. Acute confusion is uncommon.
2. Jaundice occurs in 2–4% of patients taking **chlorpromazine**, usually during the second to fourth weeks of treatment. It is due to intrahepatic cholestasis and is a hypersensitivity phenomenon associated with eosinophilia. Substitution of another phenothiazine may not reactivate the jaundice.
3. Ocular disorders during chronic administration include corneal and lens opacities and pigmentary retinopathy. This may be associated with cutaneous light sensitivity.
4. About 5% of patients develop urticarial, maculopapular or petechial rashes. These disappear on withdrawal of the drug and may not recur if the drug is reinstated. Contact dermatitis and light sensitivity are common complications. Abnormal melanin pigmentation may develop in the skin.
5. Hyperprolactinaemia.
6. Blood dyscrasias are uncommon, but may be lethal, particularly leukopenia and thrombocytopenia. These usually develop in the early days or weeks of treatment. The incidence of agranulocytosis is approximately 1 in 10 000 patients receiving **chlorpromazine**.
7. Cardiac dysrhythmia, including torsades de pointes (see Chapter 32) and arrest.
8. Malignant neuroleptic syndrome is rare but potentially fatal. Its clinical features are rigidity, hyperpyrexia, stupor or coma, and autonomic disorder. It responds to treatment with **dantrolene** (a ryanodine receptor antagonist that blocks intracellular Ca^{2+} mobilization).
9. Seizures, particularly in alcoholics. Pre-existing epilepsy may be aggravated.
10. Impaired temperature control, with hypothermia in cold weather and hyperthermia in hot weather.

Table 19.1: Conventional antipsychotic drugs

	Sedation	Extrapyramidal symptoms	Hypotension
Phenothiazines			
Chlorpromazine	++	++	++
Fluphenazine[a]	+	+++	+
Butyrophenones			
Haloperidol	+	+++	+
Thioxanthines			
Fluphenthixol[a]	+	++	+

[a]Depot preparation available.
All increase serum prolactin levels
Note: Pimozide causes a prolonged QT and cardiac arrhythmias.

The Boston Collaborative Survey indicated that adverse reactions are most common in patients receiving high doses, and that they usually occur soon after starting treatment. The most common serious reactions were fits, coma, severe hypotension, leukopenia, thrombocytopenia and cardiac arrest.

Contraindications and cautions

These include the following:

- coma due to cerebral depressants, bone marrow depression, phaeochromocytoma, epilepsy, chronic respiratory disease, hepatic impairment or Parkinson's disease;
- caution is needed in the elderly, especially in hot or cold weather;
- pregnancy, lactation;
- alcoholism.

Pharmacokinetics

The pharmacokinetics of conventional antipsychotic drugs have been little studied. They have multiple metabolites and their large apparent volumes of distribution (V_d) (e.g. for **chlorpromazine** $V_d = 22\,L/kg$) result in low plasma concentrations, presenting technical difficulties in estimation. Most is known about **chlorpromazine**, see Box 19.4.

Drug interactions

These include the following:

- alcohol and other CNS depressants – enhanced sedation;
- hypotensive drugs and anaesthetics – enhanced hypotension;
- increased risk of cardiac arrhythmias with drugs that prolong the QT interval (e.g. **amiodarone**, **sotalol**);
- tricyclic antidepressants – increased antimuscarinic actions;
- **metoclopramide** – increased extrapyramidal effects and akathisia;
- antagonism of anti-Parkinsonian dopamine agonists (e.g. L-dopa) (these are in any case contraindicated in schizophrenia).

Box 19.4: Pharmacokinetics (chlorpromazine)

- Dose regimes are largely empirical.
- There is variable absorption.
- There are >70 metabolites, some of which are active.
- Enterohepatic circulation is involved.
- There is enormous variability in plasma concentrations and $t_{1/2}$.
- There is a vast volume of distribution.
- Brain:plasma concentration is 5:1.
- Reduced doses should be prescribed in the elderly (for both pharmacokinetic and pharmacodynamic differences).

Case history

A 50-year-old woman whose schizophrenia is treated with oral haloperidol is admitted to the Accident and Emergency Department with a high fever, fluctuating level of consciousness, muscular rigidity, pallor, tachycardia, labile blood pressure and urinary incontinence.
Question 1
What is the likely diagnosis?
Question 2
How should this patient be managed?
Answer 1
Neuroleptic malignant syndrome.
Answer 2
1. Stop the haloperidol.
2. Initiate supportive therapy.
3. Bromocriptine (value uncertain).
4. Dantrolene (value uncertain).

ATYPICAL ANTIPSYCHOTIC DRUGS

The term 'atyptical antipsychotic' is used very imprecisely. 'Newer' or 'second-generation' antipsychotics are synonymous in some texts. In comparison to the conventional antipsychotics where potency is closely related to D_2 receptor blockade, atypical antipsychotics bind less tightly to D_2 receptors and have additional pharmacological activity which varies with the drug. Efficacy against negative symptoms, as well as less extrapyramidal side effects, are characteristic. These may be the result of the transient ('hit and run') binding to D_2 receptors.

Clozapine is the original 'atypical' antipsychotic and is described below. Its use is limited to resistant patients due to the risk of agranulocytosis. A variety of other atypical antipsychotic drugs are available. Features of **clozapine** are:

- $D_4 + 5HT_2$ blockade;
- $D_1 > D_2$ blockade;
- α-adrenoceptor blockade;
- effective in resistant patients;
- effective against negative and positive symptoms;
- virtually free from extrapyramidal effects;
- agranulocytosis (3%) – use is restricted to patients licensed with a monitoring service: blood count (weekly for first 18 weeks, then every two weeks till one year, then every four weeks);
- severe postural hypotension – initiate therapy under supervision;
- sedation, dizziness, hypersalivation;
- weight gain, glucose intolerance, possible intestinal obstruction;
- myocarditis and cardiomyopathy;
- pulmonary embolism;
- seizures.

Many newer alternatives, but none with the unique properties of **clozapine**, e.g. **risperidone**, **olanzapine**, **aripiprazole**, **amisulpride**, **quetiapine** and **zotepine**, have been introduced. Their pharmacology, efficacy and adverse effects vary. Although more expensive, in June 2002 NICE recommended that atypical antipsychotics should be considered in newly diagnosed schizophrenic patients and in those who have unacceptable effects from, or inadequate response to, conventional antipsychotic drugs. **Risperidone** blocks D_2, D_4 and in particular $5HT_2$ receptors. Careful dose titration reduces the risk of adverse effects, but extrapyramidal side effects are common at high doses. It is available as an intramuscular injection for acute control of agitation and disturbed behaviour. Weight gain and, more worryingly, an increased incidence of stroke in elderly patients with dementia have been reported wih both **risperidone** and **olanzapine**. **Aripiprazole** is a long-acting atypical antipsychotic which is a partial agonist at D_2 receptors, as well as blocking $5HT_2$. It is not associated with extrapyramidal effects, prolactin secretion or weight gain.

> ### Key points
> Pharmacological treatment
> - Receptor blockade:
>   - D_2, D_4, $5HT_2$.
> - Although there may be a rapid behavioural benefit, a delay (usually of the order of weeks) in reduction of many symptoms implies secondary effects (e.g. receptor up/downregulation).
> - Conventional antipsychotics (e.g. chlorpromazine, haloperidol, fluphenazine), act predominantly by D_2 blockade.
> - Atypical antipsychotics (e.g. clozapine, risperidone, olanzapine) are less likely to cause extrapyramidal side effects.

> ### Key points
> Adverse effects of antipsychotic drugs
> - Extrapyramidal motor disturbances, related to dopamine blockade.
> - Endocrine distributions (e.g. gynaecomastia), related to prolactin release secondary to dopamine blockade.
> - Autonomic effects, dry mouth, blurred vision, constipation due to antimuscarinic action and postural hypotension due to α-blockade.
> - Cardiac dysrhythmias, which may be related to prolonged QT, e.g. sertindole (an atypical antipsychotic), pimozide.
> - Sedation.
> - Impaired temperature homeostasis.
> - Weight gain.
> - Idiosyncratic reactions;
>   - jaundice (e.g. chlorpromazine);
>   - leukopenia and agranulocytosis (e.g. clozapine);
>   - skin reactions;
>   - neuroleptic malignant syndrome.

BEHAVIOURAL EMERGENCIES

MANIA

Acute attacks are managed with antipsychotics, but **lithium** is a common and well-established long-term prophylactic treatment. The control of hypomanic and manic episodes with **chlorpromazine** is often dramatic.

ACUTE PSYCHOTIC EPISODES

Patients with organic disorders may experience fluctuating confusion, hallucinations and transient paranoid delusions. Violent incidents sometimes complicate schizophrenic illness.

> ### Case history
> A 60-year-old man with schizophrenia who has been treated for 30 years with chlorpromazine develops involuntary (choreo-athetoid) movements of the face and tongue.
> *Question 1*
> What drug-induced movement disorder has developed?
> *Question 2*
> Will an anticholinergic drug improve the symptoms?
> *Question 3*
> Name three other drug-induced movement disorders associated with antipsychotic drugs.
> *Answer 1*
> Tardive dyskinesia.
> *Answer 2*
> No. Anticholinergic drugs may unmask or worsen tardive dyskinesia.
> *Answer 3*
> 1. Akathisia.
> 2. Acute dystonias.
> 3. Chronic dystonias.
> 4. Pseudo-parkinsonism.

MANAGEMENT

Antipsychotics and benzodiazepines, either separately or together, are effective in the treatment of patients with violent and disturbed behaviour. **Lorazepam** by mouth or parenteral injection is most frequently used to treat severely disturbed behaviour as an in-patient.

Haloperidol can rapidly terminate violent and psychotic behaviour, but hypotension, although uncommon, can be severe, particularly in patients who are already critically ill. Doses should be reduced in the elderly.

Intramuscular **olanzapine** or liquid **risperidone** are gradually supplanting more conventional antipsychotics in the acute management of psychosis.

When treating violent patients, large doses of antipsychotics may be sometimes needed. Consequently, extrapyramidal toxicity, in particular acute dystonias, develops in up to one-third of patients. Prophylactic anti-parkinsonian drugs, such as **procyclidine**, may be given, especially in patients who are particularly prone to movement disorders.

The combination of **lorazepam** and **haloperidol** has been successful in treating otherwise resistant delirious behaviour.

Oral medication, especially in liquid form, is the preferred mode of administration, if the patient will accept it, but intramuscular or intravenous routes may have to be used.

Antipsychotics, such as **chlorpromazine** should be avoided in alcohol withdrawal states, in alcoholics or in those dependent on benzodiazepines because of the risk of causing fits.

Ensure resuscitation facilities including those for mechanical ventilation are available. Many centres insist on the availability of **flumazenil** if (particularly i.v.) benzodiazepines are used.

FURTHER READING

Anon. Which atypical antipsychotic for schizophrenia? *Drugs and Therapeutics Bulletin* 2004; **42**: 57–60.

Freedman R. Drug therapy: schizophrenia. *New England Journal of Medicine* 2003; **334**: 1738–49.

CHAPTER 20

MOOD DISORDERS

DEPRESSIVE ILLNESSES AND ANTIDEPRESSANTS

Many forms of depression are recognized clinically and most respond well to drugs. From a biochemical viewpoint, there are probably different types of depression (which do not correspond predictably to clinical variants) depending on which neurotransmitter is involved, and these may respond differently to different drugs.

PATHOPHYSIOLOGY: INSIGHTS FROM ANTIDEPRESSANT DRUG ACTIONS

The monoamine theory of mood is mainly based on evidence from the actions of drugs.

1. **Reserpine**, which depletes neuronal stores of noradrenaline (NA) and 5-hydroxytryptamine (5HT) and α-methyltyrosine, which inhibits NA synthesis, cause depression.
2. Tricyclic antidepressants (TCA) of the amitriptyline type (which raise the synaptic concentration of NA and 5HT) are antidepressant.
3. Monoamine oxidase inhibitors (MAOIs, which increase total brain NA and 5HT) are antidepressant.

On the basis of these actions, it was suggested that depression could be due to a cerebral deficiency of monoamines. One difficulty with this theory is that **amfetamine** and **cocaine**, which act like tricyclic drugs in raising the synaptic NA content, are not antidepressive, although they do alter mood. Even worse, the tricyclic antidepressants block amine reuptake from synapses within one or two hours of administration, but take from ten days to four weeks to alleviate depression. Such a long time-course suggests a resetting of postsynaptic or presynaptic receptor sensitivity.

Another theory of depression is the serotonin-only hypothesis. This theory emphasizes the role of 5HT and downplays that of NA in the causation of depression, and is backed by the effectiveness of the selective serotonin reuptake inhibitors, or SSRI class of drugs, in the treatment of depression. However, it also

does not explain the delay in onset of the clinical effect of antidepressant drugs, including the SSRIs, and again receptor resetting has to be invoked. Also, many strands of evidence suggest that NA does indeed have an important role in depression.

The permissive hypothesis of mania/depression suggests that the control of emotional behaviour results from a balance between NA and 5HT. According to this theory, both the manic phase and the depressive phase of bipolar disorder are characterized by low central 5HT function. Evidence suggests that brain 5HT systems dampen or inhibit a range of functions involving other neurotransmitters. Mood disorders result from the removal of the serotonin damper. This hypothesis postulates that low levels of 5HT permit abnormal levels of NA to cause depression or mania. If 5HT cannot control NA and NA falls to abnormally low levels, the patient becomes depressed. On the other hand, if the level of 5HT falls and the level of NA becomes abnormally high, the patient becomes manic. According to this hypothesis, antidepressant drugs are effective to the degree that they restore the ability of 5HT to control NA, thus restoring the critical balance that controls emotional behaviour. A recently available class of antidepressant drugs, serotonin-noradrenaline reuptake inhibitors (SNRI), work by selectively blocking reuptake of both NA and 5HT, thereby increasing levels of both monoamines. The SNRIs have very little affinity for other postsynaptic receptor sites and are therefore less likely to produce some of the side effects associated with TCA.

Dysregulation of the hypothalamic–pituitary–adrenal axis is a common biological marker of depression and the value of antiglucocorticoid drugs is under investigation.

GENERAL PRINCIPLES OF MANAGEMENT

Depression is common, but under-diagnosed. It can be recognized during routine consultations, but additional time may be needed. Genetic and social factors are often relevant. Drug treatment is not usually appropriate at the mild end of the severity range. Drugs are used in more severe depression, especially if it has melancholic ('endogenous') features. Even if depression is attributable to external factors ('exogenous'), e.g. interpersonal difficulties or other life stresses (including physical illness), antidepressant drugs may be useful. Drugs used in the initial treatment of depression include TCAs and related drugs, SSRIs and SNRIs. Although clinical experience is most extensive with the TCAs, the side-effect profile of the SSRIs is usually less troublesome, and these drugs are safer in overdose. Therefore many psychiatrists and general practitioners use SSRIs rather than TCAs as first-line treatment for depression. SSRIs are more expensive than TCAs. The relative side effects of the different antidepressant drugs are summarized in Table 20.1.

In refractory depression, other drug treatment or electroconvulsive therapy (ECT) are considered. Alternative drug strategies include (1) adding **lithium** to a tricyclic to give a **lithium** blood level of 0.6–0.8 mmol/L; (2) combining antidepressants; (3) augmenting with T3 (or T4), a mood stabilizer such as **lamotrigine**, **buspirone** or **estradiol**; (4) MAOIs, usually prescribed only by psychiatrists; (5) MAOI plus a TCA – but only in expert psychiatric hands; or (6) small doses of **flupentixol** (for short-term treatment only).

Figures 20.1 and 20.2 show a treatment algorithm for management of depressive illness.

SELECTIVE SEROTONIN REUPTAKE INHIBITORS (SSRIs)

These drugs are safer in overdose than the tricyclic group. Selective serotonin reuptake inhibitors (SSRIs) do not stimulate

appetite and have much fewer antimuscarinic side effects than the tricyclics and other catecholamine-uptake inhibitors. They are also well tolerated in the elderly. Examples include **fluoxetine**, **fluvoxamine**, **paroxetine**, **sertraline**, **citalopram** and **escitalopram**.

Uses

These include the following:

1. in depression (they have similar efficacy to tricyclics, but are much more expensive);
2. in chronic anxiety, and as prophylaxis for panic attacks;
3. obsessive-compulsive states;
4. bulimia nervosa;
5. seasonal affective disorder, especially if accompanied by carbohydrate craving and weight gain;
6. possibly effective as prophylactic agents in recurrent depression.

Adverse effects

1. The most common adverse reactions to SSRIs are nausea, dyspepsia, diarrhoea, dry mouth, headache, insomnia and dizziness. Sweating, erectile dysfunction and delayed orgasm are well-recognized associations. These tend to become less severe after one to two months of treatment.
2. They have less anticholinergic and cardiotoxic actions than tricyclic drugs.

Table 20.1: Relative antidepressant side effects

Drug	Anticholinergic effects	Cardiac effects	Nausea	Sedation	Overdose risk	Pro-convulsant	Tyramine interaction
Tricyclics and related antidepressants							
Amitriptyline	+++	+++	+	+++	++	++	−
Clomipramine	+++	++	+	++	+	++	−
Dothiepin	++	++	−	+++	+++	++	−
Imipramine	++	++	+	+	++	++	−
Lofepramine	++	+	+	+	−	−	−
Trazodone	+	+	++	++	+	−	−
Selective serotonin reuptake inhibitors							
Citalopram	−	−	++	−	+	−	−
Fluoxetine	−	−	++	−	−	?	−
Paroxetine	−	−	++	−	−	?	−
Sertraline	−	−	++	−	−	?	−
Monoamine oxidase inhibitors							
Phenelzine	+	+	++	−	+	−	+++
Moclobemide	+	−	+	−	−	?	+
Others							
Venlafaxine	−	++	++	+	?	+	−

−, little or nothing reported; +, mild; ++, moderate; +++, high; ?, insufficient information available.

3. Epilepsy can be precipitated.
4. They are usually non-sedating, but may cause insomnia and do not usually cause orthostatic hypotension.
5. All antidepressants can cause hyponatraemia, probably due to induction of inappropriate antidiuretic hormone secretion, but it is reported more frequently with SSRIs than with other antidepressants.

Contraindications

These include the following:

- hepatic and renal failure;
- epilepsy;
- manic phase.

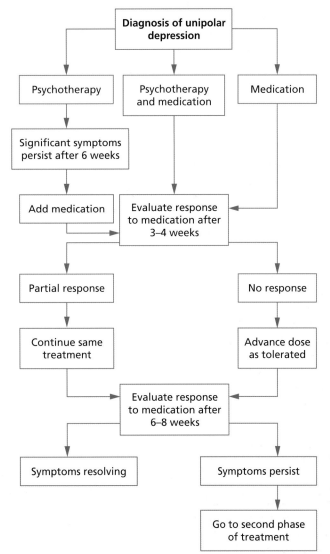

Figure 20.1: General algorithm for the initial phase of treatment of depression. When symptoms persist after first-line treatment, re-evaluate the accuracy of the diagnosis, the adequacy of the dose and the duration of treatment before moving to the second phase of treatment. (Redrawn with permission from Aronson SC and Ayres VE. 'Depression: A Treatment Algorithm for the Family Physician', *Hospital Physician* Vol 36 No 7, 2000. Copyright 2000 Turner White Communications, Inc.)

Drug interactions

- Combinations of SSRI with **lithium**, **tryptophan** or MAOIs may enhance efficacy, but are currently contraindicated because they increase the severity of 5HT-related toxicity. In the worst reactions, the life-threatening 5HT syndrome develops. This consists of hyperthermia, restlessness, tremor, myoclonus, hyperreflexia, coma and fits. After using MAOIs, it is recommended that two weeks should elapse before starting SSRIs. Avoid **fluoxetine** for at least five weeks before using MAOI because of its particularly long half-life (about two days).
- The action of **warfarin** is probably enhanced by **fluoxetine** and **paroxetine**.
- There is antagonism of anticonvulsants.
- **Fluoxetine** raises blood concentrations of **haloperidol**.

SEROTONIN-NORADRENALINE REUPTAKE INHIBITORS AND RELATED ANTIDEPRESSANTS

Venlafaxine: A potent 5HT and NA uptake inhibitor that appears to be as effective as TCAs, but without anticholinergic effects. It may have a more rapid onset of therapeutic action than other antidepressants, but this has yet to be confirmed. It is associated with more cardiac toxicity than the SSRIs.

Duloxetine inhibits NA and 5HT reuptake.

TRICYCLICS AND RELATED ANTIDEPRESSANTS (TCAs)

Uses

These include the following:

1. depressive illnesses, especially major depressive episodes and melancholic depression;
2. atypical oral and facial pain;
3. prophylaxis of panic attacks;
4. phobic anxiety;
5. obsessive–compulsive disorders;
6. **imipramine** has some efficacy in nocturnal enuresis.

Although these drugs share many properties, their profiles vary in some respects, and this may alter their use in different patients. The more sedative drugs include **amitriptyline**, **dosulepin** and **doxepin**. These are more appropriate for agitated or anxious patients than for withdrawn or apathetic patients, for whom **imipramine** or **nortriptyline**, which are less sedative, are preferred. **Protriptyline** is usually stimulant.

Only 70% of depressed patients respond adequately to TCAs. One of the factors involved may be the wide variation in individual plasma concentrations of these drugs that is obtained with a given dose. However, the relationship between plasma concentration and response is not well defined. A multicentre collaborative study organized by the World Health Organization failed to demonstrate any relationship whatsoever between plasma amitriptyline concentration and clinical effect.

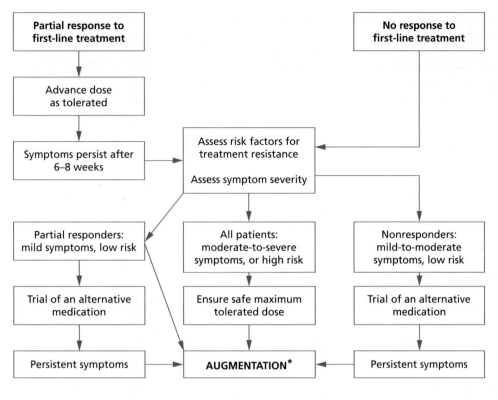

Figure 20.2: General algorithm for the second phase of treatment of depression. Augmentation* involves the use of a combination of medications to enhance the efficacy of an antidepressant. (Redrawn with permission from Aronson SC and Ayres VE, 'Depression: A Treatment Algorithm for the Family Physician', *Hospital Physician* Vol 36 No 7, 2000. Copyright 2000 Turner White Communications, Inc.)

Imipramine and **amitriptyline** (tertiary amines) have more powerful anticholinergic and cardiac toxic effects than secondary amines (e.g. **nortriptyline**).

Mechanism of action

The tricyclics block uptake-1 of monoamines into cerebral (and other) neurones. Thus, the concentration of amines in the synaptic cleft rises. As discussed above, they may also induce a slow adaptive decrease in pre- and/or postsynaptic amine receptor sensitivity.

Adverse effects

Autonomic (anticholinergic)/cardiovascular Dry mouth, constipation (rarely paralytic ileus, gastroparesis), tachycardia, paralysis of accommodation, aggravation of narrow-angle glaucoma, retention of urine, dry skin due to loss of sweating, and (due to α-blockade) postural hypotension. Rarely, sudden death due to a cardiac dysrhythmia. In overdose, a range of tachydysrhythmias and intracardiac blocks may be produced.

Central nervous system Fine tremor and sedation, but also (paradoxically) sometimes insomnia, decreased rapid eye movement (REM) sleep, twitching, convulsions, dysarthria, paraesthesia, ataxia. Increased appetite and weight gain, particularly with the sedative tricyclics, are common. On withdrawal of the drug, there may be gastro-intestinal symptoms such as nausea and vomiting, headache,

giddiness, shivering and insomnia. Sometimes anxiety, agitation and restlessness follow sudden withdrawal.

Allergic and idiosyncratic reactions These include bone marrow suppression and jaundice (both rare).

Hyponatraemia Hyponatraemia is an adverse effect due to inappropriate ADH secretion, and is more common in the elderly.

Contraindications

These include the following:

- epilepsy;
- recent myocardial infarction, heart block;
- mania;
- porphyria.

RELATED NON-TRICYCLIC ANTIDEPRESSANT DRUGS

This is a mixed group which includes 1-, 2- and 4-ring structured drugs with broadly similar properties. Characteristics of specific drugs are summarized below.

Maprotiline – sedative, with less antimuscarinic effects, but rashes are more common and fits are a significant risk.

Mianserin – blocks central α₂-adrenoceptors. It is sedative, with much fewer anticholinergic effects, but can cause postural hypotension and blood dyscrasias, particularly in the elderly. Full blood count must be monitored.

Lofepramine – less sedative, and with less cardiac toxicity, but occasionally hepatotoxic.

Mirtazapine – increases noradrenergic and serotonergic neurotransmission via central α_2 adrenoceptors. The increased release of 5HT stimulates $5HT_1$ receptors, whilst $5HT_2$ and $5HT_3$ receptors are blocked. H_1 receptors are also blocked. This combination of actions appears to be associated with antidepressant activity, anxiolytic and sedative effects. Reported adverse effects include increased appetite, weight gain, drowsiness, dry mouth and (rarely) blood dyscrasias.

Drug interactions

These include the following:

- antagonism of anti-epileptics;
- potentiation of sedation with alcohol and other central depressants;
- antihypertensives and diuretics increase orthostatic hypotension;
- hypertension and cardiac dysrhythmias with adrenaline, noradrenaline and ephedrine.

MONOAMINE OXIDASE INHIBITORS (MAOIs)

These drugs were little used for many years because of their toxicity, and particularly potentially lethal food and drug interactions causing hypertensive crises. Non-selective MAOIs should only be prescribed by specialists who are experienced in their use. They can be effective in some forms of refractory depression and anxiety states, for which they are generally reserved. The introduction of **moclobemide**, a reversible selective MAO-A inhibitor, may lead to more widespread use of this therapeutic class.

Tranylcypromine is the most hazardous MAOI because of its stimulant activity. The non-selective MAOIs of choice are **phenelzine** and **isocarboxazid**.

Uses

These include the following:

1. MAOIs can be used alone or (with close psychiatric supervision) with a TCA, in depression which has not responded to TCAs alone;
2. in phobic anxiety and depression with anxiety;
3. in patients with anxiety who have agoraphobia, panic attacks or multiple somatic symptoms;
4. hypochondria and hysterical symptoms may respond well;
5. for atypical depression with biological features such as hypersomnia, lethargy and hyperphagia.

Adverse effects

1. Common effects include orthostatic hypotension, weight gain, sexual dysfunction, headache and aggravation of migraine, insomnia, anticholinergic actions and oedema.
2. Rare and potentially fatal effects include hypertensive crisis and 5HT syndrome, psychotic reactions, hepatocellular necrosis, peripheral neuropathy and convulsions.
3. Stopping a MAOI is more likely to produce a withdrawal syndrome than is the case with tricyclics. The syndrome includes agitation, restlessness, panic attacks and insomnia.

Contraindications

These include the following:

- liver failure;
- cerebrovascular disease;
- phaeochromocytoma;
- porphyria;
- epilepsy.

Drug interactions

Many important interactions occur with MAOI. A treatment card for patients should be carried at all times, which describes precautions and lists some of the foods to be avoided. The interactions are as follows:

- hypertensive and hyperthermic reactions sufficient to cause fatal subarachnoid haemorrhage, particularly with **tranylcypromine**. Such serious reactions are precipitated by amines, including indirectly acting sympathomimetic agents such as tyramine (in cheese), dopamine (in broad bean pods and formed from levodopa), amines formed from any fermentation process (e.g. in yoghurt, beer, wine), **phenylephrine** (including that administered as nosedrops and in cold remedies), **ephedrine**, **amfetamine** (all can give hypertensive reactions), other amines, **pethidine** (excitement, hyperthermia), **levodopa** (hypertension) and tricyclic, tetracyclic and bicyclic antidepressants (excitement, hyperpyrexia). **Buspirone** should not be used with MAOIs. Hypertensive crisis may be treated with α-adrenoceptor blockade analogous to medical treatment of patients with phaeochromocytoma (see Chapter 40). Interactions of this type are much less likely to occur with **moclobemide**, as its MAO inhibition is reversible, competitive and selective for MAO-A, so that MAO-B is free to deaminate biogenic amines;
- failure to metabolize drugs that are normally oxidized, including opioids, benzodiazepines, alcohol (reactions with alcoholic drinks occur mainly because of their tyramine content). These drugs will have an exaggerated and prolonged effect;
- enhanced effects of oral hypoglycaemic agents, anaesthetics, suxamethonium, caffeine and anticholinergics (including benzhexol and similar anti-Parkinsonian drugs);
- antagonism of anti-epileptics;
- enhanced hypotension with antihypertensives;
- central nervous system (CNS) excitation and hypertension with **oxypertine** (an antipsychotic) and **tetrabenazine** (used for chorea);
- increased CNS toxicity with triptans ($5HT_1$ agonists) and with **sibutramine**.

Key points

Drug treatment of depression

- Initial drug treatment is usually with SSRIs, tricyclic antidepressants or related drugs.
- The choice is usually related to the side-effect profile of relevance to the particular patient.
- Tricyclic antidepressants are more dangerous in overdose.
- Tricyclic antidepressants commonly cause antimuscarinic and cardiac effects.
- Tricyclic antidepressants tend to increase appetite and weight, whereas SSRIs more commonly reduce appetite and weight.
- SSRIs are associated with nausea, sexual dysfunction and sleep disturbance.
- There is a variable delay (between ten days and four weeks) before therapeutic benefit is obtained.
- Following remission, antidepressant therapy should be continued for at least four to six months.

Key points

Antidepressant contraindications

- Tricyclic antidepressants – recent myocardial infarction, dysrhythmias, manic phase, severe liver disease.
- SSRIs – manic phase.
- Monamine oxidase inhibitors – acute confused state, phaeochromocytoma.
- Caution is needed – cardiac disease, epilepsy, pregnancy and breast-feeding, elderly, hepatic and renal impairment, thyroid disease, narrow-angle glaucoma, urinary retention, prostatism, porphyria, psychoses, electroconvulsive therapy (ECT) and anaesthesia.

LITHIUM, TRYPTOPHAN AND ST JOHN'S WORT

LITHIUM

Although **lithium** is widely used in affective disorders, it has a low toxic to therapeutic ratio, and serum concentration monitoring is essential. Serum is used rather than plasma because of possible problems due to lithium heparin, which is often used as an anticoagulant in blood sample tubes. Serum **lithium** levels fluctuate between doses and serum concentrations should be measured at a standard time, preferably 12 hours after the previous dose. This measurement is made frequently until steady state is attained and is then made every three months, unless some intercurrent event occurs that could cause toxicity (e.g. desal-ination or diuretic therapy).

Use

Lithium is effective in acute mania, but its action is slow (one to two weeks), so antipsychotic drugs, such as **haloperidol**, are preferred in this situation (see Chapter 19). Its main use is in prophylaxis in unipolar and bipolar affective illness

(therapeutic serum levels 0.4–1 mmol/L). **Lithium** is also used on its own or with another antidepressant in refractory depression to terminate a depressive episode or to prevent recurrences and aggressive or self-mutilating behaviour.

Patients should avoid major dietary changes that alter sodium intake and maintain an adequate water intake.

Different **lithium** preparations have different bioavailabilities, so the form should not be changed.

Mechanism of action

Lithium increases 5HT actions in the CNS. It acts as a $5HT_{1A}$ agonist and is also a $5HT_2$ antagonist. This may be the basis for its antidepressant activity and may explain why it increases the CNS toxicity of selective 5HT uptake inhibitors.

The basic biochemical activity of **lithium** is not known. It has actions on two second messengers.

1. Hormone stimulation of adenylyl cyclase is inhibited, so that hormone-stimulated cyclic adenosine monophosphate (cAMP) production is reduced. This probably underlies some of the adverse effects of **lithium**, such as goitre and nephrogenic diabetes insipidus, since thyroid-stimulating hormone (TSH) and antidiuretic hormone activate adenylyl cyclase in thyroid and collecting duct cells, respectively. The relevance of this to its therapeutic effect is uncertain.
2. **Lithium** at a concentration of 1 mmol/L inhibits hydrolysis of myoinositol phosphate in the brain, so **lithium** may reduce the cellular content of phosphatidyl inositides, thereby altering the sensitivity of neurones to neurotransmitters that work on receptors linked to phospholipase C (including muscarinic and α-adrenoceptors).

From these actions, it is clear that **lithium** can modify a wide range of neurotransmitter effects, yet its efficacy both in mania and in depression indicates a subtlety of action that is currently unexplained, but may be related to activation of the brain stem raphe nuclei.

Adverse effects

1. When monitored regularly **lithium** is reasonably safe in the medium term. However, adverse effects occur even in the therapeutic range – in particular, tremor, weight gain, oedema, polyuria, nausea and loose bowels.
2. Above the therapeutic range, tremor coarsens, diarrhoea becomes more severe and ataxia and dysarthria appear. Higher levels cause gross ataxia, coma, fits, cardiac dysrhythmias and death. Serum **lithium** concentrations greater than 1.5 mmol/L may be dangerous and if greater than 2 mmol/L, are usually associated with serious toxicity.
3. Goitre, hypothyroidism and exacerbation of psoriasis are less common.
4. Renal tubular damage has been described in association with prolonged use.

Contraindications

These include the following:

- renal disease;
- cardiac disease;
- sodium-losing states (e.g. Addison's disease, diarrhoea, vomiting);
- myasthenia gravis;
- during surgical operations;
- avoid when possible during pregnancy and breast-feeding.

Pharmacokinetics

Lithium is readily absorbed after oral administration and injectable preparations are not available. Peak serum concentrations occur three to five hours after dosing. The $t_{1/2}$ varies with age because of the progressive decline in glomerular filtration rate, being 18–20 hours in young adults and up to 36 hours in healthy elderly people. Sustained-release preparations are available, but in view of the long $t_{1/2}$ they are not kinetically justified. **Lithium** takes several days to reach steady state and the first samples for serum level monitoring should be taken after about one week unless loading doses are given. **Lithium** elimination is almost entirely renal. Like sodium, **lithium** does not bind to plasma protein, and it readily passes into the glomerular filtrate; 70–80% is reabsorbed in the proximal tubules but, unlike sodium, there is no distal tubular reabsorption and its elimination is not directly altered by diuretics acting on the distal tubule. However, states such as sodium deficiency and sodium diuresis increase **lithium** retention (and cause toxicity) by stimulating proximal tubular sodium and **lithium** reabsorption. An important implication of the renal handling of **lithium** is that neither loop diuretics, thiazides nor potassium-sparing diuretics can enhance **lithium** loss in a toxic patient, but all of them do enhance its toxicity. Dialysis reduces elevated serum **lithium** concentration effectively.

Drug interactions

- **Lithium** concentration in the serum is increased by diuretics and non-steroidal anti-inflammatory drugs.
- **Lithium** toxicity is increased by concomitant administration of **haloperidol**, serotonin uptake inhibitors, calcium antagonists (e.g. **diltiazem**) and anticonvulsants (**phenytoin** and **carbamazepine**) without a change in serum concentration.
- **Lithium** increases the incidence of extrapyramidal effects of antipsychotics.

L-TRYPTOPHAN

Tryptophan is the amino acid precursor of 5HT. On its own or with other antidepressants or **lithium** it sometimes benefits refractory forms of depression. However, L-tryptophan should only be initiated under specialist supervision because of its association with an eosinophilic myalgic syndrome characterized by intense and incapacitating fatigue, myalgia and eosinophilia. Arthralgia, fever, cough, dyspnoea and rash may also develop over several weeks. A few patients develop myocarditis.

ST JOHN'S WORT

St John's wort (*Hypericum perforatum*) is an unlicensed herbal remedy in popular use for treating depression (Chapter 17). However, it can induce drug-metabolizing enzymes, and many important drug interactions have been identified, including with antidepressant drugs, with which St John's wort should therefore not be given. The amount of active ingredient can vary between different preparations, thus changing the preparation can alter the degree of such interactions. Importantly, when St John's wort is discontinued, the concentrations of interacting drugs may increase.

SPECIAL GROUPS

THE ELDERLY

Depression is common in the elderly, in whom it tends to be chronic and has a high rate of recurrence. Treatment with drugs is made more difficult because of slow metabolism and sensitivity to anticholinergic effects. Lower doses are therefore needed than in younger patients.

Lack of response may indicate true refractoriness of the depression, or sadness due to social isolation or bereavement. The possibility of underlying disease, such as hypothyroidism (the incidence of which increases with age), should be considered.

Lofepramine and SSRIs cause fewer problems in patients with prostatism or glaucoma than do the tricyclic antidepressants because they have less antimuscarinic action. Dizziness and falls due to orthostatic hypotension are less common with **nortriptyline** than with **imipramine**. **Mianserin** has fewer anticholinergic effects, but blood dyscrasias occur in about one in 4000 patients and postural hypotension can be severe.

EPILEPSY

No currently used antidepressive is entirely safe in epilepsy, but SSRIs are less likely to cause fits than the amitriptyline group, **mianserin** or **maprotiline**.

Case history

A 75-year-old woman with endogenous depression is treated with amitriptyline. After three weeks, she appears to be responding, but then seems to become increasingly drowsy and confused. She is brought to the Accident and Emergency Department following a series of convulsions.
Question
What is the likely cause of her drowsiness, confusion and convulsions?
Answer
Hyponatraemia.
Comment
Hyponatraemia (usually in the elderly) has been associated with all types of antidepressant but most frequently with SSRIs.

Case history

A 45-year-old man with agoraphobia, anxiety and depression associated with hypochondriacal features is treated with phenelzine. He has no history of hypertension. He is seen in the Accident and Emergency Department because of a throbbing headache and palpitations. On examination he is hypertensive 260/120 mmHg with a heart rate of 40 beats/minute. He is noted to have nasal congestion.

Question 1

What is the likely diagnosis?

Question 2

What is the most appropriate treatment?

Answer 1

Hypertensive crisis, possibly secondary to taking a cold cure containing an indirectly acting sympathomimetic.

Answer 2

Phentolamine, a short-acting alpha-blocker, may be given by intravenous injection, with repeat doses titrated against response.

FURTHER READING

Aronson SC, Ayres VD. Depression: a treatment algorithm for the family physician. *Hospital Physician* 2000; **44**: 21–38.

Ebmeier KP, Donaghey C, Steele JD. Recent developments and current controversies in depression. *The Lancet* 2005; **367**: 153–67.

CHAPTER 21

MOVEMENT DISORDERS AND DEGENERATIVE CNS DISEASE

PARKINSON'S SYNDROME AND ITS TREATMENT

PATHOPHYSIOLOGY

James Parkinson first described the tremor, rigidity and bradykinesia/akinesia that characterize the syndrome known as Parkinson's disease. Most cases of Parkinson's disease are caused by idiopathic degeneration of the nigrostriatal pathway. Atherosclerotic, toxic (e.g. related to antipsychotic drug treatment, manganese or carbon monoxide poisoning) and post-encephalitic cases also occur. Treatment of parkinsonism caused by antipsychotic drugs differs from treatment of the idiopathic disease, but other aetiologies are treated similarly to the idiopathic disease. Parkinsonian symptoms manifest after loss of 80% or more of the nerve cells in the substantia nigra. The nigrostriatal projection consists of very fine nerve fibres travelling from the substantia nigra to the corpus striatum. This pathway is dopaminergic and inhibitory, and the motor projections to the putamen are more affected than either those to the cognitive areas or to the limbic and hypolimbic regions (Figure 21.1). Other fibres terminating in the corpus striatum include excitatory cholinergic nerves and noradrenergic and serotoninergic fibres, and these are also affected, but to varying extents, and the overall effect is a complex imbalance between inhibitory and excitatory influences.

Parkinsonism arises because of deficient neural transmission at postsynaptic D_2 receptors, but it appears that stimulation of both D_1 and D_2 is required for optimal response. D_1 receptors activate adenylyl cyclase, which increases intracellular cyclic adenosine monophosphate (cAMP). The antagonistic effects of dopamine and acetylcholine within the striatum have suggested that parkinsonism results from an imbalance between these neurotransmitters (Figure 21.2). The therapeutic basis for treating parkinsonism is to increase dopaminergic activity or to reduce the effects of acetylcholine. 1-Methyl-4-phenyl-1,2,5,6-tetrahydropyridine (MPTP) has been used illicitly as a drug of abuse and it causes severe parkinsonism. MPTP is converted by monoamine oxidase-B (MAO-B) in neuronal mitochondria to a toxic free-radical metabolite (MPP^+), which is specifically toxic to dopamine-producing cells. This led to the hypothesis that idiopathic Parkinson's disease may be due to chronically increased free-radical damage to the cells of the substantia nigra. However, clinical studies of anti-oxidants have so far been disappointing.

The free-radical hypothesis has raised the worrying possibility that treatment with levodopa (see below) could accelerate disease progression by increasing free-radical formation as the drug is metabolized in the remaining nigro-striatal nerve fibres. This is consistent with the clinical impression of some neurologists, but in the absence of randomized clinical trials it is difficult to tell whether clinical deterioration is due to the natural history of the disease or is being accelerated by the therapeutic agent.

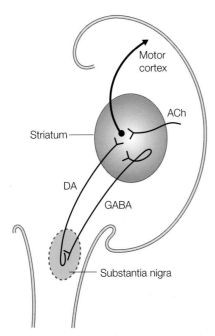

Figure 21.1: Representation of relationships between cholinergic (ACh), dopaminergic (DA) and GABA-producing neurones in the basal ganglia.

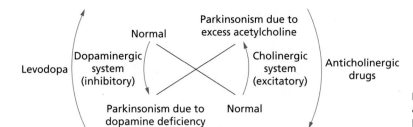

Figure 21.2: Antagonistic actions of the dopaminergic and cholinergic systems in the pathogenesis of parkinsonian symptoms.

PRINCIPLES OF TREATMENT IN PARKINSONISM

Idiopathic Parkinson's disease is a progressive disorder, and is treated with drugs that relieve symptoms and if possible slow disease progression. Treatment is usually initiated when symptoms disrupt normal daily activities. Initial treatment is often with a dopamine receptor agonist, e.g. **bromocriptine**, particularly in younger (<70) patients. A levodopa/decarboxy-lase inhibitor combination is commonly used in patients with definite disability. The dose is titrated to produce optimal results. Occasionally, **amantadine** or anticholinergics may be useful as monotherapy in early disease, especially in younger patients when tremor is the dominant symptom. In patients on levodopa the occurrence of motor fluctuations (on–off phenomena) heralds a more severe phase of the illness. Initially, such fluctuations may be controlled by giving more frequent doses of levodopa (or a sustained-release preparation). The addition of either a dopamine receptor agonist (one of the non-ergot derivatives, e.g. **ropinirole**) or one of the calechol-*O*-methyl transferase (COMT) inhibitors (e.g. **entacapone, tolcapone**) to the drug regimen may improve mobility. In addition, this usually allows dose reduction of the levodopa, while improving 'end-of-dose' effects and improving motor fluctuations. If on–off phenomena are refractory, the dopamine agonist **apomorphine** can terminate 'off' periods, but its use is complex (see below). **Selegiline**, a MAO-B inhibitor, may reduce the end-of-dose deterioration in advanced disease. Physiotherapy and psychological support are helpful. The experimental approach of implantation of stem cells into the substantia nigra of severely affected parkinsonian patients (perhaps with low-dose immunosuppression) is being investigated. The potential of stereotactic unilateral pallidotomy, for severe refractory cases of Parkinson's disease is being re-evaluated.

Drugs that cause parkinsonism, notably conventional antipsychotic drugs (e.g. **chlorpromazine, haloperidol**) (see Chapter 19) are withdrawn if possible, or substituted by the

newer 'atypical' antipsychotics (e.g. **risperidone** or **olanzapine**), since these have a lower incidence of extrapyramidal side effects. Antimuscarinic drugs (e.g. **trihexyphenidyl**) are useful if changing the drug/reducing the dose is not therapeutically acceptable, whereas drugs that increase dopaminergic transmission are contraindicated because of their effect on psychotic symptoms.

ANTI-PARKINSONIAN DRUGS

DRUGS AFFECTING THE DOPAMINERGIC SYSTEM

Dopaminergic activity can be enhanced by:

- **levodopa** with a peripheral dopa decarboxylase inhibitor;
- increasing release of endogenous dopamine;
- stimulation of dopamine receptors;
- inhibition of catechol-*O*-methyl transferase;
- inhibition of monoamine oxidase type B.

LEVODOPA AND DOPA DECARBOXYLASE INHIBITORS
Use

Levodopa (unlike dopamine) can enter nerve terminals in the basal ganglia where it undergoes decarboxylation to form dopamine. **Levodopa** is used in combination with a peripheral (extracerebral) dopa decarboxylase inhibitor (e.g. **carbidopa** or **benserazide**). This allows a four- to five-fold reduction in **levodopa** dose and the incidence of vomiting and dysrhythmias is reduced. However, central adverse effects (e.g. hallucinations) are (predictably) as common as when larger doses of **levodopa** are given without a dopa decarboxylase inhibitor.

Combined preparations (**co-careldopa** or **co-beneldopa**) are appropriate for idiopathic Parkinson's disease. (**Levodopa** is contraindicated in schizophrenia and must not be used for parkinsonism caused by antipsychotic drugs.) Combined preparations are given three times daily starting at a low dose, increased initially after two weeks and then reviewed at intervals of six to eight weeks. Without dopa decarboxylase inhibitors, 95% of **levodopa** is metabolized outside the brain. In their presence, plasma **levodopa** concentrations rise (Figure 21.3), excretion of dopamine and its metabolites falls, and the availability of **levodopa** within the brain for conversion to dopamine increases. The two available inhibitors are similar.

Adverse effects

These include the following:

- nausea and vomiting;
- postural hypotension – this usually resolves after a few weeks, but excessive hypotension may result if antihypertensive treatment is given concurrently;

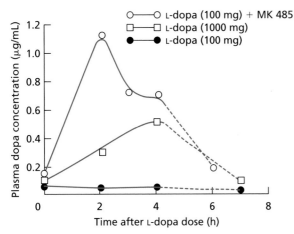

Figure 21.3: Increased plasma dopa concentrations following combination with a peripheral dopa decarboxylase inhibitor (MK 485) in one patient. (Redrawn with permission from Dunner DL et al. *Clinical Pharmacology and Therapeutics* 1971; **12**: 213.)

- involuntary movements (dystonic reactions) – these include akathisia (abnormal restlessness and inability to keep still), chorea and jerking of the limbs (myoclonus). Involuntary movements may become worse as treatment is continued, and may necessitate drug withdrawal;
- psychological disturbance, including vivid dreams, agitation, paranoia, confusion and hallucinations;
- cardiac dysrhythmias;
- endocrine effects of **levodopa**, including stimulation of growth hormone and suppression of prolactin.
- sedation and sudden onset of sleep (avoid driving at onset of treatment and if these symptoms recur).

Pharmacokinetics

Levodopa is absorbed from the proximal small intestine and is metabolized both by decarboxylases in the intestinal wall and by the gut flora. Oral absorption is variable. Absorption/bioavailability are improved by co-administration of decarboxylase inhibitors. Addition of a COMT inhibitor further increases $t_{1/2}$ and AUC.

Drug interactions

Monoamine oxidase inhibitors can produce hypertension if given concurrently with **levodopa**. The hypotensive actions of other drugs are potentiated by **levodopa**.

INCREASED RELEASE OF ENDOGENOUS DOPAMINE

AMANTADINE

Use

Amantadine has limited efficacy, but approximately 60% of patients experience some benefit. Severe toxicity is rare.

Mechanism of action

Endogenous dopamine release is stimulated by **amantadine**, which also inhibits reuptake of dopamine into nerve terminals.

Adverse effects

These include the following:

- peripheral oedema;
- gastro-intestinal upset and dry mouth;
- livedo reticularis;
- CNS toxicity – nightmares, insomnia, dizziness, hallucinations, convulsions;
- leukopenia (uncommon).

Pharmacokinetics

The $t_{1/2}$ of **amantadine** varies from 10 to 30 hours, so steady-state concentrations are reached after four to seven days of treatment. About 95% is eliminated by the kidneys and it should not be used in patients with renal failure.

DOPAMINE RECEPTOR AGONISTS

Uses

Dopamine receptor agonists are used as initial therapy or as adjuncts to levodopa–dopa decarboxylase inhibitor combinations in patients with severe motor fluctuations (on–off phenomena). Dopamine agonists share many of their adverse effects with **levodopa**, particularly nausea due to stimulation of dopamine receptors in the chemoreceptor trigger zone. This brain region is unusual in that it is accessible to drugs in the systemic circulation, so **domperidone** (a dopamine antagonist that does not cross the blood–brain barrier) prevents this symptom without blocking dopamine receptors in the striatum, and hence worsening the movement disorder. Neuropsychiatric disorders are more frequent than with **levodopa** monotherapy. (See also Chapter 42 for use in pituitary disorders, and Chapter 41 for use in suppression of lactation). Pulmonary, retroperitoneal and pericardial fibrotic reactions have been associated with some ergot-derived dopamine agonists. Dopamine receptor agonists are started at a low dose that is gradually titrated upwards depending on efficacy and tolerance. If added to **levodopa**, the dose of the latter may be reduced.

Ergot derivatives include **bromocriptine**, **lisuride**, **pergolide** and **cabergoline**. Other licensed dopamine agonists include **pramipexole**, **ropinirole** and **rotigotine**.

There is great individual variation in the efficacy of dopamine receptor agonists. The initial dose is gradually titrated upwards depending on response and adverse effects.

Adverse effects

These are primarily due to D_2 agonist activity, although $5HT_1$ and $5HT_2$ effects are also relevant.

- gastro-intestinal – nausea and vomiting, constipation or diarrhoea;
- central nervous system – headache, drowsiness, confusion, psychomotor excitation, hallucination;
- orthostatic hypotension (particularly in the elderly), syncope;
- cardiac dysrhythmias – bradycardia;

- pulmonary, retroperitoneal and pericardial fibrotic reactions have been associated with the ergot-derived dopamine agonists (**bromocriptine**, **cabergoline**, **lisuride** and **pergolide**).

APOMORPHINE

Apomorphine is a powerful dopamine agonist at both D_1 and D_2 receptors, and is used in patients with refractory motor oscillations (on–off phenomena). It is difficult to use, necessitating specialist input. The problems stem from its pharmacokinetics and from side effects of severe nausea and vomiting. The gastrointestinal side effects can be controlled with **domperidone**. **Apomorphine** is started in hospital after pretreatment with **domperidone** for at least three days, and withholding other antiparkinsonian treatment at night to provoke an 'off' attack. The subcutaneous dose is increased and when the individual dose requirement has been established, with reintroduction of other drugs if necessary, administration is sometimes changed from intermittent dosing to subcutaneous infusion via a syringe pump, with patient-activated extra boluses if needed. **Apomorphine** is extensively hepatically metabolized and is given parenterally. The mean plasma $t_{1/2}$ is approximately 30 minutes.

CATECHOL-O-METHYL TRANSFERASE INHIBITORS

Use

Tolcapone and **entacapone** are used for adjunctive therapy in patients who are already taking L-dopa/dopa decarboxylase inhibitor combinations with unsatisfactory control (e.g. end-of-dose deterioration). These agents improve symptoms with less on–off fluctuations, as well as reducing the **levodopa** dose requirement by 20–30%. Adverse effects arising from increased availability of L-dopa centrally can be minimized by decreasing the dose of **levodopa** combination treatment prospectively. Because of hepatotoxicity associated with **tolcapone** it is only used by specialists when **entacapone** is ineffective as an adjunctive treatment.

Mechanism of action

Reversible competitive inhibition of COMT, thereby reducing metabolism of L-dopa and increasing its availability within nigrostriatal nerve fibres. It is relatively specific for central nervous system (CNS) COMT, with little effect on the peripheral COMT, thus causing increased brain concentrations of L-dopa, while producing less of an increase in plasma concentration.

Adverse effects

These include the following:

- nausea, vomiting, diarrhoea and constipation;
- increased **levodopa**-related side effects;
- neuroleptic malignant syndrome;
- dizziness;
- hepatitis – rare with **entacapone**, but potentially life-threatening with **tolcapone** (liver function testing is mandatory before and during treatment);
- urine discolouration.

Pharmacokinetics

Tolcapone is rapidly absorbed and is cleared by hepatic metabolism. At recommended doses it produces approximately 80–90% inhibition of central COMT.

Drug interactions

Apomorphine is metabolized by *O*-methylation, so interaction with COMT inhibitors is to be anticipated. COMT inhibitors should not be administered with MAOIs, as blockade of both pathways of monoamine metabolism simultaneously has the potential to enhance the effects of endogenous and exogenous amines and other drugs unpredictably.

MONOAMINE OXIDASE INHIBITORS – TYPE B

SELEGILINE AND RASAGILINE

Use

Initial small controlled studies in Parkinson's disease reported that disease progression was slowed in patients treated with **selegiline** alone, delaying the need to start **levodopa**. Larger-scale studies have not confirmed this conclusion. MAO type B inhibitors, such as **selegiline** and **rasagiline**, may be used in conjunction with **levodopa** to reduce end-of-dose deterioration.

Mechanism of action

There are two forms of monoamine oxidase (MAO), namely type A (substrates include 5-hydroxytryptamine and tyramine) and type B (substrates include phenylethylamine). MAO-B, is mainly localized in neuroglia. MAO-A metabolizes endogenous adrenaline, noradrenaline and 5-hydroxytryptamine, while the physiological role of MAO-B is unclear. Both isoenzymes metabolize dopamine. Inhibition of MAO-B raises brain dopamine levels without affecting other major transmitter amines. Because **selegiline** and **rasagiline** selectively inhibit MAO-B, they are much less likely to produce a hypertensive reaction with cheese or other sources of tyramine than non-selective MAOIs, such as **phenelzine**.

Adverse effects

Selegiline is generally well tolerated, but side effects include the following:

- agitation and involuntary movements;
- confusion, insomnia and hallucinations;
- nausea, dry mouth, vertigo;
- peptic ulceration.

Pharmacokinetics

Oral **selegiline** is well absorbed (100%), but is extensively metabolized by the liver, first to an active metabolite, desmethylselegiline (which also inhibits MAO-B) and then to amphetamine and metamphetamine. Its plasma $t_{1/2}$ is long (approximately 39 h).

Drug interactions

At very high doses (six times the therapeutic dose), MAO-B selectivity is lost and pressor responses to tyramine are potentiated. Hypertensive reactions to tyramine-containing products (e.g. cheese or yeast extract) have been described, but are rare. **Amantadine** and centrally active antimuscarinic agents potenti-ate the anti-parkinsonian effects of **selegiline**. **Levodopa**-induced postural hypotension may be potentiated.

DRUGS AFFECTING THE CHOLINERGIC SYSTEM

MUSCARINIC RECEPTOR ANTAGONISTS

Use

Muscarinic antagonists (e.g. **trihexyphenidyl, benzatropine, orphenadrine, procyclidine**) are effective in the treatment of parkinsonian tremor and – to a lesser extent – rigidity, but produce only a slight improvement in bradykinesia. They are usually given in divided doses, which are increased every two to five days until optimum benefit is achieved or until adverse effects occur. Their main use is in patients with parkinsonism caused by antipsychotic agents.

Mechanism of action

Non-selective muscarinic receptor antagonism is believed to restore, in part, the balance between dopaminergic/cholinergic pathways in the striatum.

Key points

Treatment of Parkinson's disease

- A combination of levodopa and a dopa-decarboxylase inhibitor (carbidopa or benserazide) or a dopamine agonist (e.g. ropinirole) are standard first-line therapies.
- Dopamine agonists and COMT inhibitors (e.g. entacapone) are helpful as adjuvant drugs for patients with loss of effect at the end of the dose interval, and to reduce 'on–off' motor fluctuations.
- The benefit of early treatment with an MAO-B inhibitor, selegiline, to retard disease progression is unproven, and it may even increase mortality.
- Polypharmacy is almost inevitable in patients with longstanding disease.
- Ultimately, disease progression requires increasing drug doses with a regrettable but inevitable increased incidence of side effects, especially involuntary movements and psychosis.
- Anticholinergic drugs reduce tremor, but dose-limiting CNS side effects are common, especially in the elderly. These drugs are first-line treatment for parkinsonism caused by indicated (essential) antipsychotic drugs.

Adverse effects

These include the following:

- dry mouth, blurred vision, constipation;
- precipitation of glaucoma or urinary retention – they are therefore contraindicated in narrow angle glaucoma and in men with prostatic hypertrophy;
- cognitive impairment, confusion, excitement or psychosis, especially in the elderly.

Pharmacokinetics

Table 21.1 lists some drugs of this type that are in common use, together with their major pharmacokinetic properties.

SPASTICITY

Spasticity is an increase in muscle tone, for example, due to damage to upper motor neurone pathways following stroke or in demyelinating disease. It can be painful and disabling. Treatment is seldom very effective. Physiotherapy, limited surgical release procedures or local injection of botulinum toxin (see below) all have a role to play. Drugs that reduce spasticity include **diazepam, baclofen, tizanidine** and **dantrolene**, but they have considerable limitations.

Diazepam (see Chapter 18, **Hypnotics and anxiolytics**) facili-tates γ-aminobutyric acid (GABA) action. Although spasticity and flexor spasms may be diminished, sedating doses are often needed to produce this effect.

Baclofen facilitates GABA-B receptors and also reduces spasticity. Less sedation is produced than by equi-effective doses of **diazepam**, but **baclofen** can cause vertigo, nausea and hypotension. Abrupt withdrawal may precipitate hyperactivity, convulsions and autonomic dysfunction. There is specialist interest in chronic administration of low doses of **baclofen** intrathecally via implanted intrathecal cannulae in selected patients in order to maximize efficacy without causing side effects.

Dantrolene (a ryanodine receptor antagonist) is generally less useful for symptoms of spasticity than **baclofen** because muscle power is reduced as spasticity is relieved. It is used intravenously to treat malignant hyperthermia and the neuroleptic malignant syndrome, for both of which it is uniquely effective (see Chapter 24). Its adverse effects include:

- drowsiness, vertigo, malaise, weakness and fatigue;
- diarrhoea;
- increased serum potassium levels.

Table 21.1: Common muscarinic receptor antagonists, dosing and pharmacokinetics

Drug	Route of administration	Half-life (hours)	Metabolism and excretion	Special features
Trihexyphenidyl	Oral	3–7	Hepatic	
Orphenadrine	Oral	13.7–16.1	Hepatic-active metabolite	Central stimulation
Procyclidine	Oral	12.6	Hepatic	

CHOREA

The γ-aminobutyric acid content in the basal ganglia is reduced in patients with Huntington's disease. Dopamine receptor antagonists (e.g. **haloperidol**) or **tetrabenazine** suppress the choreiform movements in these patients, but dopamine antagonists are best avoided, as they themselves may induce dyskinesias. **Tetrabenazine** is therefore preferred. It depletes neuronal terminals of dopamine and serotonin. It can cause severe dose-related depression. **Diazepam** may be a useful alternative, but there is no effective treatment for the dementia and other manifestations of Huntington's disease.

DRUG-INDUCED DYSKINESIAS

- The most common drug-induced movement disorders are 'extrapyramidal symptoms' related to dopamine receptor blockade.
- The most frequently implicated drugs are the 'conventional' antipsychotics (e.g. **haloperidol** and **fluphenazine**). **Metoclopramide**, an anti-emetic, also blocks dopamine receptors and causes dystonias.
- Acute dystonias can be effectively treated with parenteral benzodiazepine (e.g. **diazepam**) or anticholinergic (e.g. **procyclidine**).
- Tardive dyskinesia may be permanent.
- Extrapyramidal symptoms are less common with the newer 'atypical' antipsychotics (e.g. **olanzapine** or **aripiprazole**).

NON-DOPAMINE-RELATED MOVEMENT DISORDERS

- 'Cerebellar' ataxia – ethanol, **phenytoin**
- Tremor
  - β-Adrenoceptor agonists, e.g. **salbutamol**;
  - caffeine;
  - **thyroxine**;
  - SSRIs, e.g. **fluoxetine**;
  - **valproate**;
  - withdrawal of alcohol and benzodiazepines.
- vestibular toxicity – aminoglycosides;
- myasthenia – aminoglycosides;
- proximal myopathy – ethanol, corticosteroids;
- myositis – lipid-lowering agents – statins, fibrates;
- tenosynovitis – fluoroquinolones.

TREATMENT OF OTHER MOVEMENT DISORDERS

TICS AND IDIOPATHIC DYSTONIAS

Botulinum A toxin is one of seven distinct neurotoxins produced by *Clostridium botulinum* and it is a glycoprotein. It is used by neurologists to treat hemifacial spasm, blepharospasm, cervical dystonia (torticollis), jaw-closing oromandibular dystonia and adductor laryngeal dysphonia. Botulinum A toxin is given by local injection into affected muscles, the injection site being best localized by electromyography. Recently, it has also proved successful in the treatment of achalasia. Injection of botulinum A toxin into a muscle weakens it by irreversibly blocking the release of acetylcholine at the neuromuscular junction. Muscles injected with botulinum A toxin atrophy and become weak over a period of 2–20 days and recover over two to four months as new axon terminals sprout and restore transmission. Repeated injections can then be given. The best long-term treatment plan has not yet been established. Symptoms are seldom abolished and adjuvant conventional therapy should be given. Adverse effects due to toxin spread causing weakness of nearby muscles and local autonomic dysfunction can occur. In the neck, this may cause dysphagia and aspiration into the lungs. Electromyography has detected evidence of systemic spread of the toxin, but generalized weakness does not occur with standard doses. Occasionally, a flu-like reaction with brachial neuritis has been reported, suggesting an acute immune response to the toxin. Neutralizing antibodies to botulinum toxin A cause loss of efficacy in up to 10% of patients. Botulinum B toxin does not cross-react with neutralizing antibodies to botulinum toxin A, and is effective in patients with torticollis who have botulinum toxin A-neutralizing antibodies. The most common use of botulinum is now cosmetic.

AMYOTROPHIC LATERAL SCLEROSIS (MOTOR NEURONE DISEASE)

Riluzole is used to extend life or time to mechanical ventilation in patients with the amyotrophic lateral sclerosis (ALS) form of motor neurone disease (MND). It acts by inhibiting the presynaptic release of glutamate. Side effects include nausea, vomiting, dizziness, vertigo, tachycardia, paraesthesia and liver toxicity.

MYASTHENIA GRAVIS

PATHOPHYSIOLOGY

Myasthenia gravis is a syndrome of increased fatiguability and weakness of striated muscle, and it results from an autoimmune process with antibodies to nicotinic acetylcholine receptors. These interact with postsynaptic nicotinic cholinoceptors at the neuromuscular junction. (Such antibodies may be passively transferred via purified immunoglobulin or across the placenta to produce a myasthenic neonate.) Antibodies vary from one patient to another, and are often directed against receptor-protein domains distinct from the acetylcholine-binding site. Nonetheless, they interfere with neuromuscular transmission by reducing available receptors, by increasing receptor turnover by activating complement and/or cross-linking adjacent receptors. Endplate potentials are reduced in amplitude, and in some fibres may be below the threshold for initiating a muscle action potential, thus reducing the force of contraction of the muscle. The precise stimulus for the production of the antireceptor antibodies is not known, although since antigens in the thymus cross-react with acetylcholine receptors, it is possible that these are responsible for autosensitization in some cases.

Diagnosis is aided by the use of **edrophonium**, a short-acting inhibitor of acetylcholinesterase, which produces a transient increase in muscle power in patients with myasthenia gravis. The initial drug therapy of myasthenia consists of oral anticholinesterase drugs, usually **neostigmine**. If the disease is non-responsive or progressive, then thymectomy or immunosuppressant therapy with glucocorticosteroids and **azathioprine** are needed. Thymectomy is beneficial in patients with associated thymoma and in patients with generalized disease who can withstand the operation. It reduces the number of circulating T-lymphocytes that are capable of assisting B-lymphocytes to produce antibody, and a fall in antibody titre occurs after thymectomy, albeit slowly. Corticosteroids and immunosuppressive drugs also reduce circulating T cells. Plasmapheresis or infusion of intravenous immunoglobulin is useful in emergencies, producing a striking short-term clinical improvement in a few patients.

ANTICHOLINESTERASE DRUGS

The defect in neuromuscular transmission may be redressed by cholinesterase inhibitors that inhibit synaptic acetylcholine breakdown and increase the concentration of transmitters available to stimulate the nictonic receptor at the motor end plate.

Neostigmine is initially given orally eight-hourly, but usually requires more frequent administration (up to two-hourly) because of its short duration of action (two to six hours). It is rapidly inactivated in the gut. Cholinesterase inhibitors enhance both muscarinic and nicotinic cholinergic effects. The former results in increased bronchial secretions, abdominal colic, diarrhoea, miosis, nausea, hypersalivation and lachrymation. Excessive muscarinic effects may be blocked by giving **atropine** or **propantheline**, but this increases the risk of overdosage and consequent cholinergic crisis.

Pyridostigmine has a more prolonged action than **neostigmine** and it is seldom necessary to give it more frequently than four-hourly. The effective dose varies considerably between individual patients.

ADJUVANT DRUG THERAPY

Remissions of myasthenic symptoms are produced by oral administration of **prednisolone**. Increased weakness may occur at the beginning of treatment, which must therefore be instituted in hospital. This effect has been minimized by the use of alternate-day therapy. **Azathioprine** (see Chapter 50) has been used either on its own or combined with glucocorticosteroids for its 'corticosteroid-sparing' effect.

MYASTHENIC AND CHOLINERGIC CRISIS

Severe weakness leading to paralysis may result from either a deficiency (myasthenic crisis) or an excess (cholinergic crisis) of acetylcholine at the neuromuscular junction. Clinically, the distinction may be difficult, but it is assisted by the **edrophonium** test.

Edrophonium, a short-acting cholinesterase inhibitor, is given intravenously, and is very useful in diagnosis and for differentiating a myasthenic crisis from a cholinergic one. It transiently improves a myasthenic crisis and aggravates a cholinergic crisis. Because of its short duration of action, any deterioration of a cholinergic crisis is unlikely to have serious consequences, although facilities for artificial ventilation must be available. In this setting, it is important that the strength of essential (respiratory or bulbar) muscles be monitored using simple respiratory spirometric measurements (FEV_1 and FVC) during the test, rather than the strength of non-essential (limb or ocular) muscles.

Myasthenic crises may develop as a spontaneous deterioration in the natural history of the disease, or as a result of infection or surgery, or be exacerbated due to concomitant drug therapy with the following agents:

- aminoglycosides (e.g. **gentamicin**);
- other antibiotics, including **erythromycin**;
- myasthenics demonstrate increased sensitivity to non-depolarizing neuromuscular-blocking drugs;
- anti-dysrhythmic drugs, which reduce the excitability of the muscle membrane, and **quinidine** (**quinine**), **lidocaine**, **procainamide** and **propranolol**, which may increase weakness;
- benzodiazepines, due to their respiratory depressant effects and inhibition of muscle tone.

TREATMENT
Myasthenic crisis

Myasthenic crisis is treated with intramuscular **neostigmine**, repeated every 20 minutes with frequent **edrophonium** tests. Mechanical ventilation may be needed.

Key points

Myasthenia gravis

- Auto-antibodies to nicotinic acetylcholine receptors lead to increased receptor degradation and neuromuscular blockade.
- Treatment is with an oral anticholinesterase (e.g. **neostigmine** or **physostigmine**). Over- or under-treatment both lead to increased weakness ('cholinergic' and 'myasthenic' crises, respectively).
- Cholinergic and myasthenic crises are differentiated by administering a short-acting anticholinesterase, intravenous **edrophonium**. This test transiently improves a myasthenic crisis while transiently worsening a cholinergic crisis, allowing the appropriate dose adjustment to be made safely.
- Immunotherapy with **azathioprine** and/or corticosteroids or thymectomy may be needed in severe cases.
- Weakness is exacerbated by aminoglycosides or **erythromycin** and patients are exquisitely sensitive to non-depolarizing neuromuscular blocking drugs (e.g. **vecuronium**).

Cholinergic crisis

Treatment of myasthenia with anticholinesterases can be usefully monitored clinically by observation of the pupil (a diameter of 2 mm or less in normal lighting suggests overdose). Overdosage produces a cholinergic crisis, and further drug should be withheld.

ALZHEIMER'S DISEASE

Alzheimer's disease (AD) is the most common cause of dementia. Its incidence increases with age. It is estimated that approximately 500 000 people in the USA are affected. The symptoms of Alzheimer's disease are progressive memory impairment associated with a decline in language, visuospatial function, calculation and judgement. Ultimately, this leads to major behavioural and functional disability. Acetylcholinesterase inhibiting drugs, e.g. **donepezil**, can slow down the progression of mild and moderate Alzheimer's disease, but the benefit is pitifully small and only temporary. Clinical trials of other drug therapy, such as oestrogens, non-steroidal anti-inflammatory drugs (NSAIDs), statins, metal chelation and vitamin E, have failed to show conclusive benefit. Depression is commonly associated with Alzheimer's disease and can be treated with a selective serotonin reuptake inhibitor (SSRI), e.g. **sertraline**. Antipsychotic drugs and benzodiazepines are sometimes indicated in demented patients for symptoms of psychosis or agitation but their use is associated with an increased risk of stroke.

PATHOPHYSIOLOGY

Specific pathological changes in the brains of patients with AD can be demonstrated, for example by positron emission tomography (PET) scanning (Figure 21.4). Forty per cent of AD patients have a positive family history. Histopathology features of AD are the presence of amyloid plaques, neurofibrillary tangles and neuronal loss in the cerebrum. Degeneration of cholinergic neurones has been implicated in the pathogenesis of Alzheimer's disease. Neurochemically, low levels of acetylcholine are related to damage in the ascending cholinergic tracts of the nucleus basalis of Meynert to the cerebal cortex. Other neurotransmitter systems have also been implicated. The brains of patients with Alzheimer's disease show a reduction in acetylcholinesterase, the enzyme in the brain that is primarily responsible for the hydrolysis of acetylcholine. This loss is mainly due to the depletion of cholinesterase-positive neurones within the cerebral cortex and basal forebrain.

These findings led to pharmacological attempts to augment the cholinergic system by means of cholinesterase inhibitors. **Donepezil**, **galantamine** and **rivastigmine** are acetylcholinesterase inhibitors that are licensed for the treatment of mild to moderate AD. **Memantine** is an NMDA receptor antagonist and inhibits glutamate transmission. It is licensed for moderate to severe dementia in AD.

DONEPEZIL, GALANTAMINE AND RIVASTIGMINE

Use

Donepezil, galantamine and rivastigmine have been licensed for the treatment of mild to moderate dementia in AD. Only specialists in management of AD should initiate treatment. Regular review through Mini-Mental State Examination with assessment of global, functional and behavioural condition of the patient is necessary to justify continued treatment (Table 21.2).

Mechanism of action

These drugs are centrally acting, reversible inhibitors of acetylcholinesterase. Galantamine is also a nicotinic receptor agonist.

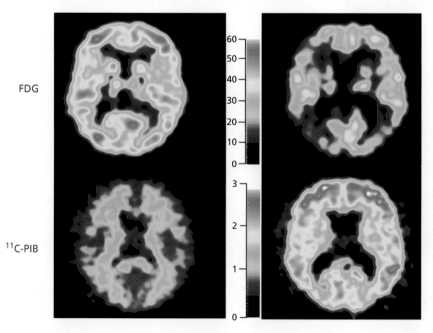

Figure 21.4: PET images of the brain of a 67-year-old healthy control subject (left) and a 79-year-old Alzheimer's disease patient (right). The top images show ^{18}FDG uptake, and the bottom images show Pittsburgh Compound-B (PIB) retention. The left column shows lack of PIB retention in the entire grey matter of the healthy subject (bottom left) and normal ^{18}FDG uptake (top left). Nonspecific PIB retention is seen in the white matter (bottom left). The right column shows high PIB retention most marked in the frontal and temporoparietal cortices of the Alzheimer patient (bottom right) and generalized ^{18}FDG hypometabolism (top right) (adapted from Klunk WE et al. *Annals of Neurology* 2004; **55**: 306–19).

Table 21.2: Pharmacokinetics of donepezil, galantamine and rivastigmine

	Donepezil	Galantamine (prolonged release preparation)	Rivastigmine
T_{max}	4 hours	4 hours	1 hour
Protein binding	90%	18%	40%
CYP3A4 metabolites	✓	✓	✓
Plasma $t_{1/2}$ unknown	70 hours	8 hours	<2 hours[a]

[a]Cholinesterase inhibition, duration 10 hours.

Adverse effects

With all three drugs, adverse effects are mainly a consequence of the cholinomimetic mechanism of action and are usually mild and transient. Nausea, vomiting and diarrhoea are common. Fatigue, dizziness, dyspepsia, urinary problems and syncope have been reported. Careful dose titration can improve tolerance. In overdose, a cholinergic crisis may develop including severe nausea, vomiting, abdominal pain, salivation, lacrimation, urination, defaecation, sweating, bradycardia, hypotension, collapse, convulsions and respiratory depression. In addition to supportive treatment, **atropine** should be administered which reverses most of the effects.

Drug interactions

Theoretically, **donepezil** might interact with a number of other drugs that are metabolized by cytochrome P450, but at present there is no clinical evidence that this is important.

MEMANTINE

Memantine is an NMDA receptor antagonist used in moderate to severe dementia in AD and Parkinson's disease. The National Institute for Clinical Excellence (NICE) does not recommend its use outside clinical trials.

Key points

Alzheimer's disease

- The prevalence of Alzheimer's disease is increasing in ageing populations.
- Currently, the principal therapeutic target is reduced cholinergic transmission.
- Placebo-controlled studies in patients with mild or moderate Alzheimer's disease of central cholinesterase inhibitors showed that scores of cognitive function were greater at three to six months in patients treated with the active drug. The clinical importance of this difference is uncertain.
- The therapeutic benefits of cholinesterase inhibitors appear to be modest and have not yet been demonstrated to be sustained. Such therapy does not appear to affect underlying disease progression or mortality.

Case history

A 21-year-old woman was treated with an anti-emetic because of nausea and vomiting secondary to viral labyrinthitis. She received an initial intramuscular dose of 10 mg of metoclopromide and then continued on oral metoclopramide 10 mg three times a day, which relieved her nausea and vomiting. Two days later she was brought into the local Accident and Emergency Department because her husband thought she was having an epileptic fit. Her arms and feet were twitching, her eyes were deviated to the left and her neck was twisted, but she opened her mouth and tried to answer questions. Muscle tone in the limbs was increased.

Question
What is the diagnosis here and what is the most appropriate and diagnostic acute drug treatment?

Answer
Her posture, dystonia and head and ocular problems all point to a major dystonia with oculogyric crisis, almost certainly caused by metoclopromide. This side effect is more common in young women on high doses (a similar syndrome can occur with neuroleptics, such as prochlorperazine, used to treat nausea). It is probably due to excessive dopamine blockade centrally in a sensitive patient. It usually resolves within several hours of discontinuing the offending drug, and in mild cases this is all that may be needed. In more severe cases, the treatment of choice is intravenous benztropine or procyclidine (anticholinergic agents), and further doses may be required, given orally. An alternative, equi-effective but less satisfactory therapy because it is not diagnostic is intravenous diazepam.

FURTHER READING

Citron M. Strategies for disease modification in Alzheimer's disease. *Nature Reviews. Neuroscience* 2004; **5**: 677–85.

Nutt JG, Wooten GF. Diagnosis and initial managements of Parkinson's disease. *New England Journal of Medicine* 2005; **353**: 1021–7.

Richman D, Agius M. Treatment of autoimmune myasthenia gravis. *Neurology* 2003; **61**: 1652–61.

CHAPTER 22

ANTI-EPILEPTICS

INTRODUCTION

Epilepsy is characterized by recurrent seizures. An epileptic seizure is a paroxysmal discharge of cerebral neurones associated with a clinical event apparent to an observer (e.g. a tonic clonic seizure), or as an abnormal sensation perceived by the patient (e.g. a distortion of consciousness in temporal lobe epilepsy, which may not be apparent to an observer but which is perceived by the patient).

'Funny turns', black-outs or apparent seizures have many causes, including hypoglycaemia, vasovagal attacks, cardiac dysrhythmias, drug withdrawal, migraine and transient ischaemic attacks. Precise differentiation is essential not only to avoid the damaging social and practical stigma associated with epilepsy, but also to ensure appropriate medical treatment. Febrile seizures are a distinct problem and are discussed at the end of this chapter.

> **Key points**
>
> - Epilepsy affects 0.5% of the population.
> - It is characterized by recurrent seizures.

MECHANISMS OF ACTION OF ANTI-EPILEPTIC DRUGS

The pathophysiology of epilepsy and the mode of action of anti-epileptic drugs are poorly understood. These agents are not all sedative, but selectively block repetitive discharges at concentrations below those that block normal impulse conduction. **Carbamazepine** and **phenytoin** prolong the inactivated state of the sodium channel and reduce the likelihood of repetitive action potentials. Consequently, normal cerebral activity, which is associated with relatively low action potential frequencies, is unaffected, whilst epileptic discharges are suppressed.

γ-Aminobutyric acid (GABA) acts as an inhibitory neurotransmitter by opening chloride channels that lead to hyperpolarization and suppression of epileptic discharges. In addition to the receptor site for GABA, the GABA receptor–channel complex includes benzodiazepine and barbiturate recognition sites which can potentiate GABA anti-epileptic activity. Vigabatrin (γ-vinyl-γ-aminobutyric acid) irreversibly inhibits GABA transaminase, the enzyme that inactivates GABA. The resulting increase in synaptic GABA probably explains its anti-epileptic activity.

Glutamate is an excitatory neurotransmitter. A glutamate receptor, the N-methyl-D-aspartate (NMDA) receptor, is important in the genesis and propagation of high-frequency discharges. **Lamotrigine** inhibits glutamate release and has anticonvulsant activity.

> **Key points**
>
> Mechanisms of action of anticonvulsants
>
> - The action of anticonvulsants is poorly understood.
> - They cause blockade of repetitive discharges at a concentration that does not block normal impulse conduction.
> - This may be achieved via enhancement of GABA action or inhibition of sodium channel function.

GENERAL PRINCIPLES OF TREATMENT OF EPILEPSY

Figure 22.1 outlines the general principles for managing epilepsy.

Before treatment is prescribed, the following questions should be asked:

- Are the fits truly epileptic and not due to some other disorder (e.g. syncope, cardiac dysrhythmia)?
- Is the epilepsy caused by a condition that requires treatment in its own right (e.g. brain tumour, brain abscess, alcohol withdrawal)?

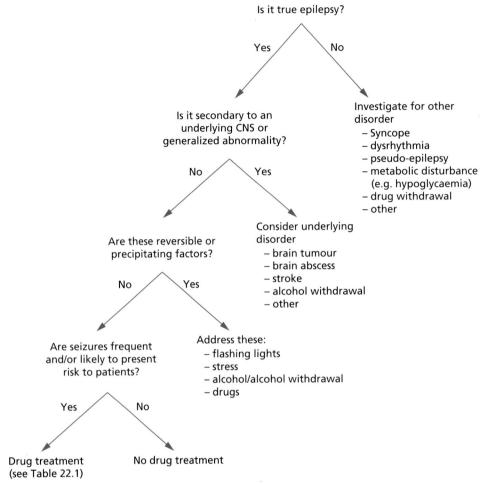

Figure 22.1: Pathway for the management of epilepsy.

- Are there remediable or reversible factors that aggravate the epilepsy or precipitate individual attacks?
- Is there a clinically important risk if the patient is left untreated?
- What type of epilepsy is present?

The ideal anti-epileptic drug would completely suppress all clinical evidence of epilepsy, while producing no immediate or delayed side effects. This ideal does not exist (the British National Formulary currently lists 23 anti-epileptic drugs), and the choice of drug depends on the balance between efficacy and toxicity and the type of epilepsy being treated. Table 22.1 summarizes the most common forms of seizure and their drug treatment.

Control should initially be attempted using a single drug which is chosen on the basis of the type of epilepsy. The dose is increased until either the seizures cease or the blood drug concentration (see Chapter 8) is in the toxic range and/or signs of toxicity appear. It should be emphasized that some patients have epilepsy which is controlled at drug blood concentrations below the usual therapeutic range, and others do not manifest toxicity above the therapeutic range. Thus, estimation of drug plasma concentration is to be regarded as a guide, but not an

Table 22.1: Choice of drug in various forms of seizure

Form of seizure	First line	Second line
Partial seizures with or without secondary generalized tonic–clonic seizures	Valproate Carbamazepine Lamotrigine	Phenytoin Topiramate Tiagabine
Generalized seizures		
Primary (tonic–clonic)	Valproate Lamotrigine	Clonazepam/ clobazam Topiramate Phenytoin
Absence seizures	Ethosuximide Valproate	Lamotrigine Clobazam/ clonazepam
Myoclonic jerks	Valproate	Lamotrigine Clonazepam

Other anti-epileptics not listed above may be useful. Refer to National Institute for Clinical Excellence (NICE) guidelines.

absolute arbiter. The availability of plasma concentration monitoring of anticonvulsant drugs has allowed the more efficient use of individual drugs, and is a crude guide to compliance. If a drug proves to be ineffective, it should not be withdrawn suddenly, as this may provoke status epilepticus. Another drug should be introduced in increasing dosage while the first is gradually withdrawn.

Few studies have investigated combined drug therapy, although empirically this is sometimes necessary. In most but not all cases, effects are additive. Combinations of three or more drugs probably do more harm than good by increasing the likelihood of adverse drug reaction without improving seizure control. Many anticonvulsant drugs are enzyme inducers, so pharmacokinetic interactions are common (e.g. **carbamazepine** reduces plasma concentrations of **phenytoin**).

Key points

Choice of anticonvulsant

- Use a single drug based on type of epilepsy.
- Generally increase the dose every two weeks until either the seizures cease or signs of toxicity appear and/or the plasma drug concentration is in the toxic range.
- If unsatisfactory, substitute another drug.
- Probably less than 10% of epileptic patients benefit from two or more concurrent anticonvulsants.

Beware drug interactions.
Beware pregnancy.

INDIVIDUAL ANTI-EPILEPTIC DRUGS

CARBAMAZEPINE

Use

Carbamazepine is structurally related to the tricyclic antidepressants. It is the drug of choice for simple and complex partial seizures and for tonic–clonic seizures secondary to a focal discharge seizure, and it is effective in trigeminal neuralgia and in the prophylaxis of mood swings in manic-depressive illness (see Chapter 20). A low starting dose is given twice daily followed by a slow increase in dose until seizures are controlled. Assays of serum concentration are a useful guide to compliance, rapid metabolism or drug failure if seizures continue. The therapeutic range is 4–12 mg/L.

Pharmacokinetics

Carbamazepine is slowly but well absorbed following oral administration. Plasma $t_{1/2}$ after a single dose is 25–60 hours, but on chronic dosing this decreases to 10 hours, because of CYP450 enzyme induction. A controlled-release preparation reduces peak plasma concentrations. It is indicated in patients with adverse effects (dizziness, diplopia and drowsiness) that occur only around peak drug concentrations, and in patients who have difficulty in complying with three or more doses per day.

Adverse effects

Adverse effects are common, but seldom severe. They are particularly troublesome early in treatment, before induction of the enzyme responsible for **carbamazepine** elimination (see above). Sedation, ataxia, giddiness, nystagmus, diplopia, blurred vision and slurred speech occur in 50% of patients with plasma levels over 8.5 mg/L. Other effects include rash and (much more rarely) blood dyscrasia, cholestatic jaundice, renal impairment and lymphadenopathy. **Carbamazepine** can cause hyponatraemia and water intoxication due to an antidiuretic action. It is contraindicated in patients with atrioventricular (AV) conduction abnormalities and a history of bone marrow depression or porphyria. Its use in pregnancy has been associated with fetal neural-tube defects and hypospadias.

Drug interactions

Carbamazepine should not be combined with monoamine oxidase inhibitors. It is a potent enzyme inducer and, in particular, it accelerates the metabolism of **warfarin**, **theophylline** and the oral contraceptive.

SODIUM VALPROATE

Use

Sodium valproate (dipropylacetate) is effective against many forms of epilepsy, including tonic–clonic, absence, partial seizures and myoclonic epilepsy. Dosage starts low and is increased every three days until control is achieved.

Adverse effects

The adverse effects involve the following:

- tremor, ataxia and incoordination (dose related);
- nausea, vomiting and abdominal pain (reduced by using enteric-coated tablets);
- enhancement of sedatives (including alcohol);
- hair loss (temporary);
- thrombocytopenia: platelet count should be checked before surgery or with abnormal bruising;
- a false-positive ketone test in urine;
- teratogenic effects (neural-tube defects and hypospadias);
- hepatic necrosis, particularly in children taking high doses and suffering from congenital metabolic disorders;
- acute pancreatitis (another rare complication).

Pharmacokinetics

Valproate is well absorbed when given orally (95–100% bioavailability). The plasma $t_{1/2}$ is seven to ten hours. Active metabolites may explain its slow onset and long time-course of action. The brain to plasma ratio is low (0.3). There is substantial inter-individual variation in metabolism. Plasma valproate concentrations do not correlate closely with efficacy.

PHENYTOIN

Use

Phenytoin is effective in the treatment of tonic–clonic and partial seizures, including complex partial seizures. Dose individualization is essential. Plasma concentration is measured after two weeks. According to clinical response and plasma concentration, adjustments should be small and no more frequent than every four to six weeks. **Phenytoin** illustrates the usefulness of therapeutic drug monitoring (see Chapter 8), but not all patients require a plasma **phenytoin** concentration within the therapeutic range of 10–20 mg/L for optimum control of their seizures. In status epilepticus, phenytoin may be given by slow intravenous infusion diluted in sodium chloride. **Fosphenytoin** is a more convenient parenteral preparation. It can cause dysrhythmia and/or hypotension, so continuous monitoring (see below) is needed throughout the infusion.

Adverse effects

These include the following:

- effects on nervous system – high concentrations produce a cerebellar syndrome (ataxia, nystagmus, intention tremor, dysarthria), involuntary movements and sedation. Seizures may paradoxically increase with **phenytoin** intoxication. High concentrations cause psychological disturbances;
- 'allergic' effects – rashes, drug fever and hepatitis may occur. Oddly, but importantly, such patients can show cross-sensitivity to **carbamazepine**;
- skin and collagen changes – coarse facial features, gum hypertrophy, acne and hirsutism may appear;
- haematological effects – macrocytic anaemia which responds to folate is common; rarely there is aplastic anaemia, or lymphadenopathy ('pseudolymphoma', which rarely progresses to true lymphoma);

- effects on fetus – (these are difficult to distinguish from effects of epilepsy). There is increased perinatal mortality, raised frequency of cleft palate, hare lip, microcephaly and congenital heart disease;
- effects on heart – too rapid intravenous injection causes dysrhythmia and it is contraindicated in heart block unless paced;
- exacerbation of porphyria.

Pharmacokinetics

Intestinal absorption is variable. There is wide variation in the handling of **phenytoin** and in patients taking the same dose, there is 50-fold variation in steady-state plasma concentrations (see Figure 22.2). **Phenytoin** metabolism is under polygenic control and varies widely between patients, accounting for most of the inter-individual variation in steady-state plasma concentration.

Phenytoin is extensively metabolized by the liver and less than 5% is excreted unchanged. The enzyme responsible for elimination becomes saturated at concentrations within the therapeutic range, and **phenytoin** exhibits dose-dependent kinetics (see Chapter 3) which, because of its low therapeutic index, makes clinical use of **phenytoin** difficult. The clinical implications include:

- Dosage increments should be small (50 mg or less) once the plasma concentration approaches the therapeutic range.
- Fluctuations above and below the therapeutic range occur relatively easily due to changes in the amount of drug absorbed, or as a result of forgetting to take a tablet.
- Clinically important interactions are common with drugs that inhibit or induce **phenytoin** metabolism (see Table 22.2).

The saturation kinetics of **phenytoin** make it invalid to calculate $t_{1/2}$, as the rate of elimination varies with the plasma

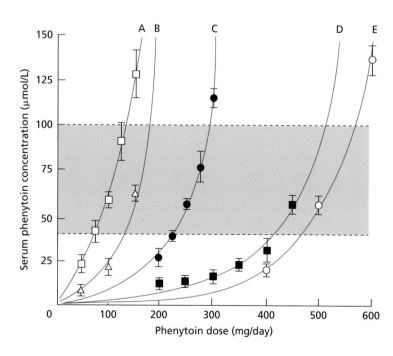

Figure 22.2: Relationship between daily dose of phenytoin and resulting steady-state serum level in five patients on several different doses of the drug. The curves were fitted by computer assuming Michaelis–Menten kinetics (Redrawn with permission from Richens A, Dunlop A. *Lancet* 1975; **ii**: 247. © The Lancet Ltd.)

Table 22.2: Metabolic interactions of anticonvulsants

Enzyme-inducing effect of anti-epileptic drugs		Drugs that inhibit the metabolism of anticonvulsants	
Anti-epileptic drug	Drugs whose metabolism is enhanced	Inhibitor	Anticonvulsant
Carbamazepine	Warfarin	Amiodarone	Phenytoin
Phenobarbitone	Oral contraceptives	Fluoxetine	Phenytoin, carbamazepine
Phenytoin	Theophylline	Diltiazem, nifedipine	Phenytoin
Primidone	Ciclosporin	Chloramphenicol	Phenytoin
Topiramate	Some tricyclic antidepressants	Disulfiram	Phenytoin
	Doxycycline	Erythromycin and clarithromycin	Carbamazepine
	Corticosteroids		
	Anticonvulsants	Cimetidine	Phenytoin
		Isoniazid	Carbamazepine, ethosuximide, phenytoin
		Metronidazole	Phenytoin
		Miconazole, fluconazole	Phenytoin
		Valproate	Lamotrigine

concentration. The time to approach a plateau plasma concentration is longer than is predicted from the $t_{1/2}$ of a single dose of the drug.

Phenytoin is extremely insoluble and crystallizes out in intramuscular injection sites, so this route should never be used. Intravenous **phenytoin** is irritant to veins and tissues because of the high pH. **Phenytoin** should be given at rates of <50 mg/min, because at higher rates of administration cardiovascular collapse, respiratory arrest and seizures may occur. Electrocardiographic monitoring with measurement of blood pressure every minute during administration is essential. If blood pressure falls, administration is temporarily stopped until the blood pressure has risen to a satisfactory level. **Fosphenytoin**, a prodrug of **phenytoin** can be given more rapidly, but still requires careful monitoring.

At therapeutic concentrations, 90% of **phenytoin** is bound to albumin and to two α-globulins which also bind **thyroxine**. In uraemia, displacement of **phenytoin** from plasma protein binding results in lower total plasma concentration and a lower therapeutic range (see Chapter 3).

Phenytoin elimination is impaired in liver disease. This can lead to increased plasma concentration and toxicity, but is not reliably predicted by liver function tests. Conversely hypoalbuminaemia from whatever cause (e.g. cirrhosis or nephrotic syndrome) can result in low total plasma concentrations, and reductions in both effective and toxic plasma concentration.

PHENOBARBITAL

Phenobarbital is an effective drug for tonic and partial seizures, but is sedative in adults and causes behavioural disturbances and hyperkinesia in children. It has been used as a second-line drug for atypical absence, atonic and tonic seizures, but is obsolete. Rebound seizures may occur on withdrawal. Monitoring plasma concentrations is less useful than with **phenytoin** because tolerance occurs, and the relationship between plasma concentration and therapeutic and adverse effects is less predictable than is the case with **phenytoin**.

Other adverse effects include dependency, rashes, anaphylaxis, folate deficiency, aplastic anaemia and congenital abnormalities.

BENZODIAZEPINES

Use

Benzodiazepines (e.g. **diazepam**, **clobazepam** and **clonazepam**) have anticonvulsant properties in addition to their anxiolytic and other actions. Tolerance to their anti-epileptic properties limits chronic use. **Clonazepam** was introduced specifically as an anticonvulsant. It is used intravenously in status epilepticus. **Clonazepam** has a wide spectrum of activity, having a place in the management of the motor seizures of childhood, particularly absences and infantile spasms. It is also useful in complex partial seizures and myoclonic epilepsy in patients who are not adequately controlled by **phenytoin** or **carbamazepine**. Oral treatment is usually started with a single dose at night. The dose is gradually titrated upwards until control is achieved or adverse effects become unacceptable.

Adverse effects

Adverse effects are common and about 50% of patients experience lethargy, somnolence and dizziness. This is minimized by starting with a low dose and then gradually increasing it. Sedation often disappears during chronic treatment. More serious effects include muscular incoordination, ataxia, dysphoria, hypotonia and muscle relaxation, increased salivary secretion and hyperactivity with aggressive behaviour.

Pharmacokinetics

Oral **clonazepam** is well absorbed and the $t_{1/2}$ is about 30 hours. Neither therapeutic nor adverse effects appear to be closely related to plasma concentrations. Control of most types of epilepsy occurs within the range 30–60 ng/mL. **Clonazepam** is extensively metabolized to inactive metabolites.

VIGABATRIN

Use

Vigabatrin, a structural analogue of GABA, increases the brain concentration of GABA (an inhibitory neurotransmitter) through irreversible inhibition of GABA transaminase. It is reserved for the treatment of epilepsy that is unsatisfactorily controlled by more established drugs. Lower doses should be used in the elderly and in those with impaired renal function. **Vigabatrin** should be avoided in those with a psychiatric history.

Adverse effects

- The most common reported adverse event (up to 30%) is drowsiness.
- Fatigue, irritability, dizziness, confusion and weight gain have all been reported.
- Behavioural side effects (e.g. ill temper) may occur.
- Psychotic reactions, including hallucinations and paranoia, are common.
- Nystagmus, ataxia, tremor, paraesthesia, retinal disorders, visual-field defects and photophobia. Regular testing of visual fields is recommended. The patient should be warned to report any visual symptoms and an urgent ophthalmological opinion should be sought if visual-field loss is suspected.

Pharmacokinetics

Absorption is not influenced by food and peak plasma concentrations occur within two hours of an oral dose. In contrast to most other anticonvulsants, **vigabatrin** is not metabolized in the liver, but is excreted unchanged by the kidney and has a plasma half-life of about five hours. Its efficacy does not correlate with the plasma concentration and its duration of action is prolonged due to irreversible binding to GABA transaminase.

LAMOTRIGINE

Lamotrigine prolongs the inactivated state of the sodium channel. It is indicated as monotherapy and adjunctive treatment of partial seizures, generalized tonic–clonic seizures that are not satisfactorily controlled with other drugs, and seizures associated with Lennox–Gastaut syndrome (a severe, rare seizure disorder of young people). It is contraindicated in hepatic and renal impairment. Side effects include rashes (rarely angioedema, Steven–Johnson syndrome and toxic epidermal necrolysis), flu-like symptoms, visual disturbances, dizziness, drowsiness, gastro-intestinal disturbances and aggression. The patient must be counselled to seek urgent medical advice if rash or influenza symptoms associated with hypersensitivity develop.

GABAPENTIN

Gabapentin is licensed as an 'add-on' therapy in the treatment of partial seizures and is also used for neuropathic pain. It is a GABA analogue, but its mechanism of action is thought to be at calcium channels. It is generally well tolerated; somnolence is the most common adverse effect. It is well absorbed after oral administration and is eliminated by renal excretion; the average half-life is five to seven hours. It does not interfere with the metabolism or protein binding of other anticonvulsants.

TOPIRAMATE

Topiramate blocks sodium channels, attenuates neuronal excitation and enhances GABA-mediated inhibition. It is licensed as monotherapy and as adjunctive therapy of generalized tonic–clonic and partial seizures. **Topiramate** induces cytochrome P450, and its own metabolism is induced by **carbamazepine** and **phenytoin**. **Topiramate** has been associated with several adverse effects on the eye. Raised intra-ocular pressure necessitates urgent specialist advice. Other adverse effects include poor concentration and memory, impaired speech, mood disorders, ataxia, somnolence, anorexia and weight loss.

TIAGABINE

Tiagabine inhibits the neuronal and glial uptake of GABA. **Tiagabine** has recently been licensed as adjunctive therapy in the UK for partial seizures with or without secondary generalization. Reported adverse events include dizziness, asthenia, nervousness, tremor, depression and diarrhoea. It has a $t_{1/2}$ of approximately seven hours, which may be halved by concurrent administration of **carbamazepine** and **phenytoin**.

ETHOSUXIMIDE

Use

Ethosuximide is a drug of choice in absence seizures. It is continued into adolescence and then gradually withdrawn over several months. If a drug for tonic–clonic seizures is being given concurrently, this is continued for a further three years. It may also be used in myoclonic seizures and in atypical absences.

Adverse effects

Apart from dizziness, nausea and epigastric discomfort, side effects are rare and it appears safe. Tonic–clonic and absence seizures may coexist in the same child. **Ethosuximide** is not effective against tonic–clonic seizures, in contrast to **valproate** which is active against both absence and major seizures and is used when these coexist.

Pharmacokinetics

Ethosuximide is well absorbed following oral administration. Its plasma $t_{1/2}$ is 70 hours in adults, but only 30 hours in children. Thus, **ethosuximide** need be given only once daily and steady-state values are reached within seven days. Plasma concentration estimations are not usually required.

FURTHER ANTI-EPILEPTICS

Other drugs licensed for use in certain forms of epilepsy in the UK include **oxcarbamazepine, pregabalin, levetiracetam, zonisamide, acetazolamide** (see also Chapter 36) and **piracetam**.

DRUG INTERACTIONS WITH ANTI-EPILEPTICS

Clinically important drug interactions occur with several anti-epileptics. The therapeutic ratio of anti-epileptics is often small and changes in plasma concentrations can seriously affect both efficacy and toxicity. In addition, anti-epileptics are prescribed over long periods, so there is a considerable likelihood that sooner or later they will be combined with another drug.

Several mechanisms are involved:

- enzyme induction, so the hepatic metabolism of the anti-epileptic is enhanced, plasma concentration lowered and efficacy reduced;
- enzyme inhibition, so the metabolism of the anti-epileptic is impaired with the development of higher blood concentrations and toxicity;
- displacement of the anti-epileptic from plasma binding sites.

In addition to this, several anti-epileptics (e.g. **phenytoin, phenobarbital, carbamazepine**) are powerful enzyme inducers and alter the metabolism of other drugs. Table 22.2 lists the effects of some drugs on the metabolism of widely used anti-epileptics, and the effects of anti-epileptics on the metabolism of other drugs.

ANTI-EPILEPTICS AND THE ORAL CONTRACEPTIVE

Phenytoin, phenobarbital, topiramate and **carbamazepine** induce the metabolism of oestrogen and can lead to unwanted pregnancy: alternative forms of contraception or a relatively high oestrogen pill may be appropriate.

ANTI-EPILEPTICS AND PREGNANCY

The risk of teratogenicity is greater if more than one drug is used (see Chapter 9).

STATUS EPILEPTICUS

Status epilepticus is a medical emergency with a mortality of about 10%, and neurological and psychiatric sequelae possible in survivors. Management is summarized in Figure 22.3. Rapid suppression of seizure activity is essential and can usually be achieved with intravenous benzodiazepines (e.g. **lorazepam**, administered i.v.). Rectal **diazepam** is useful in children and if venous access is difficult (see Chapter 10).

Intravenous **clonazepam** is an alternative. False teeth should be removed, an airway established and oxygen administered as soon as possible. Transient respiratory depression and hypotension may occur. Relapse may be prevented with intravenous **phenytoin** and/or early recommencement of regular anticonvulsants. Identification of any precipitating factors, such as hypoglycaemia, alcohol, drug overdose, low anticonvulsant plasma concentrations and non-compliance, may influence the immediate and subsequent management. If intravenous benzodiazepines and **phenytoin** fail to control the fits, transfer to an intensive care unit (ICU) and assistance from an anaesthetist are essential. Intravenous **thiopental** is sometimes used in this situation.

> **Key points**
>
> Status epilepticus
>
> If fits are <5 minutes in duration or there is incomplete recovery from fits of shorter duration, suppress seizure activity as soon as possible.
>
> - Remove false teeth, establish an airway and give oxygen at a high flow rate. Assess the patient, verify the diagnosis and place them in the lateral semi-prone position.
> - Give i.v. lorazepam, 4 mg.
> - Rectal diazepam and rectal paraldehyde are alternatives if immediate i.v. access is not possible).
> - The lorazepam may be repeated once if fits continue.
> - Take blood for anticonvulsant, alcohol and sugar analysis, as well as calcium, electrolytes and urea (if there is doubt about the diagnosis, test for prolactin).
> - If glucose levels are low, give 50% dextrose. If alcohol is a problem, give i.v. vitamins B and C.
> - If fits continue, give i.v. phenytoin by infusion, and monitor with electrocardiogram (ECG).
> - If fits continue, transfer to intensive care unit, consult anaesthetist, paralyse if necessary, ventilate, give thiopental, monitor cerebral function, check pentobarbitone levels.

WITHDRAWAL OF ANTI-EPILEPTIC DRUGS

All anti-epileptics are associated with adverse effects. Up to 70% of epileptics eventually enter a prolonged remission and do not require medication. However, it is difficult to know whether a prolonged seizure-free interval is due to efficacy of the anti-epileptic drug treatment or to true remission. Individuals with a history of adult-onset epilepsy of long duration which has been difficult to control, partial seizures and/or underlying cerebral disorder have a less favourable prognosis. Drug withdrawal itself may precipitate seizures, and the possible medical and social consequences of recurrent seizures (e.g. loss of driving licence; see Table 22.3) must be carefully discussed with the patient. If drugs are to be withdrawn, the

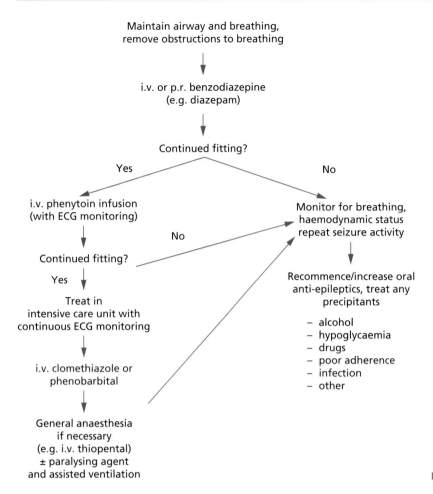

Figure 22.3: Management of status epilepticus.

Table 22.3: Driving and epilepsy

Patients with epilepsy may drive a motor vehicle (but not an
HGV[a] or public service vehicle) provided that they have been
seizure free for one year or have established a three-year
period of seizures whilst asleep.
Patients affected by drowsiness should not drive or operate
machinery.
Patients should not drive during withdrawal of anticonvulsants
or for six months thereafter.

[a]An HGV licence can be held by a person who has been seizure free and
off all anticonvulsant medication for ten years or longer.

dose should be reduced gradually (e.g. over six months or
more) with strict instructions to report any seizure activity.
Patients should not drive during withdrawal or for six months
afterwards.

FEBRILE CONVULSIONS

Febrile seizures are the most common seizures of childhood. A
febrile convulsion is defined as a convulsion that occurs in a
child aged between three months and five years with a fever,
but without any other evident cause, such as an intracranial
infection or previous non-febrile convulsions. Approximately
3% of children have at least one febrile convulsion, of whom
about one-third will have one or more recurrences and 3% will
develop epilepsy in later life.

Despite the usually insignificant medical consequences, a
febrile convulsion is a terrifying experience to parents. Most
children are admitted to hospital following their first febrile
convulsion. If prolonged, the convulsion can be terminated
with either rectal or intravenous (formulated as an emulsion)
diazepam. If the child is under 18 months old, pyogenic
meningitis should be excluded. It is usual to reduce fever by
giving **paracetamol**, removal of clothing, tepid sponging and
fanning. Fever is usually due to viral infection, but if a bacterial cause is found this should be treated.

Uncomplicated febrile seizures have an excellent prognosis, so the parents can be confidently reassured. They should
be advised how to reduce the fever and how to deal with a
subsequent fit, should this occur. There is no evidence that
prophylactic drugs reduce the likelihood of developing
epilepsy in later life, and any benefits are outweighed by
adverse effects. Rectal **diazepam** may be administered by parents as prophylaxis during a febrile illness, or to stop a prolonged convulsion.

Case history

A 24-year-old woman whose secondary generalized tonic–clonic seizures have been well controlled with carbamazepine for the previous four years develops confusion, somnolence, ataxia, vertigo and nausea. Her concurrent medication includes the oral contraceptive, Loestrin 20 (which contains norethisterone 1 mg and ethinylestradiol 20 μg) and erythromycin, which was started one week earlier for sinusitis. She has no history of drug allergy.

Question 1
What is the likely cause of her symptoms?

Question 2
Is the oral contraceptive preparation appropriate?

Answer 1
Erythromycin inhibits the metabolism of carbamazepine, and the symptoms described are attributable to a raised plasma concentration of carbamazepine.

Answer 2
This patient is not adequately protected against conception with the low-dose oestrogen pill, since carbamazepine induces the metabolism of oestrogen.

FURTHER READING

Anon. When and how to stop antiepileptic drugs in adults. *Drugs and Therapeutics Bulletin* 2003; **41**: 41–43.

Duncan JS, Sander JW, Sisodiya SM, Walker ML. Adult epilepsy. *Lancet* 2006; **367**: 1087–100.

MIGRAINE

PATHOPHYSIOLOGY

Migraine is common and prostrating, yet its pathophysiology remains poorly understood. The aura is associated with intracranial vasoconstriction and localized cerebral ischaemia. Shortly after this, the extracranial vessels dilate and pulsate in association with local tenderness and the classical unilateral headache, although it is unclear whether this or a neuronal abnormality ('spreading cortical depression') is the cause of the symptoms.

5-Hydroxytryptamine (5HT, serotonin) is strongly implicated, but this longstanding hypothesis remains unproven. 5HT is a potent vasoconstrictor of extracranial vessels in humans and also has vasodilator actions in some vascular beds. Excretion of 5-HIAA (the main urinary metabolite of 5HT) is increased following a migraine attack, and blood 5HT (reflecting platelet 5HT content) is reduced, suggesting that platelet activation and 5HT release may occur during an attack. This could contribute to vasoconstriction during the aura and either summate with or oppose the effects of kinins, prostaglandins and histamine to cause pain in the affected arteries. The initial stimulus for platelet 5HT release is unknown.

Ingestion by a migraine sufferer of vasoactive amines in food may cause inappropriate responses of intra- and extracranial vessels. Several other idiosyncratic precipitating factors are recognized anecdotally, although in some cases (e.g. precipitation by chocolate), they are not easily demonstrated scientifically. These include physical trauma, local pain from sinuses, cervical spondylosis, sleep (too much or too little), ingestion of tyramine-containing foods such as cheese, alcoholic beverages (especially brandy), allergy (e.g. to wheat, eggs or fish), stress, hormonal changes (e.g. during the menstrual cycle and pregnancy, and at menarche or menopause), fasting and hypoglycaemia.

Some of the most effective prophylactic drugs against migraine inhibit 5HT reuptake by platelets and other cells. Several of these have additional antihistamine and anti-5HT activity. Assessment of drug efficacy in migraine is bedevilled by variability in the frequency and severity of attacks both within an individual and between different sufferers. A scheme for the acute treatment and for the prophylaxis of migraine, as well as the types of medication used for each, is shown in Figure 23.1.

DRUGS USED FOR THE ACUTE MIGRAINE ATTACK

In the majority of patients with migraine, the combination of a mild analgesic with an anti-emetic and, if possible, a period of rest aborts the acute attack. $5HT_{1D}$ agonists (see below) can also be used and have largely replaced **ergotamine** in this context (although ergot-containing preparations are still available), due to better tolerability and side-effect profile. They are very useful in relieving migraine which is resistant to simple therapy.

SIMPLE ANALGESICS

Aspirin, 900 mg, or **paracetamol**, 1 g, are useful in the treatment of headache. They are inexpensive and are effective in up to 75% of patients. Other NSAIDs (see Chapter 26) can also be used. During a migraine attack, gastric stasis occurs and this impairs drug absorption. If necessary, analgesics should be used with **metoclopramide** (as an anti-emetic and to enhance gastric emptying).

ANTI-EMETICS FOR MIGRAINE

Metoclopramide, a dopamine and weak $5HT_4$ antagonist, or **domperidone**, a dopamine antagonist that does not penetrate the blood–brain barrier, are appropriate choices. Sedative anti-emetics (e.g. antihistamines, phenothiazines) should generally be avoided. **Metoclopramide** should be used with caution in adolescents and women in their twenties because of the risk of spasmodic torticollis and dystonia (see Chapter 21).

5HT₁ AGONISTS

The $5HT_1$ agonists (otherwise known as 'triptans') stimulate $5HT_{1B/1D}$ receptors, which are found predominantly in the cranial circulation, thereby causing vasoconstriction predominantly of the carotids; they are very effective in the treatment of an acute migraine attack. Examples are **rizatriptan**, **sumatriptan**

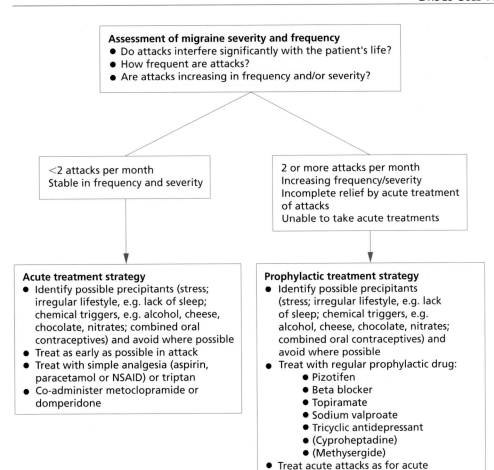

Assessment of migraine severity and frequency
- Do attacks interfere significantly with the patient's life?
- How frequent are attacks?
- Are attacks increasing in frequency and/or severity?

<2 attacks per month
Stable in frequency and severity

2 or more attacks per month
Increasing frequency/severity
Incomplete relief by acute treatment
of attacks
Unable to take acute treatments

Acute treatment strategy
- Identify possible precipitants (stress; irregular lifestyle, e.g. lack of sleep; chemical triggers, e.g. alcohol, cheese, chocolate, nitrates; combined oral contraceptives) and avoid where possible
- Treat as early as possible in attack
- Treat with simple analgesia (aspirin, paracetamol or NSAID) or triptan
- Co-administer metoclopramide or domperidone

Prophylactic treatment strategy
- Identify possible precipitants (stress; irregular lifestyle, e.g. lack of sleep; chemical triggers, e.g. alcohol, cheese, chocolate, nitrates; combined oral contraceptives) and avoid where possible
- Treat with regular prophylactic drug:
  - Pizotifen
  - Beta blocker
  - Topiramate
  - Sodium valproate
  - Tricyclic antidepressant
  - (Cyproheptadine)
  - (Methysergide)
- Treat acute attacks as for acute treatment strategy

Figure 23.1: Scheme for the acute treatment and prophylaxis of migraine.

and **zolmitriptan**. **Sumatriptan** is also of value in cluster headache. Importantly, they can cause vasoconstriction in other vascular beds, notably the coronary and pulmonary vasculature; they should therefore be avoided in patients with coronary heart disease, cerebrovascular disease or peripheral arterial disease, and should also not be used in patients with significant systemic or pulmonary hypertension. They should not be combined with other serotoninergic drugs: **ergotamine**, MAOIs, **lithium** or selective serotonin reuptake inhibitors (SSRIs).

Sumatriptan can be given subcutaneously, by mouth or as a nasal spray. Its bioavailability is only 14% when given orally due to substantial presystemic hepatic metabolism. **Rizatriptan** can be given orally, or as wafers to be dissolved on the tongue. **Zolmitriptan** can be given orally or by intranasal spray. Both **rizatriptan** and **zolmitriptan** have good oral bioavailability, but when given parenterally have a quicker onset of action. These drugs can be taken at any time during a migraine attack, but are most effective if taken early, and relieve symptoms in 65–85% of attacks.

DRUGS USED FOR MIGRAINE PROPHYLAXIS

Migraine prophylaxis should be considered in patients who:

- suffer at least two attacks a month;
- are experiencing an increasing frequency of headaches;

- are significantly symptomatic despite suitable treatment for migraine attacks;
- cannot take suitable treatment for migraine attacks.

Due to the relapsing/remitting natural history of migraine, prophylactic therapy should be given for four to six months and then withdrawn with monitoring of the frequency of attacks.

β-Adrenoreceptor antagonists (e.g. **propranolol**, **metoprolol**) have good prophylactic efficacy and can be given as a once daily dose of a long-acting preparation. The mechanism of action of the β-blockers in this regard is uncertain, but they may act by opposing dilatation of extracranial vessels. They potentiate the peripheral vasoconstriction caused by triptans or **ergotamine**, and these drugs should not be given concurrently.

Pizotifen is an appropriate choice for migraine prophylaxis, especially if β-blockers are contraindicated. It is related to the tricyclic antidepressants. It is a $5HT_2$ antagonist. It also has mild antimuscarinic and antihistaminic activity. It affords good prophylaxis, but can cause drowsiness, appetite stimulation and weight gain. It potentiates the drowsiness and sedation of sedatives, tranquillizers and antidepressants, and should not be used with monoamine oxidase inhibitors.

The anti-epileptic drugs **topiramate** and **sodium valproate** (see Chapter 22) also have good effectiveness in the prophylaxis of migraine. **Topiramate** should only be initiated under specialist supervision.

The tricyclic antidepressant **amitriptyline** (see Chapter 20) is not licensed for this indication, but can afford good prophylactic efficacy in some patients; it is given in a single dose at night.

Cyproheptadine is an antihistamine with additional 5HT-antagonist and calcium channel-antagonist activity. It can be used for prophylaxis of migraine in refractory cases.

Methysergide is a semi-synthetic ergot alkaloid and $5HT_2$ antagonist, which is sometimes used to counteract the effects of secreted 5HT in the management of carcinoid syndrome. It is highly effective as migraine prophylaxis in up to 80% of patients. It is used for severe migraine or cluster headaches refractory to other measures. It should only be used under specialist hospital supervision because of its severe toxicity (retroperitoneal fibrosis and fibrosis of the heart valves and pleura). It is only indicated in patients who, despite other attempts at control, experience such severe and frequent migraine as to interfere substantially with their work or social activities. The smallest dose that suppresses about 75% of the headaches is used for the shortest period of time possible.

Key points

Migraine and its drug treatment

- The clinical features of classical migraine consist of aura followed by unilateral and then generalized throbbing headache, photophobia and visual disturbances (e.g. fortification spectra) with nausea and vomiting.
- The pathophysiology of migraine is poorly understood. 5HT in particular, but also noradrenaline, prostaglandins and kinins, have all been implicated. Initial cranial vasoconstriction gives way to vasodilatation, and spreading neuronal depression occurs.
- Attacks may be precipitated by relaxation after stress, tyramine, caffeine or alcohol. Avoiding these and other precipitants is worthwhile for individuals with a clear history.
- Up to 70% of acute attacks are aborted with simple analgesics (e.g. paracetamol/aspirin), together with an anti-emetic (e.g. metoclopramide/domperidone) if necessary.
- Unresponsive and disabling attacks merit more specific therapy with $5HT_{1D}$ agonists (e.g. sumatriptan).
- Preferred first-line drugs for prophylaxis are pizotifen or β-adrenoceptor antagonists. Topiramate, valproate, tricyclic antidepressants, cyproheptadine and, in exceptional cases only, methysergide may also be effective.

Case history

A 29-year-old woman has suffered from migraine for many years. Her attacks are normally ameliorated by oral Cafergot tablets (containing ergotamine and caffeine) which she takes up to two at a time. One evening she develops a particularly severe headache and goes to lie down in a darkened room. She takes two Cafergot tablets. Two hours later, there has been no relief of her headache, and she takes some metoclopramide 20 mg and two further Cafergot tablets, followed about one hour later by another two Cafergot tablets as her headache is unremitting. Approximately 30 minutes later, her headache starts to improve, but she feels nauseated and notices that her fingers are turning white (despite being indoors) and are numb. She is seen in the local Accident and Emergency Department where her headache has now disappeared, but the second and fifth fingers on her left hand are now blue and she has lost sensation in the other fingers of that hand.

Question

What is the problem and how would you treat her?

Answer

The problem is that the patient has inadvertently ingested an overdose of Cafergot (ergotamine tartrate 1 mg and caffeine 100 mg). No more than four Cafergot tablets should be taken during any 24-hour period (a maximum of eight tablets per week). The major toxicity of ergotamine is related to its potent α-agonist activity, which causes severe vasoconstriction and potentially leads to digital and limb ischaemia. Cardiac and cerebral ischaemia may also be precipitated or exacerbated. Treatment consists of keeping the limb warm but not hot, together with a vasodilator – either an α-blocker to antagonize the α_1 effects of ergotamine, or another potent vasodilator such as a calcium-channel antagonist or nitroglycerin. Blood pressure must be monitored carefully, as must blood flow to the affected limb/digits. The dose of the vasodilating agents should be titrated, preferably in an intensive care unit.

FURTHER READING

Arulmozhi DK, Veeranjaneyulu A, Bodhankar SL. Migraine: current therapeutic targets and future avenues. *Current Vascular Pharmacology* 2006; **4**: 117–28.

Krymchantowski AV, Bigal ME. Polytherapy in the preventive and acute treatment of migraine: fundamentals for changing the approach. *Expert Review of Neurotherapeutics* 2006; **6**: 283–9.

CHAPTER 24

ANAESTHETICS AND MUSCLE RELAXANTS

GENERAL ANAESTHETICS

The modern practice of anaesthesia most commonly involves the administration of an intravenous anaesthetic agent to induce rapid loss of consciousness, amnesia and inhibition of autonomic and sensory reflexes. Anaesthesia is maintained conventionally by the continuous administration of an inhalational anaesthetic agent and cessation of administration results in rapid recovery. An opioid is often administered for analgesia, and in many cases a muscle relaxant is given in order to produce paralysis. A combination of drugs is normally used and the concept of a 'triad of anaesthesia' (Figure 24.1) describes general anaesthesia as a combination of relaxation, hypnosis and analgesia.

INHALATIONAL ANAESTHETICS

UPTAKE AND DISTRIBUTION

A few inhalational general anaesthetics are gases (e.g. nitrous oxide), but most are volatile liquids (e.g. sevoflurane) which are administered as vapours from calibrated vaporizers. None of the drugs in current use is flammable (unlike ether!). The anaesthetic vapours are carried to the patient in a mixture of nitrous oxide and oxygen or oxygen-enriched air. The concentration of an individual gas in a mixture of gases is proportional to its partial pressure. It is the partial pressure of an anaesthetic agent in the brain that determines the onset of anaesthesia, and this equates with the alveolar partial pressure of that agent. The rate of induction and recovery from anaesthesia depends on factors that determine the rate of transfer of the anaesthetic agent from alveoli to arterial blood and from arterial blood to brain (Figure 24.2):

- *Anaesthetic concentration in the inspired air* – increases in the inspired anaesthetic concentration increase the rate of induction of anaesthesia by increasing the rate of transfer into the blood.
- *Relative solubility in blood* – the blood:gas solubility coefficient defines the relative affinity of an anaesthetic for blood compared to air. Anaesthetic agents that are not very soluble in blood have a low blood:gas solubility coefficient, and the alveolar concentration during inhalation will rise rapidly, as little drug is taken up into the circulation. Agents with low blood solubility rapidly produce high arterial tensions and therefore large concentration gradients between the blood and brain. This leads to rapid induction and, on discontinuing administration, rapid recovery. Agents with higher solubility in blood are associated with slower induction and slower recovery.

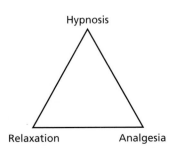

Figure 24.1: Triad of anaesthesia.

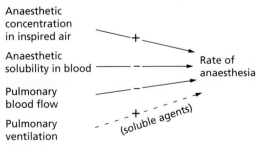

Figure 24.2: Factors determining the onset of action of inhalational anaesthetics.

- *Pulmonary blood flow* – an increase in cardiac output results in an increase in pulmonary blood flow and more agent is removed from the alveoli, thereby slowing the rate of increase in arterial tension and slowing induction. A fall in pulmonary blood flow, as occurs in shock, hastens induction.
- *Pulmonary ventilation* – changes in minute ventilation have little influence on induction with insoluble agents, as the alveolar concentration is always high. However, soluble agents show significant increases in alveolar tension with increased minute ventilation.
- *Arteriovenous concentration gradient* – the amount of anaesthetic in venous blood returning to the lungs is dependent on the rate and extent of tissue uptake. The greater the difference in tension between venous and arterial blood, the more slowly equilibrium will be achieved.

PHARMACODYNAMICS

MECHANISM OF ACTION AND MEASURE OF POTENCY

The molecular mechanism of action of anaesthetics is still incompletely understood. All general anaesthetics depress spontaneous and evoked activity of neurones, especially synaptic transmission in the central nervous system. They cause hyperpolarization of neurones by activating potassium and chloride channels, and this leads to an increase in action potential threshold and decreased firing. Progressive depression of ascending pathways in the reticular activating system produces complete but reversible loss of consciousness. The probable principal site of action is a hydrophobic site on specific neuronal membrane protein channels, rather than bulk perturbations in the neuronal lipid plasma membrane. This is consistent with classical observations that anaesthetic potency is strongly correlated with lipid solubility which were originally interpreted as evidence that general anaesthetics act on lipid rather than on proteins.

The relative potencies of different anaesthetics are expressed in terms of their minimum alveolar concentration (MAC), expressed as a percentage of alveolar gas mixture at atmospheric pressure. The MAC of an anaesthetic is defined as the minimum alveolar concentration that prevents reflex response to a standard noxious stimulus in 50% of the population. MAC represents one point on the dose–response curve, but the curve for anaesthetic agents is steep, and 95% of patients will not respond to a surgical stimulus at 1.2 times MAC. Nitrous oxide has an MAC of 105% (MAC of 52.5% at 2 atmospheres, calculated using volunteers in a hyperbaric chamber) and is a weak anaesthetic agent, whereas halothane is a potent anaesthetic with an MAC of 0.75%. If nitrous oxide is used with halothane, it will have an addi-tive effect on the MAC of halothane, 60% nitrous oxide reducing the MAC of halothane by 60%. Opioids also reduce MAC. MAC is reduced in the elderly and is increased in neonates.

HALOTHANE

Use

Halothane is a potent inhalational anaesthetic. It is a clear, colourless liquid. It is a poor analgesic, but when co-administered with nitrous oxide and oxygen, it is effective and convenient. It is inexpensive and used world-wide, although only infrequently in the UK. Although apparently simple to use, its therapeutic index is relatively low and overdose is easily produced. Warning signs of overdose are bradycardia, hypotension and tachypnoea. Halothane produces moderate muscular relaxation, but this is rarely sufficient for major abdominal surgery. It potentiates most non-depolarizing muscle relaxants, as do other volatile anaesthetics.

Adverse effects

- *Cardiovascular*:
  - ventricular dysrhythmias;
  - bradycardia mediated by the vagus;
  - hypotension;
  - cerebral blood flow is increased, which contraindicates its use where reduction of intracranial pressure is desired (e.g. head injury, intracranial tumours).
- *Respiratory*: respiratory depression commonly occurs, resulting in decreased alveolar ventilation due to a reduction in tidal volume, although the rate of breathing increases.
- *Hepatic*. There are two types of hepatic dysfunction following halothane anaesthesia: mild, transient subclinical hepatitis due to the reaction of halothane with hepatic macromolecules, and (very rare) massive hepatic necrosis due to formation of a hapten–protein complex and with a mortality of 30–70%. Patients most at risk are middle-aged, obese women who have previously (within the last 28 days) had halothane anaesthesia. Halothane anaesthesia is contraindicated in those who have had jaundice or unexplained pyrexia following halothane anaesthesia, and repeat exposure is not advised within three months.
- *Uterus*: halothane can cause uterine atony and postpartum haemorrhage.

Pharmacokinetics

Because of the relatively low blood:gas solubility, induction of anaesthesia is rapid but slower than that with isoflurane, sevoflurane and desflurane. Excretion is predominantly by exhalation, but approximately 20% is metabolized by the liver. Metabolites can be detected in the urine for up to three weeks following anaesthesia.

ISOFLURANE

Isoflurane has a pungent smell and the vapour is irritant, making gas induction difficult. Compared with halothane, it has a lower myocardial depressant effect and reduces systemic vascular resistance through vasodilation. It is popular in hypotensive anaesthesia and cardiac patients, although there is the theoretical concern of a 'coronary steal' effect in patients with ischaemic heart disease. Cerebral blood flow is little affected, and uterine tone is well preserved. Isoflurane has muscle-relaxant properties and potentiates non-depolarizing muscle relaxants. The rate of induction is limited by the pungency of the vapour. Fluoride accumulation is rare, but may occur during prolonged administration (e.g. when used for sedation in intensive care).

SEVOFLURANE

Sevoflurane is a volatile liquid used for induction and maintenance of general anaesthesia. It has a blood:gas solubility coefficient of 0.6 and an MAC of 2%. Cardiovascular stability during administration is a feature and it has gained popularity for rapid and smooth gaseous induction, with rapid recovery. A theoretical disadvantage is that it is 3% metabolized producing fluoride. It may also react with soda lime. In many centres in the UK it is the inhalational anaesthetic of first choice for most indications.

DESFLURANE

Desflurane is an inhalational anaesthetic. It has an MAC of 6% and a boiling point of 23.5°C, so it requires a special heated vaporizer. It has a blood:gas coefficient of 0.42 and therefore induction and recovery are faster than with any other volatile agents, allowing rapid alteration of depth of anaesthesia. Cardiovascular stability is good. It cannot be used for inhalational induction because it is irritant to the respiratory tract.

NITROUS OXIDE

Use

Nitrous oxide is a non-irritant gas which is compressed and stored in pressurized cylinders. It is analgesic, but only a weak anaesthetic. It is commonly used in the maintenance of general anaesthetic in concentrations of 50–70% in oxygen in combination with other inhalational or intravenous agents. It can reduce the MAC value of the volatile agent by up to 65%.

A 50:50 mixture of nitrous oxide and oxygen is useful as a self-administered analgesic in labour, for emergency paramedics and to cover painful procedures, such as changing surgical dressings and removal of drainage tubes.

Adverse effects

- When nitrous oxide anaesthesia is terminated, nitrous oxide diffuses out of the blood into the alveoli faster than nitrogen is taken up. This dilutes the concentration of gases in the alveoli, including oxygen, and causes hypoxia. This effect is known as diffusion hypoxia, and it is countered by the administration of 100% oxygen for 10 minutes.
- Nitrous oxide in the blood equilibrates with closed gas-containing spaces inside the body, and if the amount of nitrous oxide entering a space is greater than the amount of nitrogen leaving, the volume of the space will increase. Thus pressure can increase in the gut, lungs, middle ear and sinuses. Ear complications and tension pneumothorax may occur.

- Prolonged use may result in megaloblastic anaemia due to interference with vitamin B12 and agranulocytosis.
- Nitrous oxide is a direct myocardial depressant, but this effect is countered indirectly by sympathetic stimulation.

Pharmacokinetics

Nitrous oxide is eliminated unchanged from the body, mostly via the lungs. Despite its high solubility in fat, most is eliminated within minutes of ceasing administration.

Key points

Inhaled anaesthetics

Volatile liquid anaesthetics administered via calibrated vaporizers using carrier gas (air, oxygen or nitrous oxygen mixture):

- halothane;
- isoflurane;
- sevoflurane;
- desflurane.

Gaseous anaesthetic

- nitrous oxide.

Key points

Volatile liquid anaesthetics

- All cause dose-dependent cardiorespiratory depression.
- Halothane is convenient, inexpensive and widely used, but due to association with severe hepatotoxicity it has been superseded by sevoflurane (which is also associated with less cardiac depression) in the UK.

Key points

Commission on Human Medicines (CHM) advice (halothane hepatoxicity)
    Recommendations prior to use of halothane

- A careful anaesthetic history should be taken to determine previous exposure and previous reactions to halothane.
- Repeated exposure to halothane within a period of at least three months should be avoided unless there are overriding clinical circumstances.
- A history of unexplained jaundice or pyrexia in a patient following exposure to halothane is an absolute contraindication to its future use in that patient.

OCCUPATIONAL HAZARDS OF INHALATIONAL ANAESTHETICS

There is evidence to suggest that prolonged exposure to inhalational agents is hazardous to anaesthetists and other theatre personnel. Some studies have reported an increased incidence of spontaneous abortion and low-birth-weight infants among female operating department staff. Although much of the evidence is controversial, scavenging of expired or excessive anaesthetic gases is now standard practice.

INTRAVENOUS ANAESTHETICS

UPTAKE AND DISTRIBUTION

There is a rapid increase in plasma concentration after administration of a bolus dose of an intravenous anaesthetic agent; this is followed by a slower decline. Anaesthetic action depends on the production of sufficient brain concentration of anaesthetic. The drug has to diffuse across the blood–brain barrier from arterial blood, and this depends on a number of factors, including protein binding of the agent, blood flow to the brain, degree of ionization and lipid solubility of the drug, and the rate and volume of injection. Redistribution from blood to viscera is the main factor influencing recovery from anaesthesia following a single bolus dose of an intravenous anaesthetic. Drug diffuses from the brain along the concentration gradient into the blood. Metabolism is generally hepatic and elimination may take many hours.

THIOPENTAL

Use and pharmacokinetics

Thiopental is a potent general anaesthetic induction agent with a narrow therapeutic index which is devoid of analgesic properties. Recovery of consciousness occurs within five to ten minutes after an intravenous bolus injection. The alkaline solution is extremely irritant. The plasma $t_{1/2\beta}$ of the drug is six hours, but the rapid course of action is explained by its high lipid solubility coupled with the rich cerebral blood flow which ensures rapid penetration into the brain. The short-lived anaesthesia results from the rapid fall (α phase) of the blood concentration (short $t_{1/2\alpha}$), which occurs due to the distribution of drug into other tissues. When the blood concentration falls, the drug diffuses rapidly out of the brain. The main early transfer is into the muscle. In shock, this transfer is reduced and sustained high concentrations in the brain and heart produce prolonged depression of these organs.

Relatively little of the drug enters fat initially because of its poor blood supply, but 30 minutes after injection the **thiopental** concentration continues to rise in this tissue. Maintainance of anaesthesia with **thiopental** is therefore unsafe, and its use is in induction.

Metabolism occurs in the liver, muscles and kidneys. The metabolites are excreted via the kidneys. Reduced doses are used in the presence of impaired liver or renal function. **Thiopental** has anticonvulsant properties and may be used in refractory status epilepticus (see Chapter 22).

Adverse effects

- *Central nervous system* – many central functions are depressed, including respiratory and cardiovascular centres. The sympathetic system is depressed to a greater extent than the parasympathetic system, and this can result in bradycardia. **Thiopental** is not analgesic and at subanaesthetic doses it actually reduces the pain threshold. Cerebral blood flow, metabolism and intracranial pressure are reduced (this is turned to advantage when **thiopental** is used in neuroanaesthesia).
- *Cardiovascular system* – cardiac depression: cardiac output is reduced. There is dilatation of capacitance vessels. Severe hypotension can occur if the drug is administered in excessive dose or too rapidly, especially in hypovolaemic patients in whom cardiac arrest may occur.
- *Respiratory system* – respiratory depression and a short period of apnoea is common. There is an increased tendency to laryngeal spasm if anaesthesia is light and there is increased bronchial tone.
- *Miscellaneous adverse effects* – urticaria or anaphylactic shock due to histamine release. Local tissue necrosis and peripheral nerve injury can occur due to accidental extravascular administration. Accidental arterial injection causes severe burning pain due to arterial constriction, and can lead to ischaemia and gangrene. Post-operative restlessness and nausea are common.
- **Thiopental** should be avoided or the dose reduced in patients with hypovolaemia, uraemia, hepatic disease, asthma and cardiac disease. In patients with porphyria, **thiopental** (like other barbiturates) can precipitate paralysis and cardiovascular collapse.

PROPOFOL

Uses

Propofol has superseded **thiopental** as an intravenous induction agent in many centres, owing to its short duration of action, anti-emetic effect and the rapid clear-headed recovery. It is formulated as a white emulsion in soya-bean oil and egg phosphatide. It is rapidly metabolized in the liver and extra-hepatic sites, and has no active metabolites. Its uses include:

- *Intravenous induction* – **propofol** is the drug of choice for insertion of a laryngeal mask, because it suppresses laryngeal reflexes.
- *Maintenance of anaesthesia* – **propofol** administered as an infusion can provide total intravenous anaesthesia (TIVA). It is often used in conjunction with oxygen or oxygen-enriched air, opioids and muscle relaxants. Although recovery is slower than that following a single dose, accumulation is not a problem. It is particularly useful in middle-ear surgery (where nitrous oxide is best avoided) and in patients with raised intracranial pressure (in whom volatile anaesthetics should be avoided).
- *Sedation* – for example, in intensive care, during investigative procedures or regional anaesthesia.

Adverse effects

- *Cardiovascular system* – **propofol** causes arterial hypotension, mainly due to vasodilation although there is some myocardial depression. It should be administered particularly slowly and cautiously in patients with hypovolaemia or cardiovascular compromise. It can also cause bradycardia, responsive to a muscarinic antagonist.

- *Respiratory system* – apnoea following injection may require assisted ventilation. If opioids are also administered, as with other agents, the respiratory depression is more marked.
- *Pain on injection* – this is common, and the incidence is reduced if a larger vein is used or **lidocaine** mixed with **propofol**.
- Involuntary movements and convulsions (which can be delayed).

KETAMINE

Use and pharmacokinetics

Ketamine is chemically related to **phencyclidine** (still used as an animal tranquillizer, but no longer for therapeutic use in humans because of its psychogenic effects and potential for abuse), and produces dissociative anaesthesia, amnesia and profound analgesia. It is a relatively safe anaesthetic from the viewpoint of acute cardiorespiratory effects since, unlike other intravenous anaesthetics, it is a respiratory and cardiac stimulant. A patent airway is maintained and it is a bronchodilator. Because of its ease of administration and safety, its use is widespread in countries where there are few skilled anaesthetists. It has been used for management of mass casualties or for anaesthesia of trapped patients to carry out amputations, etc. It is used in shocked patients, because unlike other intravenous anaesthetics it raises rather than lowers blood pressure.

An intravenous dose produces anaesthesia within 30–60 seconds, which lasts for 10–15 minutes. An intramuscular dose is effective within three to four minutes, and has a duration of action of 15–25 minutes. There is a high incidence of hallucinations, nightmares and transient psychotic effects. Children cannot articulate such symptoms and it is disturbing that it is still used particularly in this age group.

Adverse effects

- Psychosis and hallucinations are common.
- Intracranial pressure is increased by ketamine.
- Blood pressure and heart rate are increased.
- Salivation and muscle tone are increased.
- Recovery is relatively slow.

> **Key points**
>
> - Intravenous anaesthetics may cause apnoea and hypotension.
> - Adequate resuscitation facilities must be available.

OTHER AGENTS

Etomidate has a rapid onset and duration of action and has been used for induction. Its use has declined because it causes pain on injection, nausea and vomiting, and excitatory phenomena including extraneous muscle movements. **Etomidate** can suppress synthesis of cortisol (see below) and it should not be used for maintenance of anaesthesia.

> **Key points**
>
> Intravenous induction agents
>
> All have a rapid onset of action, with **propofol** gradually replacing **thiopental** in the UK as the usual agent of choice.
> - **Propofol** – rapid recovery, pain on injection, bradycardia which may be avoided by use of an antimuscarinic agent, rarely anaphylaxic and causing convulsions.
> - **Thiopental** – smooth induction but narrow therapeutic index, cardiorespiratory depression, awakening usually rapid due to redistribution, but metabolism slow and sedative effects prolonged, very irritant injection.
> - **Methohexitone** – barbiturate similar to **thiopental**, less smooth induction, less irritant, may cause hiccup, tremor and involuntary movements.
> - **Etomidate** – rapid recovery and less hypotensive effect than **propofol** and **thiopental**, but painful on injection. Extraneous muscle movements and repeated doses cause adrenocortical suppression.
> - **Ketamine** – good analgesic, increases cardiac output and muscle tone. Due to unpleasant psychological effects (e.g. nightmares and hallucinations) it is restricted to high-risk patients. Useful in children (in whom central nervous system (CNS) effects are less problematic), particularly when repeated doses may be required, and in mass disasters (relatively wide therapeutic index, may be used intramuscularly, slow recovery, safer than other agents in less experienced hands).

SUPPLEMENTARY DRUGS

BENZODIAZEPINES

See Chapters 18 and Chapter 22.

Midazolam is a water-soluble benzodiazepine and useful intravenous sedative. It has a more rapid onset of action than **diazepam** and a shorter duration of action, with a plasma half-life of 1.5–2.5 hours. Dose is titrated to effect. **Midazolam** causes amnesia, which is useful for procedures such as endoscopy or dentistry. The use of benzodiazepines for induction of anaesthesia is usually confined to slow induction of poor-risk patients. Prior administration of a small dose of **midazolam** decreases the dose of intravenous anaesthetic required for induction. Large doses can cause cardiovascular and respiratory depression. Repeated doses of **midazolam** accumulate and recovery is prolonged.

Diazepam is used for premedication (oral), sedation (by slow intravenous injection) and as an anticonvulsant (intravenously). A preparation formulated as an emulsion in soyabean oil has reduced thrombophlebitis from intravenous **diazepam**.

OPIOIDS

High-dose opioids (see Chapter 25) are used to induce and maintain anaesthesia in poor-risk patients undergoing major surgery. Opioids such as **fentanyl** provide cardiac stability.

Onset is slow and the duration of action prolonged so that ventilatory support is required post-operatively. Addition of a small dose of volatile anaesthetic, benzodiazepine or **propofol** is required to avoid awareness during anaesthesia. High-dose opioids can cause chest wall rigidity interfering with mechanical ventilation. This can be prevented by muscle relaxants.

FENTANYL

Fentanyl is a synthetic opioid and is the most commonly employed analgesic supplement during anaesthesia. It is very lipid soluble and has an onset time of one to two minutes. It has approximately 100 times the analgesic activity of **morphine**. **Fentanyl** is rapidly and extensively metabolized, the $t_{1/2}$ being two to four hours, the short duration of action (the peak effect lasts only 20–30 minutes) being explained by redistribution from brain to tissues. Particular care should be taken after multiple injections because of saturation of tissue stores. Depression of ventilation can occur for several minutes. **Fentanyl** and the other potent opioids must not be used in situations where ventilation cannot be controlled. **Fentanyl** has little cardiovascular effect, but bradycardia may occur.

Neuroleptanalgesia is produced by a combination of a butyrophenone (**droperidol**) and an opioid (**fentanyl**). It is a state of inactivity and reduced response to external stimuli, sometimes used for complex diagnostic procedures.

ALFENTANIL

Alfentanil is a highly lipid-soluble derivative of **fentanyl** that acts in one arm–brain circulation time. It has a short duration of action of five to ten minutes, and is often used as an infusion, but causes marked respiratory depression for some minutes.

REMIFENTANIL

Remifentanil is a μ agonist with a rapid onset and short duration. It has an ester linkage, making it susceptible to rapid hydrolysis by a number of non-specific esterases in blood and tissues. It is administered as an infusion and does not accumulate even after a three-hour infusion. Its $t_{1/2}$ is five to seven minutes. It is a useful adjunct to anaesthetics, particularly in patients with renal or hepatic impairment.

α_2-ADRENOCEPTOR AGONISTS

Clonidine has analgesic, anxiolytic and sedative properties. It potentiates inhalational and intravenous anaesthetics. The reduction of MAC of anaesthetics is more marked with the more specific α_2-adrenoceptor agonist **dexmetomidine**, but this is not currently available in the UK. Adverse effects include hypotension and bradycardia.

SEDATION IN THE INTENSIVE CARE UNIT

Patients in the intensive care unit frequently require sedative/analgesic drugs to facilitate controlled ventilation, to provide sedation and analgesia during painful procedures, to allay anxiety and psychological stress and to manage confusional states. The choice of agent(s) used is tailored to meet the needs of the individual patient and must be frequently reviewed. Most sedative and analgesic drugs are given by continuous intravenous infusion both for convenience of administration and for control. Opioids are often used to provide analgesia. They also suppress the cough reflex and are respiratory depressants, which is useful in ventilated patients. **Morphine** and **fentanyl** have been used for long-term sedation. **Alfentanil** has a short half-life and is given by infusion. Opioids are often combined with benzodiazepines (e.g. **midazolam**). Monitoring the level of sedation is particularly important in cases where long-acting opioids or benzodiazepines are being used whose action may be prolonged due to accumulation of drug and active metabolites. **Propofol** is increasingly used where short-term sedation or regular assessment is required, because its lack of accumulation results in rapid recovery. It is not recommended in children. **Etomidate** was used for intensive care sedation before it was shown to increase mortality by adrenocortical suppression. Inhalational agents, such as **isoflurane**, have also been successfully used to provide sedation. Occasionally, muscle relaxants are indicated in critically ill patients to facilitate ventilation. **Atracurium** is then the drug of choice and sedation must be adequate to avoid awareness.

PREMEDICATION FOR ANAESTHESIA

Premedication was originally introduced to facilitate induction of anaesthesia with agents, such as chloroform and ether, that are irritant and produce copious amounts of secretions. Modern induction methods are simple and not unpleasant, and the chief aim of premedication is now to allay anxiety in the patient awaiting surgery. Oral **temazepam** is often the only premedication used before routine surgery. Adequate premedication leads to the administration of smaller doses of anaesthetic than would otherwise have been required, thereby resulting in fewer side effects and improved recovery. Intravenous **midazolam**, which causes anxiolysis and amnesia, can be used. Opioids such as **morphine**, phenothiazines and muscarinic receptor antagonists (e.g. **hyoscine**) are also used. Gastric prokinetic agents, anti-emetics and H_2-receptor antagonists are used to enhance gastric emptying, decrease the incidence of nausea and vomiting, and reduce gastric acidity and volume in certain situations.

MUSCLE RELAXANTS

Muscle relaxants are neuromuscular blocking drugs which cause reversible muscle paralysis (Figure 24.3). They are grouped as follows:

- non-depolarizing agents (competitive blockers), such as **vecuronium** and **atracurium**, which bind reversibly to the post-synaptic nicotinic acetylcholine receptors on the motor end-plate, competing with acetylcholine and thereby preventing end-plate depolarization and blocking neuromuscular transmission;
- **suxamethonium**, a depolarizing agent which also binds acetylcholine receptors at the neuromuscular junction,

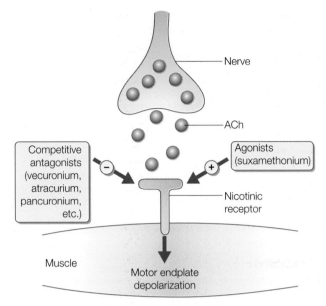

Figure 24.3: Mode of action of muscle relaxants.

but is an agonist. It causes depolarization and initial uncoordinated contractions ('fasciculation'), followed by block.

All muscle relaxants are highly charged molecules and do not readily pass through plasma membranes into cells. They are usually administered intravenously and are distributed throughout the body by blood flow and diffusion. Changes in muscle blood flow or cardiac output can thus alter the speed of onset of neuromuscular blockade. At the end of a procedure, the concentration of relaxant at the end-plate decreases as the drug diffuses down a concentration gradient into the plasma. At this point, the effect of non-depolarizing drugs can be reversed by the injection of an anticholinesterase, such as **neostigmine**, which increases the amount of acetylcholine at the end-plate by preventing its breakdown by acetylcholinesterase. **Atropine** or **glycopyrronium bromide** is administered before **neostigmine**, to prevent the parasympathetic effects of acetylcholine by blocking muscarinic receptors.

Respiratory acidosis, myasthenic syndromes and several drugs (including some β-adrenoceptor blockers, aminoglycosides, **furosemide**, volatile anaesthetics and some tetracyclines) potentiate neuromuscular blockade. The muscle relaxants have poor penetration of the placental barrier, and normal doses do not affect the fetus or cross the blood–brain barrier.

Key points

Muscle relaxants in anaesthesia

- Neuromuscular blocking drugs:
    - non-depolarizing (e.g. atracurium);
    - depolarizing (e.g. suxamethonium).
- Used to:
    - facilitate tracheal intubation;
    - relax muscles of the abdomen and diaphragm during surgery.
- Following administration, respiration must be assisted or controlled until the effects have subsided.

NON-DEPOLARIZING AGENTS

Pancuronium has a peak effect at three to four minutes following an intubating dose, and duration of action of 60–90 minutes. It is partly metabolized by the liver, but 60% is eliminated unchanged by the kidneys, so patients with reduced renal or hepatic function show reduced elimination and prolonged neuromuscular blockade. **Pancuronium** has a direct vagolytic effect, as well as sympathomimetic effects, which can cause tachycardia and slight hypertension. This may prove useful when it is used in cardiovascularly compromised patients.

Vecuronium has an onset of action within three minutes, following an intubating dose. The duration of action is approximately 30 minutes, and can usually be reversed by anticholinesterases after only 15–20 minutes. It has little or no effect on heart rate and blood pressure, and does not liberate histamine. **Vecuronium** undergoes hepatic de-acetylation and the kidneys excrete 30% of the drug.

Rocuronium bromide is a steroid muscle relaxant. Good intubating conditions are achieved within 60–90 seconds. **Rocuronium bromide** has the most rapid onset of any nondepolarizing muscle relaxant, and is only slightly slower than **suxamethonium**. Its duration of action is 30–45 minutes, but it is otherwise similar to **vecuronium**.

Atracurium is a non-depolarizing muscle relaxant with a rapid onset time (2.0–2.5 minutes) and duration of 20–25 minutes. Histamine release may cause flushing of the face and chest, local wheal and flare at the site of injection and, more rarely, bronchospasm and hypotension. **Atracurium** does not accumulate and hence continuous infusion is popular in intensive care to facilitate intermittent positive pressure ventilation (IPPV). During long surgical cases it can provide stable and readily reversible muscle relaxation. It is unique in that it is inactivated spontaneously at body temperature and pH by Hoffman elimination, a chemical process that requires neither hepatic metabolism nor renal excretion. This makes it the agent of choice for use in patients with significant hepatic and renal impairment. **Cisatracurium**, a stereoisomer of **atracurium**, has the advantage of causing less histamine release.

Mivacurium has an onset time and propensity for histamine release similar to **atracurium**. Because it is metabolized

---

Key points

Non-depolarizing muscle relaxants

- These compete with acetylcholine at the neuromuscular junction.
- Action is reversed by anticholinesterases (e.g. neostigmine) (note that atropine or glycopyrrolate is required to prevent dangerous bradycardia and hypersalivation).
- They may cause histamine release.
- Allergic cross-reactivity has been reported.
- There is a prolonged effect in myasthenia gravis and hypothermia.
- Examples include atracurium, vecuronium and pancuronium (longer duration of action).

by plasma cholinesterase, reversal with an anticholinesterase may not always be necessary, and recovery occurs within 20 minutes. It is useful for short procedures requiring muscle relaxation (e.g. oesophagoscopy) and avoids the side effects of **suxamethonium**.

DEPOLARIZING AGENTS

SUXAMETHONIUM

Use

Suxamethonium (known as succinylcholine in the USA) is the dicholine ester of succinic acid and thus structurally resembles two molecules of acetylcholine linked together. Solutions of **suxamethonium** are unstable at room temperature and must be stored at 4°C. **Suxamethonium** administered intravenously produces paralysis within one minute with good tracheal intubating conditions. Therefore **suxamethonium** is particularly useful when it is important to intubate the trachea rapidly, as in patients at risk of aspiration of gastric contents and patients who may be difficult to intubate for anatomical reasons. **Suxamethonium** is also used to obtain short-duration muscle relaxation as needed during bronchoscopy, orthopaedic manipulation and electroconvulsive therapy. The drug is metabolized rapidly by plasma cholinesterase, and recovery begins within three minutes and is complete within 15 minutes. The use of an anticholinesterase, such as **neostigmine**, is contraindicated because it inhibits plasma cholinesterase, reducing the rate of elimination of **suxamethonium**.

Adverse reactions

- In about 1 in 2800 of the population, a genetically determined abnormal plasma pseudocholinesterase is present which has poor metabolic activity (see Chapter 14). **Suxamethonium** undergoes slow hydrolysis by non-specific esterases in these patients, producing prolonged apnoea, sometimes lasting for several hours. Acquired deficiency of cholinesterase may be caused by renal disease, liver disease, carcinomatosis, starvation, pregnancy and cholinesterase inhibitors. However, unlike the genetic poor metabolizers, these acquired disorders only prolong **suxamethonium** apnoea by several minutes rather than several hours.
- Muscle fasciculations are often produced several seconds after injection of **suxamethonium**, and are associated with muscular pains after anaesthesia.
- Malignant hyperthermia is a rare disorder, see below.
- Muscarinic effects involve bradycardia or asystole.
- An increase in intragastric pressure occurs, but seldom causes regurgitation of stomach contents provided the lower oesophageal sphincter is normal and there is no history of oesophageal reflux.
- There is increased intra-ocular pressure and should not be used in glaucoma and open eye injuries.
- Increased plasma K^+ concentration, due to potassium released from muscle. This is increased if the muscle cells

are damaged: **suxamethonium** is contraindicated in patients with neuropathies, muscular dystrophy, myopathies or severe burns in whom fatal dysrhythmias have been reported.
- Anaphylactic reactions are rare.

Key points

Suxamethonium is a depolarizing muscle relaxant.

- It has the most rapid onset of action.
- Its action is not reversed by anticholinesterases.
- Paralysis is usually preceded by painful muscle fasciculations. Therefore it should be given immediately after induction. Myalgia after surgery may occur.
- Premedication with atropine reduces bradycardia and hypersalivation.
- Prolonged paralysis occurs in patients with low plasma cholinesterase (genetically determined).
- It is contraindicated in patients with neuropathies, myopathies or severe burns, due to risk of hyperkalaemia.

MALIGNANT HYPERTHERMIA

This is a rare complication of anaesthesia. Predisposition is inherited as an autosomal dominant, the protein abnormality residing in a sarcoplasmic reticulum calcium channel (the 'ryanodine receptor'). If untreated, the mortality is 80%. All of the volatile anaesthetic agents and suxamethonium have been implicated in its causation. It consists of a rapid increase in body temperature of approximately 2°C per hour accompanied by tachycardia, increased carbon dioxide production and generalized muscle rigidity. Severe acidosis, hypoxia, hypercarbia and hyperkalaemia can lead to serious dysrhythmias.

Treatment includes the following:

- Anaesthetic should be discontinued and 100% oxygen administered via a vapour-free breathing system.
- **Dantrolene** should be administered intravenously. This blocks the ryanodine receptor, preventing intracellular calcium mobilization and relieving muscle spasm.
- Hyperkalaemia should be corrected.
- Employ cooling measures such as tepid sponging, ice packs and cold fluids.

LOCAL ANAESTHETICS

INTRODUCTION

Local and regional techniques can be used to provide anaesthesia for many surgical procedures. They can also provide good-quality post-operative analgesia, especially when using continuous epidural infusions. A local anaesthetic may be the method of choice for patients with severe cardiorespiratory disease, as the risks of general anaesthesia and systemic narcotic analgesics are avoided. Local anaesthetic techniques have also proved useful in combination with general anaesthesia. Local anaesthetics reversibly block impulse transmission in peripheral nerves. They consist of an aromatic group joined by an intermediate chain to an amine and are injected in their ionized water-soluble form. In tissues a proportion of the drug dissociates to lipid-soluble free base. The free base is able to cross neuronal lipid membrane. Ionized drug enters and blocks sodium channels blocking nerve action potentials. Local anaesthetics depress small unmyelinated fibres first and larger myelinated fibres last. The order of loss of function is therefore as follows:

* pain;
* temperature;
* touch;
* motor function.

SYSTEMIC TOXICITY

Inadvertent intravascular injection is the most common cause of systemic toxicity: gentle suction to check that blood does not enter the syringe is vital before injection. Even when injected by the correct route, toxicity may result from overdose, so recommended safe doses should not be exceeded. Early signs of toxicity are circumoral numbness and tingling, which may be followed by drowsiness, anxiety and tinnitus. In severe cases there is loss of consciousness, and there may be convulsions with subsequent coma, apnoea and cardiovascular collapse. The addition of a vasoconstrictor such as adrenaline to a local anaesthetic solution slows the rate of absorption, prolongs duration and reduces toxicity. The concentration of adrenaline should not be greater than 1:200 000. Preparations containing adrenaline are contraindicated for injection close to end-arteries ('ring' blocks of the digits and penis) because of the risk of vasospasm and consequent ischaemia.

LIDOCAINE

Lidocaine is the most widely used local anaesthetic in the UK (its use as an anti-dysrhythmic drug is discussed in Chapter 32). It has a quick onset and medium duration of action. In addition to injection, **lidocaine** can be administered topically as a gel or aerosol. It is used in all forms of local anaesthesia. Absorption following topical application can be rapid (e.g. from the larynx, bronchi or urethra). Systemic allergy is uncommon.

PRILOCAINE

Prilocaine is similar to **lidocaine**, but its clearance is more rapid, so it is less toxic. It is most useful when a large total amount of local anaesthetic is needed or a high plasma concentration is likely (e.g. injection into vascular areas, such as the perineum), or for use in intravenous regional anaesthesia

(e.g. Biers' block). **EMLA** is a 'eutectic mixture of local anaesthetic' and is a combination of prilocaine and lidocaine in the form of a cream. If applied topically for 30–60 minutes and covered with an occlusive dressing, it provides reliable anaesthesia for venepuncture (important, especially for children). In dental procedures, **prilocaine** is often used with the peptide vasoconstrictor **felypressin**. Excessive doses can lead to systemic toxicity, dependent on plasma concentration.

Prilocaine is metabolized by amidases in the liver, kidney and lungs. The rapid production of oxidation products may rarely give rise to methaemoglobinaemia.

BUPIVACAINE

Bupivacaine is a long-acting amide local anaesthetic commonly used for epidural and spinal anaesthesia. Although it has a slow onset, peripheral nerve and plexus blockade can have a duration of 5–12 hours. Epidural blockade is much shorter, at about two hours, but is still longer than for **lidocaine**. The relatively short duration of epidural block is related to the high vascularity of the epidural space and consequent rapid uptake of anaesthetic into the bloodstream. **Bupivacaine** is the agent of choice for continuous epidural blockade in obstetrics, as the rise in maternal (and therefore fetal) plasma concentration occurs less rapidly than with **lidocaine**. The acute central nervous system toxicity of **bupivacaine** is similar to that of **lidocaine**, it is thought to be more toxic to the myocardium. The first sign of toxicity can be cardiac arrest from ventricular fibrillation, which is often resistant to defibrillation. For this reason, it should not be used in intravenous regional anaesthesia.

ROPIVACAINE

Ropivacaine is a propyl analogue of **bupivacaine**, and is the only local anaesthetic that occurs in a single enantiomeric form. It is marginally less potent than **bupivacaine**, with a slightly shorter duration of action. Its advantages are that it produces less motor block and less cardiac toxicity if inadvertently administered intravenously.

COCAINE

The use of **cocaine** (see also Chapter 53) as a local anaesthetic is restricted to topical application in ear, nose and throat (ENT) procedures because of its adverse effects and potential for abuse. Acute intoxication can occur, consisting of restlessness, anxiety, confusion, tachycardia, angina, cardiovascular collapse, convulsions, coma and death. In the central nervous system, initial stimulation gives rise to excitement and raised blood pressure followed by vomiting. This may be followed by fits and CNS depression. It causes vasoconstriction, so adrenaline must not be added.

BENZOCAINE

Benzocaine is a topical anaesthetic which is comparatively non-irritant and has low toxicity. Compound **benzocaine** lozenges (containing 10 mg **benzocaine**) are used to alleviate the pain of local oral lesions, such as aphthous ulcers, lacerations and carcinoma of the mouth.

TETRACAINE

The use of **tetracaine** in the UK is restricted to topical application, especially in ophthalmic surgery. However, it is popular in the USA for use in spinal anaesthesia because of its potency and long duration of action.

CHLOROPROCAINE

Chloroprocaine is claimed to have the most rapid onset of all and has low toxicity. Although not available in the UK, it is widely used in North America.

Key points

Toxicity of local anaesthetics

- Inadvertent intravenous injection may lead to convulsions and cardiovascular collapse.
- Initial symptoms of overdose (excess local dose resulting in high plasma concentrations and systemic toxicity) may include light-headedness, sedation, circumoral paraesthesia and twitching.
- The total dose of lidocaine should not exceed 200 mg (or 500 mg if given in solutions containing adrenaline).

Case history

An 18-year-old white South African girl who had recently commenced the oral contraceptive was admitted with abdominal pain and proceeded to have a laparotomy. Anaesthesia was induced using **thiopental** and **suxamethonium**, and was maintained with isoflurane. A normal appendix was removed. Post-operatively, the patient's abdominal pain worsened and was not significantly improved with a **morphine** injection. A nurse reported that the patient's urine appeared dark in colour and her blood pressure was high.

Question

What is the likely post-operative diagnosis and what may have precipitated this?

Answer

Acute intermittent porphyria in association with:

- oral contraceptive pill;
- thiopental.

Opiates, such as **morphine** and **pethidine**, are thought to be safe in porphyria. (Ectopic pregnancies should always be considered in sexually active female patients with abdominal pain.)

FURTHER READING

Allman KG, Wilson IH. *Oxford handbook of anaesthesia*, 2nd edn. Oxford: Oxford University Press, 2006.

Saseda M, Smith S. *Drugs in anaesthesia and intensive care*. Oxford: Oxford Publications, 2003.

CHAPTER 25

ANALGESICS AND THE CONTROL OF PAIN

INTRODUCTION

Pain is a common symptom and is important because it both signals 'disease' (in the broadest sense) and aids diagnosis. Irrespective of the cause, its relief is one of the most important duties of a doctor. Fortunately, pain relief was one of the earliest triumphs of pharmacology, although clinicians have only recently started to use the therapeutic armamentarium that is now available adequately and rationally.

PATHOPHYSIOLOGY AND MECHANISM OF PAIN

Pain is usually initiated by a harmful (tissue-damaging, noxious) stimulus. The perception of such stimuli is termed 'nociception' and is not quite the same as the subjective experience of pain, which contains a strong central and emotional component. Consequently, the intensity of pain is often poorly correlated with the intensity of the nociceptive stimulus, and many clinical states associated with pain are due to a derangement of the central processing such that a stimulus that is innocuous is perceived as painful. Trigeminal neuralgia is an example where a minimal mechanical stimulus triggers excruciating pain.

The main pathways are summarized in Figure 25.1. The afferent nerve fibres involved in nociception consist of slowly conducting non-myelinated C-fibres that are activated by stimuli of various kinds (mechanical, thermal and chemical) and fine myelinated (Aδ) fibres that conduct more rapidly but respond to similar stimuli. These afferents synapse in the dorsal horn of grey matter in the spinal cord in laminae I, V and II (the substantia gelatinosa). The cells in laminae I and V cross over and project to the contralateral thalamus, whereas cells in the substantia gelatinosa have short projections to laminae I and V and function as a 'gate', inhibiting transmission of impulses from the primary afferent fibres. The gate provided by the substantia gelatinosa can also be activated centrally by descending pathways. There is a similar gate mechanism in the thalamus. Descending inhibitory controls are very important, a key

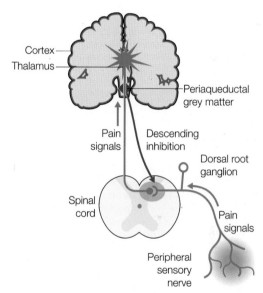

Figure 25.1: Neural pain pathways.

component being the small region of grey matter in the midbrain known as the periaqueductal grey (PAG) matter. Electrical stimulation of the PAG causes profound analgesia. The main pathway from this area runs to the nucleus raphe magnus in the medulla and thence back to the dorsal horn of the cord connecting with the interneurones involved in nociception.

Key mediators of nociception are summarized in Figure 25.2. Stimulation of nociceptive endings in the periphery is predominantly chemically mediated. Bradykinin, prostaglandins and various neurotransmitters (e.g. 5-hydroxytryptamine, 5HT) and metabolites (e.g. lactate) or ions (e.g. K$^+$) released from damaged tissue are implicated. **Capsaicin**, the active principle of red peppers, potently stimulates and then desensitizes nociceptors. The neurotransmitters of the primary nociceptor fibres include fast neurotransmitters – including glutamate and probably adenosine triphosphate (ATP) – and various neuropeptides, including substance P and calcitonin gene-related peptide (CGRP). Neurotransmitters involved in modulating the pathway include opioid peptides (e.g. endorphins), endocannabinoids (e.g. anandamide), 5HT and noradrenaline.

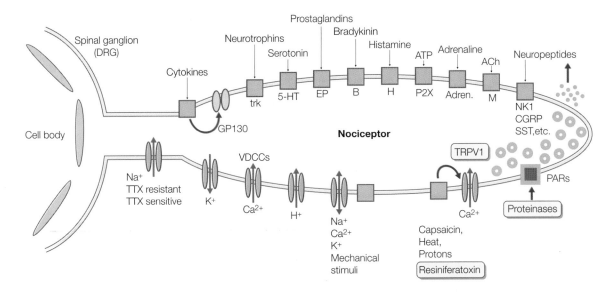

Figure 25.2: Influence of inflammatory mediators on activity of a C-fibre nociceptor. DRG, dorsal root ganglion, TTX, tetrodotoxin; GP130, glycoprotein 130; trk, tyrosine kinase; 5-HT, 5-hydroxytryptamine (serotonin) receptor; EP, prostaglandin EP receptor; B, bradykinin receptor; H, histamine receptor; P2X, purinergic P2X receptor; Adren, adrenoceptor; M, muscarinic receptor; NKT, neokyotorphine; CGRP, calcitonin gene-related peptide; SST, somatostatin; PARs protease activated receptors; TRPV1, transient receptor potential vanilloid 1 receptor; VDCCs, voltage-dependent calcium channels.

Key points

Mechanisms of pain and actions of analgesic drugs

- Nociception and pain involve peripheral and central mechanisms; 'gating' mechanisms in the spinal cord and thalamus are key features.
- Pain differs from nociception because of central mechanisms, including an emotional component.
- Many mediators are implicated, including prostaglandins, various peptides that act on μ-receptors (including endorphins), 5HT, noradrenaline and anandamide.
- Analgesics inhibit, mimic or potentiate natural mediators (e.g. aspirin inhibits prostaglandin biosynthesis, morphine acts on μ-receptors, and tricyclic drugs block neuronal amine uptake).

SITES OF ACTION OF ANALGESICS

Drugs can prevent pain:

- at the site of injury (e.g. NSAIDs);
- by blocking peripheral nerves (local anaesthetics);
- by closing the 'gates' in the dorsal horn and thalamus (one action of opioids and of tricyclic antidepressants that inhibit axonal re-uptake of 5HT and noradrenaline);
- by altering the central appreciation of pain (another effect of opioids).

DRUGS USED TO TREAT MILD OR MODERATE PAIN

PARACETAMOL

Uses

Paracetamol is an antipyretic and mild analgesic with few, if any, anti-inflammatory properties and no effect on platelet aggregation. It has no irritant effect on the gastric mucosa and can be used safely and effectively in most individuals who are intolerant of **aspirin**. It is the standard analgesic/antipyretic in paediatrics since, unlike **aspirin**, it has not been associated with Reye's syndrome and can be formulated as a stable suspension. The usual adult dose is 0.5–1 g repeated at intervals of four to six hours if needed.

Mechanism of action

Paracetamol inhibits prostaglandin biosynthesis under some circumstances (e.g. fever), but not others. The difference from other NSAIDs is still under investigation.

Adverse effects

The most important toxic effect is hepatic necrosis leading to liver failure after overdose, but renal failure in the absence of liver failure has also been reported after overdose. There is no convincing evidence that **paracetamol** causes chronic liver disease when used regularly in therapeutic doses (<4 g/24 hours). **Paracetamol** is structurally closely related to **phenacetin** (now withdrawn because of its association with analgesic nephropathy) raising the question of whether long-term abuse of **paracetamol** also causes analgesic nephropathy, an issue which is as yet unresolved.

Pharmacokinetics, metabolism and interactions

Absorption of **paracetamol** following oral administration is increased by **metoclopramide**, and there is a significant relationship between gastric emptying and absorption. **Paracetamol** is rapidly metabolized in the liver. The major sulphate and glucuronide conjugates (which account for approximately 95% of a **paracetamol** dose) are excreted in the urine. When **paracetamol** is taken in overdose (Chapter 54), the capacity of the conjugating mechanisms is exceeded and a toxic metabolite, *N*-acetyl benzoquinone imine (NABQI), is formed via metabolism through the CYP450 enzymes.

ASPIRIN (ACETYLSALICYLATE)

Use

Antiplatelet uses of **aspirin** are described in Chapters 29 and 30. As an antipyretic and mild analgesic it has similar efficacy to **paracetamol**. However, unlike **paracetamol** it also has anti-inflammatory properties when used in high doses. Various preparations are available, including regular as well as buffered, soluble and enteric-coated forms. Enteric coating is intended to reduce local gastric irritation, but much of the gastric toxicity is due to inhibition of gastric mucosal prostaglandin biosynthesis (see below), rather than to direct gastric irritation. Consequently, slow-release preparations do not eliminate the adverse effects of **aspirin** on the gastric mucosa.

Mechanism of action

Aspirin inhibits prostaglandin biosynthesis, irreversibly acetylating a serine residue in the active site of cyclo-oxygenase (COX). There are two main isoforms, COX-1 and COX-2. COX-1 is a constitutive enzyme which is present in platelets and other cells under basal conditions. COX-2 is an inducible form, which is produced in response to cytokine stimulation in areas of inflammation and produces large amounts of prostaglandins. Acetylation of the serine in COX-1 active site prevents access of the endogenous substrate (arachidonic acid) to the active site, very effectively blocking thromboxane formation in platelets, as well as prostaglandin formation.

Adverse effects and contraindications

These include:

- *Salicylism* – toxic doses of salicylates, including **aspirin**, cause tinnitus, deafness, nausea, vomiting, abdominal pain and flushing and fever.
- *Dyspepsia* is common as is mild gastric blood loss. Severe blood loss from the stomach can be life-threatening. The mechanism is inhibition of gastric prostaglandin (PGE_2) biosynthesis. PGE_2 is the main prostaglandin made by the human stomach, which it protects in several ways:
  - inhibition of acid secretion;
  - stimulation of mucus secretion;
  - increased clearance of acid from the submucosa via local vasodilatation.

  Aspirin and other NSAIDs damage the stomach by impairing these protective mechanisms. **Aspirin** should not be given to patients with active peptic ulceration.
- *Aspirin-sensitive asthma* occurs in approximately 5% of asthmatics (Chapter 33). It is associated with nasal polyps. Reactions to other chemically unrelated NSAIDs commonly occur in such individuals. Abnormal leukotriene (Chapter 33) production and sensitivity are implicated. In addition, **aspirin** and similar drugs can directly activate eosinophils and mast cells in these patients through IgE-independent mechanisms.
- *Reye's syndrome*, a rare disease of children, with high mortality, is characterized by hepatic failure and encephalopathy, often occurring in the setting of a viral illness (Figure 25.3).

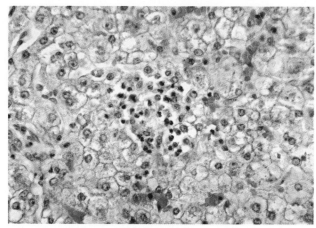

Figure 25.3: Histopathology of autopsy liver from child who died of Reye's syndrome as a result of taking asprin. Hepatocytes are pale-staining due to intracellular fat droplets.

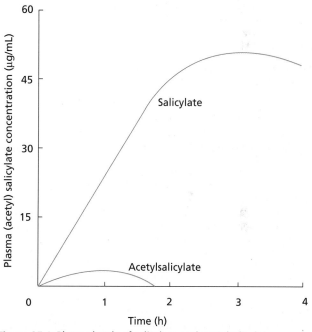

Figure 25.4: Plasma levels of salicylate and acetylsalicylate following 640 mg aspirin given orally, demonstrating rapid conversion of acetylsalicylate to salicylate.

Pharmacokinetics

Gastro-intestinal absorption is rapid. **Aspirin** is subject to considerable presystemic metabolism (to salicylate), so the plasma concentration of **aspirin** (acetyl salicylic acid) is much lower than that of salicylate following an oral dose (Figure 25.4). Some of the selectivity of aspirin for platelet cyclo-oxygenase is probably due to exposure of platelets to high concentrations of aspirin in portal blood, whereas tissues are exposed to the lower concentrations present in the systemic circulation. Salicylate is metabolized in the liver by five main parallel pathways, two of which are saturable (Michaelis–Menten kinetics) and is also excreted unchanged in the urine by a first-order process. This is summarized in Figure 25.5. The formation of salicylurate (in mitochondria) is easily saturable. Consequently,

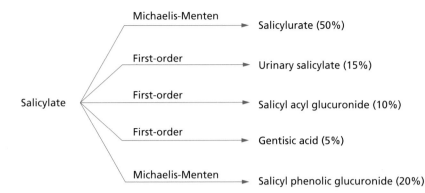

Figure 25.5: The main pathways of salicylate metabolism and excretion.

salicylate has dose-dependent (non-linear) kinetics (Chapter 3) at high therapeutic doses or after overdose. Urinary elimination of salicylate is considerably influenced by pH, being more rapid in alkaline urine, which favours the charged (polar) anionic form that is not reabsorbed, rather than the free acid (Chapter 6). This property is utilized in the treatment of salicylate overdose by urine alkalinization and demonstrates the principle of ion trapping. (Chapter 54).

Drug interactions

Aspirin increases the risk of bleeding in patients receiving anticoagulants via effects on platelets, gastrotoxicity and, in overdose, by a hypoprothrombinaemic effect. **Aspirin** should not be given to neonates with hyperbilirubinaemia because of the risk of kernicterus as a result of displacement of bilirubin from its binding site on plasma albumin (Chapter 13).

IBUPROFEN

Ibuprofen has an approximately similar analgesic potency to **paracetamol** and, in addition, has useful anti-inflammatory activity, so it is an alternative to **aspirin** for painful conditions with an inflammatory component (e.g. sprains and minor soft tissue injury). It is also useful in dysmenorrhoea. It is a reversible cyclo-oxygenase inhibitor, but causes rather less gastric irritation than **aspirin** and other NSAIDs at normal doses, and is available over the counter in the UK and in many other countries. A suspension is available for use in children. It can cause other adverse reactions common to the NSAIDs, including reversible renal impairment in patients who are elderly or have cirrhosis, nephrotic syndrome or heart failure. It reduces the efficacy of antihypertensive medication and of diuretics by blocking formation of vasodilator and natriuretic prostaglandins in the kidney.

For more detailed discussion of other common NSAIDs, which are widely used, see Chapter 26.

TOPICAL NON-STEROIDAL ANTI-INFLAMMATORY DRUGS

Several NSAIDs (including **ibuprofen** and **piroxicam**) are available as topical preparations. Systemic absorption does occur, but is modest. Their effectiveness in soft tissue injuries and other localized inflammatory conditions is also modest. They occasionally cause local irritation of the skin, but adverse effects are otherwise uncommon.

NEFOPAM

Use

Nefopam is chemically and pharmacologically unrelated to other analgesics. It is intermediate in potency between **aspirin** and **morphine**. Unlike NSAIDs, it does not injure the gastric mucosa. It is less of a respiratory depressant than the opioids and does not cause dependence. It is useful when opioid-induced respiratory depression is unacceptable. Neither tolerance nor drug dependence occur.

Mechanism of action

Nefopam is a potent inhibitor of amine uptake and potentiates descending pathways that operate the gate mechanism described above.

Adverse effects and contraindications

Nefopam has few severe (life-threatening) effects, although convulsions, cerebral oedema and fatality can result from massive overdose. It is contraindicated in patients with epilepsy, and also in patients receiving monoamine oxidase inhibitors (see below). It should not be used in acute myocardial infarction, as it increases myocardial oxygen demand and may be pro-dysrhythmogenic. **Nefopam** causes a high incidence of minor adverse effects, especially after parenteral use. These include sweating, nausea, headache, dry mouth, insomnia, dizziness and anorexia. **Nefopam** is contraindicated in glaucoma, and can cause urinary retention in men with prostatic hypertrophy.

Pharmacokinetics

Nefopam is rapidly absorbed following oral administration. It is extensively metabolized by the liver to inactive compounds excreted in the urine. Presystemic metabolism is substantial.

Drug interactions

Nefopam can cause potentially fatal hypertension with monoamine oxidase inhibitors (MAOIs) and potentiates the dysrhythmogenic effect of halothane.

OPIOIDS

Opium is derived from the dried milky juice exuded by incised seed capsules of a species of poppy, *Papaver somniferum*, that is grown in Turkey, India and South-East Asia. Homer refers to it in the *Odyssey* as 'nepenthes', a drug given to Odysseus and his followers 'to banish grief or trouble of the mind'. Osler referred to it as 'God's own medicine'. A number of notably discreditable events, including the Opium Wars, ensued from the commercial, social, moral and political interests involved in its world-wide trade and use. Opium is a complex mixture of alkaloids, the principal components being **morphine**, **codeine** and **papaverine**. The main analgesic action of **opium** is due to **morphine**. **Papaverine** is a vasodilator without analgesic actions.

Until 1868, **opium** could be purchased without prescription from grocers' shops in the UK. Much work has gone into synthesizing **morphine** analogues in the hope of producing a drug with the therapeutic actions of **morphine**, but without its disadvantages. **Morphine** was introduced as a 'non-addictive' alternative to **opium** and this in turn was superseded by **diamorphine**, which was also believed to be non-addicting! Synthetic drugs such as **pethidine**, **dextropropoxyphene** and **pentazocine** were originally incorrectly thought to lack potential for abuse.

Morphine is active when given by mouth and a more rapid effect can be obtained if it is administered intravenously, but the potential for abuse is also greatly increased. Some anaesthetists give synthetic high potency opioids, such as **fentanyl**, either intravenously or epidurally, for obstetric surgery (e.g. Caesarean section).+

OPIOID RECEPTORS

Stereospecific receptors with a high affinity for opioid analgesics are present in neuronal membranes. They are found in high concentrations in the PAG, the limbic system, the thalamus, the hypothalamus, medulla oblongata and the substantia gelatinosa of the spinal cord. Several endogenous peptides with analgesic properties are widely distributed throughout the nervous system. They can be divided into the following three groups:

1. encephalins (leu-encephalin and met-encephalin) are pentapeptides;
2. dynorphins are extended forms of encephalins;
3. endorphins (e.g. β-endorphin).

These peptides are derived from larger precursors (pro-opiomelanocortin, pro-encephalin and pro-dynorphin) and act as neurotransmitters or neuromodulators (neurotransmitters convey information from an axon terminal to a related nerve cell, whereas neuromodulators influence the responsiveness of one or more neurons to other mediators, see Figure 25.6).

There are three types of opioid receptor, named μ, δ and κ. All belong to the G-protein coupled receptor family, and μ is the most important. A fourth category, σ, is now not classified as an opioid receptor because they bind non-opioid psychotomimetic drugs of abuse, such as **phencyclidine** and the only opioids that bind appreciably to them are drugs like **pentazocine** that have psychotomimetic adverse effects.

Blocking opioid receptors with **naloxone** (see below) has little effect in normal individuals, but in patients suffering from chronic pain it produces hyperalgesia. Electrical stimulation of areas of the brain that are rich in encephalins and opioid receptors elicits analgesia which is abolished by **naloxone**, implying

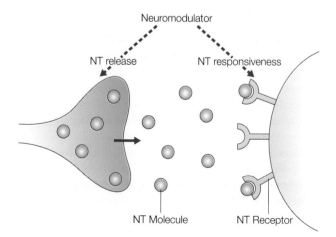

Figure 25.6: Role of neurotransmitter and neuromodulator at synapse. -->, Stimulatory or inhibitory action; NT, neurotransmitter.

that it is caused by liberation of endogenous opioids. Pain relief by acupuncture may also be mediated by encephalin release, because it is antagonized by **naloxone**.

Narcotic analgesics exert their effects by binding to opioid receptors. The resulting pattern of pharmacological activity depends on their affinity for the various receptors and whether they are full or partial agonists. The affinity of narcotic analgesics for μ-receptors parallels their analgesic potency. In addition to their involvement in brain function, the opioid peptides play a neuroendocrine role. Administration in humans suppresses the pituitary–gonadal and pituitary–adrenal axis and stimulates the release of prolactin, thyroid-stimulating hormone (TSH) and growth hormone. High concentrations of opioid peptides are also present in sympathetic ganglia and the adrenal medulla. Their function at these sites has not been elucidated, but they may play an inhibitory role in the sympathetic system.

Following repeated administration of an exogenous opioid, the sensitivity of the receptors decreases, necessitating an increased dose to produce the same effect ('tolerance'). On withdrawal of the drug, endogenous opioids are not sufficient to stimulate the insensitive receptors, resulting in a withdrawal state characterized by autonomic disturbances, e.g. pallor, sweating and piloerection ('cold turkey') and abdominal pain.

MORPHINE

Use

- The most important use of **morphine** is for pain relief. The effective dose is highly variable. Previous analgesic requirements (if known) should be taken into account when selecting a dose.
- **Morphine** may be given as an intravenous bolus if rapid relief is required (e.g. during myocardial infarction).
- Alternatively, **morphine** can be given continuously by an infusion pump (e.g. post-operatively), either intravenously or subcutaneously.
- **Morphine** is effective orally, although larger doses are needed due to presystemic metabolism. **Morphine** is given by mouth initially every four hours, giving additional doses as needed between the regular doses as a 'top-up', the daily dose being reviewed and titrated. Once the dose requirement is established, sustained-release morphine (12-hourly) is substituted, which should still be supplemented by immediate release morphine, for breakthrough pain.
- Spinal (epidural or intrathecal) administration of **morphine** is effective at much lower doses than when given by other routes and causes fewer systemic side effects. It is useful in those few patients with opioid-responsive pain who experience intolerable side effects when morphine is administered by other routes.
- Continuous subcutaneous infusions by pump are useful in the terminally ill. There is an advantage in using **diamorphine** rather than **morphine** for this purpose, since its greater solubility permits smaller volumes of more concentrated solution to be used.

- **Morphine** is effective in the relief of acute left ventricular failure, via dilatation of the pulmonary vasculature and the great veins.
- **Morphine** inhibits cough, but **codeine** is preferred for this indication.
- **Morphine** relieves diarrhoea, but **codeine** is preferred for this indication.

Mechanism of action

Morphine relieves both the perception of pain and the emotional response to it.

Adverse effects

Certain patients are particularly sensitive to the pharmacological actions of **morphine**. These include the very young, the elderly and those with chronic lung disease, untreated hypothyroidism, chronic liver disease and chronic renal failure. Overdose leads to coma. **Morphine** depresses the sensitivity of the respiratory centre to carbon dioxide, thus causing a progressively decreased respiratory rate. Patients with decreased respiratory reserve due to asthma, bronchitis, emphysema or hypoxaemia of any cause are more sensitive to the respiratory depressant effect of opioids. Bronchoconstriction occurs via histamine release, but is usually mild and clinically important only in asthmatics, in whom **morphine** should be used with care and only for severe pain. **Morphine** causes vomiting in 20–30% of patients by stimulation of the chemoreceptor trigger zone. Dopamine receptors are important and opioid-induced emesis is responsive to dopamine-receptor antagonists (e.g. **prochlorperazine**). **Morphine** increases smooth muscle tone throughout the gastro-intestinal tract, which is combined with decreased peristalsis. The result is constipation with hard dry stool. The increase in muscle tone also involves the sphincter of Oddi and **morphine** increases intrabiliary pressure. Dependence (both physical and psychological) is particularly likely to occur if **morphine** is used for the pleasurable feeling it produces, rather than in a therapeutic context. In common with most other opioids it causes pupillary constriction. This provides a useful diagnostic sign in narcotic overdosage or chronic abuse. Patients with prostatic hypertrophy may suffer acute retention of urine, as **morphine** increases the tone in the sphincter of the bladder neck.

Pharmacokinetics

Morphine can be given orally or by subcutaneous, intramuscular or intravenous injection. **Morphine** is metabolized by combination with glucuronic acid and also by *N*-dealkylation and oxidation, about 10% being excreted in the urine as morphine and 60–70% as a mixture of glucuronides. Metabolism occurs in the liver and gut wall, with extensive presystemic metabolism. The dose–plasma concentration relationships for **morphine** and its main metabolite are linear over a wide range of oral dosage. Morphine-6-glucuronide has analgesic properties and contributes substantially to the analgesic action of **morphine**. Only low concentrations of this active metabolite appear in the blood after a single oral dose. With repeated dosing the concentration of morphine-6-glucuronide increases, correlating with the high efficacy of repeated-dose oral **morphine**. Morphine-6-glucuronide is eliminated in the urine, so patients with renal impairment may experience severe and prolonged respiratory depression. The birth of opiate-dependent babies born to addicted mothers demonstrates the ability of **morphine** and its glucuronide to cross the placenta.

Drug interactions

- **Morphine** augments other central nervous system depressants.
- Morphine should not be combined with MAOIs.
- Opioid (μ) receptor antagonists (e.g. **naloxone**) are used in overdose.

DIAMORPHINE ('HEROIN')
Use

Diamorphine is diacetylmorphine. Its actions are similar to those of **morphine**, although it is more potent as an analgesic when given by injection. **Diamorphine** has a reputation for having a greater addictive potential than **morphine** and is banned in the USA. The more rapid central effect of intravenous **diamorphine** than of **morphine** (the faster 'buzz'), due to rapid penetration of the blood–brain barrier, makes this plausible (see below). **Diamorphine** is used for the same purposes as **morphine**. It is more soluble than **morphine**, and this may be relevant to limit injection volume (e.g. in epidural analgesia).

Adverse effects

The adverse effects of **diamorphine** are the same as those for **morphine**.

Pharmacokinetics

Diamorphine is hydrolysed (deacetylated) rapidly to form 6-acetylmorphine and morphine, and if given by mouth owes its effect entirely to **morphine**. **Diamorphine** crosses the blood–brain barrier even more rapidly than **morphine**. This accounts for its rapid effect when administered intravenously and hence increased abuse potential compared with **morphine**.

PETHIDINE
Use

The actions of **pethidine** are similar to those of **morphine**. It causes similar respiratory depression, vomiting and gastro-intestinal smooth muscle contraction to **morphine**, but does not constrict the pupil, release histamine or suppress cough. It produces little euphoria, but does cause dependence. It can cause convulsions. **Pethidine** is sometimes used in obstetrics because it does not reduce the activity of the pregnant uterus, but **morphine** is often preferred. Delayed gastric emptying (common to all opioids) is of particular concern in obstetrics, as gastric aspiration is a leading cause of maternal morbidity.

Pharmacokinetics

Hepatic metabolism is the main route of elimination. Norpethidine is an important metabolite since it is proconvulsant. The $t_{1/2}$ of **pethidine** is three to four hours in healthy individuals, but this is increased in the elderly and in patients with liver disease. **Pethidine** crosses the placenta and causes respiratory depression of the neonate. This is exacerbated by the prolonged elimination $t_{1/2}$ in neonates of about 22 hours.

Drug interactions

- When **pethidine** is given with monoamine oxidase inhibitors, rigidity, hyperpyrexia, excitement, hypotension and coma can occur.
- **Pethidine**, like other opiates, delays gastric emptying, thus interfering with the absorption of co-administered drugs.

ALFENTANYL, FENTANYL AND REMIFENTANYL
Use

These are derivatives of pethidine. They are more potent but shorter-acting and are used to treat severe pain or as an adjunct to anaesthesia. **Fentanyl** is available as a transdermal patch which is changed every 72 hours. They can be given intrathecally and via patient-controlled devices.

TRAMADOL
Use

Tramadol is widely used for moderate to severe pain, including post-operative pain. It can be administered by mouth, or by intramuscular or intravenous injection

Mechanism of action

Tramadol works partly through an agonist effect at μ receptors (opioid action) and partly by enhancing amine (5HT and catecholamine) transmission (and hence gating mechanism) by blocking neuronal amine re-uptake.

Adverse effects

These differ from pure opioid agonists, including less respiratory depression, constipation and abuse potential. Diarrhoea, abdominal pain, hypotension, psychiatric reactions, as well as seizures and withdrawal syndromes have been reported.

METHADONE
Use

Methadone has very similar actions to **morphine**, but is less sedating and longer acting. Its main use is by mouth to replace **morphine** or **diamorphine** when these drugs are being withdrawn in the treatment of drug dependence. **Methadone** given once daily under supervision is preferable to leaving addicts to seek **diamorphine** illicitly. Many of the adverse effects of opioid abuse are related to parenteral administration, with its attendant risks of infection (e.g. endocarditis, human immunodeficiency virus or hepatitis). The object is to reduce craving by occupying opioid receptors, simultaneously reducing the 'buzz' from any additional dose taken. The slower onset following oral administration reduces the reward and reinforcement of dependence. The relatively long half-life reduces the intensity of withdrawal and permits once-daily dosing under supervision. **Methadone** is also becoming more widely used in the treatment of chronic or terminal pain patients where its additional property of being an NMDA antagonist may be helpful.

Pharmacokinetics

After oral dosage, the peak blood concentration is achieved within about four hours, and once-daily dosing is practicable because of its long half-life.

CODEINE

Use

Codeine is the methyl ether of **morphine**, but has only about 10% of its analgesic potency. (**Dihydrocodeine** is similar, and is a commonly prescribed alternative.) Although **codeine** is converted to **morphine**, it produces little euphoria and has low addiction potential. As a result, it has been used for many years as an analgesic for moderate pain, as a cough suppressant and for symptomatic relief of diarrhoea.

Adverse effects

Common adverse effects involve constipation, nausea and vomiting.

Pharmacokinetics

Free **morphine** also appears in plasma following **codeine** administration, and **codeine** acts as a prodrug, producing a low but sustained concentration of **morphine**. Individuals who are CYP2D6 poor metabolizers convert much less **codeine** to **morphine**, and consequently experience less, if any, analgesic effect.

PENTAZOCINE

Pentazocine is a partial agonist on opioid receptors (especially κ-receptors, with additional actions on σ-receptors, which result in hallucinations and thought disturbance). It also increases pulmonary artery pressure. Its use is not recommended.

BUPRENORPHINE

Use

Buprenorphine is a partial agonist. It is given sublingually. It antagonizes full agonists and can precipitate pain and cause withdrawal symptoms in patients who are already receiving **morphine**. It has recently (in the USA, as well as in the UK) become more widely used in the treatment of opiate withdrawal as an alternative to **methadone**.

Pharmacokinetics

Like other opiates, **buprenorphine** is subject to considerable pre-systemic and hepatic first-pass metabolism (via glucuronidation to inactive metabolites), but this is circumvented by sublingual administration.

OPIOID ANTAGONISTS

Minor alterations in the chemical structure of opioids result in drugs that are competitive antagonists.

NALOXONE

Naloxone is a pure competitive antagonist of opioid agonists at μ-receptors. It is given intravenously, the usual dose being 0.8–2.0 mg for the treatment of poisoning with full opiate agonists (e.g. **morphine**), higher doses (up to ten times the recommended dose, depending on clinical response) being required for overdosage with partial agonists (e.g. **buprenorphine**, **pentazocine**). Its effect has a rapid onset and if a satisfactory response has not been obtained within three minutes, the dose may be repeated. The action of many opioids outlasts that of **naloxone**, which has a $t_{1/2}$ of one hour, and a constant-rate infusion of **naloxone** may be needed in these circumstances. **Naloxone** is used in the management of the apnoeic infant after birth when the mother has received opioid analgesia during labour. **Naloxone** can precipitate acute withdrawal symptoms in opiate-dependent patients.

NALTREXONE

Naltrexone is an orally active opioid antagonist that is used in specialized clinics as adjunctive treatment to reduce the risk of relapse in former opioid addicts who have been detoxified. Such patients who are receiving **naltrexone** in addition to supportive therapy, are less likely to resume illicit opiate use (detected by urine measurements) than those receiving placebo plus supportive therapy. However, the drop-out rate is high due to non-compliance. **Naltrexone** has weak agonist activity, but this is not clinically important, and withdrawal symptoms do not follow abrupt cessation of treatment. Treatment should not be started until the addict has been opioid-free for at least seven days for short-acting drugs (e.g. **diamorphine** or **morphine**), or ten days for longer-acting drugs (e.g. **methadone**), because it can precipitate a severe and prolonged abstinence syndrome. **Naltrexone** has not been extensively studied in non-addicts, and most of the symptoms that have been attributed to it are those that arise from opioid withdrawal. Its major side effects are various type of rash.

ANALGESICS IN TERMINAL DISEASE

The relief of pain in terminal disease, usually cancer, requires skilful use of analgesic drugs. There are several important principles:

- Non-opioid analgesics minimize opioid requirement. The World Health Organization (WHO) has endorsed a simple stepwise approach (WHO 'pain ladder'), moving from non-opioid to weak opioid to strong opioid. For mild pain, **paracetamol**, **aspirin** or **codeine** (a weak opioid) or a combined preparation (e.g. **cocodamol**) is usually satisfactory.
- **Morphine** (or a congener) is the key treatment for severe pain. It is important to use a large enough dose, if necessary given intravenously, to relieve the pain completely. There is a wide range in dose needed to suppress pain in different individuals.
- Drug dependence is not a problem in this type of patient.
- It is much easier to prevent pain before it has built up than to relieve pain when it has fully developed.

- If possible, use oral medications. Once pain control is established (e.g. with frequent doses of **morphine** orally), change to a slow-release **morphine** preparation. This produces a smoother control of pain, without peaks and troughs of analgesia, which can still be supplemented with shorter duration **morphine** formulations for breakthrough pain.

Tolerance is not a problem in this setting, the dose being increased until pain relief is obtained.

Adverse effects of opioids should be anticipated. **Prochlorperazine** or **metoclopramide** can be used to reduce nausea and vomiting, and may increase analgesia. Stimulant laxatives, such as senna, and/or glycerine suppositories should be used routinely to reduce constipation. Spinal administration of opioids is not routinely available, but is sometimes useful for those few patients with opioid-responsive pain who experience intolerable systemic side effects when **morphine** is given orally.

Bone pain is often most effectively relieved by local radiotherapy rather than by drugs, but bisphosphonates (see Chapter 39) and/or NSAIDs are useful.

Key points

Analgesics in terminal care

- Stepwise use of non-opioid to opioid analgesics as per the WHO analgesic ladder (e.g. paracetomol)/weak opioid (e.g. codeine)/strong opioid (e.g. morphine) is rational when the patient presents with mild symptoms.
- In cases where severe pain is already established, parenteral morphine is often needed initially, followed by regular frequent doses of morphine by mouth with additional ('top-up'–'breakthrough') doses prescribed as needed, followed by conversion to an effective dose of long-acting (slow-release) oral morphine, individualized to the patient's requirements.
- Chronic morphine necessitates adjunctive treatment with:
  - anti-emetics: prochloperazine, metoclopramide;
  - laxative: senna.
- Additional measures that are often useful include:
  - radiotherapy (for painful metastases);
  - a cyclo-oxygenase inhibitor (especially with bone involvement);
  - bisphosphonates are also effective in metastatic bone pain
  - an antidepressant.

MANAGEMENT OF POST-OPERATIVE PAIN

Post-operative pain provides a striking demonstration of the importance of higher functions in the perception of pain. When patients are provided with devices that enable them to control their own analgesia (see below), they report superior pain relief but use less analgesic medication than when this is administered intermittently on demand. Unfortunately, post-operative pain has traditionally been managed by analgesics prescribed by the most inexperienced surgical staff and administered at the discretion of nursing staff. Recently, anaesthetists have become more involved in the management of post-operative pain and

pain teams have led to notable improvements. There are several general principles:

- Surgery results in pain as the anaesthetic wears off. This causes fear, which makes the pain worse. This vicious circle can be avoided by time spent on pre-operative explanation, giving reassurance that pain is not a result of things having gone wrong, will be transient and will be controlled.
- Analgesics are always more effective in preventing the development of pain than in treating it when it has developed. Regular use of mild analgesics can be highly effective. Non-steroidal anti-inflammatory drugs (e.g. **ketorolac**, which can be given parenterally) can have comparable efficacy to opioids when used in this way. They are particularly useful after orthopaedic surgery.
- Parenteral administration is usually only necessary for a short time post-operatively, after which analgesics can be given orally. The best way to give parenteral opioid analgesia is often by intravenous or subcutaneous infusion under control of the patient (patient-controlled analgesia (PCA)). Opioids are effective in visceral pain and are especially valuable after abdominal surgery. Some operations (e.g. cardiothoracic surgery) cause both visceral and somatic pain, and regular prescription of both an opioid and a non-opioid analgesic is appropriate. Once drugs can be taken by mouth, slow-release morphine, or **buprenorphine** prescribed on a regular basis, are effective. Breakthrough pain can be treated by additional oral or parenteral doses of **morphine**.
- **Tramadol** is useful when respiratory depression is a particular concern.
- Anti-emetics (e.g. **metoclopramide**, **prochlorperazine**) should be routinely prescribed to be administered on an 'as-needed' basis. They are only required by a minority of patients, but should be available without delay when needed.
- A nitrous oxide/oxygen mixture (50/50) can be self-administered and is useful during painful procedures, such as dressing changes or physiotherapy, and for childbirth. It should not be used for prolonged periods (e.g. in intensive care units), as it can cause vitamin B_{12} deficiency in this setting.

Key points

Analgesia and post-operative pain

- Pre-operative explanation minimizes analgesic requirements.
- Prevention of post-operative pain is initiated during anaesthesia (e.g. local anaesthetics, parenteral cyclo-oxygenase inhibitor).
- Patient-controlled analgesia using morphine is safe and effective.
- The switch to oral analgesia should be made as soon as possible.
- Anti-emetics should be prescribed 'as needed', to avoid delay if they are required.

Key points

Opioids

- The main drug is morphine, which is a full agonist at μ-receptors.
- The effects of morphine include:
  - analgesia;
  - relief of left ventricular failure;
  - miosis (pupillary constriction);
  - suppression of cough ('antitussive' effect);
  - constipation;
  - nausea/vomiting;
  - liberation of histamine (pruritus, bronchospasm);
  - addiction;
  - tolerance;
  - withdrawal symptoms following chronic use.
- Diamorphine ('heroin'):
  - is metabolized rapidly to morphine;
  - gains access to the central nervous system (CNS) more rapidly than morphine (when given i.v. or snorted);
  - for this reason gives a rapid 'buzz';
  - may therefore have an even higher potential for abuse than morphine;
  - is more soluble than morphine.
- Codeine and dihydrocodeine are:
  - weak opioid prodrugs;
  - slowly metabolized to morphine;
  - used in combination with paracetamol for moderate pain;
  - used for diarrhoea or as antitussives.
- Pethidine:
  - is a strong synthetic opioid;
  - metabolized to normeperidine which can cause seizures;
  - does not inhibit uterine contraction;
  - is widely used in obstetrics;
  - can cause respiratory depression in neonates;
  - is less liable than morphine to cause bronchial constriction;
  - does not cause miosis;
  - has potential for abuse.
- Buprenorphine and dextropropoxyphene are partial agonists.
  - Buprenorphine is used sublingually in severe chronic pain.
  - Dextropropoxyphene is combined with paracetamol for moderately severe chronic pain. This combination is no more effective than paracetamol alone for acute pain and is very dangerous in overdose. The March 2007 British National Formulary states 'co-proxamol (dextropropoxyphene + paracetamol) is to be withdrawn from the market and the CSM has advised that co-proxamol treatment should *no longer* (their emphasis) be prescribed'.
- Opioid effects are antagonized competitively by naloxone: very large doses are needed to reverse the effects of partial opiate agonists, e.g. buprenorphine, pentazocine.

Case history

A 55-year-old retired naval officer presents to the Accident and Emergency Department with sudden onset of very severe back pain. A chest x-ray reveals a mass, and plain spine films shows a crush fracture. He is admitted at 9 a.m. for further management and investigation. On examination he is pale, sweaty and distressed. The doctor on call prescribes morphine 10 mg subcutaneously, four-hourly as needed, and the pain responds well to the first dose, following which the patient falls into a light sleep.

That evening his wife, scarcely able to contain her anger, approaches the consultant on the Firm's round and strongly advocates that her husband be given some more analgesic.

Comment

Communication is key in managing pain. There are often difficulties when, as in the present case, the diagnosis is probable but not confirmed, and when the patient is admitted to a general ward which may be short of nursing staff. The Senior House Officer was concerned not to cause respiratory depression, so did not prescribe regular analgesia, but unfortunately neither medical nor nursing staff realized that the patient had awoken with recurrent severe pain. He had not himself asked for additional analgesia (which was prescribed) because his personality traits would lead him to lie quietly and 'suffer in silence'. The good initial response suggests that his pain will respond well to regular oral morphine, and this indeed proved to be the case. A subsequent biopsy confirmed squamous-cell carcinoma, and a bone scan demonstrated multiple metastases, one of which had led to a crush fracture of a vertebral body visible on plain x-ray. A non-steroidal drug (e.g. ibuprofen or ketorolac) reduced his immediate requirement for morphine, and radiotherapy resolved his back pain completely. Morphine was discontinued. He remained pain-free at home for the next four months and was then found dead in bed by his wife. Autopsy was not performed. One of several possibilities is that he died from pulmonary embolism.

FURTHER READING

Ballantyne JC, Mao JR. Opioid therapy for chronic pain. *New England Journal of Medicine* 2003; **349**: 1943–53.

Dahl JB, Kehlet H. The value of pre-emptive analgesia in the treatment of post-operative pain. *British Journal of Anaesthesia* 1993; **70**: 434–9.

Holdgate A, Pollock T. Systematic review of the relative efficacy of non-steroidal anti-inflammatory drugs and opioids in the treatment of acute renal colic. *British Medical Journal* 2004; **328**: 1401–4.

McMahon S, Koltzenburg M. *Wall and Melzack's textbook of pain*, 5th edn. Edinburgh: Churchill Livingstone, 2005.

PART III

THE MUSCULOSKELETAL SYSTEM

CHAPTER 26

ANTI-INFLAMMATORY DRUGS AND THE TREATMENT OF ARTHRITIS

INTRODUCTION: INFLAMMATION

Inflammation plays a major role in the pathophysiology of a wide spectrum of diseases. It is primarily a protective response, but if excessive or inappropriately prolonged can contribute adversely to the disease process. Consequently anti-inflammatory drugs are very widely used. Some are safe enough to be available over the counter, but they are a two-edged sword and potent anti-inflammatory drugs can have severe adverse effects.

Inflammatory cells: many different cells are involved in different stages of different kinds of inflammatory response, including neutrophils (e.g. in acute bacterial infections), eosinophils, mast cells and lymphocytes (e.g. in asthma, see Chapter 33), monocytes, macrophages and lymphocytes (for example, in autoimmune vasculitic disease, including chronic joint diseases, such as rheumatoid arthritis and atherothrombosis, where platelets are also important, see Chapter 27).

Inflammatory mediators: include prostaglandins, complement- and coagulation-cascade-derived peptides, and cytokines (for example, interleukins, especially IL-2 and IL-6, and tumour necrosis factor (TNF)). The mediators orchestrate and amplify the inflammatory cell responses. Anti-inflammatory drugs work on different aspects of the inflammatory cascade including the synthesis and action of mediators, and in the case of immunosuppressants on the amplification of the response (see Chapter 50).

NON-STEROIDAL ANTI-INFLAMMATORY DRUGS

Non-steroidal anti-inflammatory drugs (NSAIDs) inhibit prostaglandin biosynthesis by inhibiting cyclo-oxygenase (COX), see Figure 26.1. This is the basis of most of their therapeutic, as well as their undesired actions. COX is a key enzyme in the synthesis of prostaglandins and thromboxanes (see also Chapters 25 and 30), important medi-ators of the erythema, oedema, pain and fever of inflammation. There are two main isoforms of the enzyme, namely a constitutive form (COX-1) that is present in platelets, stomach, kidneys and other tissues, and an inducible form, (COX-2), that is expressed in inflamed tissues as a result of stimulation by cytokines and is also present to a lesser extent in healthy organs, including the kidneys. (A third form, COX-3, is a variant of COX-1 of uncertain importance in humans.) Selective inhibitors of COX-2 were developed with the potential of reduced gastric toxicity. This was at least partly realized, but several of these drugs increased atherothrombotic events, probably as a class effect related to inhibition of basal prostacyclin biosynthesis.

Use

NSAIDs provide symptomatic relief in acute and chronic inflammation, but do not improve the course of chronic inflammatory conditions, such as rheumatoid arthritis as regards disability and deformity. There is considerable variation in clinical response. Other types of pain, both mild (e.g. headaches, dysmenorrhoea, muscular sprains and other soft tissue injuries) and severe (e.g. pain from metastatic deposits in bone) may respond to NSAID treatment (Chapter 25). Aspirin is a special case in that it irreversibly inhibits COX-1 and has a unique role as an antiplatelet drug (Chapters 29 and 30), as well as retaining a place as a mild analgesic in adults.

Adverse effects and interactions common to NSAIDs

The main adverse effects of NSAIDs are predominantly in the following tissues:

- *gastro-intestinal tract*: gastritis and gastric mucosal ulceration and bleeding;
- *kidneys*: vasoregulatory renal impairment, hyperkalaemia, nephritis, interstitial nephritis and nephrotic syndrome;
- *airways*: bronchospasm;
- *heart*: cardiac failure with fluid retention and myocardial infarction (COX-2);
- *liver*: biochemical hepatitis.

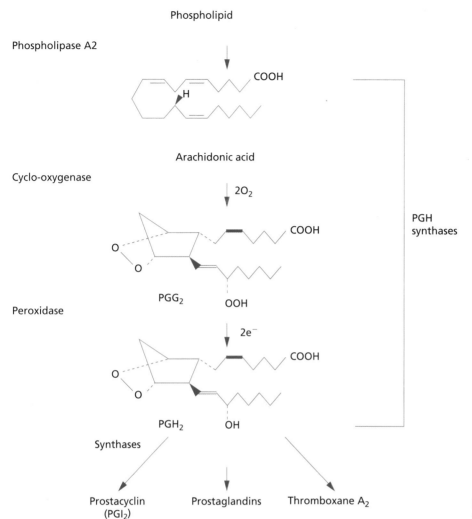

Figure 26.1: The arachidonic acid cascade.

Adverse effects of NSAID on the stomach are covered in Chapter 25. They can be reduced by co-administration of a proton pump inhibitor, such as **omeprazole** (Chapter 34).

The main prostaglandins produced in human kidneys are prostacyclin (PGI_2) and prostaglandin E_2. NSAIDs predictably cause functional renal impairment in patients with pre-existing glomerular disease (e.g. lupus nephritis), or with systemic diseases in which renal blood flow is dependent on the kidneys' ability to synthesize these vasodilator prostaglandins. These include heart failure, salt and water depletion, cirrhosis and nephrotic syndrome. The elderly, with their reduced glomerular filtration rate and reduced capacity to eliminate NSAIDs, are especially at risk. Renal impairment is reversible within a few days if the NSAID is stopped promptly. All NSAIDs can cause this effect, but it is less common with **aspirin** or low doses of **sulindac**. This is because **sulindac** is a prodrug that acts through an active sulphide metabolite; the kidney converts the sulphide back into the inactive sulphone. **Sulindac** is therefore relatively 'renal sparing', although, at higher doses, inhibition of renal prostaglandin biosynthesis and consequent renal impairment in susceptible patients do occur. For the same reason (inhibition of renal prostaglandin biosynthesis), NSAIDs all interact non-specifically with antihypertensive medication, rendering them less effective. NSAIDs are a common cause of loss of control of blood pressure in treated hypertensive patients. Again and for the same reasons, **aspirin** and **sulindac** are less likely to cause this problem.

PGE_2 and PGI_2 are natriuretic as well as vasodilators, and NSAIDs consequently cause salt and water retention, antagonize the effects of diuretics and exacerbate heart failure. (Some of their interaction with diuretics also reflects competition for the renal tubular weak acid secretory mechanism.) As well as reducing sodium excretion, NSAIDs reduce lithium ion clearance and plasma concentrations of lithium should be closely monitored in patients on maintenance doses of lithium in whom treatment with an NSAID is initiated. NSAIDs increase plasma potassium ion concentration.

In addition to these predictable effects on the kidney, NSAIDs can cause acute interstitial nephritis, presenting as nephrotic syndrome or renal impairment that resolves after withdrawing the drug. This is an idiosyncratic effect, unique to a particular drug within one susceptible individual. NSAIDs worsen bronchospasm in **aspirin**-sensitive asthmatics (who sometimes have a history of nasal polyps and urticaria, see

Chapter 33). All NSAIDs cause wheezing in **aspirin**-sensitive individuals.

COX-2 inhibitors increase cardiovascular events, limiting their usefulness. Unfortunately, they were aggressively marketed to elderly people many of whom were not at high risk for gastro-toxicity and this has led to the withdrawal of agents that would have been valuable for a more carefully targeted patient population. It is unclear how much, if any, cardiovascular risk is associated with conventional NSAIDs, but it is possible that this is, at a maximum, similar to certain COX-2-selective drugs.

NSAIDs cause hepatitis in some patients. The mechanism is not understood, but the elderly are particularly susceptible. Different NSAIDs vary in how commonly they cause this problem. (Hepatotoxicity was one of the reasons for the withdrawal of one such drug, **benoxaprofen**, from the market.) **Aspirin** is a recognized cause of hepatitis, particularly in patients with systemic lupus erythematosus.

Aspirin and ibuprofen are covered in Chapter 25). Other important NSAIDs are covered below.

INDOMETACIN

Use

Indometacin has a powerful anti-inflammatory action, but only a weak analgesic action. It is used to treat rheumatoid arthritis and associated disorders, ankylosing spondylitis and acute gout. Adverse effects are common (approximately 25% of patients).

Adverse effects

Gastric intolerance and toxicity, renal and pulmonary toxicities occur, as with other NSAIDs (see above). Headache is also common; less often light-headedness, confusion or hallucinations arise.

Pharmacokinetics

Indometacin is readily absorbed by mouth or from suppositories. It undergoes extensive hepatic metabolism. Both the parent drug and inactive metabolites are excreted in the urine.

Drug interactions

The actions of antihypertensive drugs and diuretics are opposed by **indometacin**. **Triamterene**, in particular, should be avoided, because of hyperkalaemia.

NAPROXEN

Use

Naproxen is used rheumatic and musculoskeletal diseases, acute gout and dysmenorrhoea.

Mechanism of action

Naproxen is approximately 20 times as potent an inhibitor of COX as **aspirin**. An additional property is inhibition of leukocyte migration, with a potency similar to **colchicine**.

Adverse effects

Naproxen causes all of the adverse effects common to NSAIDs.

> **Key points**
>
> NSAIDs
>
> - Inhibit cyclo-oxygenase (COX).
> - Examples include indometacin, naproxen and ibuprofen.
> - Uses:
>   - short term: analgesia/anti-inflammatory;
>   - chronic: symptomatic relief in arthritis.
> - Adverse effects:
>   - gastritis and other gastrointestinal inflammation/bleeding;
>   - reversible renal impairment (haemodynamic effect);
>   - interstitial nephritis (idiosyncratic);
>   - asthma in 'aspirin-sensitive' patients;
>   - hepatitis (idiosyncratic).
> - Interactions:
>   - antihypertensive drugs (reduced effectiveness);
>   - diuretics: reduced effectiveness
> - COX-2-selective drugs may have reduced gastric toxicity, but increase cardiovascular thrombotic events.

GLUCOCORTICOIDS

Glucocorticoids are discussed in Chapters 40 and 50. Despite their profound effects on inflammation (they were the original 'wonder drugs' of the 1950s), they have such severe long-term effects that their use is now much more circumscribed. **Prednisolone** is generally preferred for systemic use when a glucocorticoid is specifically indicated (e.g. for giant-cell arteritis, where steroid treatment prevents blindness). A brief course of high-dose **prednisolone** is usually given to suppress the disease, followed if possible by dose reduction to a maintenance dose, given first thing in the morning when endogenous glucocorticoids are at their peak. A marker of disease activity, such as C-reactive protein (CRP), is followed as a guide to dose reduction. Intra-articular steroid injections are important to reduce pain and deformity. It is essential to rule out infection before injecting steroids into a joint, and meticulous aseptic technique is needed to avoid introducing infection. A suspension of a poorly soluble drug, such as **triamcinolone**, is used to give a long-lasting effect. The patient is warned to avoid over-use of the joint should the desired improvement materialize, to avoid joint destruction. Repeated injections can cause joint destruction and bone necrosis.

DISEASE-MODIFYING ANTIRHEUMATIC DRUGS

Disease-modifying antirheumatic drugs (DMARDs) are not analgesic and do not inhibit COX, but they do suppress the inflammatory process in inflammatory arthritis. Their mechanisms are generally poorly understood. They are used in patients with progressive disease. Response (though unpredictable) is usually maximal in four to ten weeks. Unlike NSAIDs, DMARDs reduce inflammatory markers (historically, it was this effect that led to them being referred to as 'disease-modifying'). It is difficult to prove that a drug influences the natural history of a relapsing/remitting and unpredictably progressing disease, such as rheumatoid arthritis, but immunosuppressants retard the radiological progression of bony erosions. DMARDs are toxic, necessitating careful patient monitoring, and are best used by physicians experienced in rheumatology. Rheumatologists use them earlier than in the past, with close monitoring for toxicity, with the patient fully informed about toxic, as well as desired, effects. This is especially important since many of these drugs are licensed for quite different indications to arthritis. In terms of efficacy, **methotrexate**, **gold**, D-**penicillamine**, **azathioprine** and **sulfasalazine** are similar, and are all more potent than **hydroxychloroquine**. **Methotrexate** (Chapter 48) is better tolerated than the other DMARDs, and is usually the first choice. **Sulfasalazine** (Chapter 34) is the second choice. Alternative DMARDs, and some of their adverse effects, are summarized in Table 26.1.

GOLD SALTS

Use

Gold was originally introduced to treat tuberculosis. Although ineffective, it was found to have antirheumatic properties and has been used to treat patients with rheumatoid arthritis since the 1920s. **Sodium aurothiomalate** is administered weekly by deep intramuscular injection. About 75% of patients improve, with a reduction in joint swelling, disappearance of rheumatoid nodules and a fall in C-reactive protein (CRP) levels. Urine must be tested for protein and full blood count (with platelet count and differential white cell count) performed before each injection. **Auranofin** is an oral gold preparation with less toxicity, but less efficacy than **aurothiomalate**. Treatment should be stopped if there is no response within six months.

Mechanism of action

The precise mechanism of gold salts is unknown. Several effects could contribute. Gold–albumin complexes are phagocytosed by macrophages and polymorphonuclear leukocytes and concentrated in their lysosomes, where **gold** inhibits lysosomal enzymes that have been implicated in causing joint damage. **Gold** binds to sulphhydryl groups and inhibits sulphhydryl–disulphide interchange in immunoglobulin and complement, which could influence immune processes.

Adverse effects

Adverse effects are common and severe:

- Rashes are an indication to stop treatment, as they can progress to exfoliation.
- Photosensitive eruptions and urticaria are often preceded by itching.
- Glomerular injury can cause nephrotic syndrome. Treatment must be withheld if more than a trace of proteinuria is present, and should not be resumed until the urine is protein free.
- Blood dyscrasias (e.g. neutropenia) can develop rapidly.

Table 26.1: Disease-modifying antirheumatic drugs (DMARDs)

Drug	Adverse effects	Comments
Immunosuppressants: azathioprine, methotrexate, ciclosporin	Blood dyscrasias, carcinogenesis, opportunistic infection, alopecia, nausea; methotrexate also causes mucositis and cirrhosis; ciclosporin causes nephrotoxicity, hypertension and hyperkalaemia	Methotrexate is usually the first-choice DMARD
Sulfasalazine	Blood dyscrasias, nausea, rashes, colours urine/tears orange	First introduced for arthritis, now used mainly in inflammatory bowel disease (Chapter 34)
Gold salts	Rashes, nephrotic syndrome, blood dyscrasias, stomatitis, diarrhoea	Oral preparation (auranofin) more convenient, less toxic, but less effective than intramuscular aurothiomalate
Penicillamine	Blood dyscrasias, proteinuria, urticaria	
Antimalarials: chloroquine, hydroxychloroquine	Retinopathy, nausea, diarrhoea, rashes, pigmentation of palate, bleaching of hair	See Chapter 47

- Stomatitis suggests the possibility of neutropenia.
- Diarrhoea is uncommon, but **gold** colitis is life-threatening.

Pharmacokinetics

The plasma half-life of **gold** increases with repeated administration and ranges from one day to several weeks. **Gold** is bound to plasma proteins and is concentrated in inflamed areas. It is excreted in urine and a small amount is lost in the faeces. **Gold** continues to be excreted in the urine for up to one year after a course of treatment.

PENCILLAMINE

Use

Penicillamine is a breakdown product of **penicillin**. Penicillamine should only be used by clinicians with experience of the drug and with meticulous monitoring, because of its toxicity (see below). Its effect in rheumatoid arthritis is similar to **gold**. Clinical improvement is anticipated only after 6–12 weeks. Treatment is discontinued if there is no improvement within one year. If improvement occurs, the dose is gradually reduced to the minimum effective maintenance dose. Full blood count and urine protein determination are performed regularly, initially weekly and then monthly during maintenance treatment.

Mechanism of action

Penicillamine acts by several mechanisms, including metal ion chelation and dissociation of macroglobulins. It inhibits release of lysosomal enzymes from cells in inflamed connective tissue.

Adverse effects

Penicillamine commonly causes taste disturbance, anorexia and weight loss. Other effects are more serious, and are more common in patients with poor sulphoxidation.

- Bone marrow hypoplasia, thrombocytopenia and leukopenia can be fatal. They are indications to stop treatment.
- Immune-complex glomerulonephritis causes mild proteinuria in 30% of patients. The drug should be stopped until proteinuria resolves and treatment then resumed at a lower dose. Heavy proteinuria is an indication to stop treatment permanently.
- Other symptoms include hypersensitivity reactions with urticaria.
- Systemic lupus erythematosus-like and myasthenia gravis-like syndromes can also be involved.

Contraindications

Penicillamine is contraindicated in patients with systemic lupus erythematosus, and should be used with caution, if at all, in individuals with renal or hepatic impairment.

Pharmacokinetics

Penicillamine is well absorbed. A number of hepatic metabolites are formed and rapidly excreted renally.

Drug interactions

Penicillamine should not be used with **gold**, **chloroquine** or immunosuppressive treatment, because of increased toxicity. It chelates metals and should not be given with iron preparations for this reason.

Key points

Disease-modifying antirheumatic drugs (DMARDs)

- Mechanisms are poorly understood; these drugs are often licensed for indications other than arthritis. Examples include:
  - methotrexate;
  - sulfasalazine;
  - gold;
  - D-penicillamine;
  - hydroxychloroquine;
  - cytokine (TNF) inhibitors.
- Uses: these drugs are used by rheumatologists to treat patients with progressive rheumatoid or psoriatic arthritis. A trial should be considered before a patient becomes disabled.
- All of these drugs can have severe adverse effects, and informed consent should be obtained before they are prescribed (especially those that are unlicensed for this indication).
- Their action is slow in onset.
- In contrast to NSAIDs, these drugs:
  - reduce erythrocyte sedimentation rate (ESR);
  - retard progression of bony erosions on x-ray.
- Close monitoring for toxicity (blood counts, urinalysis and serum chemistry) is essential.

CYTOKINE (TNF) INHIBITORS

Adalimumab, **infliximab** and **etanercerpt** are all engineered proteins which directly or indirectly inhibit tumour necrosis factor (TNF) signaling, by various mechanisms (blockade of TNF receptors or binding to, and hence inactivating, circulating TNF). They are a major advance in treating various immune diseases (see Chapter 50), including rheumatoid arthritis, but have serious adverse effects, including infusion reactions and reactivation of tuberculosis. Increased risk of malignancy is a theoretical concern. They are currently used by rheumatologists for adults with active disease which has not responded to two standard DMARD drugs, usually including **methotrexate** (Chapter 48). They are not continued if a response has not occurred within three months. Combinations of these proteins with **methotrexate** are being investigated for refractory disease, with encouraging results.

HYPERURICAEMIA AND GOUT

Uric acid is the end-product of purine metabolism in humans and gives rise to problems because of its limited solubility. Crystals of uric acid evoke a severe inflammatory response

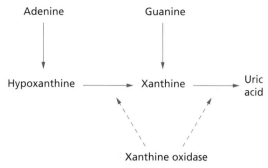

Figure 26.2: The final stages of the production of uric acid.

(acute gout), cause chalky deposits (tophi) and cause renal stones and/or renal tubular obstruction. The final enzymatic reactions in the production of uric acid are shown in Figure 26.2. Two of these stages are dependent on xanthine oxidase. In most mammals, uricase converts uric acid to allantoin, which is rapidly eliminated by the kidneys, but humans lack uricase, so the less soluble uric acid must be excreted. It is more soluble in an alkaline urine (Chapter 6). Plasma uric acid concentration is lowered either by increasing renal excretion or, more often, by inhibiting synthesis.

Hyperuricaemia often occurs in the setting of obesity and excessive ethanol consumption. Genetically determined defects of metabolism causing overproduction of uric acid are rare. Increased breakdown of nuclear material occurs in malignancies, particularly when treated by cytotoxic drugs, and is extremely important because it can lead to acute renal failure if measures are not taken to reduce urate formation and enhance its excretion in this setting (see below). Hyperuricaemia also occurs when excretion is decreased, for example, in renal failure or when tubular excretion is diminished by diuretics, **pyrazinamide** (Chapter 44) or low doses of **salicylate** (Chapter 25).

ACUTE GOUT

The acute attack is treated with anti-inflammatory analgesic agents (e.g. **indometacin**). **Aspirin** is contraindicated because of its effect on reducing urate excetion. **Colchicine** (derived from the autumn crocus) is relatively specific in relieving the symptoms of acute gout and is an alternative to an NSAID. It does not inhibit COX, so it lacks the side effects of NSAIDs, but commonly causes diarrhoea.

COLCHICINE
Use

Colchicine is a useful alternative to NSAIDs in patients with gout in whom NSAIDs are contraindicated. Its efficacy is similar to **indometacin**. It is also used in patients with familial Mediterranean fever and Behçet's disease. Unlike many NSAIDs, it does not interact with **warfarin**. For acute attacks, it is given up to four times a day. A low dose can be used prophylactically. It is relatively contraindicated in the elderly and in those with renal or gastro-intestinal disease.

Mechanism of action

Colchicine binds to the tubulin protein of microtubules and impairs their function This has important results:

- toxic concentrations cause arrest of cell division (exploited in making chromosome preparations ex vivo);
- inhibition of leukocyte migration and hence reduced inflammation.

Adverse effects

Adverse effects include the following:

- nausea, vomiting and diarrhoea;
- gastro-intestinal haemorrhage;
- rashes;
- renal failure;
- peripheral neuropathy;
- alopecia;
- blood dyscrasias.

Pharmacokinetics

Colchicine is well absorbed from the gastro-intestinal tract. It is partly metabolized, and a major portion is excreted via the bile and undergoes enterohepatic circulation, contributing to its gastro-intestinal toxicity.

PROPHYLAXIS FOR RECURRENT GOUT

ALLOPURINOL
Use

Allopurinol is used as long-term prophylaxis for patients with recurrent gout, especially tophaceous gout, urate renal stones, gout with renal failure and acute urate nephropathy, and to prevent this complication in patients about to undergo treatment with cytotoxic drugs, especially patients with haematological malignancies. The plasma uric acid concentration should be kept below 0.42 mmol/L. **Allopurinol** may provoke acute gout during the first few weeks of treatment. It must not be commenced till several weeks after an acute attack has completely resolved. Concurrent **indometacin** or **colchicine** is given during the first month of treatment.

Mechanism of action

Allopurinol is a xanthine oxidase inhibitor and decreases the production of uric acid (Figure 26.2). This reduces the concentration of uric acid in extracellular fluid, thereby preventing precipitation of crystals in joints or elsewhere. Uric acid is mobilized from tophaceous deposits which slowly disappear.

Adverse effects

Precipitating an acute attack (see above) is common if the above precautions are not adhered to. Mild dose-related rashes and life-threatening hypersensitivity reactions (including Stevens Johnson syndrome) can occur. Malaise, nausea, vertigo, alopecia and hepatotoxicity are uncommon toxicities.

Pharmacokinetics

Allopurinol is well absorbed. Hepatic metabolism yields **oxypurinol**, itself a weak xanthine oxidase inhibitor.

Drug interactions

- **Allopurinol** decreases the breakdown of 6-mercaptopurine (the active metabolite of **azathioprine**) with a potential for severe toxicity (haematopoietic and mucosal).
- Metabolism of **warfarin** is inhibited.

URICOSURIC DRUGS

Use

These drugs (e.g. **sulfinpyrazone**, **probenecid**) have been largely superseded by **allopurinol**, but are useful for patients who require prophylactic therapy and who have severe adverse reactions to **allopurinol**. Uricosuric drugs inhibit active transport of organic acids by renal tubules (Chapter 6). Their main effect on the handling of uric acid by the kidney is to prevent the reabsorption of filtered uric acid by the proximal tubule, thus greatly increasing excretion. **Probenecid** can precipitate an acute attack of gout. **Sulfinpyrazone** is a weak NSAID in its own right, and a flare of gout is less likely to occur when using it. Unlike other NSAIDs, there is also evidence that it has a clinically useful antiplatelet action. The patient should drink enough water to have a urine output of 2 L/day during the first month of treatment and a sodium bicarbonate or potassium citrate mixture should be given to keep the urinary pH above 7.0 to avoid precipitation of uric acid stones. Other adverse effects include rashes and gastro-intestinal upsets.

RASBURICASE

Rasburicase, a recently introduced preparation of recombinant xanthine oxidase, is used to prevent complications of acute hyperuricaemia in leukaemia therapy, especially in children.

Key points

Gout

- Gout is caused by an inflammatory reaction to precipitated crystals of uric acid.
- Always consider possible contributing factors, including drugs (especially diuretics) and ethanol.
- Treatment of the acute attack:
  - NSAIDs (e.g. ibuprofen);
  - colchicine (useful in cases where NSAIDs are contraindicated).
- prophylaxis (for recurrent disease or tophaceous gout):
  - allopurinol (xanthine oxidase inhibitor) is only started well after the acute attack has resolved and with NSAID cover to prevent a flare;
  - uricosuric drugs (e.g. sulfinpyrazone, which has additional NSAID and antiplatelet actions) are less effective than allopurinol. They are a useful alternative when allopurinol causes severe adverse effects (e.g. rashes). A high output of alkaline urine should be maintained to prevent stone formation.

Case history

A 45-year-old publican presents to a locum GP with symptoms of a painful, swollen and red big toe. There is a history of essential hypertension, and he has had a similar but less severe attack three months previously which settled spontaneously. Following this, serum urate concentrations were determined and found to be within the normal range. His toe is now inflamed and exquisitely tender. His blood pressure is 180/106 mmHg, but the examination is otherwise unremarkable. The locum is concerned that treatment with an NSAID might increase the patient's blood pressure, and that, since his uric acid was recently found to be normal, he might not have gout. He therefore prescribes cocodamol for the pain and repeated the serum urate measurement. The patient returns the following day unimproved, having spent a sleepless night, and you see him yourself for the first time. The examination is as described by your locum, and serum urate remains normal. What would you do?

Comment

Normal serum urate does not exclude gout. The patient requires treatment with an NSAID, such as ibuprofen. Review his medication (is he on a diuretic for his hypertension?) and enquire about his alcohol consumption. Blood pressure is commonly increased by acute pain. Despite his occupation, the patient does not drink alcohol and he was receiving bendroflumethiazide for hypertension. This was discontinued, amlodipine was substituted and his blood pressure fell to 162/100 mmHg during treatment with ibuprofen. A short period of poor antihypertensive control in this setting is not of great importance. After the pain has settled and ibuprofen stopped, the patient's blood pressure decreases further to 140/84 mmHg on amlodipine. He did not have any recurrence of gout. (Only if recurrent gout was a problem would prophylactic treatment with allopurinol be worth considering.)

FURTHER READING

Boers M. NSAIDs and selective COX-2 inhibitors: competition between gastroprotection and cardioprotection. *Lancet* 2001; **357**: 1222–3.

De Broe ME, Elseviers MM. Analgesic nephropathy. *New England Journal of Medicine* 1998; **338**: 446–42.

Emmerson BT. The management of gout. *New England Journal of Medicine* 1996; **334**: 445–51.

Feldmann M. Development of anti-TNF therapy for rheumatoid arthritis. *Nature Reviews. Immunology* 2002; **2**: 364–71.

FitzGerald GA, Patrono C. The coxibs, selective inhibitors of cyclooxygenase-2. *New England Journal of Medicine* 2001; **345**: 433–42.

Graham DJ, Campen D, Hui R et al. Risk of acute myocardial infarction and sudden cardiac death in patients treated with cyclo-oxygenase 2 selective and non-selective non-steroidal anti-inflammatory drugs: nested case control study. *Lancet* 2005; **365**: 475–81.

Klippel JHK. Biologic therapy for rheumatoid arthritis. *New England Journal of Medicine* 2000; **343**: 1640–1.

Maini RN, Taylor PC. Anti-cytokine therapy for rheumatoid arthritis. *Annual Review of Medicine* 2000; **51**: 207–29.

O'Dell JR, Haire CE, Erikson N et al. Treatment of rheumatoid arthritis with methotrexate alone, sulfasalazine and hydroxychloroquine or a combination of all three medications. *New England Journal of Medicine* 1996; **334**: 1287–91.

Rongean JC, Kelly JP, Naldi L. Medication use and the risk of Stevens-Johnson syndrome or toxic epidermal necrolysis. *New England Journal of Medicine* 1995; **333**: 1600–7.

Vane JR, Bakhle YS, Botting RM. Cyclo-oxygenases 1 and 2. *Annual Review of Pharmacology and Toxicology* 1998; **38**: 97–120.

PART IV

THE CARDIOVASCULAR SYSTEM

CHAPTER 27

PREVENTION OF ATHEROMA: LOWERING PLASMA CHOLESTEROL AND OTHER APPROACHES

INTRODUCTION

Atheroma is the most common cause of ischaemic heart disease, stroke and peripheral vascular disease. Since these are the major causes of morbidity and mortality among adults in industrialized societies, its prevention is of great importance. An important practical distinction is made between preventive measures in healthy people (called 'primary prevention') and measures in people who have survived a stroke or a heart attack, or who are symptomatic, e.g. from angina or claudication (called 'secondary prevention'). The absolute risk per unit time is greatest in those with clinical evidence of established disease, so secondary prevention is especially worthwhile (and cost-effective, since the number needed to treat to prevent a further event is lower than with primary prevention). Primary prevention inevitably involves larger populations who are at relatively low absolute risk per unit time, so interventions must be inexpensive and have a low risk of adverse effects.

A family history of myocardial infarction confers an increased risk of ischaemic heart disease and genetic factors are important in the development of atheroma. Epidemiological observations, including the rapid change in incidence of coronary disease in Japanese migrants from Japan (low risk) to Hawaii (intermediate risk) to the west coast of the USA (high risk), and the recent substantial decline in coronary risk in the USA population, indicate that environmental factors are also of paramount importance in the pathogenesis of atheroma.

PATHOPHYSIOLOGY

Atheromatous plaques are focal lesions of large- and medium-sized arteries (Figure 27.1). They start as fatty streaks in the intima and progress to proliferative fibro-fatty growths that can protrude into the vascular lumen and limit blood flow.

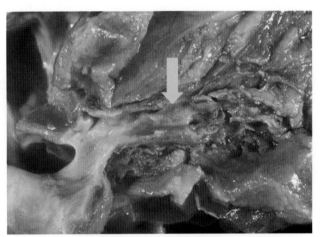

Figure 27.1: A coronary artery dissected open longitudinally, with a severe stenosis (arrowed) caused by an atheromatous plaque.

These plaques are rich in both extracellular and intracellular cholesterol. During their development, they do not initially give rise to symptoms, but as they progress they may cause angina pectoris, intermittent claudication or other symptoms depending on their anatomical location. They may rupture or ulcerate, in which event the subintima acts as a focus for thrombosis: platelet-fibrin thrombi propagate and can occlude the artery, causing myocardial infarction or stroke.

Epidemiological observations (e.g. the Framingham study) have shown that there is a strong positive relationship between the concentration of circulating cholesterol, specifically of the low-density lipoprotein (LDL) fraction, and the risk of atheroma. This relationship is non-linear and depends strongly on the presence or absence of other risk factors, including male sex, arterial hypertension, cigarette smoking, diabetes mellitus, and left ventricular hypertrophy (Figure 27.2).

Figure 27.3 summarizes metabolic pathways involved in lipid transport. Approximately two-thirds of cholesterol circulating in the blood is synthesized in the liver. Hepatocytes synthesize cholesterol and bile acids from acetate, and secrete them

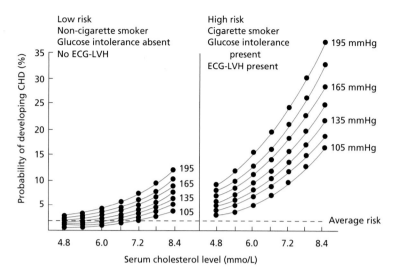

Figure 27.2: Probability of developing coronary heart disease in six years: 40-year-old men in the Framingham Study during 16 years follow up. The numbers to the right of the curves show the systolic blood pressure (mmHg).

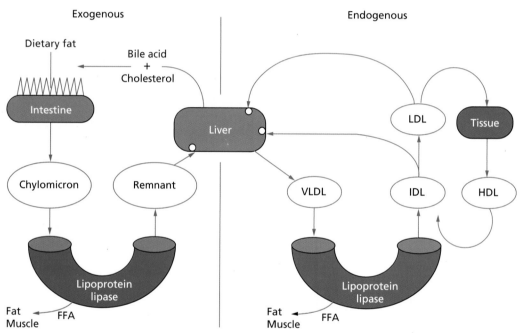

Figure 27.3: Lipoprotein transport. FFA, free fatty acids; VLDL, very-low-density lipoprotein; IDL, intermediate-density lipoprotein; HDL, high-density lipoprotein.

in bile into the intestine, where they are involved in fat absorption. The rate-limiting enzyme in cholesterol biosynthesis is 3-hydroxyl 3-methylglutaryl coenzyme A reductase (HMG CoA reductase). Fat is absorbed in the form of triglyceride-rich chylomicra. Free fatty acid is cleaved from triglyceride in these particles by lipoprotein lipase, an enzyme on the surface of endothelial cells. Free fatty acids are used as an energy source by striated muscle or stored as fat in adipose tissue. Chylomicron remnants are taken up by hepatocytes to complete the exogenous cycle. The endogenous cycle consists of the secretion of triglyceride-rich (and hence very-low-density) lipoprotein particles (VLDL) by the liver into the blood, followed by removal of free fatty acid by lipoprotein lipase. This results in progressive enrichment of the particles with cholesterol, with an increase in their density through intermediate-density to low-density

lipoprotein (LDL). Low-density-lipoprotein particles bind to receptors (LDL receptors) located in coated pits on the surface of hepatocytes, so the plasma concentration of LDL is determined by a balance between LDL synthesis and hepatic uptake. Low-density lipoprotein that enters arterial walls at sites of endothelial damage can be remobilized in the form of high-density lipoprotein (HDL), or may become oxidized and be taken up by macrophages as part of atherogenesis (see below).

Transgenic mice deficient in specific key enzymes and receptors in lipoprotein metabolism are useful models, but most of our understanding of atheroma comes from human pathology and from experimental studies in primates. Intimal injury initiates atherogenesis, which is a chronic inflammatory process. Rheological factors (e.g. turbulence) are believed to be responsible for the strong predilection for certain sites (e.g. at the low-shear side of the origin of arteries branching from the aorta). The injury may initially be undetectable morphologically, but results in focal endothelial dysfunction. Blood monocytes adhere to adhesion molecules expressed by injured endothelium and migrate into the vessel wall, where they become macrophages. These possess receptors for oxidized (but not native) LDL, which they ingest to become 'foam cells'.

Lesions become infiltrated with extracellular as well as intracellular cholesterol. Lymphocytes and platelets adhere to the injured intima and secrete growth factors and cytokines, which cause migration, proliferation and differentiation of vascular smooth muscle cells and fibroblasts from the underlying media and adventitia. These processes result in the formation of fibro-fatty plaques.

Atheromatous lesions are not necessarily irreversible. Cholesterol is mobilized from tissues in the form of HDL particles. These are not atherogenic – indeed, epidemiological studies have identified HDL as being strongly negatively correlated with coronary heart disease. There is a close relationship between an apolipoprotein, apo(a), and plasminogen, linking atherogenesis to thrombosis. Apo(a) is present in a lipoprotein known as Lp(a). The plasma concentration of Lp(a) varies over a 100-fold range and is strongly genetically determined. Most drugs have little effect (nicotinic acid is an exception). Apo(a) contains multiple repeats of one of the kringles of plasminogen (a kringle is a doughnut-shaped loop of amino acids held together by three internal disulphide bonds). This leads to interference by Lp(a) with the function of plasminogen, which is the precursor of the endogenous fibrinolytic plasmin, and hence to a predisposition to thrombosis on atheromatous plaques.

Key points

Atherogenesis

- Endothelial injury initiates the process. The distribution of lesions is influenced by turbulence (e.g. at branch points) in the arterial circulation.
- Monocytes in the blood bind to ICAM/integrin receptors on injured endothelium and migrate into the vessel wall, where they become macrophages.
- LDL is oxidized by free radicals generated by activated cells (including macrophages and endothelial cells). Oxidized LDL is taken into macrophages via scavenger receptors.
- This sets up a chronic inflammatory process in which chemical messengers are released by lipid-laden macrophages ('foam cells'), T-lymphocytes and platelets. These interleukins and growth factors cause the migration and proliferation of vascular smooth muscle cells and fibroblasts, which form a fibro-fatty plaque.
- Cigarette smoking promotes several of these processes (e.g. platelet aggregation).
- If the plaque ruptures, thrombosis occurs on the subendothelium, and may occlude the vessel, causing stroke, myocardial infarction, etc., depending on the anatomical location.

PREVENTION OF ATHEROMA

Modifiable risk factors are potentially susceptible to therapeutic intervention. These include smoking, obesity, sedentary habits, dyslipidaemia, glucose intolerance (Chapter 37) and hypertension (Chapter 28). Disappointingly hopes, based on epidemiological observations, that hormone replacement treatment of post-menopausal women (Chapter 41) would prevent atheromatous disease were disproved by randomized controlled trials (Figure 27.4).

SMOKING

Cigarette smoking (Chapter 53) is a strong risk factor for vascular disease. It causes vasoconstriction via activation of the sympathetic nervous system and platelet activation/aggregation with a consequent increase in thromboxane A_2 biosynthesis (see Figure 27.2), although the precise mechanism whereby smoking promotes atheroma is unknown. Stopping smoking is of substantial and rapid benefit. Smoking is addictive and attempts to give up are often unsuccessful. The use of **nicotine**, **bupropion** and **varenicline** (partial agonist at the nicotinic receptor) in conjunction with counselling in smoking cessation programmes are covered in Chapter 53.

DIET AND EXERCISE

Obesity is increasingly common and is a strong risk factor, partly via its associations with hypertension, diabetes and dyslipidaemia. Treatment (Chapter 34) is notoriously difficult. Sedentary habit is a risk factor and regular exercise reduces cardiovascular risk, partly by reducing resting systolic blood pressure and increasing HDL.

DYSLIPIDAEMIA

Most patients with dyslipidaemia have a combination of genetic and dietary factors. Secondary forms of dyslipidaemia are listed in Table 27.1. Reducing the total plasma cholesterol concentration reduces the risk of coronary heart disease and can cause regression of atheroma. Dietary advice focuses on reducing saturated fat and correcting obesity rather than reducing cholesterol intake per se. In people without clinical evidence of atheromatous disease, the decision as to whether to initiate drug treatment at any given level of serum lipids should be informed by the risk of coronary events. This is calculated from cardiovascular risk prediction charts (e.g. at the back of the British National Formulary) or algorithms or calculators available on--line, e.g. via the British Hypertension Society website (www.bhsoc.org/Cardiovascular_Risk_Charts_and_Calculators.stm). An approach to therapy is summarized in Figure 27.5.

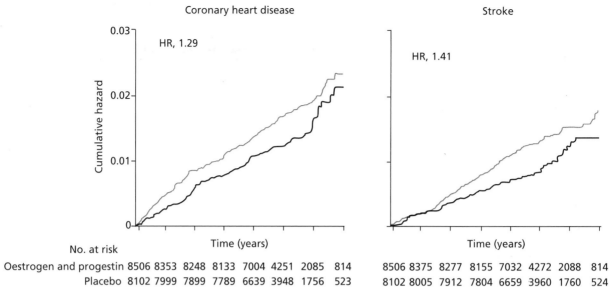

Figure 27.4: Kaplan–Meier plots of cumulative hazards for coronary heart disease and stroke in the Women's Health Initiative study, in healthy postmenopausal women taking hormone replacement therapy or placebo. Blue line, oestrogen and progestin; black line, placebo. (Redrawn with permission from Writing Group for the Women's Health Initiative Investigators, *Journal of the American Medical Association* 2002; 288: 321–33.)

Table 27.1: Secondary dyslipidaemia

Disorder	Main lipid disturbance
Diabetes	Mixed
Hypothyroidism	Cholesterol
Ethanol excess	Triglyceride
Nephrotic syndrome	Cholesterol
Renal failure	Mixed
Primary biliary cirrhosis	Cholesterol

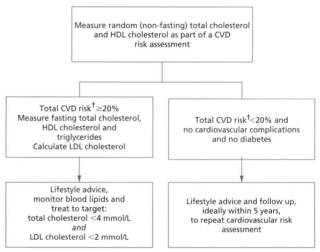

†Assessed with CVD risk chart.
Statins are first line drugs for reducing total and LDL cholesterol. Other classes of lipid lowering drugs (fibrates, bile acid sequestrants, cholesterol absorption inhibitors, nicotinic acid, omega-3 (n-3) fatty acids) should be considered in addition to a statin if the total and LDL cholesterol targets have not been achieved, or if other lipid parameters such as HDL cholesterol or triglycerides need to be addressed.

Figure 27.5: Risk thresholds and targets for blood cholesterol in asymptomatic people without cardiovascular disease (CVD). (*Source*: JBS 2. Joint British Societies' guidelines on prevention of cardiovascular disease in clinical practice. *Heart* 2005; 91(Suppl. 5): v1–v52. Reproduced with permission from the BMJ Publishing Group.)

DRUGS USED TO TREAT DYSLIPIDAEMIA

The three main classes of drugs used to treat dyslipidaemia are the statins (HMG CoA reductase inhibitors), drugs that block cholesterol absorption and fibrates (Figure 27.6). Additional drugs (see Table 27.2) are useful in special situations.

STATINS

Use

Simvastatin, **pravastatin**, **atorvastatin** and **rosuvastatin** are available in the UK. Randomized controlled trials have shown that **simvastatin**, **atorvastatin** and **pravastatin** reduce cardiac events and prolong life, and are safe. **Pravastatin** is distributed selectively to the liver and is tolerated even by some individuals who develop mylagia on other statins, but is less potent. **Rosuvastatin** lacks clinical end-point data, but is more potent. Another highly potent statin, **cerivastatin**, was withdrawn because of rhabdomyolysis and drug interactions.

Mechanism of action

HMG CoA reductase is the rate-limiting step in cholesterol biosynthesis. Statins inhibit this enzyme, lowering cytoplasmic cholesterol. Hepatocytes respond by increasing the synthesis of LDL receptors. This increases hepatic LDL uptake from the plasma, further reducing the plasma LDL concentration.

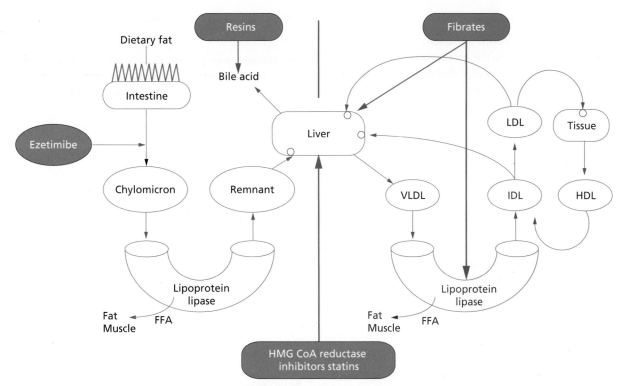

Figure 27.6: Sites of action of lipid-lowering drugs (see **Figure 27.3** for abbreviations).

Table 27.2: Drugs used in dyslipidaemia

Class/drug	Biochemical effect	Effect on coronary artery disease	Effect on longevity	Adverse effects	Special situations
Statin/simvastin, pravastatin	LDL ↓ ↓	↓ ↓	↑ (4S,WOSCOPS)	Rare: myositis ↑ liver transaminase	Contraindicated in pregnancy, caution in children
Resin/cholestyramine	LDL ↓ TG ↑	↓	NP	Constipation, flatulence, nausea	Contraindicated in biliary obstruction
Fibrate/gemfibrozil, bezafibrate	TG ↓ ↓ LDL ↓ HDL ↑	↓	NP	Myocitis; gastro-intestinal symptoms	Contraindicated in alcoholics, renal/liver impairment
Nicotinic acid derivatives/high-dose nicotinic acid, acipimox	TG ↓ ↓ LDL ↓ HDL ↑	↓	NP	Flushing (PGD$_2$-mediated); diarrhoea; urticaria; epigastric pain; hyperuricaemia; hyperglycaemia	Useful in familial hypercholesterolaemia; PG-related adverse effects ameliorated by aspirin before the dose
Fish oil/eicosapentanoic acid-rich supplements	TG ↓	NP	NP	Belching with a fishy after-taste	Used in patients with pancreatitis caused by raised TG. Contraindicated in patients with familial hypercholesterolaemia, in whom it increases cholesterol levels
Ezetimibe	LDL ↓	NP	NP	Mild GI effects, myalgia	Adjunct to statin in resistant dyslipidaemia

LDL, low-density lipoprotein; TG, triglycerides; HDL, high-density lipoprotein; NP, not proven.

Adverse effects and contraindications

Mild and infrequent side effects include nausea, constipation, diarrhoea, flatulence, fatigue, insomnia and rash. More serious adverse events are rare, but include rhabdomyolysis, hepatitis and angioedema. Liver function tests should be performed before starting treatment and at intervals thereafter, and patients should be warned to stop the drug and report at once for determination of creatine kinase if they develop muscle aches. HMG CoA reductase inhibitors should be avoided in alcoholics and patients with active liver disease, and are contraindicated during pregnancy.

Pharmacokinetics

Statins are well absorbed, extracted by the liver (their site of action) and are subject to extensive presystemic metabolism by CYP3A4 or CYP2D6. **Simvastatin** is an inactive lactone prodrug which is metabolized in the liver to its active form, the corresponding β-hydroxy fatty acid.

Drug interactions

The risk of rhabdomyolysis is increased by concurrent use of a fibrate or inhibitors of statin metabolism, e.g. azoles (Chapter 45), macrolides (Chapter 43). Their potency is increased by concurrent use of a drug that interferes with cholesterol absorption (see below).

DRUGS THAT REDUCE CHOLESTEROL ABSORPTION

EZETIMIBE

Use

Ezetimibe is most often used in combination with diet and statins for severe hypercholesterolaemia; also in occasional patients who cannot tolerate statins or where statins are contraindicated, and in (rare) cases of homozygous sitosterolaemia.

Mechanism of action

It blocks the NPLC1L sterol transporter in the brush border of enterocytes, preventing cholesterol and plant sterols (phytosterols) transport from the intestinal lumen. This mechanism is distinct from that of phytosterol and phytostanol esters (present in 'health' foods such as Benecol™) which interfere with the micellar presentation of sterols to the cell surface, or of resins (see below) which bind bile acids in the gut lumen.

Pharmacokinetics

Ezetimibe is administered by mouth and is absorbed into intestinal epithelial cells, where it localizes to the brush border. It is metabolized, followed by enterohepatic recycling and slow elimination. It enters breast milk.

Adverse effects and contraindications

Diarrhoea, abdominal pain or headaches are occasional problems; rash and angioedema have been reported. It is contraindicated in breast-feeding.

ANION-EXCHANGE RESINS

Use

Colestyramine or **colestipol** were used for hypercholesterolaemia, but have been almost completely superseded by statins. Resins retained an important niche as add-in treatment in severe disease (e.g. heterozygous familial hypercholesterolaemia (FH)) which was inadequately responsive to statin monotherapy. This role has now been taken by **ezetimibe** (see above) which is effective and well tolerated in milligram doses in contrast to resins which are administered in doses of several grams, are unpalatable and commonly cause abdominal bloating and diarrhoea. They retain a highly limited usefulness in children and in breast-feeding women. Completely separate indications include bile salt diarrhoea and pruritus in incomplete biliary obstruction. (They are ineffective in patients with complete biliary obstruction, in whom there are no bile salts to bind in the gut lumen.) They cause malabsorption of fat soluble vitamins and interfere with the absorption of many drugs (Chapter 13).

FIBRATES

Use

Bezafibrate, **gemfibrozil** and **fenofibrate** are available in the UK and are used mainly for patients with mixed dyslipidaemia with severely raised triglycerides especially if they are poorly responsive to statins. **Clofibrate**, which was used in a World Health Organization (WHO) trial, is less often used because it increases biliary cholesterol secretion and predisposes to gallstones. Its use is therefore limited to patients who have had a cholecystectomy. Furthermore, while it reduced the number of myocardial infarctions in the WHO trial, this was offset by an increased number of cancers of various kinds. The meaning of this has been extensively debated, but remains obscure. This issue is clouded by an effect of malignancy of lowering serum cholesterol. The original observations with **clofibrate** may have been a statistical accident and there is no excess of cancers in patients treated with **gemfibrozil** in other trials (e.g. the Helsinki Heart Study). These studies have shown that fibrates have a marked effect in lowering plasma triglycerides (TG), with a modest (approximately 10%) reduction in LDL and increase in HDL. **Fenofibrate** has an additional uricosuric effect.

Mechanism of action

Fibrates are agonists at a nuclear receptor (peroxisome proliferator-activated receptor α (PPARα)) which is present in many tissues including fat. The ensuing effects are incompletely understood. They stimulate lipoprotein lipase (hence their marked effect on TG) and increase LDL uptake by the liver. In addition to their effects on plasma lipids, fibrates lower fibrinogen.

Adverse effects

Fibrates can cause myositis (in severe cases rhabdomyolysis with acute renal failure), especially in alcoholics (in whom they should not be used) and in patients with impaired renal function (in whom elimination is prolonged and protein binding reduced). The risk of muscle damage is increased if they are taken with a statin, although lipid specialists sometimes employ this combination. They can cause a variety of gastrointestinal side effects, but are usually well tolerated.

Contraindications

Fibrates should be used with caution, if at all, in patients with renal or hepatic impairment. They should not be used in patients with gall-bladder disease or with hypoalbuminaemia. They are contraindicated in pregnancy and in alcoholics (this is particularly important because alcohol excess causes hypertriglyceridaemia; see Table 27.1).

Pharmacokinetics

Bezafibrate and **gemfibrozil** are completely absorbed when given by mouth, highly protein bound, and excreted mainly by the kidneys.

OTHER DRUGS

Other drugs sometimes used by lipidologists are summarized in Table 27.2. These include **nicotinic acid** which needs to be administered in much larger doses than needed for its effect as a B vitamin (Chapter 35). Its main effects on lipids are distinctive, namely to increase HDL, reduce TG and reduce Lp(a). Unfortunately, it has troublesome adverse effects including flushing (mediated by release of vasodilator prostaglandin D_2) which is reduced by giving the dose 30 minutes after a dose of **aspirin**.

Key points

Treatment of dyslipidaemia

* Treatment goals must be individualized according to absolute risk. Patients with established disease need treatment irrespective of LDL.
* Dietary measures involve maintaining ideal body weight (by caloric restriction if necessary) and reducing consumption of saturated fat – both animal (e.g. red meat, dairy products) and vegetable (e.g. coconut oil) – as well as cholesterol (e.g. egg yolk).
* Drug treatment is usually with a statin (taken once daily at night) which is effective, well tolerated and reduces mortality. Consider the possibility of secondary dyslipidaemia.
* Ezetimibe is well tolerated. It is a useful adjunct to a statin in severely dyslipidaemic patients who show an inadequate response to a statin alone, and has almost completely replaced bile acid binding resins for this indication.
* Fibrates are useful as a first-line treatment in patients with primary mixed dyslipidaemias with high triglyceride concentrations, as well as high LDL (and often low HDL). Avoid in alcoholics.
* Other reversible risk factors for atheroma (e.g. smoking, hypertension) should be sought and treated.
* Consideration should be given to adjunctive use of aspirin as an antiplatelet/antithrombotic drug.

Case history

A 36-year-old male primary-school teacher was seen because of hypertension at the request of the surgeons following bilateral femoral artery bypass surgery. His father had died at the age of 32 years of a myocardial infarct, but his other relatives, including his two children, were healthy. He did not smoke or drink alcohol. He had been diagnosed as hypertensive six years previously, since which time he had been treated with slow-release nifedipine, but his serum cholesterol level had never been measured. He had been disabled by claudication for the past few years, relieved temporarily by angioplasty one year previously. There were no stigmata of dyslipidaemia, his blood pressure was 150/100 mmHg and the only abnormal findings were those relating to the peripheral vascular disease and vascular surgery in his legs. Serum total cholesterol was 12.6 mmol/L, triglyceride was 1.5 mmol/L and HDL was 0.9 mmol/L. Serum creatinine and electrolytes were normal. The patient was given dietary advice and seen in clinic four weeks after discharge from hospital. He had been able to run on the games field for the first time in a year, but this had been limited by the new onset of chest pain on exertion. His cholesterol level on the diet had improved to 8.0 mmol/L. He was readmitted.
Questions
Decide whether each of the following statements is true or false.

(a) This patient should receive a statin.
(b) Coronary angiography is indicated.
(c) Renal artery stenosis should be considered.
(d) The target for total cholesterol should be 6.0 mmol/L.
(e) Ezetimibe would be contraindicated.
(f) An α_1-blocker for his hypertension could coincidentally improve his dyslipidaemia.
(g) His children should be screened for dyslipidaemia and cardiovascular disease.

Answer

(a) True.
(b) True.
(c) True.
(d) False.
(e) False.
(f) True.
(g) True.

Comment
It was unfortunate that this young man's dyslipidaemia was not recognized earlier. Coronary angiography revealed severe inoperable triple-vessel disease. The target total cholesterol level should be <5.0 mmol/L and was achieved with a combination of diet, a statin at night and ezetimibe in the morning. Renal artery stenosis is common in the setting of peripheral vascular disease, but renal angiography was negative. This patient's relatively mild hypertension was treated with doxazosin (a long-acting α_1-blocker, see Chapter 28) which increases HDL, as well as lowering blood pressure. He probably has heterozygous monogenic familial hypercholesterolaemia and his children should be screened. One of his sons is hypercholesterolaemic and is currently being treated with a combination of diet and a statin.

FURTHER READING

Durrington PN. Dyslipidaemia. *Lancet* 2003; **362**: 717–31.

Durrington PN. *Hyperlipidaemia: diagnosis and management*, 3rd edn. London: Hodder Arnold, 2005.

Feher MD, Richmond W. *Lipids and lipid disorders*. London: Gower Medical Publishing, 1991.

Hansson GK. Mechanisms of disease: inflammation, atherosclerosis, and coronary artery disease. *New England Journal of Medicine* 2005; **352**: 1685–95.

Kosoglou T, Statkevich P, Johnson-Levonas AO et al. Ezetimibe – A review of its metabolism, pharmacokinetics and drug interactions. *Clinical Pharmacokinetics* 2005; **44**: 467–94.

Ross R. Atherosclerosis – an inflammatory disease. *New England Journal of Medicine* 1999; **340**: 115–26.

Scandinavian Simvastatin Survival Study Group. Randomised trial of cholesterol lowering in 4444 patients with coronary heart disease: the Scandinavian Simvastatin Survival Study (4S). *Lancet* 1994; **344**: 1383–9.

Shepherd J, Cobbe SM, Ford I et al. Prevention of coronary heart disease with pravastatin in men with hypercholesterolemia. *New England Journal of Medicine* 1995; **333**: 1301–7.

CHAPTER 28

HYPERTENSION

INTRODUCTION

Systemic arterial hypertension is one of the strongest known modifiable risk factors for ischaemic heart disease, stroke, renal failure and heart failure. It remains poorly treated. As an asymptomatic disorder, people are understandably reluctant to accept adverse drug effects in addition to the inconvenience of long-term treatment. In this regard, modern drugs represent an enormous improvement.

Figure 28.1 shows the relationship between the usual mean diastolic blood pressure and the risks of coronary heart disease and of stroke. A meta-analysis of published randomized controlled trials showed that the reduction in diastolic blood pressure achieved by drug treatment reduced the risk of stroke by the full extent predicted, and reduced the risk of coronary disease by about 50% of the maximum predicted, within approximately 2.5 years. These impressive results form a secure clinical scientific evidence base for the value of treating hypertension adequately.

PATHOPHYSIOLOGY AND SITES OF DRUG ACTION

Hypertension is occasionally secondary to some distinct disease. However, most patients with persistent arterial hypertension have essential hypertension.

Arterial blood pressure is determined by cardiac output, peripheral vascular resistance and large artery compliance. Peripheral vascular resistance is determined by the diameter of resistance vessels (small muscular arteries and arterioles) in the various tissues (see Figure 28.2). One or more of a 'mosaic' of interconnected predisposing factors (including positive family history, obesity and physical inactivity among others) are commonly present in patients with essential hypertension, some of which are amenable to changes in diet and other habits. The importance of intrauterine factors (the 'Barker hypothesis') is supported by the finding that hypertension in adult life is strongly associated with low birth weight.

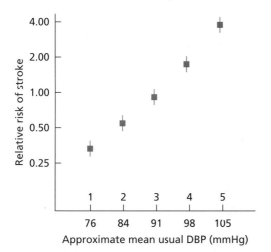

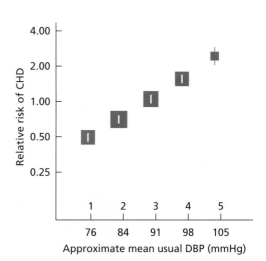

Figure 28.1: Risks of stroke and coronary heart disease (CHD) in relation to diastolic blood pressure (DBP). (Redrawn with permission from MacMahon et al. *Lancet* 1990; **335**: 765–4. © The Lancet Ltd.)

Cardiac output may be increased in children or young adults during the earliest stages of essential hypertension, but by the time hypertension is established in middle life the predominant haemodynamic abnormality is an elevated peripheral vascular resistance. With ageing, elastic fibres in the aorta and conduit arteries are replaced by less compliant collagen causing arterial stiffening and systolic hypertension, which is common in the elderly.

The kidney plays a key role in the control of blood pressure and in the pathogenesis of hypertension. Excretion of salt and water controls intravascular volume. Secretion of renin influences vascular tone and electrolyte balance via activation of the renin–angiotensin–aldosterone system. Renal disease (vascular, parenchymal or obstructive) is a cause of arterial hypertension. Conversely, severe hypertension causes glomerular sclerosis, manifested clinically by proteinuria and reduced glomerular filtration, leading to a vicious circle of worsening blood pressure and progressive renal impairment. Renal cross-transplantation experiments in several animal models of hypertension, as well as observations following therapeutic renal transplantation in humans, both point to the importance of the kidney in the pathogenesis of hypertension.

The sympathetic nervous system is also important in the control of blood pressure, providing background α receptor-mediated vasoconstrictor tone and β receptor-mediated cardiac stimulation. Sympathetic activity varies rapidly to adjust for changes in cardiovascular demand with alterations in posture and physical activity. It is also activated by emotional states such as anxiety, and this can result in 'white-coat' hypertension. A vasoconstrictor peptide, endothelin, released by the endothelium contributes to vasoconstrictor tone. Conversely, endothelium-derived nitric oxide provides background active vasodilator tone.

Cardiovascular drugs work by augmenting or inhibiting these processes, see Figure 28.3. The main such drugs for treating hypertension can usefully be grouped as:

A angiotensin-converting enzyme inhibitors (ACEI) and angiotensin AT$_1$ receptor antagonists (sartans);
B beta-adrenoceptor antagonists;
C calcium channel antagonists;
D diuretics.

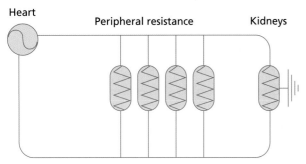

Figure 28.2: Arterial blood pressure is controlled by the force of contraction of the heart and the peripheral resistance (resistances in parallel though various vascular beds). The fullness of the circulation is controlled by the kidneys, which play a critical role in essential hypertension.

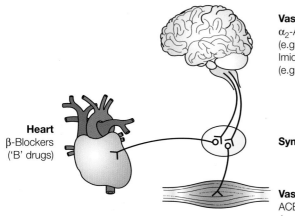
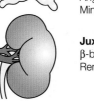

Figure 28.3: Classes of antihypertensive drugs and their sites of action.

Each of these classes of drug reduces clinical end-points such as stroke, but in uncomplicated hypertension B drugs may be less effective than other classes. Other antihypertensive drugs useful in specific circumstances include α-adrenoceptor antagonists, aldosterone antagonists and centrally acting antihypertensive drugs.

Key points

Pathophysiology of hypertension

- Few patients with persistent systemic arterial hypertension have a specific aetiology (e.g. renal disease, endocrine disease, coarctation of aorta). Most have essential hypertension (EH), which confers increased risk of vascular disease (e.g. thrombotic or haemorrhagic stroke, myocardial infarction). Reducing blood pressure reduces the risk of such events.
- The cause(s) of EH is/are ill-defined. Polygenic influences are important, as are environmental factors including salt intake and obesity. The intrauterine environment (determined by genetic/environmental factors) may be important in determining blood pressure in adult life.
- Increased cardiac output may occur before EH becomes established.
- Established EH is characterized haemodynamically by normal cardiac output but increased total systemic vascular resistance. This involves both structural (remodelling) and functional changes in resistance vessels.
- EH is a strong independent risk factor for atheromatous disease and interacts supra-additively with other such risk factors.

GENERAL PRINCIPLES OF MANAGING ESSENTIAL HYPERTENSION

- Consider blood pressure in the context of other risk factors: use cardiovascular risk to make decisions about whether to start drug treatment and what target to aim for. (Guidance, together with risk tables, is available, for example, at the back of the British National Formulary).
- Use non-drug measures (e.g. salt restriction) in addition to drugs.
- Explain goals of treatment and agree a plan the patient is comfortable to live with (concordance).
- Review the possibility of co-existing disease (e.g. gout, angina) that would influence the choice of drug.
- The 'ABCD' rule provides a useful basis for starting drug treatment. A (and B) drugs inhibit the renin–angiotensin–aldosterone axis and are effective when this is active – as it usually is in young white or Asian people. An A drug is preferred for these unless there is some reason to avoid it (e.g. in a young woman contemplating pregnancy) or some additional reason

(e.g. co-existing angina) to choose a B drug. Older people and people of Afro-Caribbean ethnicity often have a low plasma renin and in these patients a class C or D drug is preferred.

- Use a low dose and, except in emergency situations, titrate this upward gradually.
- Addition of a second drug is often needed. A drug of the other group is added, i.e. an A drug is added to patients started on a C or D drug, a C or D drug is added to a patient started on an A drug. A third or fourth drug may be needed. It is better to use such combinations than to use very high doses of single drugs: this seldom works and often causes adverse effects.
- Loss of control – if blood pressure control, having been well established, is lost, there are several possibilities to be considered:
  - non-adherence;
  - drug interaction – e.g. with non-steroidal anti-inflammatory drugs (NSAIDs) – see Chapter 26;
  - intercurrent disease – e.g. renal impairment, atheromatous renal artery stenosis.

DRUGS USED TO TREAT HYPERTENSION

A DRUGS

ANGIOTENSIN-CONVERTING ENZYME INHIBITORS

Use

Several angiotensin-converting enzyme inhibitors (ACEI) are in clinical use (e.g. **ramipril**, **trandolapril**, **enalapril**, **lisinopril**, **captopril**). These differ in their duration of action. Longer-acting drugs (e.g. **trandolapril**, **ramipril**) are preferred. They are given once daily and produce good 24-hour control. Their beneficial effect in patients with heart failure (Chapter 31) or following myocardial infarction (Chapter 29) makes them or a sartan (below) particularly useful in hypertensive patients with these complications. Similarly an ACEI or sartan is preferred over other anti-hypertensives in diabetic patients because they slow the progression of diabetic nephropathy.

Treatment is initiated using a small dose given last thing at night, because of the possibility of first-dose hypotension. If possible, diuretics should be withheld for one or two days before the first dose for the same reason. The dose is subsequently usually given in the morning and increased gradually if necessary, while monitoring the blood-pressure response.

Mechanism of action

ACE catalyses the cleavage of a pair of amino acids from short peptides, thereby 'converting' the inactive decapeptide angiotensin I to the potent vasoconstrictor angiotensin II (Figure 28.4). As well as activating the vasoconstrictor angiotensin in this way, it also inactivates bradykinin – a vasodilator peptide. ACEI lower blood pressure by reducing angiotensin II and perhaps also by increasing vasodilator

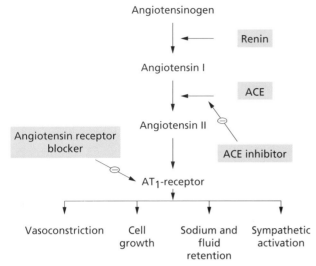

Figure 28.4: Generation of angiotensin II, and mode of action of ACE inhibitors and of angiotensin receptor blockers.

peptides, such as bradykinin. Angiotensin II causes aldosterone secretion from the zona glomerulosa of the adrenal cortex and inhibition of this contributes to the antihypertensive effect of ACE inhibitors.

Metabolic effects

ACEI cause a mild increase in plasma potassium which is usually unimportant, but may sometimes be either desirable or problematic depending on renal function and concomitant drug therapy (see Adverse effects and Drug interactions below).

Adverse effects

ACE inhibitors are generally well tolerated. Adverse effects include:

- First-dose hypotension.
- Dry cough – this is the most frequent symptom (5–30% of cases) during chronic dosing. It is often mild, but can be troublesome. The cause is unknown, but it may be due to kinin accumulation stimulating cough afferents. Sartans (see below) do not inhibit the metabolism of bradykinin and do not cause cough.
- Functional renal failure – this occurs predictably in patients with haemodynamically significant bilateral renal artery stenosis, and in patients with renal artery stenosis in the vessel supplying a single functional kidney. Plasma creatinine and potassium concentrations should be monitored and the possibility of renal artery stenosis considered in patients in whom there is a marked rise in creatinine. Provided that the drug is stopped promptly, such renal impairment is reversible. The explanation of acute reduction in renal function in this setting is that glomerular filtration in these patients is critically dependent on angiotensin-II-mediated efferent arteriolar

vasoconstriction, and when angiotensin II synthesis is inhibited, glomerular capillary pressure falls and glomerular filtration ceases. This should be borne in mind particularly in ageing patients with atheromatous disease.

- Hyperkalaemia is potentially hazardous in patients with renal impairment and great caution must be exercised in this setting. This is even more important when such patients are also prescribed potassium supplements and/or potassium-sparing diuretics.
- Fetal injury – ACEI cause renal agenesis/failure in the fetus, resulting in oligohydramnios. ACEI are therefore contraindicated in pregnancy and other drugs are usually preferred in women who may want to start a family.
- Urticaria and angio-oedema – increased kinin concentration may explain the urticarial reactions and angioneurotic oedema sometimes caused by ACEI.
- Sulphhydryl group-related effects – high-dose **captopril** causes heavy proteinuria, neutropenia, rash and taste disturbance, attributable to its sulphhydryl group.

Pharmacokinetics

Currently available ACE inhibitors are all active when administered orally, but are highly polar and are eliminated in the urine. A number of these drugs (e.g. **captopril**, **lisinopril**) are active per se, while others (e.g. **enalapril**) are prodrugs and require metabolic conversion to active metabolites (e.g. **enalaprilat**). In practice, this is of little or no importance. None of the currently available ACEI penetrate the central nervous system. Many of these agents have long half-lives permitting once daily dosing; **captopril** is an exception.

Drug interactions

The useful interaction with diuretics has already been alluded to above. Diuretic treatment increases plasma renin activity and the consequent activation of angiotensin II and aldosterone limits their efficacy. ACE inhibition interrupts this loop and thus enhances the hypotensive efficacy of diuretics, as well as reducing thiazide-induced hypokalaemia. Conversely, ACEI have a potentially adverse interaction with potassium-sparing diuretics and potassium supplements, leading to hyperkalaemia, especially in patients with renal impairment, as mentioned above. As with other antihypertensive drugs, NSAIDs increase blood pressure in patients treated with ACE inhibitors.

ANGIOTENSIN RECEPTOR BLOCKERS

Several angiotensin receptor blockers (ARB or 'sartans') are in clinical use (e.g. **losartan**, **candesartan**, **irbesartan**, **valsartan**).

Use

Sartans are pharmacologically distinct from ACEI, but clinically similar in hypotensive efficacy. However, they lack the common ACEI adverse effect of dry cough. Long-acting drugs (e.g. **candesartan**, which forms a stable complex with the

AT$_1$ receptor) produce good 24-hour control. Their beneficial effect in patients with heart failure (Chapter 31) or following myocardial infarction (Chapter 29) makes them or an ACEI (above) useful in hypertensive patients with these complications. Similarly, an ACEI or a sartan is preferred over other anti-hypertensive drugs in diabetic patients where they slow the progression of nephropathy. Head to head comparison of **losartan** versus **atenolol** in hypertension (the LIFE study) favoured the sartan. Their excellent tolerability makes them first choice 'A' drugs for many physicians, but they are more expensive than ACEI.

First-dose hypotension can occur and it is sensible to apply similar precautions as when starting an ACEI (first dose at night, avoid starting if volume contracted).

Mechanism of action

Most of the effects of angiotensin II, including vasoconstriction and aldosterone release, are mediated by the angiotensin II subtype 1 (AT$_1$) receptor. The pharmacology of sartans differs predictably from that of ACEI, since they do not inhibit the degradation of bradykinin (Figure 28.5). This difference probably explains the lack of cough with sartans.

Adverse effects

Adverse effects on renal function in patients with bilateral renal artery stenosis are similar to an ACEI, as is hyperkalaemia and fetal renal toxicity. Angio-oedema is much less common than with ACEI, but can occur.

Pharmacokinetics

Sartans are well absorbed after oral administration. **Losartan** has an active metabolite. Half-lives of most marketed ARB are long enough to permit once daily dosing.

Drug interactions

There is a rationale for combining a sartan with an ACEI (not all angiotensin II is ACE-derived, and some useful effects of ACEI could be kinin-mediated); clinical experience suggests that this has little additional effect in hypertensive patients, however. Clinical trial data on this combination in heart failure are discussed in Chapter 31.

B DRUGS

β-ADRENOCEPTOR ANTAGONISTS
Use

See Chapter 32 for use of β-adrenoceptor antagonists in cardiac dysrhythmias.

Examples of β-adrenoceptor antagonists currently in clinical use are shown in Table 28.1. Beta-blockers lower blood pressure and reduce the risk of stroke in patients with mild essential hypertension, but in several randomized controlled

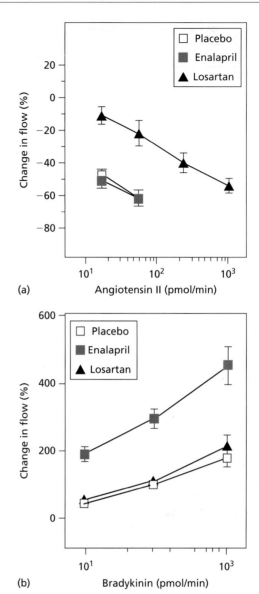

Figure 28.5: Differential effects of angiotensin converting enzyme inhibition (enalapril) and of angiotensin receptor blockade (losartan) on angiotensin II and bradykinin vasomotor actions in the human forearm vasculature. (Redrawn with permission from Cockcroft JR et al. *Journal of Cardiovascular Pharmacology* 1993; **22**: 579–84.)

trials (particularly of **atenolol**) have performed less well than comparator drugs. The explanation is uncertain, but one possibility is that they have less effect on central (i.e. aortic) blood pressure than on brachial artery pressure. 'B' drugs are no longer preferred over 'A' drugs as first line in situations where an A or B would previously have been selected, as explained above.

They are, however, useful in hypertensive patients with an additional complication such as ischaemic heart disease (Chapter 29) or heart failure (Chapter 31). The negative inotropic effect of beta-blocking drugs is particularly useful for stabilizing patients with dissecting aneurysms of the thoracic aorta, in whom it is desirable not only to lower the

Table 28.1: Examples of β-adrenoceptors in clinical use

Drug	Selectivity	Pharmacokinetic features	Comment
Propranolol	Non-selective	Non-polar; substantial presystematic metabolism; variable dose requirements; multiple daily dosing	First beta-blocker in clinical use
Atenolol	β_1-selective	Polar; renal elimination; once daily dosing	Widely used; avoid in renal failure
Metoprolol	β_1-selective	Non-polar; cytochrome P450 (2D6 isoenzyme)	Widely used
Esmolol	β_1-selective	Short acting given by i.v. infusion; renal elimination of acid metabolite	Used in intensive care unit/theatre (e.g. dissecting aneurysm)
Sotalol	Non-selective (L-isomer)	Polar; renal elimination	A racemate: the D-isomer has class III anti-dysrhythmic actions (see Chapter 31)
Labetolol	Non-selective	Hepatic glucuronidation	Additional alpha-blocking and partial β_2-agonist activity. Used in the latter part of pregnancy
Oxprenolol	Non-selective	Hepatic hydroxylation/glucuronidation	Partial agonist

mean pressure, but also to reduce the rate of rise of the arterial pressure wave.

Classification of β-adrenoceptor antagonists

β-Adrenoceptors are subdivided into β_1-receptors (heart), β_2-receptors (blood vessels, bronchioles) and β_3-receptors (some metabolic effects, e.g. in brown fat). Cardioselective drugs (e.g. **atenolol**, **metoprolol**, **bisoprolol**, **nebivolol**) inhibit β_1-receptors with less effect on bronchial and vascular β_2-receptors. However, even cardioselective drugs are hazardous for patients with asthma.

Some beta-blockers (e.g. **oxprenolol**) are partial agonists and possess intrinsic sympathomimetic activity. There is little hard evidence supporting their superiority to antagonists for most indications although individual patients may find such a drug acceptable when they have failed to tolerate a pure antagonist (e.g. patients with angina and claudication).

Beta-blockers with additional vasodilating properties are available. This is theoretically an advantage in treating patients with hypertension. Their mechanisms vary. Some (e.g. **labetolol**, **carvedilol**) have additional α-blocking activity. **Nebivolol** releases endothelium-derived nitric oxide.

Mechanism of action

β-Adrenoceptor antagonists reduce cardiac output (via negative chronotropic and negative inotropic effects on the heart), inhibit renin secretion and some have additional central actions reducing sympathetic outflow from the central nervous system (CNS).

Adverse effects and contraindications

- *Intolerance* – fatigue, cold extremities, erectile dysfunction; less commonly vivid dreams.
- *Airways obstruction* – asthmatics sometimes tolerate a small dose of a selective drug when first prescribed, only to suffer an exceptionally severe attack subsequently, and β-adrenoceptor antagonists should ideally be avoided altogether in asthmatics and used only with caution in COPD patients, many of whom have a reversible component.
- *Decompensated heart failure* – β-adrenoceptor antagonists are contraindicated (in contrast to stable heart failure, Chapter 31).
- *Peripheral vascular disease and vasospasm* – β-adrenoceptor antagonists worsen claudication and Raynaud's phenomenon.
- *Hypoglycaemia* – β-adrenoceptor antagonists can mask symptoms of hypoglycaemia and the rate of recovery is slowed, because adrenaline stimulates gluconeogenesis.
- *Heart block* – β-adrenoceptor antagonists can precipitate or worsen heart block.
- *Metabolic disturbance* – β-adrenoreceptor antagonists worsen glycaemic control in type 2 diabetes mellitus.

Pharmacokinetics

β-Adrenoceptor antagonists are well absorbed and are only given intravenously in emergencies. Lipophilic drugs (e.g. **propranolol**) are subject to extensive presystemic metabolism in the gut wall and liver by CYP450. Lipophilic beta-blockers enter the brain more readily than do polar drugs and so

Table 28.2: Examples of calcium-channel blocking drugs in clinical use

Class	Drug	Effect on heart rate	Adverse effects	Comment
Dihydropyridine	Nifedipine	↑	Headache, flushing, ankle swelling	Slow-release preparations for once/twice daily use
	Amlodipine	0	Ankle swelling	Once daily use in hypertension, angina
	Nimodipine	↑	Flushing, headache	Prevention of cerebral vasospasm after subarachnoid haemorrhage
Benzothiazepine	Diltiazem	0	Generally mild	Prophylaxis of angina, hypertension
Phenylalkylamine	Verapamil	↓	Constipation; marked negative inotropic action	See Chapter 32 for use in dysrhythmias. Slow-release preparation for hypertension, angina

central nervous system side effects (e.g. nightmares) occur more commonly. Polar (water-soluble) beta-blockers (e.g. **atenolol**) are excreted by the kidneys and accumulate in patients with renal impairment/failure.

Drug interactions

- *Pharmacokinetic interactions*: β-adrenoceptor antagonists inhibit drug metabolism indirectly by decreasing hepatic blood flow secondary to decreased cardiac output. This causes accumulation of drugs such as **lidocaine** that have such a high hepatic extraction ratio that their clearance reflects hepatic blood flow.
- *Pharmacodynamic interactions*: Increased negative inotropic and atrioventricular (AV) nodal effects occur with **verapamil** (giving both intravenously can be fatal), **lidocaine** and other negative inotropes.

C DRUGS

CALCIUM-CHANNEL BLOCKERS

Drugs that block voltage-dependent Ca^{2+} channels are used to treat angina (see Chapter 29) and supraventricular tachydys-rhythmias (see Chapter 32), as well as hypertension. There are three classes: dihydropyridines, benzothiazepines and pheny-lalkylamines. Examples are listed in Table 28.2.

Use

Dihydropyridine calcium-channel blockers. **Amlodipine** has been compared directly with a diuretic (**chlortalidone**) and an ACEI (**lisinopril**), in a very large end-point trial (ALLHAT) and as a basis for treatment in another large trial, ASCOT. It is a good choice, especially in older patients and Afro-Caribbeans, although more expensive than **chlortalidone**. **Amlodipine** is taken once daily. The daily dose can be increased if needed,

usually after a month or more. Slow-release preparations of **nifedipine** provide an alternative to **amlodipine**.

Mechanism of action

Calcium-channel blockers inhibit Ca^{2+} influx through volt-age-dependent L-type calcium channels. Cytoplasmic Ca^{2+} concentrations control the contractile state of actomyosin. Calcium-channel blockers therefore relax arteriolar smooth muscle, reduce peripheral vascular resistance and lower arterial blood pressure.

Adverse effects

Calcium-channel blocking drugs are usually well tolerated.

- Short-acting preparations (e.g. **nifedipine** capsules) cause flushing and headache. Baroreflex activation causes tachycardia, which can worsen angina. These formulations of **nifedipine** should be avoided in the treatment of hypertension and never used sublingually.
- Ankle swelling (oedema) is common, often troublesome, but not sinister.
- The negative inotropic effect of **verapamil** exacerbates cardiac failure.
- Constipation is common with **verapamil**.

Pharmacokinetics

Calcium-channel antagonists are absorbed when given by mouth. **Nifedipine** has a short half-life and many of its adverse effects (e.g. flushing, headache) relate to the peak plasma concentration. Slow-release preparations improve its profile in this regard. **Amlodipine** is renally eliminated and has a half-life of two to three days and produces a persistent antihypertensive effect with once daily administration.

Drug interactions

Intravenous **verapamil** can cause circulatory collapse in patients treated concomitantly with β-adrenoceptor antagonists.

D DRUGS

DIURETICS

For more information, see Chapters 31 and 36.

Use in hypertension

A low dose of a **thiazide**, or related diuretic, e.g. **chlortalidone**, remains the best first choice for treating older patients and Afro-Caribbeans with uncomplicated mild essential hypertension, unless contraindicated by some co-existent disease (e.g. gout). They are also essential in more severe cases, combined with other drugs. Diuretics reduced the risk of stroke in several large clinical trials and in the Medical Research Council (MRC) trial they did so significantly more effectively than did beta-blockade. **Chlortalidone** performed at least as well as **amlodipine** and **lisinopril** in ALLHAT and thiazides are much less expensive than all other antihypertensive drugs. The dose–response curve of diuretics on blood pressure is remarkably flat. However, adverse metabolic effects (see below) are dose related, so increasing the dose is seldom appropriate. Thiazides (e.g. **bendroflumethiazide**) are preferred to loop diuretics for uncomplicated essential hypertension. They are given by mouth as a single morning dose. They begin to act within one to two hours and work for 12–24 hours. Loop diuretics are useful in hypertensive patients with moderate or severe renal impairment, and in patients with hypertensive heart failure.

Mechanism of action

Thiazide diuretics inhibit reabsorption of sodium and chloride ions in the proximal part of the distal convoluted tubule. Excessive salt intake or a low glomerular filtration rate interferes with their antihypertensive effect. Natriuresis is therefore probably important in determining their hypotensive action. However, it is not the whole story since although plasma volume falls when treatment is started, it returns to normal with continued treatment, despite a persistent effect on blood pressure. During chronic treatment, total peripheral vascular resistance falls slowly, suggesting an action on resistance vessels. Responsiveness to pressors (including **angiotensin II** and **noradrenaline**) is reduced during chronic treatment with thiazides.

Adverse effects

- Metabolic and electrolyte changes involve:
  - hyponatraemia – sometimes severe, especially in the elderly;
  - hypokalaemia – kaliuretis is a consequence of increased sodium ion delivery to the distal nephron where sodium and potassium ions are exchanged. Mild hypokalaemia is common but seldom clinically important in uncomplicated hypertension;
  - hypomagnesaemia;
  - hyperuricaemia – most diuretics reduce urate clearance, increase plasma urate and can precipitate gout;
  - hyperglycaemia – thiazides reduce glucose tolerance: high doses cause hyperglycaemia in type 2 diabetes;
  - hypercalcaemia – thiazides reduce urinary calcium ion clearance (unlike loop diuretics, which increase it) and can aggravate hypercalcaemia in hypertensive patients with hyperparathyroidism;
  - hypercholesterolaemia – high-dose thiazides cause a small increase in plasma LDL cholesterol concentration.
- Erectile dysfunction which is reversible on stopping the drug.
- Increased plasma renin, limiting the antihypertensive effect.
- Idiosyncratic reactions, including rashes (which may be photosensitive) and purpura, which may be thrombocytopenic or non-thrombocytopenic.

Contraindications

The effects of thiazide diuretics described above contraindicate their use in patients with severe renal impairment (in whom they are unlikely to be effective), and in patients with a history of gout. They should not be used in pre-eclampsia, which is associated with a contracted intravascular volume. Diuretics should be avoided in men with prostatic symptoms. It is prudent to discontinue diuretics temporarily in patients who develop intercurrent diarrhoea and/or vomiting, to avoid exacerbating fluid depletion.

Drug interactions

In addition to the non-specific adverse interaction with NSAIDs (see above and Chapter 26), all diuretics interact with **lithium**. Li^+ is similar to Na^+ in many respects, and is reabsorbed mainly in the proximal convoluted tubule (Chapter 20). Diuretics indirectly increase Li^+ reabsorption in the proximal tubule, by causing volume contraction. This results in an increased plasma concentration of Li^+ and increased toxicity. Diuretic-induced hypokalaemia and hypomagnesaemia increase the toxicity of digoxin (Chapters 31 and 32). Combinations of a thiazide with a potassium-sparing diuretic, such as **amiloride (co-amilozide)**, **triamterene** or **spironolactone** can prevent undue hypokalaemia, and are especially useful in patients who require simultaneous treatment with **digoxin**, **sotalol** (Chapter 32) or other drugs that prolong the electrocardiographic QT-interval.

Key points

Drugs used in essential hypertension

- *Diuretics*: thiazides (in low dose) are preferred to loop diuretics unless there is renal impairment. They may precipitate gout and worsen glucose tolerance or dyslipidaemia, but they reduce the risk of stroke and other vascular events. Adverse effects include hypokalaemia, which is seldom problematic, and impotence. They are suitable first-line drugs, especially in black patients, who often have low circulating renin levels and respond well to salt restriction and diuretics.
- *Beta-blockers* reduce the risk of vascular events, but are contraindicated in patients with obstructive pulmonary disease. Adverse events (dose-related) include fatigue and cold extremities. Heart failure, heart block or claudication can be exacerbated in predisposed patients. They are particularly useful in patients with another indication for them (e.g. angina, post-myocardial infarction). Patients of African descent tend to respond poorly to them as single agents.
- *ACE inhibitors* are particularly useful as an addition to a thiazide in moderately severe disease. The main adverse effect on chronic use is cough; losartan, an angiotensin-II receptor antagonist, lacks this effect but is otherwise similar to ACE inhibitors.
- *Calcium-channel antagonists* are useful, especially in moderately severe disease. Long-acting drugs/preparations are preferred. The main adverse effect in chronic use is ankle swelling.
- α_1-Blockers are useful additional agents in patients who are poorly controlled on one or two drugs. Long-acting drugs (e.g. doxazosin) are preferred. Effects on vascular event rates are unknown. Unlike other antihypertensives, they improve the lipid profile.
- *α-Methyldopa* is useful in patients with hypertension during pregnancy.
- Other drugs that are useful in occasional patients with severe disease include **minoxidil**, **hydralazine** and **nitroprusside**.

OTHER ANTIHYPERTENSIVE DRUGS

Other important drugs (aldosterone antagonists, other vasodilators and centrally acting drugs) are summarized in Table 28.3.

ALDOSTERONE ANTAGONISTS

Neither **spironolactone** nor the more selective (and much more expensive) **eplerenone** is licensed for treating essential hypertension. They are used to treat Conn's syndrome, but are also effective in essential hypertension (especially low renin essential hypertension) and are recommended as add-on treatment for resistant hypertension by the British Hypertension Society

(BHS) guidelines. The main adverse effects are hyperkalaemia (especially in patients with renal impairment) and, with **spironolactone**, oestrogen-like effects of gynaecomastia, breast tenderness and menstrual disturbance.

OTHER VASODILATORS

α-ADRENOCEPTOR ANTAGONISTS

There are two main types of α-adrenoceptor, α_1- and α_2. α_1-Adrenoceptor antagonists lower blood pressure.

Use

Phenoxybenzamine irreversibly alkylates α-receptors. It is uniquely valuable in preparing patients with phaeochromocytoma for surgery, but has no place in the management of essential hypertension. **Prazosin** is a selective α_1-blocker, but its use is limited by severe postural hypotension, especially following the first dose. It has a short elimination half-life. **Doxazosin** is closely related to **prazosin**, but is longer lasting, permitting once daily use and causing fewer problems with first-dose hypotension. It did not compare well with diuretic, Ca^{2+} antagonist or ACEI as first-line agent in ALLHAT, but is useful as add-on treatment in patients with resistant hypertension. It is given last thing at night.

Doxazosin improves symptoms of bladder outflow tract obstruction (Chapter 36), and is useful in men with mild symptoms from benign prostatic hypertrophy.

Mechanism of action

Noradrenaline activates α_1-receptors on vascular smooth muscle, causing tonic vasoconstriction. α_1-Antagonists cause vasodilatation by blocking this tonic action of **noradrenaline**.

Adverse effects

- First-dose hypotension and postural hypotension are adverse effects.
- Nasal stuffiness, headache, dry mouth and pruritus have been reported, but are relatively infrequent.
- α-Blockers can cause urinary incontinence, especially in women with pre-existing pelvic pathology.

Metabolic effects

α_1-Adrenoceptor antagonists have a mild favourable effect on plasma lipids, with an increase in HDL and a reduction in LDL cholesterol.

Pharmacokinetics

Doxazosin has an elimination half-life of approximately 10–12 hours and provides acceptably smooth 24-hour control if used once daily.

Table 28.3: Additional antihypertensive drugs used in special situations

Drug	Mechanism of action	Uses	Side-effects/limitations
Minoxidil	Minoxidil sulphate (active metabolite) is a K$^+$-channel activator	Very severe hypertension that is resistant to other drugs	Fluid retention; reflex tachycardia; hirsutism; coarsening of facial appearance. Must be used in combination with other drugs (usually a loop diuretic and β-antagonist)
Nitroprusside	Breaks down chemically to NO, which activates guanylyl cyclase in vascular smooth muscle	Given by intravenous infusion in intensive care unit for control of malignant hypertension	Short term IV use only: prolonged use causes cyanide toxicity (monitor plasma thiocyanate); sensitive to light; close monitoring to avoid hypotension is essential
Hydralazine	Direct action on vascular smooth muscle; biochemical mechanism not understood	Previously used in 'stepped-care' approach to severe hypertension: β-antagonist in combination with diuretic. Retains a place in severe hypertension during pregnancy	Headache; flushing; tachycardia; fluid retention. Long-term high-dose use causes systemic lupus-like syndrome in susceptible individuals
α-Methyldopa	Taken up by noradrenergic nerve terminals and converted to α-methylnoradrenaline, which is released as a false transmitter. This acts centrally as an α$_2$-agonist and reduces sympathetic outflow	Hypertension during pregnancy. Occasionally useful in patients who cannot tolerate other drugs	Drowsiness (common); depression; hepatitis; immune haemolytic anaemia; drug fever

MINOXIDIL

Minoxidil works via a sulphate metabolite which activates K$^+$ channels. This relaxes vascular smooth muscle, reducing peripheral vascular resistance and lowering blood pressure. It is a powerful vasodilator and is used in very severe hypertension unresponsive to other drugs, combined with a β-adrenoceptor antagonist to block reflex tachycardia and a loop diuretic because of the severe fluid retention it causes. It increases hair growth (indeed the sulphate metabolite is licensed as a topical cream for male baldness) and coarsens facial features, so is unacceptable to most women.

HYDRALAZINE

Hydralazine has a direct vasodilator action that is not fully understood. It used to be widely used as part of 'triple therapy' with a β-adrenoceptor antagonist and a diuretic in patients with severe hypertension, but has been rendered largely obsolete by better tolerated drugs such as Ca^{2+} antagonists (see above). Large doses are associated with a lupus-like syndrome with positive antinuclear antibodies. It has been widely and safely used in pregnancy and retains a use for severe hypertension in this setting although **nifedipine** is now preferred by many obstetric physicians.

NITROPRUSSIDE

Nitroprusside is given by intravenous infusion in hypertensive emergencies (e.g. hypertensive encephalopathy), in an intensive care unit. It is a rapid acting inorganic nitrate which degrades to NO. Co-administration of a β-adrenoceptor antagonist is usually required. Prolonged use is precluded by the development of cyanide toxicity and its use requires specialist expertise.

CENTRALLY ACTING DRUGS

α-**Methyldopa** has been extensively used in pregnancy and is a preferred agent when drug treatment is needed in this setting. Drowsiness is common, but often wears off. A positive Coombs' test is also not uncommon: rarely this is associated with haemolytic anaemia. Other immune effects include drug fever and hepatitis. Its mechanism is uptake into central neurones and metabolism to false transmitter (α-**methylnoradrenaline**) which is an α$_2$-adrenoceptor agonist. Activating central α$_2$-adrenoceptors inhibits sympathetic outflow from the CNS. **Moxonidine** is another centrally acting drug: it acts on imidazoline receptors and is said to be better tolerated than **methyldopa**.

OTHER ANTIHYPERTENSIVE DRUGS **195**

Case history

A 72-year-old woman sees her general practitioner because of an *Escherichia coli* urinary infection. Her blood pressure is 196/86 mmHg. She had had a small stroke two years previously, which was managed at home, and from which she made a complete recovery. At that time, her blood pressure was recorded as 160/80 mmHg. She looks after her husband (who has mild dementia) and enjoys life, particularly visits from her grandchildren. She smokes ten cigarettes/day, does not drink any alcohol and takes no drugs. The remainder of the examination is unremarkable. Serum creatinine is normal, total cholesterol is 5.6 mmol/L and HDL is 1.2 mmol/L. The urinary tract infection resolves with a short course of amoxicillin. This patient's blood pressure on two further occasions is 176/84 and 186/82 mmHg, respectively. An ECG is normal. She is resistant to advice to stop smoking (on the grounds that she has been doing it for 55 years and any harm has been done already) and the suggestion of drug treatment (on the grounds that she feels fine and is 'too old for that sort of thing').

Questions
Decide whether each of the following statements is true or false.

(a) This patient's systolic hypertension is a reflection of a 'stiff' circulation, and drug treatment will not improve her prognosis.
(b) Drug treatment of the hypertension should not be contemplated unless she stops smoking first.
(c) If she agrees to take drugs such as thiazides for her hypertension, she will be at greater risk of adverse effects than a younger woman.
(d) Attempts to discourage her from smoking are futile.
(e) An α_1-blocker would be a sensible first choice of drug, as it will improve her serum lipid levels.
(f) Aspirin treatment should be considered.

Answer

(a) False
(b) False
(c) True
(d) False
(e) False
(f) True.

Comment
Treating elderly patients with systolic hypertension reduces their excess risk of stroke and myocardial infarction. The absolute benefit of treatment is greatest in elderly people (in whom events are common). Treatment is particularly desirable as this patient made a good recovery from a stroke. She was strongly discouraged from smoking (by explaining that this would almost immediately reduce the risk of a further vascular event), but she was unable to stop. Continued smoking puts her at increased risk of stroke and she agreed to take bendroflumethiazide 2.5 mg daily with the goal of staying healthy so that she could continue to look after her husband and enjoy life. She tolerated this well and her blood pressure fell to around 165/80 mmHg. The addition of a long-acting ACE inhibitor (trandolapril, 0.5 mg in the morning) led to a further reduction in blood pressure to around 150/80 mmHg. α_1-Antagonists can cause postural hypotension, which is particularly undesirable in the elderly.

FURTHER READING

Dahlof B, Sever PS, Poulter NR et al. Prevention of cardiovascular events with an antihypertensive regimen of amlodipine adding perindopril as required versus atenolol adding bendroflumethiazide as required, in the Anglo-Scandinavian Cardiac Outcomes Trial-Blood Pressure Lowering Arm (ASCOT-BPLA): a multicentre randomised controlled trial. *Lancet* 2005; **366**: 895–906.

Furberg CD, Wright JT, Davis BR et al. Major cardiovascular events in hypertensive patients randomized to doxazosin vs chlorthalidone – The Antihypertensive and Lipid-Lowering Treatment to Prevent Heart Attack Trial (ALLHAT). *Journal of the American Medical Association* 2000; **283**: 1967–75.

Furberg CD, Wright JT, Davis BR et al. Major outcomes in high-risk hypertensive patients randomized to angiotensin-converting enzyme inhibitor or calcium channel blocker vs diuretic – The Antihypertensive and Lipid-Lowering Treatment to Prevent Heart Attack Trial (ALLHAT). *Journal of the American Medical Association* 2002; **288**: 2981–97.

Goodfriend TL, Elliott ME, Catt KJ. Angiotensin receptors and their antagonists. *New England Journal of Medicine* 1996; **334**: 1649–54.

Palmer BF. Current concepts: Renal dysfunction complicating the treatment of hypertension. *New England Journal of Medicine* 2002; **347**: 1256–61.

Setaro JF, Black HR. Refractory hypertension. *New England Journal of Medicine* 1992; **327**: 543–7.

Sibai BM. Treatment of hypertension in pregnant women. *New England Journal of Medicine* 1996; **335**: 257–65.

Staessen JA, Li Y, Richart T. Oral renin inhibitors. *Lancet* 2006; **368**: 1449–56.

Swales JD (ed.). *Textbook of hypertension*. Oxford: Blackwell Science, 1994.

van Zwieten PA. Central imidazoline (I1) receptors as targets of centrally acting antihypertensives: moxonidine and rilmenidine. *Journal of Hypertension* 1997; **15**: 117–25.

ISCHAEMIC HEART DISEASE

PATHOPHYSIOLOGY

Ischaemic heart disease is nearly always caused by atheroma (Chapter 27) in one or more of the coronary arteries. Such disease is very common in western societies and is often asymptomatic. When the obstruction caused by an uncomplicated atheromatous plaque exceeds a critical value, myocardial oxygen demand during exercise exceeds the ability of the stenosed vessel to supply oxygenated blood, resulting in chest pain brought on predictably by exertion and relieved within a few minutes on resting ('angina pectoris'). Drugs that alter haemodynamics can reduce angina.

Most patients with angina pectoris experience attacks of pain in a constant stable pattern, but in some patients attacks occur at rest, or they may occur with increasing frequency and severity on less and less exertion ('unstable angina'). Unstable angina may be a prelude to myocardial infarction, which can also occur unheralded. Both unstable angina and myocardial infarction occur as a result of fissuring of an atheromatous plaque in a coronary artery. Platelets adhere to the underlying subendothelium and white thrombus, consisting of platelet/fibrinogen/fibrin aggregates, extends into the lumen of the artery. Myocardial infarction results when thrombus occludes the coronary vessel.

In addition to mechanical obstruction caused by atheroma, with or without adherent thrombus, spasm of smooth muscle in the vascular media can contribute to ischaemia. The importance of such vascular spasm varies both among different patients and at different times in the same patient, and its contribution is often difficult to define clinically. The mechanism of spasm also probably varies and has been difficult to establish. A variety of vasoconstrictive mediators released from formed elements of blood (e.g. platelets or white cells) or from nerve terminals may contribute to coronary spasm. Its importance or otherwise in the majority of patients with acute coronary syndromes is a matter of considerable debate.

Treatment of patients with ischaemic heart disease is directed at the three pathophysiological elements identified above, namely atheroma, haemodynamics and thrombosis. New onset of chest pain at rest or crescendo symptoms should raise suspicion of unstable angina or myocardial infarction,

and emergency referral to a hospital with coronary care unit. The general management of stable angina is illustrated in Figure 29.1 and detailed further below.

MANAGEMENT OF STABLE ANGINA

MODIFIABLE RISK FACTORS

Modifiable risk factors include smoking, hypertension, hypercholesterolaemia, diabetes mellitus, obesity and lack of exercise. The object of defining these factors is to improve them in individual patients, thereby preventing progression (and hopefully causing regression) of coronary atheroma. This is discussed in Chapters 27, 28 and 37.

PAIN RELIEF

An attack of angina is relieved by **glyceryl trinitrate** (GTN), which is given by sublingual administration. However, in patients with chronic stable angina, pain usually resolves within a few minutes of stopping exercise even without treatment, so prophylaxis is usually more important than relief of an attack. In patients hospitalized with acute coronary syndrome, GTN is often administered by intravenous infusion; its short half-life allows rapid titration, thus permitting effective pain relief whilst promptly averting any adverse haemodynamic consequences (in particular, hypotension).

PROPHYLAXIS

Figure 29.2 outlines the drug treatment of stable angina. Antithrombotic therapy with **aspirin** reduces the incidence of myocardial infarction; its use and mechanism of action as an antiplatelet agent are discussed further in Chapter 30. Prophylaxis is also directed at reducing the frequency of attacks of angina. In this context, **GTN** is best used for 'acute' prophylaxis. A dose is taken immediately before undertaking activity that usually brings on pain (e.g. climbing a hill), in

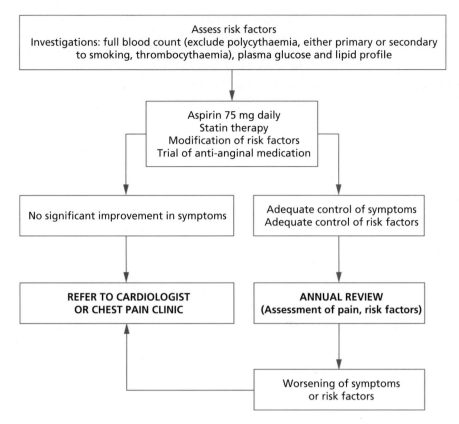

Figure 29.1: General management of stable angina.

order to prevent pain. Alternatively, long-acting nitrates (e.g. **isosorbide mononitrate**) may be taken regularly to reduce the frequency of attacks. Beta-blockers (usually of the 'cardioselective' type, e.g. **atenolol**, **metoprolol** or **bisoprolol**) or calcium-channel blockers (most commonly **diltiazem**, less commonly **verapamil** or one of the dihydropyridine drugs, such as **nifedipine** or **amlodipine**) are also useful for chronic prophylaxis (see below). **Nicorandil** combines nitrate-like with K^+-channel-activating properties and relaxes veins and arteries. It is used in acute and long-term prophylaxis of angina, usually as an add-on to nitrates, beta-blockers and/or calcium-channel blockers where these have been incompletely effective, poorly tolerated or contraindicated. Statins (e.g. **simvastatin** or **atorvastatin**) should be prescribed routinely for cholesterol lowering unless there is a contraindication, regardless of serum cholesterol (unless it is already very low: total cholesterol <4 mmol/L and/or LDL cholesterol <2 mmol/L), as numerous large studies have shown prognostic benefit in terms of prevention of cardiac events and reduction in mortality.

CONSIDERATION OF SURGERY/ANGIOPLASTY

Cardiac catheterization identifies patients who would benefit from coronary artery bypass graft (CABG) surgery or percutaneous coronary intervention (PCI, which most commonly involves balloon angioplasty of the affected coronary arteries with concomitant stent insertion). Coronary artery disease is progressive and there are two roles for such interventions:

1. symptom relief;
2. to improve outcome.

CABG and PCI are both excellent treatments for relieving the symptoms of angina, although they are not a permanent cure and symptoms may recur if there is restenosis, if the graft becomes occluded, or if the underlying atheromatous disease progresses. Restenosis following PCI is relatively common, occurring in 20–30% of patients in the first four to six months following the procedure, and various strategies are currently under investigation for reducing the occurrence of restenosis; one very promising strategy involves the use of 'drug-eluting' stents (stents which are coated with a thin polymer containing a cytotoxic drug, usually **sirolimus** or **paclitaxel**, which suppresses the hypertrophic vascular response to injury). PCI as currently performed does not improve the final outcome in terms of survival or myocardial infarction, whereas CABG can benefit some patients. Those with significant disease in the left main coronary artery survive longer if they are operated on and so do patients with severe triple-vessel disease. Patients with strongly positive stress cardiograms have a relatively high incidence of such lesions, but unfortunately there is no foolproof method of making such anatomical diagnoses non-invasively, so the issue of which patients to subject to the low risks of invasive study remains one of clinical judgement and of cost.

Surgical treatment consists of coronary artery grafting with saphenous vein or, preferably, internal mammary artery (and sometimes other artery segments, e.g. radial artery) to bypass diseased segment(s) of coronary artery. Arterial bypass grafts have a much longer patency life than vein grafts, the latter usually becoming occluded after 10–15 years (and often after much shorter periods). PCI has yet to be shown to prolong life in the setting of stable angina, but can be valuable as a less demanding alternative to surgery in patients with accessible

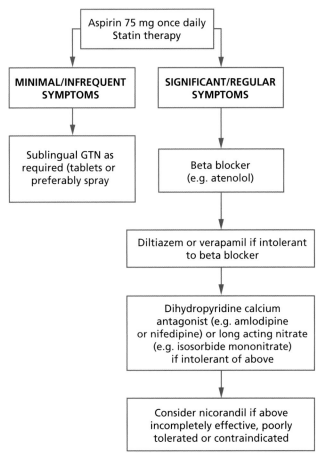

Figure 29.2: Drug therapy of stable angina.

lesions whose symptoms are not adequately controlled by medical therapy alone. Several antiplatelet drugs are given at the time of PCI, including oral **aspirin** and **clopidogrel**, and a glycoprotein IIb/IIIa inhibitor given intravenously such as **abciximab**, **eptifibatide** or **tirofiban** (Chapter 30). **Aspirin** is usually continued indefinitely and **clopidogrel** is usually continued for at least one month following the procedure.

MANAGEMENT OF UNSTABLE CORONARY DISEASE

ACUTE CORONARY SYNDROME

Acute coronary syndrome (ACS) is a blanket term used to describe the consequences of coronary artery occlusion, whether transient or permanent, partial or complete. These different patterns of coronary occlusion give rise to the different types of ACS, namely unstable angina (where no detectable myocardial necrosis is present), non-ST-segment-elevation myocardial infarction (NSTEMI) and ST-segment-elevation myocardial infarction (STEMI, usually larger in extent and fuller in thickness of myocardial wall affected than NSTEMI). A flow chart for management of ACS is given in Figure 29.3. Unstable angina and NSTEMI are a continuum of disease, and usually only distinguishable by the presence of

a positive serum troponin test in NSTEMI (troponin now being the gold standard serum marker of myocardial damage); their management is similar and discussed further here. Management of STEMI is discussed separately below. All patients with ACS must stop smoking. This is more urgent than in other patients with coronary artery disease, because of the acute pro-thrombotic effect of smoking.

Patients with ACS require urgent antiplatelet therapy, in the form of **aspirin** and **clopidogrel** (Chapter 30), plus antithrombotic therapy with **heparin** (nowadays most often **low-molecular-weight heparin** administered subcutaneously; see Chapter 30). Data from the CURE trial suggest that combined **aspirin** and **clopidogrel** treatment is better than **aspirin** alone, and that this combination should be continued for several months, and preferably for up to a year, following which **aspirin** alone should be continued. This antiplatelet/antithrombotic regime approximately halves the likelihood of myocardial infarction, and is the most effective known treatment for improving outcome in pre-infarction syndromes. By contrast, **GTN**, while very effective in relieving pain associated with unstable angina, does not improve outcome. It is usually given as a constant-rate intravenous infusion for this indication. A β-blocker is prescribed if not contraindicated. If β-blockers are contraindicated, a long-acting Ca^{2+}-antagonist is a useful alternative. **Diltiazem** is often used as it does not cause reflex tachycardia and is less negatively inotropic than **verapamil**. β-Blockers and Ca^{2+}-antagonists are often prescribed together, but there is disappointingly little evidence that their effects are synergistic or even additive. Moreover, there is a theoretical risk of severe bradycardia or of precipitation of heart failure if β-blockers are co-administered with these negatively chronotropic and inotropic drugs, especially so for **verapamil**; where concomitant β-blockade and calcium-channel blockade is desired, it is probably safest to use a dihydropyridine calcium-channel blocker (e.g. **nifedipine** or **amlodipine**) rather than **verapamil** or **diltiazem**. **Nicorandil** is now often added as well, but again there is not much evidence of added benefit. Coronary angiography is indicated in patients who are potentially suitable for PCI or CABG, and should be considered as an emergency in patients who fail to settle on medical therapy.

ST-ELEVATION-MYOCARDIAL INFARCTION (STEMI)

ACUTE MANAGEMENT
Oxygen

This is given in the highest concentration available (unless there is coincident pulmonary disease with carbon dioxide retention) delivered by face mask (FiO_2 approximately 60%) or by nasal prongs if a face mask is not tolerated.

Pain relief

This usually requires an intravenous opiate (**morphine** or **diamorphine**; see Chapter 25) and concurrent treatment with an anti-emetic (e.g. **promethazine** or **metoclopramide**; see Chapter 34).

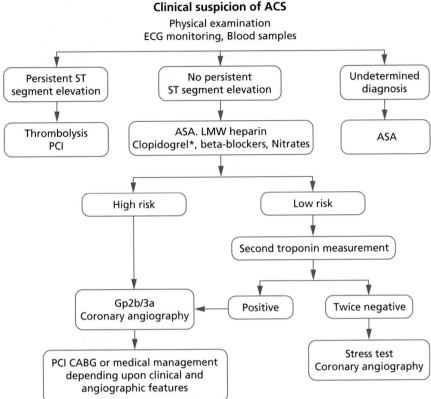

Figure 29.3: Recommended strategy for management of acute coronary syndrome. ASA, acetylsalicylic acid (aspirin); LMW heparin, low-molecular-weight heparin. (Adapted from the European Society of Cardiology guidelines, 2002).

Infarct limitation

In centres where immediate access is available to the cardiac catheterization laboratory, the treatment of choice for limitation of infarct size and severity is generally considered to be primary angioplasty. However, at the present time, many hospitals do not have such immediate access available, and in such cases, since prevention of death and other serious complications is directly related to the speed with which opening of the infarct-related artery can be achieved, antithrombotic/fibrinolytic treatment should be instituted. **Aspirin** and thrombolytic therapy both reduce infarct size and improve survival – each to a similar extent. Examples of thrombolytic drugs commonly used are **streptokinase, alteplase** (also known as recombinant tissue plasminogen activator, or rtPA), **reteplase** and **tenecteplase**. Their beneficial effects are similar to one another and additive with **aspirin**. Early fears about toxicity of the combination proved unfounded, so they are used together. **Heparin** or, more commonly **low-molecular-weight heparin** administered subcutaneously, is needed to maintain patency of a vessel opened by **aspirin** plus thrombolysis when **alteplase, reteplase** or **tenecteplase** are used; this is not the case, however, for **streptokinase**. Recent evidence suggests that the additional use of **clopidogrel** in the early course of myocardial infarction improves outcome further, over and above the benefit seen with **aspirin** and thrombolysis or primary angioplasty.

Haemodynamic treatment has less impact than opening of the infarct-related artery, but is also potentially important. The intravenous use of β-blockers within the first few hours of

infarction has a modest short-term benefit. The International Study of Infarct Survival (ISIS-1) (in patients who did not receive the thrombolytic treatment or angioplasty which is now standard) showed that the seven-day mortality in patients treated early with intravenous atenolol was 3.7%, compared to 4.3% in controls. This small absolute benefit was not maintained (there were more deaths in the **atenolol** group than in the control group at one year) and does not warrant routine use of β-blockers for this indication (as opposed to their use in secondary prevention, five days or more after acute infarction, which is discussed below). A rationale has been developed for the use of angiotensin-converting enzyme inhibitors (ACEI) in acute myocardial infarction, in terms of possible improvements in cardiac work load and prevention of deleterious cardiac remodelling. Trials with ACEI have almost universally been positive in this context, showing benefit in terms of mortality, haemodynamics and morbidity/hospitalizations from heart failure in patients with evidence of left ventricular dysfunction (e.g. on echocardiography) or of clinically evident heart failure post-myocardial infarction. Moreover, the magnitude of this benefit from ACEI treatment increases with increasing ventricular dysfunction, whilst there is little or no evidence of benefit in patients with normal left ventricular ejection post-infarct. Examples of ACEI commonly used in this context are **enalapril, lisinopril, trandolapril** and **ramipril**. Moreover, recent trial evidence (e.g. from the VALIANT study, using **valsartan**) suggests that angiotensin receptor blockade may be a useful alternative to ACEI in patients post-myocardial infarction with left ventricular dysfunction or heart failure.

Treatable complications

These may occur early in the course of myocardial infarction, and are best recognized and managed with the patient in a coronary-care unit. Transfer from the admission room should therefore not be delayed by obtaining x-rays, as a portable film can be obtained on the unit if necessary. Complications include cardiogenic shock (Chapter 31) as well as acute tachy- or brady-dysrhythmias (Chapter 32). Prophylactic treatment with anti-dysrhythmic drugs (i.e. before significant dysrhythmia is documented) has not been found to improve survival.

LONG-TERM MEASURES POST-ACUTE CORONARY SYNDROME

Modifiable factors should be sought and attended to as for patients with angina (see above). Drugs are used prophylactically following recovery from myocardial infarction to prevent sudden death or recurrence of myocardial infarction. Aspirin and β-adrenoceptor antagonists each reduce the risk of recurrence or sudden death. Meta-analysis of the many clinical trials of aspirin has demonstrated an overwhelmingly significant effect of modest magnitude (an approximately 30% reduction in the risk of reinfarction), and several individual trials of β-adrenoceptor antagonists have also demonstrated conclusive benefit. Statins should routinely be prescribed, as discussed under Management of stable angina above, because of their clear prognostic benefit in this situation. In addition, numerous trials have now demonstrated that long-term use of ACEI in patients post-myocardial infarction with either overt heart failure or clinically silent left ventricular dysfunction prevents cardiac remodelling and subsequent development/ worsening of heart failure; and recent trials suggest that the same is likely to be true of the angiotensin receptor blockers. Finally, recent evidence from the EPHESUS trial has shown that early treatment of patients with left ventricular dysfunction post-myocardial infarction (within a few days) with the aldosterone antagonist **eplerenone**, continued long term (at least 18 months), prevents development/progression of heart failure and improves mortality.

Consideration of surgery/angioplasty

Ideally all patients who are potentially operative candidates would have angiography at some stage, even if they have not undergone early angiography/angioplasty as an in-patient. In practice, the same considerations apply as for patients with angina (see above), and in the UK angiography is currently usually undertaken on the basis of a clinical judgement based on age, co-existing disease, presence or absence of post-infarction angina, and often on a stress test performed after recovery from the acute event (patients with a negative stress test are considered to be at low risk of subsequent cardiac events).

Psychological and social factors

After recovery from myocardial infarction, patients require an explanation of what has happened, advice about activity in the short and long term, and about work, driving and sexual activity, as well as help in regaining self-esteem. Cardiac rehabilitation includes attention to secondary prevention, as well as to psychological factors. A supervised graded exercise programme is often valuable. Neglect of these unglamorous aspects of management may cause prolonged and unnecessary unhappiness.

DRUGS USED IN ISCHAEMIC HEART DISEASE

Drugs that are used to influence atherosclerosis are described in Chapter 27. In the present chapter, we briefly describe those drugs that are used to treat ischaemic heart disease either because of their haemodynamic properties or because they inhibit thrombosis.

DRUGS THAT INFLUENCE HAEMODYNAMICS

ORGANIC NITRATES

Use and administration

GTN is used to relieve anginal pain. It is generally best used as 'acute' prophylaxis, i.e. immediately before undertaking strenuous activity. It is usually given sublingually, thereby ensuring rapid absorption and avoiding presystemic metabolism (Chapter 5), but in patients with unstable angina it may be given as an intravenous infusion. The spray has a somewhat more rapid onset of action and a much longer shelf-life than tablets, but is more expensive. **GTN** is absorbed transdermally and is available in a patch preparation for longer prophylaxis than the short-term benefit provided by a sublingual dose. Alternatively, a longer-acting nitrate, such as **isosorbide mononitrate**, may be used prophylactically to reduce the frequency of attacks; it is less expensive than **GTN** patches and is taken by mouth. In patients whose pattern of pain is predominantly during the daytime, it is prescribed to be taken in the morning and at lunch-time, thereby 'covering' the day, but avoiding development of tolerance by omitting an evening dose. Longer-acting controlled-release preparations are available for once daily use, and these usually provide nitrate cover during most of the day, but leave a small 'nitrate-free' window of a few hours, thereby again preventing the development of nitrate tolerance. Long-acting nitrates are also used in combination with **hydralazine** in patients with heart failure who are unable to take ACE inhibitors and, especially, in patients of African origin (Chapter 31).

GTN is volatile, so the tablets have a limited shelf-life (around six weeks after the bottle is opened) and they need to be stored in a cool place in a tightly capped dark container, without cotton wool or other tablets. Adverse effects can be minimized by swallowing the tablet after strenuous activity is completed (a more genteel alternative to spitting it out!), because of the lower systemic bioavailability from gut than from buccal mucosa.

Mechanism of action

GTN works by relaxing vascular smooth muscle. It is metabolized by smooth-muscle cells with generation of nitric oxide (NO). This combines with a haem group in the soluble isoform of guanylyl cyclase, activating this enzyme and thereby increasing the cytoplasmic concentration of the second messenger cGMP. cGMP causes sequestration of Ca^{2+} within the sarcoplasmic reticulum, thus relaxing smooth muscle. NO is also synthesized from endogenous substrate (L-arginine) under physiological conditions by a constitutive enzyme in vascular endothelial cells and is Furchgott's 'endothelium-derived relaxing factor'. This endogenous NO is responsible for the resting vasodilator tone present in human resistance arterioles under basal conditions. Nitrovasodilator drugs provide NO in an endothelium-independent manner, and are therefore effective even if endothelial function is severely impaired, as in many patients with coronary artery disease.

Haemodynamic and related effects

GTN is relatively selective for venous rather than arteriolar smooth muscle. Venodilatation reduces cardiac preload. Reduced venous return reduces ventricular filling and hence reduces ventricular diameter. Ventricular wall tension is directly proportional to chamber diameter (the Laplace relationship), so ventricular wall tension is reduced by **GTN**. This reduces cardiac work and oxygen demand. Coronary blood flow (which occurs during diastole) improves due to the decreased left ventricular end-diastolic pressure. Spasm is opposed by NO-mediated coronary artery relaxation. Reduced arterial tone reduces diastolic blood pressure and arterial wave reflection hence reducing cardiac afterload and myocardial oxygen demand. Nitrates relax some non-vascular smooth muscles and therefore sometimes relieve the pain of oesophageal spasm and biliary or renal colic, causing potential diagnostic confusion.

Adverse effects

Organic nitrates are generally very safe, although they can cause hypotension in patients with diminished cardiac reserve. Headache is common and **GTN** patches have not fared well when evaluated by 'quality of life' questionnaires for this reason. Tolerance is another problem. This can be minimized by omitting the evening dose of isosorbide mononitrate (or by removing a patch at night).

β-ADRENOCEPTOR ANTAGONISTS

For more information, see also Chapters 28, 31 and 32.

Use in ischaemic heart disease

The main uses of beta-blockers in patients with ischaemic heart disease are:

- prophylaxis of angina;
- reduction of the risk of sudden death or reinfarction following myocardial infarction ('secondary prevention');
- treatment of heart failure (Chapter 31).

ANGIOTENSIN-CONVERTING ENZYME INHIBITORS (ACEI) AND ANGIOTENSIN RECEPTOR BLOCKERS

Use in ischaemic heart disease

As well as their well established uses in hypertension (see Chapter 28) and in heart failure, including chronic heart failure caused by ischaemic heart disease (see Chapter 31), there is also substantial evidence to support the use of ACEI and angiotensin antagonists in the early stages of myocardial infarction (see above). The evidence suggests that any benefit is very small (or non-existent) in patients with completely normal ventricular function, but that with increasing ventricular dysfunction there is increasing benefit. Treatment should be started with small doses with dose titration up to doses that have been demonstrated to improve survival.

CALCIUM ANTAGONISTS

Use in ischaemic heart disease

Apart from their use in hypertension (Chapter 28) and in the treatment of cardiac dysrhythmias (see Chapter 32), the main use of calcium-channel antagonists in patients with ischaemic heart disease is for the prophylaxis of angina. They are particularly useful in patients in whom beta-blockers are contraindicated. Disappointingly, despite having quite different pharmacological actions to beta-blockers, these classes of drugs do not appear to act synergistically in angina and should not be routinely co-administered as prophylaxis to such patients. They may be particularly useful in the rare patients in whom spasm is particularly prominent (spasm can be worsened by β-blockers). Short-acting dihydropyridines should be avoided because they cause reflex tachycardia. **Diltiazem** or a long-acting dihydropyridine (e.g. **amlodipine** or a controlled-release preparation of **nifedipine**) are often used in this setting. Unlike β-adrenoceptor antagonists and ACEI, Ca^{2+} antagonists have not been found to prolong survival when administered early in the course of myocardial infarction.

DRUGS THAT INFLUENCE THROMBOSIS

ASPIRIN AND CLOPIDOGREL

The use of **aspirin** as a mild analgesic is described in Chapter 25, and the antiplatelet uses of **aspirin** and **clopidogrel** are discussed in Chapter 30. There is no evidence that the efficacy of **aspirin** varies with dose over the range 75–320 mg/day during chronic use, but there is evidence that the adverse effect of peptic ulceration and major upper gastro-intestinal haemorrhage is dose related over this range. Accordingly, the lower dose should be used routinely for chronic prophylaxis. At the onset of ACS it is appropriate to use a higher dose (e.g. 300 mg) to obtain rapid and complete inhibition of platelet cyclo-oxygenase (COX). There has been considerable interest in the possibility that very low doses of **aspirin** (40 mg/day or less) may provide the highest degree of selectivity for inhibition of platelet TXA_2 biosynthesis as opposed to endothelial prostacyclin (PGI_2) biosynthesis in blood vessels, thereby maximizing its cardiovascular benefits. **Aspirin** acetylates platelet COX as platelets circulate through portal venous blood (where the acetylsalicylic acid concentration is high during absorption of **aspirin** from the gastro-intestinal tract), whereas systemic endothelial cells are exposed to much lower concentrations because at low doses hepatic esterases result in little or no **aspirin** entering systemic blood. This has been demonstrated experimentally, but the strategy has yet to be shown to result in increased antithrombotic efficacy of very low doses. In practice, even much higher doses given once daily or every other day achieve considerable selectivity for platelet vs. endothelial COX, because platelets (being anucleate) do not synthesize new COX after their existing supply has been irreversibly inhibited by covalent acetylation by **aspirin**, whereas endothelial cells regenerate new enzyme rapidly (within six hours in healthy human subjects). Consequently, there is selective inhibition of platelet COX for most of the dose interval if a regular dose of **aspirin** is administered every 24 or 48 hours.

FIBRINOLYTIC DRUGS

Several fibrinolytic drugs are used in acute myocardial infarction, including **streptokinase**, **alteplase**, **reteplase** and **tenecteplase**. **Streptokinase** works indirectly, combining with plasminogen to form an activator complex that converts the remaining free plasminogen to plasmin which dissolves fibrin clots. **Alteplase**, **reteplase** and **tenecteplase** are direct-acting plasminogen activators. Fibrinolytic therapy is indicated, when angioplasty is not available, for STEMI patients with ST-segment elevation or bundle-branch block on the ECG. The maximum benefit is obtained if treatment is given within 90 minutes of the onset of pain. Treatment using **streptokinase** with **aspirin** is effective, safe and relatively inexpensive. **Alteplase**, **reteplase** and **tenecteplase**, which do not produce a generalized fibrinolytic state, but selectively dissolve recently formed clot, are also safe and effective; **reteplase** and **tenecteplase** can be given by bolus injection (two injections intravenously separated by 30 minutes for **reteplase**, one single intravenous injection for **tenecteplase**), whereas **alteplase** has to be given by intravenous infusion. Despite their higher cost than **streptokinase**, such drugs have been used increasingly over **streptokinase** in recent years, because of the occurrence of immune reactions and of hypotension with **streptokinase**. Being a streptococcal protein, individuals who have been exposed to it synthesize antibodies that can cause allergic reactions or (much more commonly) loss of efficacy due to binding to and neutralization of the drug. Individuals who have previously received **streptokinase** (more than a few days ago) should not be retreated with this drug if they reinfarct. The situation regarding previous streptococcal infection is less certain. Such infections (usually in the form of sore throats) are quite common and often go undiagnosed; the impact that such infections (along with more severe streptococcal infections, such as cellullitis or septicaemia) have on the efficacy of **streptokinase** treatment is uncertain, but likely to be significant. Hypotension may occur during infusion of **streptokinase**, partly as a result of activation of kinins and other vasodilator peptides. The important thing is tissue perfusion rather than the blood pressure per se, and as long as the patient is warm and well perfused, the occurrence of hypotension is not an absolute contraindication to the use of fibrinolytic therapy, although it does indicate the need for particularly careful monitoring and perhaps for changing to an alternative (non-streptokinase) fibrinolytic agent.

Key points

Ischaemic heart disease: pathophysiology and management

- Ischaemic heart disease is caused by atheroma in coronary arteries. Primary and secondary prevention involves strict attention to dyslipidaemia, hypertension and other modifiable risk factors (smoking, obesity, diabetes).
- Stable angina is caused by narrowing of a coronary artery leading to inadequate myocardial perfusion during exercise. Symptoms may be relieved or prevented (prophylaxis) by drugs that alter the balance between myocardial oxygen supply and demand by influencing haemodynamics. Organic nitrates, nicorandil and Ca^{2+}-antagonists do this by relaxing vascular smooth muscle, whereas β-adrenoceptor antagonists slow the heart.
- In most cases, the part played by coronary spasm is uncertain. Organic nitrates and Ca^{2+}-antagonists oppose such spasm.
- Unstable angina and NSTEMI are caused by fissuring of an atheromatous plaque leading to thrombosis, in the latter case causing some degree of myocardial necrosis. They are treated with aspirin, clopidogrel and heparin (usually low-molecular-weight heparin nowadays), which improve outcome, and with intravenous glyceryl trinitrate if necessary for relief of anginal pain; most cases should undergo coronary angiography at some stage to delineate the extent/degree of disease and suitability for PCI or CABG, and this should be done early in patients who fail to settle on medical therapy.
- STEMI is caused by complete occlusion of a coronary artery by thrombus arising from an atheromatous plaque, and is more extensive and/or involves a greater thickness of the myocardium than NSTEMI. It is treated by early (primary) angioplasty where this is available; where not available, fibrinolytic drugs (with or without heparin/low-molecular-weight heparin) should be given. Important adjunctive therapy includes aspirin and clopidogrel, inhaled oxygen and opoids. Angiotensin-converting enzyme inhibition, angiotensin receptor blockade and aldosterone antagonism (with eplerenone) each improve outcome in patients with ventricular dysfunction; whether the use of all three of these treatment modalities in combination confers additional benefit over maximal dosage with one of these agents remains a matter of debate.
- After recovery from myocardial infarction, secondary prophylaxis is directed against atheroma, thrombosis (aspirin) and dysrhythmia (β-adrenoceptor antagonists, which also prevent re-infarction) and in some patients is used to improve haemodynamics (angiotensin-converting enzyme inhibitors, angiotensin receptor blockers and/or eplerenone).

Because of the risks of haemorrhage, patients are not generally treated with fibrinolytic drugs if they have recently (within the last three months) undergone surgery, are pregnant, have evidence of recent active gastro-intestinal bleeding, symptoms of active peptic ulcer disease or evidence of severe liver disease (especially if complicated by the presence of varices), have recently suffered a stroke or head injury, have severe uncontrolled hypertension, have a significant bleeding diathesis, have suffered recent substantial trauma (including vigorous chest compression during resuscitation) or require invasive monitoring (e.g. for cardiogenic shock). The position regarding diabetic or other proliferative retinopathy is controversial. If ophthalmological advice is locally and immediately available, this is no longer universally regarded as an absolute contraindication to fibrinolysis.

Case history

A 46-year-old advertising executive complains of exercise-related pain when playing his regular daily game of squash for the past three months. Ten years ago he had a gastric ulcer, which healed with ranitidine, and he had experienced intermittent indigestion subsequently, but was otherwise well. His father died of a myocardial infarct at the age of 62 years. He smokes 20 cigarettes per day and admits that he drinks half a bottle of wine a day plus 'a few gins'. Physical examination is notable only for obesity (body mass index 30 kg/m^2) and blood pressure of 152/106 mmHg. Resting ECG is normal and exercise ECG shows significant ST depression at peak exercise, with excellent exercise tolerance. Serum total cholesterol is 6.4 mmol/L, triglycerides are 3.8 mmol/L and HDL is 0.6 mmol/L. γ-Glutamyl transpeptidase is elevated, as is the mean corpuscular volume (MCV). Cardiac catheterization shows a significant narrowing of the left circumflex artery, but the other vessels are free from disease.

Question

Decide whether each of the following statements is true or false.

Immediate management could reasonably include:

(a) an ACE inhibitor;
(b) GTN spray to be taken before playing squash;
(c) no reduction in alcohol intake, as this would be dangerous;
(d) referral for angioplasty;
(e) isosorbide mononitrate;
(f) a low dose of aspirin;
(g) nicotine patches;
(h) dexfenfluramine.

Answer

(a) False
(b) False
(c) False
(d) False
(e) True
(f) True
(g) False
(h) False

Comment

This patient has single-vessel disease and should be started on medical management with advice regarding diet, smoking and reduction of alcohol consumption. He should continue to exercise, but would be wise to switch to a less extreme form of exertion. Taking a GTN spray before playing squash could have unpredictable effects on his blood pressure. A long-acting nitrate may improve his exercise tolerance, and low-dose aspirin will reduce his risk of myocardial infarction. In view of the history of ulcer and indigestion, consideration should be given to checking for *Helicobacter pylori* (with treatment if present) and/or reinstitution of prophylactic acid suppressant treatment. His dyslipidaemia is a major concern, especially the low HDL despite his high alcohol intake and regular exercise. It will almost certainly necessitate some form of drug treatment in addition to diet. His blood pressure should improve with weight reduction and reduced alcohol intake. However, if it does not and if the angina persists despite the above measures, a β-adrenoceptor antagonist may be useful despite its undesirable effect on serum lipids. If angina is no longer a problem, but hypertension persists, a long-acting α-blocker (which increases HDL) would be worth considering.

FURTHER READING

Carbajal EV, Deedwania P. Treating non-ST-segment elevation ACS. Pros and cons of current strategies. *Postgraduate Medicine* 2005; **118**: 23–32.

Opie LH, Commerford PJ, Gersh BJ. Controversies in stable coronary artery disease. *Lancet* 2006; **367**: 69–78.

Sura AC, Kelemen MD. Early management of ST-segment elevation myocardial infarction. *Cardiology Clinics* 2006; **24**: 37–51.

CHAPTER 30

ANTICOAGULANTS AND ANTIPLATELET DRUGS

INTRODUCTION

The treatment and prevention of thrombosis involves three classes of drugs, namely anticoagulants, antiplatelet drugs and fibrinolytics. Fibrinolytics are discussed in Chapter 29. The clinical pharmacology of the anticoagulants and antiplatelet drugs is described in the present chapter. Anticoagulants inhibit the coagulation cascade. Their main use is to treat and prevent venous thrombosis ('red thrombus') and its major complication, pulmonary embolism, whereas antiplatelet drugs are mainly used in the treatment of platelet-rich coronary and other arterial thrombi ('white thrombus'). Nevertheless, there are many links between platelet activation and the coagulation cascade, so it is not surprising that anticoagulants can also have beneficial effects in the prevention of coronary artery disease, or that antiplatelet drugs have some (albeit a minor) effect on venous thrombosis.

PATHOPHYSIOLOGY OF THROMBOSIS

Haemostasis is achieved by an exquisitely balanced series of interlocking control systems involving both positive feedbacks – permitting very rapid responses to the threat of haemorrhage following sharp injury – and negative feedbacks – to prevent the clotting mechanism from running out of control and causing thrombus to propagate throughout the circulation following haemostasis at a site of injury. In addition there is an endogenous fibrinolytic system that dissolves thrombus that has done its job. Not surprisingly, these systems sometimes go wrong, resulting in bleeding disorders, such as haemophilia or thrombocytopenic purpura, or in thrombosis.

Thrombosis is caused by injury to the vessel wall, stasis and activation of coagulation processes (platelets and the coagulation cascade), these three processes being referred to as Virchow's triad (Figure 30.1). Coagulation involves the sequential activation of a cascade of clotting factors which amplifies a small initial event to produce a macroscopic plug of fibrin. Each factor is present in blood as an inactive zymogen. Several of these factors (II, VII, IX and X) are glycoproteins which contain γ carboxyglutamic acid residues introduced by post-translational modification. This process requires vitamin K. After activation (indicated by the letter 'a' after the Roman numeral that designates the zymogen), several of the factors acquire proteolytic activity. Thrombin and factors IXa, Xa, XIa and XIIa are all serine proteases. Oestrogens increase

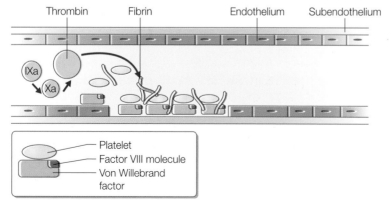

Figure 30.1: Interactions between the clotting system, platelets and the blood vessel wall.

Intrinsic pathway

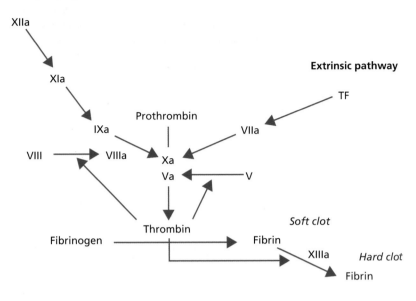

Figure 30.2 Clotting factor cascade. An 'a' indicates activation of appropriate clotting factor. TF, tissue factor. (Redrawn with permission from Dahlback B. Blood coagulation. *Lancet* 2000; **355**: 1627–32.)

the activity of the coagulation pathway and there is an increased risk of venous thrombosis associated with pregnancy, oral contraception (especially preparations containing higher doses of oestrogen), and with postmenopausal hormone replacement therapy.

Two limbs of the coagulation pathway (intrinsic and extrinsic) converge on factor X (Figure 30.2).

ANTICOAGULANTS

HEPARINS

Heparin is a sulphated acidic mucopolysaccharide that is widely distributed in the body. The unfractionated preparation is extracted from the lung or intestine of ox or pig, and is a mixture of polymers of varying molecular weights. Since the structure is variable, the dosage is expressed in terms of units of biological activity. Low-molecular-weight heparins (LMWH) are fragments or short synthetic sequences of **heparin** with much more predictable pharmacological effects, and monitoring of their anticoagulant effect is seldom needed. They have largely replaced unfractionated **heparin** in therapy.

The main indications for a **heparin** (LMWH or unfractionated) are:

- to prevent formation of thrombus (e.g. thromboprophylaxis during surgery);
- to prevent extension of thrombus (e.g. treatment of deep-vein thrombosis, following pulmonary embolism);
- prevention of thrombosis in extracorporeal circulations (e.g. haemodialysis, haemoperfusion, membrane oxygenators, artificial organs) and intravenous cannulae;
- treatment of unstable angina, non-ST elevation myocardial infarction (NSTEMI) (Chapter 29);

- following thrombolysis with some fibrinolytic drugs used for ST-elevation myocardial infarction (STEMI) (Chapter 29);
- arterial embolism;
- disseminated intravascular coagulation (DIC): as an adjunct, by coagulation specialists.

LOW-MOLECULAR-WEIGHT HEPARINS

Low-molecular-weight heparins (LMWH) preferentially inhibit factor Xa. They do not prolong the APTT, and monitoring (which requires sophisticated factor Xa assays) is not needed in routine clinical practice, because their pharmacokinetics are more predictable than those of unfractionated preparations. LMWH (e.g. **enoxaparin** and **dalteparin**) are at least as safe and effective as unfractionated products, except in patients with renal impairment. Thrombocytopenia and related thrombotic events and antiheparin antibodies are less common than with unfractionated preparations. Once-daily dosage makes them convenient, and patients can administer them at home, reducing hospitalization.

LMWH prevent deep-vein thrombosis (about one-third the incidence of venographically confirmed disease compared with unfractionated **heparin** in a meta-analysis of six trials) and pulmonary embolism (about one-half the incidence) in patients undergoing orthopaedic surgery, but with a similar incidence of major bleeds. They are at least as effective as unfractionated **heparin** in the treatment of established deep-vein thrombosis and pulmonary embolism, and for myocardial infarction. In view of their effectiveness, relative ease of use and the lack of need for blood monitoring, they have largely supplanted unfractionated **heparin** for the prophylaxis and treatment of venous thromboembolism, in unstable angina and NSTEMI and for use with some fibrinolytics in STEMI (Chapter 29).

LMWH are eliminated solely by renal excretion, unlike unfractionated **heparin**; as a consequence, unfractionated

heparin should be used rather than low-molecular-weight preparations in patients with significant renal dysfunction.

UNFRACTIONATED HEPARIN

Unfractionated **heparin** has been replaced by LMWH for most indications (see above), but remains important for patients with impaired or rapidly changing renal function. It is administered either as an intravenous infusion (to treat established disease) or by subcutaneous injection (as prophylaxis). Intramuscular injection must not be used because it causes haematomas. Intermittent bolus intravenous injections cause a higher frequency of bleeding complications than does constant intravenous infusion. For prophylaxis, a low dose is injected subcutaneously into the fatty layer of the lower abdomen 8- or 12-hourly. Coagulation times are not routinely monitored when **heparin** is used prophylactically in this way. Continuous intravenous infusion is initiated with a bolus followed by a constant infusion in saline or 5% glucose. Treatment is monitored by measuring the activated partial thromboplastin time (APTT) four to six hours after starting treatment and then every six hours, until two consecutive readings are within the target range, and thereafter at least daily. Dose adjustments are made to keep the APTT ratio (i.e. the ratio between the value for the patient and the value of a control) in the range 1.5–2.5.

Mechanism of action

The main action of **heparin** is on the coagulation cascade. It works by binding to antithrombin III, a naturally occurring inhibitor of thrombin and other serine proteases (factors IXa, Xa, XIa and XIIa), and enormously potentiating its inhibitory action. Consequently it is effective in vitro, as well as in vivo, but is ineffective in (rare) patients with inherited or acquired deficiency of antithrombin III. A lower concentration is required to inhibit factor Xa and the other factors early in the cascade than is needed to antagonize the action of thrombin, providing the rationale for low-dose **heparin** in prophylaxis. Heparin also has complex actions on platelets. As an antithrombin drug, it inhibits platelet activation by thrombin, but it can also cause platelet activation and paradoxical thrombosis by an immune mechanism (see below).

Adverse effects

Adverse effects include:

- bleeding – the chief side effect;
- thrombocytopenia and thrombosis – a modest decrease in platelet count within the first two days of treatment is common (approximately one-third of patients), but clinically unimportant. By contrast, severe thrombocytopenia (usually occurring between two days and two weeks) is rare and autoimmune in origin;
- osteoporosis and vertebral collapse – this is a rare complication described in young adult patients receiving **heparin** for longer than ten weeks (usually longer than three months);
- skin necrosis at the site of subcutaneous injection after several days treatment;
- alopecia;

- hypersensitivity reactions, including chills, fever, urticaria, bronchospasm and anaphylactoid reactions, occur rarely;
- hypoaldosteronism – **heparin** inhibits aldosterone biosynthesis. This is seldom clinically significant.

Management of heparin-associated bleeding

- Administration should be stopped and the bleeding site compressed.
- Protamine sulphate is given as a slow intravenous injection (rapid injection can cause anaphylactoid reactions). It is of no value if it is more than three hours since **heparin** was administered and is only partly effective for LMWH.

Pharmacokinetics

Heparin is not absorbed from the gastro-intestinal tract. The elimination half-life ($t_{1/2}$) of unfractionated **heparin** is in the range 0.5–2.5 hours and is dose dependent, with a longer $t_{1/2}$ at higher doses and wide inter-individual variation. The short $t_{1/2}$ probably reflects rapid uptake by the reticulo-endothelial system and there is no reliable evidence of hepatic metabolism. **Heparin** also binds non-specifically to endothelial cells, and to platelet and plasma proteins, and with high affinity to platelet factor 4, which is released during platelet activation. The mechanism underlying the dose-dependent clearance is unknown. The short $t_{1/2}$ means that a stable plasma concentration is best achieved by a constant infusion rather than by intermittent bolus administration. Neither unfractionated **heparin** nor LMWH cross the placental barrier and **heparin** is used in pregnancy in preference to the coumadins because of the teratogenic effects of **warfarin** and other oral anticoagulants. There is a paucity of evidence on entry of LMWH to milk and breast-feeding is currently contraindicated.

FONDAPARINUX

Fondaparinux is a synthetic pentasaccharide that selectively binds and inhibits factor Xa. It is more effective than low-molecular-weight **heparin** in preventing venous thromboembolism in patients undergoing orthopaedic surgery, and is as effective as **heparin** or LMWH in patients with established deep vein thrombosis or pulmonary embolism. In the setting of acute coronary syndrome, **fondaparinux** may be as effective in reducing ischaemic events, and at the same time safer in terms of bleeding complications, as compared with LMWH (the OASIS-5 trial). It is administered by subcutaneous injection once a day, at a dose that depends on body weight. Its precise place as compared with LMWH outside of the orthopaedic setting, is currently debated.

HIRUDIN

Hirudin is the anticoagulant of the leech and can now be synthesized in bulk by recombinant DNA technology. It is a direct inhibitor of thrombin and is more specific than **heparin**. Unlike **heparin**, it inhibits clot-associated thrombin and is not dependent on antithrombin III. Early human studies showed that the pharmacodynamic response is closely related to plasma concentration and its pharmacokinetics are more predictable than those of **heparin**. Other **hirudin** analogues have also been synthesized. The place of **hirudin** and its analogues in therapeutics is currently being established in clinical trials.

ORAL ANTICOAGULANTS

Warfarin, a racemic mixture of R and S stereoisomers, is the main oral anticoagulant. **Phenindione** is an alternative, but has a number of severe and distinct adverse effects (see below), so it is seldom used except in rare cases of idiosyncratic sensitivity to **warfarin**.

Use

The main indications for oral anticoagulation are:

- deep vein thrombosis and pulmonary embolism;
- atrial fibrillation (see Chapter 32);
- mitral stenosis;
- prosthetic valve replacements.

Treatment of deep-vein thrombosis and pulmonary embolus is started with a **heparin** to obtain an immediate effect. This is usually continued for up to seven days to allow stabilization of the **warfarin** dose. The effect of **warfarin** is monitored by measuring the international normalized ratio (INR). (The INR is the prothrombin time corrected for an international standard for thromboplastin reagents. Prothrombin time varies from laboratory to laboratory, but the INR in Oxford should be the same as that in, say, Boston, facilitating dose adjustment in these days of international travel.) Before starting treatment, a baseline value of INR is determined. Provided that the baseline INR is normal, anticoagulation is started by administering two consecutive doses 24 hours apart at the same time of day (most conveniently in the evening). If the baseline INR is prolonged or the patient has risk factors for bleeding (e.g. old age or debility, liver disease, heart failure, or recent major surgery), treatment is started with a lower dose. The INR is measured daily, and on the morning of day 3 about 50% of patients will be within the therapeutic range and the **heparin** can be discontinued.

Once the situation is stable, the INR is checked weekly for the first six weeks and then monthly or two-monthly if control is good. The patient is warned to report immediately if there is evidence of bleeding, to avoid contact sports or other situations that put them at increased risk of trauma, to avoid alcohol (or at least to restrict intake to a moderate and unvarying amount), to avoid over-the-counter drugs (other than paracetamol) and to check that any prescription drug is not expected to alter their anticoagulant requirement. Women of childbearing age should be warned of the risk of teratogenesis and given advice on contraception. Appropriate target ranges for different indications reflect the relative risks of thrombosis/haemorrhage in various clinical situations. Table 30.1 lists the suggested ranges of INR that are acceptable for various indications.

Table 30.1: Suggested acceptable INR ranges for various indications

Clinical state	Target INR range
Prophylaxis of DVT, including surgery on high-risk patients	2.0–2.5
Treatment of DVT/PE/systemic embolism/ mitral stenosis with embolism	2.0–3.0
Recurrent DVT/PE while on warfarin; mechanical prosthetic heart valve	3.0–4.5

Mechanism of action

Oral anticoagulants interfere with hepatic synthesis of the vitamin K-dependent coagulation factors II, VII, IX and X. Preformed factors are present in blood so, unlike **heparin**, oral anticoagulants are not effective in vitro and are only active when given in vivo. Functional forms of factors II, VII, IX and X contain residues of γ-carboxyglutamic acid. This is formed by carboxylation of a glutamate residue in the peptide chain of the precursor. This is accomplished by cycling of vitamin K between epoxide, quinone and hydroquinone forms. This cycle is interrupted by **warfarin**, which is structurally closely related to vitamin K, and inhibits vitamin K epoxide reductase.

Adverse effects

1. *Haemorrhage* If severe, vitamin K is administered intravenously, but its effect is delayed and it renders the patient resistant to re-warfarinization. Life-threatening bleeding requires administration of fresh frozen plasma, or specific coagulation factor concentrates, with advice from a haematologist.
2. Other adverse actions of **warfarin** include:
   - *teratogenesis*;
   - *rashes*;
   - *thrombosis* is a rare but severe paradoxical effect of **warfarin** and can result in extensive tissue necrosis. Vitamin K is involved in the biosynthesis of anticoagulant proteins C and S. Protein C has a short elimination half-life, and when **warfarin** treatment is started, its plasma concentration declines more rapidly than that of the vitamin K-dependent coagulation factors, so the resulting imbalance can temporarily favour thrombosis.
3. Adverse effects of **phenindione**:
   - interference with iodine uptake by the thyroid;
   - renal tubular damage;
   - hepatitis;
   - agranulocytosis;
   - dermatitis;
   - secretion into breast milk.

Pharmacokinetics

Following oral administration, absorption is almost complete and maximum plasma concentrations are reached within two to eight hours. Approximately 97% is bound to plasma albumin. **Warfarin** does gain access to the fetus, but does not appear in breast milk in clinically relevant amounts. There is substantial variation between individuals in **warfarin** $t_{1/2}$. The R and S enantiomers are metabolized differently in the liver. The (active) S enantiomer is metabolized to 7-hydroxywarfarin by a cytochrome P450-dependent mixed function oxidase, while the less active R enantiomer is metabolized by soluble enzymes to warfarin alcohols. Hepatic metabolism is followed by conjugation and excretion into the gut in the bile. Deconjugation and reabsorption then occur, completing the enterohepatic cycle.

Knowledge of the plasma concentration of **warfarin** is not useful in routine clinical practice because the pharmacodynamic response (INR) can be measured accurately, but it is valuable in the investigation of patients with unusual resistance to **warfarin**, in whom it helps to distinguish poor compliance, abnormal pharmacokinetics and abnormal sensitivity. Since **warfarin** acts by inhibiting synthesis of active vitamin K-dependent clotting factors, the onset of anticoagulation following dosing depends on the catabolism of preformed factors. Consequently, the delay between dosing and effect cannot be shortened by giving a loading dose.

Drug interactions

Potentially important pharmacodynamic interactions with **warfarin** include those with antiplatelet drugs. **Aspirin** not only influences haemostasis by its effect on platelet function, but also increases the likelihood of peptic ulceration, displaces **warfarin** from plasma albumin, and in high doses decreases prothrombin synthesis. Despite these potential problems, recent clinical experience suggests that with close monitoring the increased risk of bleeding when low doses of **aspirin** are taken regularly with **warfarin** may be more than offset by clinical benefits to patients at high risk of thromboembolism following cardiac valve replacement. Broad-spectrum antibiotics potentiate **warfarin** by suppressing the synthesis of vitamin K_1 by gut flora.

Several pharmacokinetic interactions with **warfarin** are of clinical importance. Several non-steroidal anti-inflammatory drugs (NSAIDs) and **dextropropoxyphene** inhibit **warfarin** metabolism. The gastrotoxic and platelet-inhibitory actions of the NSAIDs further increase the risk of serious haemorrhage. **Cimetidine** (but not **ranitidine**) and **amiodarone** also potently inhibit **warfarin** metabolism and potentiate its effect, as do other inhibitors of hepatic cytochrome P450, such as **erythromycin**, **ciprofloxacin** and **omeprazole** (Chapter 5). Drugs that induce hepatic microsomal enzymes, including **rifampicin**, **carbamazepine** and **phenobarbital**, increase **warfarin** metabolism and increase the dose required to produce a therapeutic effect; furthermore, if the dose is not reduced when such concurrent therapy is discontinued, catastrophic over-anticoagulation and haemorrhage may ensue.

ANTIPLATELET DRUGS

ASPIRIN

Aspirin is the main antiplatelet drug in clinical use. It works by inhibiting the synthesis of thromboxane A_2 (TXA$_2$), and its use

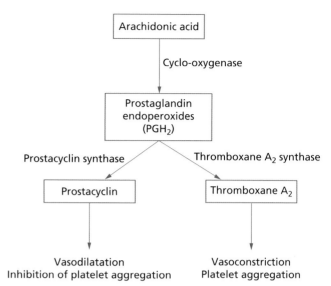

Figure 30.3: Formation of prostacyclin and thromboxane A$_2$ in vivo. These two products of arachidonic acid metabolism exert competing and opposite physiological effects.

in the treatment and prevention of ischaemic heart disease is described in Chapter 29. Numerous clinical trials have demonstrated its efficacy. Efficacy is not directly related to dose and low doses cause less adverse effects. TXA$_2$ is synthesized by activated platelets and acts on receptors on platelets (causing further platelet activation) and on vascular smooth muscle (causing vasoconstriction). Figure 30.3 shows the pathway of its biosynthesis from arachidonic acid. **Aspirin** inhibits thromboxane synthesis – it acetylates a serine residue in the active site of constitutive (type I) cyclo-oxygenase (COX-1) in platelets, irreversibly blocking this enzyme. The most common side effect is gastric intolerance and the most common severe adverse reaction is upper gastro-intestinal bleeding. Both effects stem from inhibition of COX-1 in the stomach, resulting in decreased production of the gastroprotective PGE$_2$.

EPOPROSTENOL (PROSTACYCLIN)

Epoprostenol is the approved drug name for synthetic prostacyclin, the principal endogenous prostaglandin of large artery endothelium. It acts on specific receptors on the plasma membranes of platelets and vascular smooth muscle. These are coupled by G-proteins to adenylyl cyclase. Activation of this enzyme increases the biosynthesis of cyclic adenosine monophosphate (cAMP), which inhibits platelet aggregation and relaxes vascular smooth muscle. **Epoprostenol** relaxes pulmonary as well as systemic vasculature, and this underpins its use in patients with primary pulmonary hypertension. It (or a related synthetic prostanoid, **iloprost**) is administered chronically to such patients while awaiting heart–lung transplantation. **Epoprostenol** inhibits platelet activation during haemodialysis. It can be used with **heparin**, but is also effective as the sole anticoagulant in this setting, and is used for haemodialysis in patients in whom **heparin** is contraindicated. It has also been used in other types of extracorporeal circuit (e.g. during cardiopulmonary bypass). **Epoprostenol** has been used with apparent benefit in acute retinal vessel thrombosis and in patients with critical limb ischaemia and with platelet consumption due to multiple organ failure, especially those with meningococcal sepsis. Rigorous proof of efficacy is difficult to provide in such settings. **Epoprostenol** is infused intravenously (or, in the case of haemodialysis, into the arterial limb supplying the dialyzer). It is administered with frequent monitoring of blood pressure and heart rate during the period of dose titration. A modest reduction in diastolic pressure with an increase in systolic pressure (i.e. increased pulse pressure) and reflex tachycardia is the expected and desired haemodynamic effect. If bradycardia and hypotension occur, the infusion should be temporarily discontinued. The short half-life of **epoprostenol** (approximately three minutes) allows for its rapid titration according to haemodynamic response. Bleeding complications are unusual.

DIPYRIDAMOLE
Use

Dipyridamole was introduced as a vasodilator, but provokes rather than prevents angina (via a steal mechanism). It is used acutely as in stress tests for ischaemic heart disease (e.g. combined with nuclear medicine myocardial perfusion scanning). It is also used chronically, combined with **aspirin**, for its antiplatelet effect in patients with cerebrovascular disease on the basis of the European Stroke Prevention Study 2.

Mechanism of action

Dipyridamole inhibits phosphodiesterase which leads to reduced breakdown of cAMP, and inhibits adenosine uptake with consequent enhancement of the actions of this mediator on platelets and vascular smooth muscle.

Drug interactions

Dipyridamole increases the potency and duration of action of adenosine. This may be clinically important in patients receiving **dipyridamole** in whom adenosine is considered for treatment of dysrhythmia.

CLOPIDOGREL
Use

Clopidogrel is combined with **aspirin** to treat patients with acute coronary syndromes/myocardial infarction and following percutaneous coronary intervention with stent placement (Chapter 29). It is also used instead of **aspirin** in patients with a contraindication to **aspirin** and may be marginally superior to **aspirin** for primary prevention (CAPRIE study).

Mechanism of action

Clopidogrel is an inactive prodrug that is converted in the liver to an active metabolite that binds to, and irreversibly inhibits, platelet ADP receptors. Like **aspirin**, the antiplatelet effect of **clopidogrel** is prolonged and lasts for the life of the platelet.

Adverse effects

Adverse effects include:

- haemorrhage (including intracranial, especially in patients with uncontrolled hypertension);
- nausea, vomiting, constipation or diarrhoea;
- headache;
- dizziness, vertigo;
- rash, pruritus.

Contraindications

Contraindications include the following:

- active bleeding;
- breast-feeding;
- use with caution in liver impairment, renal impairment and pregnancy.

INHIBITORS OF GLYCOPROTEIN IIb/IIIa

Abciximab, a monoclonal antibody to glycoprotein IIb/IIIa, when used as an adjunct to **heparin** and **aspirin** reduces occlusion following angioplasty, but can cause bleeding. Its use is currently restricted to patients undergoing angioplasty in whom there is a high risk of acute coronary thrombosis. Hypersensitivity reactions can occur. Alternative small molecule inhibitors of glycoprotein IIb/IIIa are **eptifibatide** and **tirofiban**; they are used under cardiology supervision in patients with early myocardial infarction.

ANTICOAGULANTS IN PREGNANCY AND PUERPERIUM

There is an increased risk of thromboembolism in pregnancy and women at risk (e.g. those with prosthetic heart valves) must continue to be anticoagulated. However, **warfarin** crosses the placenta and when taken throughout pregnancy will result in complications in about one-third of cases (16% of fetuses will be spontaneously aborted or stillborn, 10% will have post-partum complications (usually due to bleeding) and 7% will suffer teratogenic effects).

Heparin (both unfractionated and LMWH) does not cross the placenta and may be self-administered subcutaneously. Long-term **heparin** may cause osteoporosis and there is an increased risk of retroplacental bleeding. One approach to the management of pregnancy in women on anticoagulants is to change to subcutaneous **low-molecular-weight heparin** from the time of the first missed period and remain on this until term, maintaining a high intake of elemental calcium, as well as adequate but not excessive intake of vitamin D. Around the time of delivery, it may be withheld and restarted immediately post-partum, together with **warfarin** and continued until the full effect of **warfarin** is re-established. **Warfarin** does not enter breast milk to a significant extent and mothers may nurse their babies while anticoagulated on **warfarin** (in contrast to those on **phenindione**).

Thrombosis

- Thrombosis occurs when excessive clotting occurs in blood vessels, thereby occluding them, and thrombi consist of platelets and fibrin.
- In general, arterial thrombosis is prevented by antiplatelet therapy and can be treated by fibrinolytic therapy with or without concomitant anticoagulation.
- The principal antiplatelet agents in clinical use are aspirin and clopidogrel. Aspirin inhibits platelet thromboxane A_2 formation (by inhibition of cyclo-oxygenase), clopidogrel (through hepatic formation of its active metabolite) inhibits platelet ADP receptors.
- The main adverse effects of aspirin are on the gastro-intestinal tract, the most severe of these being gastro-intestinal bleeding. These effects are dose related and can be countered by suppression of acid secretion by the stomach if necessary.
- Venous and cardiac thromboembolic disease (e.g. in the context of atrial fibrillation) are best prevented by anticoagulant therapy.
- The principal anticoagulants used clinically are heparin or, more commonly nowadays low-molecular-weight heparin, and warfarin. Heparin and low-molecular-weight heparin are given parenterally, warfarin is administered orally.
- Low-molecular-weight heparins are effective and convenient. They do not require routine haematological monitoring (unlike heparin, which requires frequent monitoring of the APTT), can be given subcutaneously once a day and patients can be taught to administer them at home.
- Warfarin and other coumadins work by interfering with the action of vitamin K on factors II, VII, IX and X. Monitoring is by measurement of the international normalized ratio (INR). There is very wide variation in individual dosage requirements.
- Drug interactions with warfarin are common and important, and include interactions with anticonvulsants, antibiotics, sulphonylureas and non-steroidal anti-inflammatory drugs.

FURTHER READING

Hirsh J, O'Donnell M, Weitz JI. New anticoagulants. *Blood* 2005; **105**: 453–63.

Patrono C, Coller B, FitzGerald GA, Hirsh J, Roth G. Platelet-active drugs: The relationships among dose, effectiveness, and side effects. *Chest* 2004; **126**: 234S-64S.

Pengo V. New trends in anticoagulant treatments. *Lupus* 2005; **14**: 789–93.

Ringleb PA. Thrombolytics, anticoagulants, and antiplatelet agents. *Stroke* 2006; **37**: 312–13.

Steinhubl SR, Moliterno DJ. The role of the platelet in the pathogenesis of atherothrombosis. *American Journal of Cardiovascular Drugs* 2005; **5**: 399–408.

HEART FAILURE

INTRODUCTION

Heart failure occurs when the heart fails to deliver adequate amounts of oxygenated blood to the tissues during exercise or, in severe cases, at rest. Such failure of the pump function may be chronic, in which case symptoms of fatigue, ankle swelling, effort dyspnoea and orthopnoea predominate, or it may be acute, with sudden onset of shortness of breath due to pulmonary oedema (Figure 31.1). Both acute and chronic heart failure severely reduce life expectancy (Figure 31.2). The most severe form of heart failure (low cardiac output circulatory failure, 'cardiogenic shock') is managed with pressor drugs (e.g. **adrenaline**) or with mechanical support (e.g. intra-aortic balloon pump), in an intensive care unit. Such treatment is highly individualized (and specialized) and mortality even with the best treatment is very high. In this chapter, we cover the more common syndrome of chronic congestive heart failure and discuss the treatment of acute pulmonary oedema, since this is a common emergency.

PATHOPHYSIOLOGY AND IMPLICATIONS FOR TREATMENT

Heart failure is an end result of many diseases (not only of the myocardium, pericardium and valves, but also of extracardiac disorders, including systemic or pulmonary hypertension, fluid overload, vascular shunts, anaemia and thyrotoxicosis). The most common of these are ischaemic heart disease (Chapter 29), idiopathic congestive cardiomyopathy and cor pulmonale (Chapter 33). Specific measures are needed in each case and these are covered in other chapters. Here,

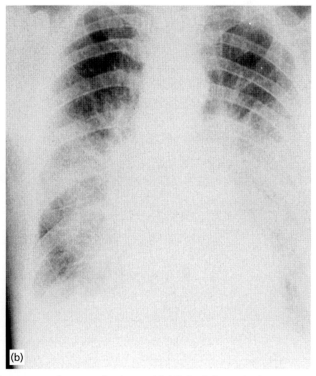

(a)

(b)

Figure 31.1: Peripheral oedema with evidence of pitting (left) and pulmonary oedema on chest x-ray (right), both important consequences of uncontrolled and inadequately treated heart failure.

we focus on aspects common to heart failure irrespective of aetiology.

Heart failure triggers 'counter-regulatory' responses (Figure 31.3), which make the situation worse, not better. Our ancestors encountered low cardiac output during haemorrhage rather than as a result of heart failure. Mechanisms to conserve blood volume and maintain blood pressure would have provided selective advantage. However, reflex and endocrine changes that are protective in the setting of haemorrhage (volume depletion 'shock') negatively impact patients with low cardiac output due to pump failure.

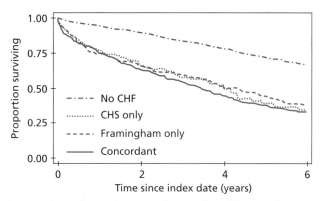

Figure 31.2: Kaplan–Meier survival curves for subjects in the Cardiovascular Health Study (CHS), United States, 1989–2000. Subjects either had no congestive heart failure (CHF) or had CHF diagnosed by different criteria (Framingham only, CHS only or both, i.e. concordant). (Redrawn with permission from Schellenbaum GD et al. *American Journal of Epidemiology* 2004; **160**: 628–35.)

Treatment of heart failure is aimed at reversing these counter-regulatory changes, which include:

- activation of the renin–angiotensin–aldosterone system;
- activation of the sympathetic nervous system;
- release of vasopressin (an antidiuretic hormone, see Chapter 42).

Cardiac performance is determined by preload, afterload, myocardial contractility and heart rate. Treatment targets these aspects, often by blocking one or other of the counter-regulatory mechanisms.

PRELOAD

Cardiac preload, the cardiac filling pressure, is determined by blood volume – increased by salt and water retention – and capacitance vessel tone, increased by sympathetic nervous system activation. Drugs can reduce blood volume (diuretics) and reduce capacitance vessel tone (venodilators).

AFTERLOAD

Afterload is determined by the systemic vascular resistance and by aortic stiffness. Drugs that relax arterial smooth muscle reduce cardiac afterload.

MYOCARDIAL CONTRACTILITY

Positive inotropes (i.e. drugs that increase the force of contraction of the heart) can improve cardiac performance temporarily by increasing contractility, but at the expense of increased oxygen consumption and risk of dysrhythmia.

HEART RATE

Cardiac function deteriorates as heart rate increases beyond an optimum, due to insufficient time for filling during diastole. Heart rate can usefully be slowed by negative chronotropes (i.e. drugs that slow the heart).

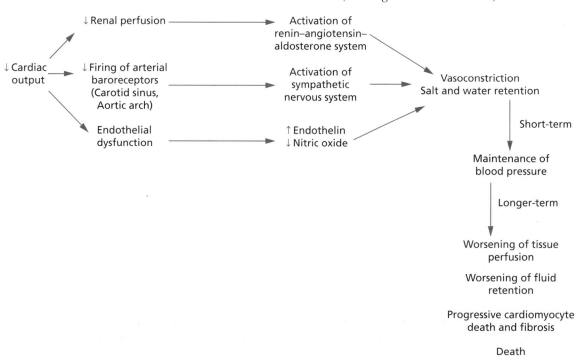

Figure 31.3: Compensatory counter-regulatory responses in heart failure and their consequences.

The drugs that are most effective in prolonging survival in chronic heart failure work indirectly, by reducing preload, afterload or heart rate, rather than directly by increasing the force of contraction.

THERAPEUTIC OBJECTIVES AND GENERAL MEASURES FOR CHRONIC HEART FAILURE

Therapeutic objectives in treating heart failure are

- to improve symptoms and
- to prolong survival.

  General principles of treating heart failure:

- restrict dietary salt;
- if there is hyponatraemia, restrict fluid;
- review prescribed drugs and if possible withdraw drugs that aggravate cardiac failure:
  - some negative inotropes (e.g. **verapamil**)
  - cardiac toxins (e.g. **daunorubicin, ethanol, imatinib, gefitinib, trastuzumab**)
  - drugs that cause salt retention (e.g. NSAID).
- consider anticoagulation on an individual basis.

DRUGS FOR HEART FAILURE

DIURETICS

For more information, see Chapter 28 for use of diuretics in hypertension and Chapter 36, for mechanisms, adverse effects and pharmacokinetics.

Use in heart failure

Chronic heart failure: a diuretic is used to control symptomatic oedema and dyspnoea in patients with heart failure. A thiazide (see Chapters 28 and 36) may be adequate in very mild cases, but a loop diuretic (e.g. **furosemide**) is usually needed. Unlike several of the drugs described below, there has been no randomized controlled trial investigating the influence of loop diuretics on survival in heart failure, but the other treatments were added to a loop diuretic and this is usually the starting point of drug treatment. **Spironolactone** improves survival in patients with cardiac failure and counters diuretic-induced hypokalaemia. Diuretic-induced hypokalaemia increases the toxicity of **digoxin**. Conversely, **spironolactone** and other K$^+$-retaining diuretics (e.g. **amiloride, triamterene**) can cause severe hyperkalaemia, especially if given with ACEI or sartans (see below) to patients with renal impairment. It is therefore important to monitor plasma K$^+$ during treatment with all diuretic therapy.

Acute heart failure: acute pulmonary oedema is treated by sitting the patient upright, administering oxygen (FiO$_2$, 28–40%) and intravenous **furosemide** which is often effective within a matter of minutes. Intravenous **morphine** (Chapter 25) is also useful. A slow intravenous infusion of **furosemide** by syringe pump may be useful in resistant cases. Once the acute situation has resolved the situation is re-assessed and drugs used for chronic heart failure (see below), including oral diuretics, are usually indicated.

ANGIOTENSIN-CONVERTING ENZYME INHIBITORS

For the mechanism of action and other aspects of angiotensin-converting enzyme inhibitors, see Chapter 28.

Use in heart failure

The first approach shown to reduce mortality in heart failure was combined **hydralazine** and **nitrate** therapy (see below). Soon after, an angiotensin-converting enzyme inhibitor (ACEI) (**captopril**) was shown to do better. Other ACEI were also shown to improve survival and ACEI treatment for heart failure was rapidly adopted. When symptoms are mild, diuretics can be temporarily discontinued a day or two before starting an ACEI, reducing the likelihood of first-dose hypotension. In these circumstances, treatment with an ACE inhibitor can be started as an out-patient, as for hypertension (see Chapter 28). A small starting dose is used and the first dose is taken last thing before retiring at night, with advice to sit on the side of the bed before standing if the patient needs to get up in the night. The dose is gradually increased to one that improves symptoms (and survival) with careful monitoring of blood pressure. Serum potassium and creatinine are checked after one to two weeks. Hypotension is more of a problem when starting treatment in heart failure patients than when treating hypertension, especially with short-acting drugs (e.g. **captopril**). Not only is the blood pressure lower to start with, but concentrations of circulating renin are high and increased further by diuretics. ACEI cause 'first-dose' hypotension most severely in patients with the greatest activation of the renin–angiotensin system. These are consequently those most likely to benefit from an ACEI in the long term. Long-acting drugs (e.g. **ramipril, trandolapril**) cause less first-dose hypotension and can be given once daily. ACEI are usually well tolerated during chronic treatment, although dry cough is common and occasionally unacceptable (see Chapter 28 for other adverse effects). Important drug–drug interactions can occur with NSAIDs (Chapter 26), which may cause renal failure and severe hyperkalaemia, especially in heart failure patients treated with ACEI.

ANGIOTENSIC RECEPTOR ANTAGONISTS, SARTANS

See Chapter 28 for the mechanism of action.

Use in heart failure

As in hypertension, the pharmacodynamics of sartans are similar to those of ACEI apart from a lower incidence of some adverse effects, including, particularly, dry cough. Several of these drugs (e.g. **candesartan, valsartan**) have been shown to prolong life in randomized controlled trials, the magnitude of the effect being similar to ACEI. It is possible that they have some additive effect when combined with ACEI, but this is hard to prove at doses that are not supramaximal. Because of the greater experience with ACEI and the lower cost, many physicians prefer to use an ACEI, unless this is not tolerated.

Precautions in terms of first-dose hypotension and monitoring creatinine and electrolytes are similar to those for ACEI.

β-ADRENOCEPTOR ANTAGONISTS

For more information, see Chapter 28 for use in hypertension, Chapter 29 for use in ischaemic heart disease and Chapter 32 for use as antidysrhythmic drugs.

Classification of β-adrenoceptor antagonists

Adrenoceptors are classified as α or β, with a further subdivision of the latter into β_1, mainly in the heart, β_2 which are present in, for example, bronchioles and β_3, which mediate metabolic effects in brown fat.

Cardioselective beta-blockers (e.g. **atenolol**, **metoprolol**) inhibit β_1-receptors relatively selectively, but are nonetheless hazardous for patients with asthma.

Some beta-blockers (e.g. **oxprenolol**) are partial agonists and possess intrinsic sympathomimetic activity. This is seldom important in practice.

Vasodilating beta-blockers include drugs (e.g. **labetolol**, **carvedilol**) with additional α-blocking activity. **Celiprolol** has additional agonist activity at β_2-receptors. **Nebivolol** releases endothelium-derived nitric oxide, as well as being a highly selective β_1-adrenoceptor blocker.

Use in heart failure

Beta-blockers are negative inotropes and so intuitively would be expected to worsen heart failure. There is, however, a rationale for their use in terms of antagonizing counter-regulatory sympathetic activation and several randomized controlled trials have demonstrated improved survival when a β-adrenoceptor antagonist is added to other drugs, including an ACEI. Several β-adrenoceptor antagonists have been shown to be of benefit including **bisoprolol**, **metoprolol** and **carvedilol**. **Bisoprolol** and **metoprolol** are cardioselective β_1 antagonists, whereas **carvedilol** is non-selective and has additional α antagonist properties. **Carvedilol** may be more effective than **bisoprolol** in heart failure, but is less well tolerated because of postural hypotension. Treatment is started with a low dose when the patient is stable and the patient reviewed regularly at short intervals (e.g. every two weeks or more frequently if needed), often by a heart failure nurse, with dose titration as tolerated.

Adverse effects

- *Intolerance* Fatigue and cold extremities are common and dose related. Erectile dysfunction occurs, but is less common than with thiazide diuretics. Central nervous system (CNS) effects (e.g. vivid dreams) can occur.
- *Airways obstruction* β-adrenoceptor antagonists predispose to severe airways obstruction in patients with pre-existing obstructive airways disease, especially asthma.
- *Peripheral vascular disease and vasospasm* β-adrenoceptor antagonists worsen claudication in patients with symptomatic atheromatous peripheral vascular disease and worsen Raynaud's phenomenon.

- *Hypoglycaemia* β-adrenoceptor antagonists mask symptoms of hypoglycaemia, and slow the rate of recovery from it, because adrenaline stimulates gluconeogenesis via β_2-adrenoceptors.
- *Heart block*.

ALDOSTERONE ANTAGONISTS

For more information, see Chapter 36.

Spironolactone (or the newer expensive agent, **eplerenone**), when added to conventional therapy with loop diuretic, ACEI and β-adrenoceptor antagonist, further improves survival. Concerns regarding hyperkalaemia in such patients may have been overstated, at least provided patients with appreciably impaired renal function are excluded from such treatment.

COMBINED HYDRALAZINE WITH ORGANIC NITRATE THERAPY

There is renewed interest in combined therapy with **hydralazine** (Chapter 28) and a long-acting **nitrate** (Chapter 29). The pharmacologic basis for investigating this was that **hydralazine** reduced afterload and the **nitrate** reduced pre-load. As mentioned above, this improved survival in one randomized controlled trial, but performed less well overall in a direct comparison with an ACEI. However, a subgroup analysis suggested that African-American patients did better with the **hydralazine/nitrate** combination, whereas Caucasians did better with ACEI. This observation led to a further study in African-Americans which confirmed the efficacy of **hydralazine–nitrate** treatment. It is now often used for patients of African origin. Hopefully, genetic testing will further improve the targeting of appropriate therapy ('personalized medicine') in future.

DIGOXIN

For more information on the use of **digoxin**, refer to Chapter 32.

William Withering described an extract of foxglove as a 'cure' for 'dropsy' (congestive cardiac failure) in 1785. **Digoxin** remains useful for symptoms.

Use in heart failure

Rapid atrial fibrillation can worsen heart failure and **digoxin** can be used to control the ventricular response, which it does by stimulating vagal efferents to the heart (Chapter 32). Its positive inotropic action is an added benefit. Heart failure patients in sinus rhythm who remain symptomatic despite optimal treatment with life-prolonging medications also benefit. Addition of **digoxin** to diuretics and ACEI reduces hospitalization and improves symptoms, without prolonging life. It is usually given orally, but can be given i.v. if a rapid effect is required. Since the half-life is approximately 30–48 hours, repeated administration of a once-daily maintenance dose results in a plateau concentration in about five to ten days. The dose may be adjusted based on plasma concentration determinations once steady state has been reached (Chapter 8). Such determinations are also useful if toxicity is suspected (e.g. because of nausea, bradycardia or ECG changes). In urgent situations, a therapeutic plasma concentration can be obtained more rapidly by administering a loading dose (Chapter 3).

Mechanism of action

Digoxin inhibits Na^+/K^+ adenosine triphosphatase (Na^+/K^+ ATPase). This causes accumulation of intracellular Na^+ and increased intracellular $[Ca^{2+}]$ concentrations via reduced Na^+/Ca^{2+} exchange. The rise in availability of intracellular Ca^{2+} accounts for the positive inotropic effect of **digoxin**. Excessive inhibition of Na^+/K^+ ATPase causes numerous non-cardiac as well as cardiac (dysrhythmogenic) toxic effects. Ventricular slowing results from increased vagal activity on the AV node. Slowing of ventricular rate improves cardiac output in patients with atrial fibrillation by improving ventricular filling during diastole. Clinical progress is assessed by measuring heart rate (at the apex): apical rates of 70–80 per minute can be achieved at rest. Unfortunately, since vagal activity is suppressed during exercise (when heart rate is controlled by sympathetic activation), control of rate during exercise is not usually achievable.

Pharmacokinetics

Approximately 80% is excreted unchanged in the urine in patients with normal renal function with a half-life of 30–48 hours. It is eliminated mainly by glomerular filtration, although small amounts are secreted and reabsorbed. A small amount (5–10%) undergoes metabolism to inactive products or excretion via the bile and elimination in faeces. The proportion eliminated by these non-renal clearance mechanisms increases in patients with renal impairment, being 100% in anephric patients, in whom the half-life is approximately 4.5 days.

Blood for **digoxin** concentration determination should be sampled more than six hours after an oral dose or immediately before the next dose is due (trough level) to allow its tissue distribution to be complete. The usual therapeutic range is 1–2 ng/mL, although toxicity can occur at concentrations of less than 1.5 ng/mL in some individuals.

Drug interactions

Digoxin has a steep dose–response curve and a narrow therapeutic range, and clinically important interactions are common (see Chapters 13 and 32). Pharmacokinetic interactions with **digoxin** include combined pharmacokinetic effects involving displacement from tissue-binding sites and reduced renal elimination (e.g. **digoxin** toxicity due to concurrent treatment with **amiodarone** or **quinidine**).

Pharmacodynamic interactions are also important. In particular, drugs that cause hypokalaemia (e.g. diuretics, β-agonists, glucocorticoids) predispose to **digoxin** toxicity by increasing its binding to (and effect on) Na^+/K^+ ATPase.

OTHER POSITIVE INOTROPES

Positive inotropes for intravenous infusion (e.g. **adrenaline**) have a place in treating acute shock, but not for chronic heart failure. Orally active positive inotropes other than **digoxin** include phosphodiesterase inhibitors, e.g. **milrinone**. These increase cardiac output and may bring some symptomatic benefit, but they worsen survival.

Key points

Heart failure: pathophysiology and principles of therapeutics

- Heart failure has diverse aetiologies; ischaemic and idiopathic cardiomyopathy are especially important.
- Neurohumoral activation (e.g. of sympathetic and renin–angiotensin systems) may have adverse consequences.
- Treatment is sometimes specific (e.g. valve replacement), but is also directed generally at:
  - reducing preload (diuretics, nitrates, ACE inhibitors and sartans);
  - reducing afterload (ACE inhibitors and hydralazine);
  - increasing contractility (digoxin);
  - reducing heart rate (rapid rates do not permit optimal filling; rapid atrial fibrillation is slowed by digoxin).

Treatment of chronic heart failure

- Dietary salt should be restricted.
- Drugs that improve survival usually reduce preload, afterload or heart rate by interrupting counter-regulatory hormonal mechanisms. They comprise:
  - diuretics (e.g. furosemide);
  - ACEI (e.g. captopril acutely, then ramipril, trolandopril);
  - sartans (e.g. candesartan);
  - β-adrenoceptor antagonists (e.g. bisoprolol, carvedilol);
  - aldosterone antagonists (e.g. spironolactone);
  - hydralazine plus an organic nitrate in African-American patients.
- Digoxin does not influence survival, but can improve symptoms.
- Other positive inotropes (e.g. phosphodiesterase inhibitors, milrinone) worsen survival.

Case history

A 62-year-old physician has developed symptoms of chronic congestive cardiac failure in the setting of treated essential hypertension. He had had an angioplasty to an isolated atheromatous lesion in the left anterior descending coronary artery two years previously, since when he had not had angina. He also has a past history of gout. He is taking bendroflumethiazide for his hypertension and takes meclofenamate regularly to prevent recurrences of his gout. He disregarded his cardiologist's advice to take aspirin because he was already taking another cyclo-oxygenase inhibitor (in the form of the meclofenamate). On examination, he has a regular pulse of 88 beats/minute, blood pressure of 160/98 mmHg, a 4–5 cm raised jugular venous pressure, mild pretibial oedema and cardiomegaly. Routine biochemistry tests are unremarkable except for a serum urate level of 0.76 mmol/L, a total cholesterol concentration of 6.5 mmol/L, a triglyceride concentration of 5.2 mmol/L and γ-glutamyltranspeptidase twice the upper limit of normal. An echocardiogram shows a diffusely poorly contracting myocardium.
Question
Decide whether each of the following would be appropriate as immediate measures.

(a) Digitalization
(b) Intravenous furosemide

(c) A detailed personal/social history
(d) Substitution of allopurinol for the meclofenamate
(e) Hold the bendroflumethiazide temporarily and start an ACE inhibitor
(f) Start bezafibrate.

Answer

(a) False
(b) False
(c) True
(d) False
(e) True
(f) False.

Comment
The aetiology of the heart failure in this case is uncertain. Although ischaemia and hypertension may be playing a part, the diffusely poorly contracting myocardium suggests the possibility of diffuse cardiomyopathy, and the raised γ-glutamyltranspeptidase and triglyceride levels point to the possibility of alcohol excess. If this is the case, and if it is corrected, this could improve the blood pressure, dyslipidaemia and gout, as well as cardiac function. In the long term, allopurinol should be substituted for the NSAID, but if done immediately this is likely to precipitate an acute attack. Aspirin should be taken (for its antiplatelet effect, which may not be shared by all other NSAIDs). Treatment with a fibrate would be useful for this pattern of dyslipidaemia, but only after establishing that it was not alcohol-induced.

FURTHER READING

Brater DC. Diuretic therapy. *New England Journal of Medicine* 1998; **339**: 387–95.

Cohn JN. The management of chronic heart failure. *New England Journal of Medicine* 1996; **335**: 490–8.

Frishman WH. Carvedilol. *New England Journal of Medicine* 1998; **339**: 1759–65.

Jessup M, Brozena S. 2003 Medical progress: heart failure. *New England Journal of Medicine* 2003; **348**: 2007–18.

McMurray JJV, Pfeffer MA. Heart failure. *Lancet* 2005; **365**: 1877–89.

Nabel EG. Cardiovascular disease. *New England Journal of Medicine* 2003; **349**: 60–72.

Palmer BF. Managing hyperkalemia caused by inhibitors of the renin–angiotensin–aldosterone system. *New England Journal of Medicine* 2004; **351**: 585–92.

Pfeffer MA, Stevenson LW. β-Adrenergic blockers and survival in heart failure. *New England Journal of Medicine* 1996; **334**: 1396–7.

Schrier RW, Abraham WT. Mechanisms of disease – hormones and hemodynamics in heart failure. *New England Journal of Medicine* 1999; **341**: 577–85.

Weber KT. Mechanisms of disease – aldosterone in congestive heart failure. *New England Journal of Medicine* 2001; **345**: 1689–97.

CARDIAC DYSRHYTHMIAS

COMMON DYSRHYTHMIAS

SUPRAVENTRICULAR

ARISING FROM THE SINUS NODE

Sinus tachycardia

In sinus tachycardia, the rate is 100–150 beats per minute with normal P-waves and PR interval. It may be physiological, for example in response to exercise or anxiety, or pathological, for example in response to pain, left ventricular failure, asthma, thyrotoxicosis or iatrogenic causes (e.g. β-agonists). If pathological, treatment is directed at the underlying cause.

Sinus bradycardia

In sinus bradycardia, the rate is less than 60 beats per minute with normal complexes. This is common in athletes, in young healthy individuals especially if they are physically fit, and patients taking beta-blockers. It also occurs in patients with raised intracranial pressure or sinoatrial (SA) node disease ('sick-sinus syndrome'), and is common during myocardial infarction, especially inferior territory myocardial infarction, since this area contains the SA node. It only requires treatment if it causes or threatens haemodynamic compromise.

ATRIAL DYSRHYTHMIAS

Atrial fibrillation

The atrial rate in atrial fibrillation is around 350 beats per minute, with variable AV conduction resulting in an irregular pulse. If the AV node conducts rapidly, the ventricular response is also rapid. Ventricular filling is consequently inadequate and cardiac output falls. The method of treating atrial fibrillation is either to convert it to sinus rhythm, or to slow conduction through the AV node, slowing ventricular rate and improving cardiac output even though the rhythm remains abnormal.

Atrial flutter

Atrial flutter has a rate of 250–350 per minute and ventricular conduction can be fixed (for example, an atrial rate of 300 per minute with 3:1 block gives a ventricular rate of 100 per minute) or variable.

NODAL AND OTHER SUPRAVENTRICULAR DYSRHYTHMIAS

Atrioventricular block

- *First degree*: This consists of prolongation of the PR interval.
- *Second degree*: There are two types, namely Mobitz I, in which the PR interval lengthens progressively until a P-wave fails to be conducted to the ventricles (Wenckebach phenomenon), and Mobitz II, in which there is a constant PR interval with variable failure to conduct to the ventricles.
  The importance of first- and second-degree block is that either may presage complete (third-degree) heart block. This is especially so in the case of Mobitz II block.
- *Third degree*: There is complete AV dissociation with emergence of an idioventricular rhythm (usually around 50 per minute, although the rhythm may be slower, e.g. 30–40 per minute). Severe cerebral underperfusion with syncope sometimes followed by convulsions (Stokes–Adams attacks) often results.

SUPRAVENTRICULAR TACHYCARDIAS

Supraventricular tachycardia (SVT) leads to rapid, narrow complex tachycardias at rates of approximately 150 per minute. Not uncommonly in older patients the rapid rate leads to failure of conduction in one or other bundle and 'aberrant' conduction with broad complexes because of the rate-dependent bundle-branch block. This can be difficult to distinguish electrocardiographically from ventricular tachycardia, treatment of which is different in important respects. SVT can be intra-nodal or extranodal.

Intranodal supraventricular tachycardia

Fibre tracts in the AV node are arranged longitudinally, and if differences in refractoriness develop between adjacent fibres then an atrial impulse may be conducted antegradely through one set of fibres and retrogradely through another, leading to a re-entry ('circus') tachycardia.

Extranodal supraventricular tachycardia

An anatomically separate accessory pathway is present through which conduction is faster and the refractory period shorter than in the AV node. The cardiogram usually shows a shortened PR interval (because the abnormal pathway conducts more rapidly from atria to ventricle than does the AV node), sometimes with a widened QRS complex with a slurred upstroke or delta wave, due to arrival of the impulse in part of the ventricle where it must pass through unspecialized slowly conducting ventricular myocytes instead of through specialized Purkinje fibres (Wolff–Parkinson–White or WPW syndrome). Alternatively, there may be a short PR interval but a normal QRS complex (Lown–Ganong–Levine syndrome), if the abnormal pathway connects with the physiological conducting system distal to the AV node.

VENTRICULAR DYSRHYTHMIAS

- *Ventricular ectopic beats*: Abnormal QRS complexes originating irregularly from ectopic foci in the ventricles. These may occur in an otherwise healthy heart or may occur as a consequence of organic heart disease, e.g. coronary heart disease, hypertrophic cardiomyopathy, heart failure from other causes. Multifocal ectopics (ectopic beats of varying morphology, arising from more than one focus) are likely to be pathological.
- *Ventricular tachycardia*: The cardiogram shows rapid, wide QRS complexes (0.14 seconds or greater) and the patient is usually, but not always, hypotensive and poorly perfused. This rhythm may presage ventricular fibrillation.
- *Ventricular fibrillation*: The cardiogram is chaotic and circulatory arrest occurs immediately.

GENERAL PRINCIPLES OF MANAGEMENT

1. Anti-dysrhythmic drugs are among the most dangerous at the clinician's disposal. Always think carefully before prescribing one.
2. If the patient is acutely ill on account of a cardiac dysrhythmia, the most appropriate treatment is almost never a drug. In bradydysrhythmia, consider pacing, and in tachydysrhythmia consider direct current (DC) cardioversion. Consider the possibility of hyperkalaemia or other electrolyte disorder, especially in renal disease, as a precipitating cause and treat accordingly.
3. It is important to treat the patient, not the cardiogram. Remember that several anti-dysrhythmic drugs can themselves cause dysrhythmias and shorten life. When

dysrhythmias are prognostically poor, this often reflects severe underlying cardiac disease which is not improved by an anti-dysrhythmic drug but which may be improved by, for example, an ACE inhibitor (for heart failure), **aspirin** or oxygen (for ischaemic heart disease) or operation (for left main coronary artery disease and valvular heart disease).
4. In an acutely ill patient, consider the possible immediate cause of the rhythm disturbance. This may be within the heart (e.g. myocardial infarction, ventricular aneurysm, valvular or congenital heart disease) or elsewhere in the body (e.g. pulmonary embolism, infection or pain, for example from a distended bladder in a stuporose patient).
5. Look for reversible processes that contribute to the maintenance of the rhythm disturbance (e.g. hypoxia, acidosis, pain, electrolyte disturbance, including Mg^{2+} as well as K^+ and Ca^{2+}, thyrotoxicosis, excessive alcohol or caffeine intake or pro-dysrhythmic drugs) and correct them.
6. Avoid 'cocktails' of drugs.

Key points

Cardiac dysrhythmias: general principles

- In emergencies consider:
  DC shock (tachydysrhythmias);
  pacing (bradydysrhythmias).
- Correct pro-dysrhythmogenic metabolic disturbances:
  electrolytes (especially K^+, Mg^{2+});
  hypoxia/acid-base;
  drugs.
- Clinical trials have shown that correcting a dysrhythmia does not necessarily improve the prognosis – anti-dysrhythmic drugs can themselves cause dysrhythmias.

CLASSIFICATION OF ANTI-DYSRHYTHMIC DRUGS

The classification of anti-dysrhythmic drugs is not very satisfactory. The Singh–Vaughan–Williams classification (classes I–IV; see Table 32.1), which is based on effects on the cardiac action potential, is widely used, but unfortunately does not reliably predict which rhythm disturbances will respond to which drug. Consequently, selection of the appropriate anti-dysrhythmic drug to use in a particular patient remains largely empirical. Furthermore, this classification does not include some of the most clinically effective drugs used to treat certain dysrhythmias, some of which are listed in Table 32.2.

CARDIOPULMONARY RESUSCITATION AND CARDIAC ARREST: BASIC AND ADVANCED LIFE SUPPORT

The European Resuscitation Council provides guidelines for basic and advanced life support (Figures 32.1 and 32.2).

Table 32.1: Anti-dysrhythmic drugs: the Vaughan–Williams/Singh classification

Class	Example	Mode of action	Comment
I		Rate-dependent block of Na^+ conductance	
a	Quinidine Procainamide Disopyramide	Intermediate kinetics between b and c	Prolong cardiac action potential
b	Lidocaine Mexiletine	Rapid dissociation from Na^+ channel	Useful in ventricular tachydysrhythmias
c	Flecainide Propafenone	Slow dissociation from Na^+ channel	Prolong His–Purkinje conduction: worsen survival in some instances
II	Atenolol	Beta blockers: slow pacemaker depolarization	Improve survival following myocardial infarction
III	Amiodarone Sotalol Dofetilide Ibutilide	Prolong cardiac action potential	Effective in supra-, as well as ventricular tachydysrhythmias. Predispose to torsades de pointes (a form of ventricular tachycardia)
IV	Verapamil Diltiazem	Calcium antagonists: block cardiac voltage-dependent Ca^{2+} conductance	Used in prophylaxis of recurrent SVT. Largely superseded by adenosine for treating acute attacks. Negatively inotropic

Table 32.2: Drugs/ions not classified primarily as anti-dysrhythmic, but used to treat important dysrhythmias

Digoxin (rapid atrial fibrillation)

Atropine (symptomatic sinus bradycardia)

Adenosine (supraventricular tachycardia)

Adrenaline (cardiac arrest)

Calcium chloride (ventricular tachycardia caused by hyperkalaemia)

Magnesium chloride (ventricular fibrillation)

BASIC LIFE SUPPORT

When a person is found to have collapsed, make a quick check to ensure that no live power lines are in the immediate vicinity. Ask them, 'Are you all right?', and if there is no response, call for help. Do not move the patient if neck trauma is suspected. Otherwise roll them on their back (on a firm surface if possible) and loosen the clothing around the throat. Assess airway, breathing and circulation (ABC).

Tilt the head and lift the chin, and sweep an index finger through the mouth to clear any obstruction (e.g. dentures). Tight-fitting dentures need not be removed and may help to maintain the mouth sealed during assisted ventilation.

If the patient is not breathing spontaneously, start mouth-to-mouth (or, if available, mouth-to-mask) ventilation. Inflate the lungs with two expirations (over about 2 seconds each)

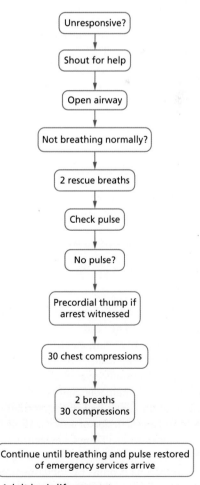

Figure 32.1: Adult basic life support.

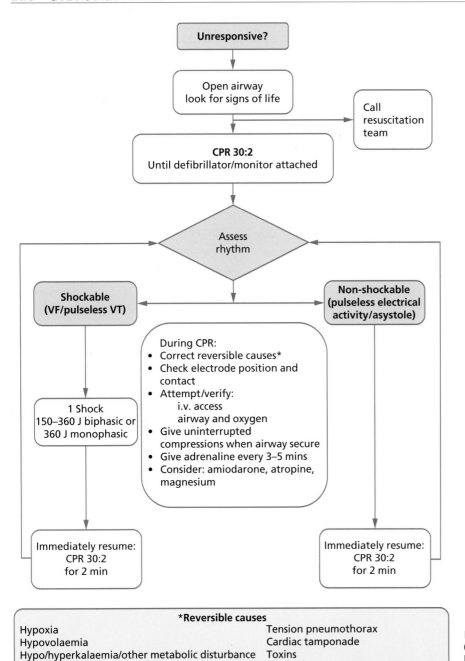

Figure 32.2: Adult advanced life support. (Redrawn with permission from the European Resuscitation Council Guidelines, 2005.)

and check that the chest falls between respirations. If available, 100% oxygen should be used.

Check for a pulse by feeling carefully for the carotid or femoral artery before diagnosing cardiac arrest. If the arrest has been witnessed, administer a single thump to the precordium. If no pulse is palpable, start cardiac compression over the middle of the lower half of the sternum at a rate of 100 per minute and an excursion of 4–5 cm. Allow two breaths per 30 chest compressions. Drugs can cause fixed dilated pupils, so do not give up on this account if drug overdose is a possibility. Hypothermia is protective of tissue function, so do not abandon your efforts too readily if the patient is severely hypothermic (e.g. after being pulled out of a freezing lake). Mobilize facilities for active warming.

ADVANCED LIFE SUPPORT

Basic cardiopulmonary resuscitation is continued throughout as described above, and it should not be interrupted for more than 10 seconds (except for palpation of a pulse or for administration of DC shock, when personnel apart from the operator must stand well back). 'Advanced' life support refers to the treatment of cardiac dysrhythmias in the setting of cardiopulmonary arrest. The electrocardiogram is likely to show asystole, severe bradycardia or ventricular fibrillation. Occasionally narrow complexes are present, but there is no detectable cardiac output ('electromechanical dissociation'). The doses given below are for an average-sized adult. During the course of an arrest, other rhythm disturbances are frequently encountered (e.g. sinus bradycardia) and these are considered in the next section on other specific dysrhythmias. If intravenous access cannot be established, the administration of double doses of **adrenaline** (or other drugs as appropriate) via an endotracheal tube can be life-saving.

ASYSTOLE

Make sure ECG leads are attached properly and that the rhythm is not ventricular fibrillation, which is sometimes mistaken for asystole if the fibrillation waves are of low amplitude. If there is doubt, DC counter-shock (200 J). Once the diagnosis is definite, administer **adrenaline** (otherwise known as **epinephrine**), 1 mg intravenously, followed by **atropine**, 3 mg intravenously. Further doses of **adrenaline** 1 mg can be given every three minutes as necessary. If P-waves (or other electrical activity) are present, but the intrinsic rate is slow or there is high grade heart block, consider pacing.

VENTRICULAR FIBRILLATION

The following sequence is used until a rhythm (hopefully sinus) is achieved that sustains a cardiac output. DC counter-shock (200 J) is delivered as soon as a defibrillator is available and then repeated (200 J, then 360 J) if necessary, followed by **adrenaline**, 1 mg intravenously, and further defibrillation (360 J) repeated as necessary. Consider varying the paddle positions and also consider **amiodarone** 300 mg, if ventricular fibrillation persists. A further dose of 150 mg may be required in refractory cases, followed by an infusion of 1 mg/min for six hours and then 0.5 mg/min, to a maximum of 2 g. Magnesium (8 mmol) is recommended for refractory VF if there is a suspicion of hypomagnesaemia, e.g. patients on potassium-losing diuretics. **Lidocaine** and **procainamide** are alternatives if **amiodarone** is not available, but should not be given in addition to **amiodarone**. During prolonged resuscitation, **adrenaline** (1 mg i.v.) every three minutes is recommended.

ELECTROMECHANICAL DISSOCIATION

When the pulse is absent, but the ECG shows QRS complexes, this is known as electromechanical dissociation. It may be the result of severe global damage to the left ventricle, in which case the outlook is bleak. If it is caused by some potentially reversible pathology such as hypovolaemia, pneumothorax, pericardial tamponade or pulmonary embolus, volume replacement or other specific measures may be dramatically effective. If pulseless electrical activity is associated with a bradycardia, atropine, 3 mg intravenously or 6 mg via the endotracheal tube, should be given. High-dose **adrenaline** is no longer recommended in this situation.

TREATMENT OF OTHER SPECIFIC DYSRHYTHMIAS

TACHYDYSRHYTHMIAS

SUPRAVENTRICULAR
Atrial fibrillation

See also Figure 32.3, which outlines a useful algorithm for the general treatment of tachydysrhythmias including atrial fibrillation.

Patients who have not been in atrial fibrillation for too long and in whom the left atrium is not irreversibly distended may 'spontaneously' revert to sinus rhythm. If this does not occur, such patients benefit from elective DC cardioversion, following which many remain in sinus rhythm. DC cardioversion is unlikely to achieve or to maintain sinus rhythm in patients with longstanding atrial fibrillation, or with atrial fibrillation secondary to mitral stenosis, especially if the left atrium is significantly enlarged; in such cases, it is quite acceptable to aim for rate control rather than rhythm conversion. Indeed, trials have demonstrated no difference in prognosis between patients with atrial fibrillation treated with a rate control vs. a rhythm control strategy, although patients who remain in atrial fibrillation are more likely to be persistently symptomatic. The main hazard of cardioversion is embolization of cerebral or peripheral arteries from thrombus that may have accumulated in the left atrial appendage. Patients should therefore be anticoagulated before elective cardioversion (usually for four to six weeks) to prevent new and friable thrombus from accumulating and to permit any existing thrombus to organize, thereby reducing the risk of embolization. An alternative is to perform early cardioversion provided that transoesophageal echocardiography can be performed and shows no evidence of thrombus in the left atrial appendage. Anticoagulation is continued for one month if the patient remains in sinus rhythm. Anticoagulation should be continued long term if fibrillation persists or intermittent episodes of dysrhythmia recur.

Atrial flutter

Atrial flutter is treated with the same drugs as are effective in atrial fibrillation, but tends to be more resistant to drug treatment. However, it is very responsive to DC cardioversion. As with atrial fibrillation, atrial flutter carries a risk of systemic embolization.

Paroxysmal supraventricular tachycardias

As discussed above, although supraventricular tachycardia is generally a narrow complex QRS tachycardia, the presence of rate-induced aberrant conduction can cause the QRS complexes to be wide, thus making it difficult to distinguish from ventricular tachycardia. Criteria exist for distinguishing broad complex supraventricular and ventricular tachycardias, but these are beyond the scope of this book, and in practice are often difficult to apply precisely. Figure 32.3 therefore

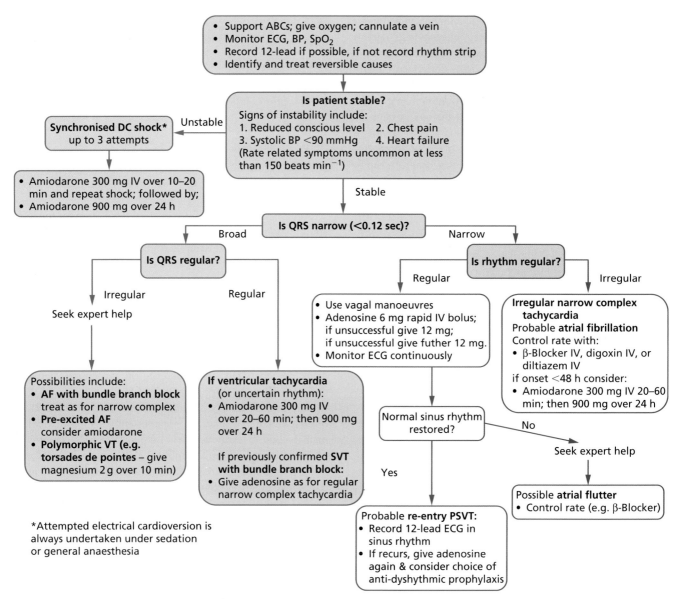

Figure 32.3: Scheme for the management of tachydysrhythmias. (Adapted with permission from the European Resuscitation Council Guidelines, 2005).

provides a simple and practical algorithm for the management of tachydysrhythmias in general.

Catheter ablation therapy is now possible for supraventricular tachycardias, atrial flutter and fibrillation. Advice from a consultant cardiac electrophysiologist should be sought regarding the suitability of a patient for this procedure.

Ventricular dysrhythmias

Ventricular ectopic beats: Electrolyte disturbance, smoking, alcohol abuse and excessive caffeine consumption should be sought and corrected if present. The only justification for treating patients with anti-dysrhythmic drugs in an attempt to reduce the frequency of ventricular ectopic (VE) beats in a chronic setting is if the ectopic beats cause intolerable palpitations, or if they precipitate attacks of more serious tachydysrhythmia (e.g. ventricular tachycardia or fibrillation). If palpitations are so unpleasant as to warrant treatment despite

the suspicion that this may shorten rather than prolong life, an oral class I agent, such as **disopyramide**, may be considered. **Sotalol** with its combination of class II and III actions is an alternative, although a clinical trial with the D-isomer (which is mainly responsible for its class III action) showed that this worsened survival (the 'SWORD' trial).

In an acute setting (most commonly the immediate aftermath of myocardial infarction), treatment to suppress ventricular ectopic beats may be warranted if these are running together to form brief recurrent episodes of ventricular tachycardia, or if frequent ectopic beats are present following cardioversion from ventricular fibrillation. **Lidocaine** is used in such situations and is given as an intravenous bolus, followed by an infusion in an attempt to reduce the risk of sustained ventricular tachycardia or ventricular fibrillation.

Ventricular tachycardia: This is covered in Figure 32.3 (management of tachydysrhythmias). In the longer term, consideration should be given to insertion of an implantable cardioverter defibrillator (ICD), if the patient is considered at high risk of further episodes and/or serious ventricular dysrhythmias remain inducible on electrophysiological testing.

Ventricular fibrillation: See above under Advanced life support. As discussed above for ventricular tachycardia, implantation of an ICD should be considered.

BRADYDYSRHYTHMIAS

ASYSTOLE

See above under Advanced life support.

Sinus bradycardia

1. Raising the foot of the bed may be successful in increasing cardiac output and cerebral perfusion.
2. Give atropine (see below).
3. Discontinue **digoxin**, beta-blockers, **verapamil** or other drugs that exacerbate bradycardia.
4. Pacemaker insertion is indicated if bradycardia is unresponsive to **atropine** and is causing significant hypotension.

Sick sinus syndrome (tachycardia–bradycardia syndrome)

Treatment is difficult. Drugs that are useful for one rhythm often aggravate the other and a pacemaker is often needed.

Atrioventricular conduction block

- First-degree heart block by itself does not require treatment.
- Second-degree Mobitz type I block (Wenckebach block) is relatively benign and often transient. If complete block occurs, the escape pacemaker is situated relatively high up in the bundle so that the rate is 50–60 per minute with narrow QRS complexes. Atropine (0.6–1.2 mg intravenously) is usually effective. Mobitz type II block is more serious and may progress unpredictably to complete block with a slow ventricular escape rate. The only reliable treatment is a pacemaker.
- Third-degree heart block (complete AV dissociation) can cause cardiac failure and/or attacks of unconsciousness (Stokes–Adams attacks). Treatment is by electrical pacing; if delay in arranging this is absolutely unavoidable, low-dose **adrenaline** intravenous infusion is sometimes used as a temporizing measure. Congenital complete heart block, diagnosed incidentally, does not usually require treatment.

SELECTED ANTI-DYSRHYTHMIC DRUGS

LIDOCAINE

For more information about **lidocaine**, see Chapter 24.

Use

Lidocaine is important in the treatment of ventricular tachycardia and fibrillation, often as an adjunct to DC cardioversion. An effective plasma concentration is rapidly achieved by giving a bolus intravenously followed by a constant rate infusion.

Mechanism of action

Lidocaine is a class Ib agent that blocks Na^+ channels, reducing the rate of increase of the cardiac action potential and increasing the effective refractory period. It selectively blocks open or inactivated channels and dissociates very rapidly.

Adverse effects

These include the following:

1. central nervous system – drowsiness, twitching, paraesthesia, nausea and vomiting; focal followed by generalized seizures;
2. cardiovascular system – bradycardia, cardiac depression (negative inotropic effect) and asystole.

Pharmacokinetics

Oral bioavailability is poor because of presystemic metabolism and **lidocaine** is given intravenously. It is metabolized in the liver, its clearance being limited by hepatic blood flow. Heart failure reduces **lidocaine** clearance, predisposing to toxicity unless the dose is reduced. The difference between therapeutic and toxic plasma concentrations is small. Monoethylglycylxylidide (MEGX) and glycylxylidide (GX) are active metabolites with less anti-dysrhythmic action than **lidocaine**, but with central nervous system toxicity. The mean half-life of **lidocaine** is approximately two hours in healthy subjects.

Drug interactions

Negative inotropes reduce **lidocaine** clearance by reducing hepatic blood flow and consequently predispose to accumulation and toxicity.

OTHER CLASS I DRUGS

Other class I drugs have been widely used in the past, but are now used much less frequently. Some of these drugs are shown in Table 32.1.

β-ADRENORECEPTOR ANTAGONISTS

For more information, see also Chapters 28, 29 and 31.

Use

Anti-dysrhythmic properties of β-adrenoceptor antagonists are useful in the following clinical situations:

- patients who have survived myocardial infarction (irrespective of any ECG evidence of dysrhythmia); β-adrenoceptor antagonists prolong life in this situation;

- inappropriate sinus tachycardia (e.g. in association with panic attacks);
- paroxysmal supraventricular tachycardias that are precipitated by emotion or exercise;
- rapid atrial fibrillation that is inadequately controlled by **digoxin**;
- tachydysrhythmias of thyrotoxicosis;
- tachydysrhythmias of phaeochromocytoma, after adequate α-receptor blockade.

Atenolol is available for intravenous use after myocardial infarction. **Esmolol** is a cardioselective β-adrenoceptor antagonist for intravenous use with a short duration of action (its elimination half-life is approximately 10 minutes). β-Adrenoceptor antagonists are given more commonly by mouth when used for the above indications.

Contraindications and cautions

Contraindications include the following;

- asthma, chronic obstructive pulmonary disease;
- peripheral vascular disease;
- Raynaud's phenomenon;
- uncompensated heart failure (β-blockers are actually beneficial in stable patients (see Chapter 31), but have to be introduced cautiously).

Drug interactions

- Beta-blockers inhibit drug metabolism indirectly by decreasing hepatic blood flow secondary to decreased cardiac output. This causes accumulation of drugs such as **lidocaine** that have such a high hepatic extraction ratio that their clearance reflects hepatic blood flow.
- Pharmacodynamic interactions include increased negative inotropic effects with **verapamil** (if given intravenously this can be fatal), **lidocaine**, **disopyramide** or other negative inotropes. Exaggerated and prolonged hypoglycaemia occurs with **insulin** and oral hypoglycaemic drugs.

AMIODARONE

Use

Amiodarone is highly effective, but its use is limited by the severity of its adverse effects during chronic administration. It is effective in a wide variety of dysrhythmias, including:

- *supraventricular dysrhythmias* – resistant atrial fibrillation or flutter, re-entrant tachycardias (e.g. WPW syndrome);
- *ventricular dysrhythmias* – recurrent ventricular tachycardia or fibrillation.

It can be given intravenously, via a central intravenous line, in emergency situations as discussed above, or orally if rapid dysrhythmia control is not required.

Mechanism of action

Amiodarone is a class III agent, prolonging the duration of the action potential but with no effect on its rate of rise.

Adverse effects and contraindications

Adverse effects are many and varied, and are common when the plasma **amiodarone** concentration exceeds 2.5 mg/L.

1. *Cardiac effects* – the ECG may show prolonged QT, U-waves or deformed T-waves, but these are not in themselves an indication to discontinue treatment. **Amiodarone** can cause ventricular tachycardia of the variety known as torsades de pointes. Care is needed in patients with heart failure and the drug is contraindicated in the presence of sinus bradycardia or AV block.
2. *Eye* – **Amiodarone** causes corneal microdeposits in almost all patients during prolonged use. Patients may report coloured haloes without a change in visual acuity. The deposits are only seen on slit-lamp examination and gradually regress if the drug is stopped.
3. *Skin* – photosensitivity rashes occur in 10–30% of patients. Topical application of compounds which reflect both UV-A and visible light can help (e.g. zinc oxide), whereas ordinary sunscreen does not; and patients should be advised to avoid exposure to direct sunlight and to wear a broad-brimmed hat in sunny weather. Patients sometimes develop blue-grey pigmentation of exposed areas. This is a separate phenomenon to phototoxicity.
4. *Thyroid* – **amiodarone** contains 37% iodine by weight and therefore may precipitate hyperthyroidism in susceptible individuals; or conversely it can cause hypothyroidism, due to alterations in thyroid hormone metabolism, with a rise in thyroxine (T_4) and reverse tri-iodothyronine (rT_3), a normal or low T_3 and a flat thyroid-stimulating hormone (TSH) response to thyrotropin-releasing hormone (TRH). Thyroid function (T_3, T_4 and TSH) should be assessed before starting treatment and annually thereafter, or more often if the clinical picture suggests thyroid dysfunction.
5. *Pulmonary fibrosis* – may develop with prolonged use. This potentially serious problem usually but not always improves on stopping the drug.
6. *Hepatitis* – transient elevation of hepatic enzymes may occur and occasionally severe hepatitis develops. It is idiosyncratic and non-dose-related.
7. *Peripheral neuropathy* – occurs in the first month of treatment and reverses on stopping dosing. Proximal muscle weakness, ataxia, tremor, nightmares, insomnia and headache are also reported.

Pharmacokinetics

Amiodarone is variably absorbed (20–80%) when administered orally. However, both the parent drug and its main metabolite, desethyl amiodarone (the plasma concentration of which exceeds that of the parent drug), are highly lipid soluble. This is reflected in a very large volume of distribution (approximately 5000 L). It is highly plasma protein bound (over 90%) and accumulates in all tissues, particularly the heart. It is only slowly eliminated via the liver, with a $t_{1/2}$ of 28–45 days. Consequently, anti-dysrhythmic activity may continue for several months after dosing has been stopped, and a loading dose is needed if a rapid effect is needed.

Drug interactions

Amiodarone potentiates **warfarin** by inhibiting its metabolism. It can precipitate **digoxin** toxicity (the **digoxin** dose should be reduced by 50% when **amiodarone** is added) and can cause severe bradycardia if used with β-adrenoceptor antagonists or **verapamil**.

SOTALOL

Use

Sotalol has uses similar to **amiodarone**, but a different spectrum of adverse effects. The plasma K^+ concentration should be monitored during chronic use and corrected if it is low in order to reduce the risk of torsades de pointes (see below).

Mechanism of action

Sotalol is unique among β-adrenoceptor antagonists in possessing substantial class III activity. It is a racemate, the D-isomer possessing exclusively class III activity. A clinical trial of D-**sotalol** (the 'SWORD' study) indicated that it reduces survival in patients with ventricular ectopic activity. The racemate is preferred.

Adverse effects and contraindications

Since it prolongs the cardiac action potential (detected on the ECG as a prolonged QT interval) it can cause ventricular tachycardia of the torsades de pointes variety, like **amiodarone**. Hypokalaemia predisposes to this effect. The beta-blocking activity of **sotalol** contraindicates its use in patients with obstructive airways disease, unstable heart failure, peripheral vascular disease or heart block.

Drug interactions

Diuretics predispose to torsades de pointes by causing electrolyte disturbance (hypokalaemia/hypomagnesaemia). Similarly, other drugs that prolong the QT interval should be avoided. These include class Ia anti-dysrhythmic drugs (**quinidine**, **disopyramide**), which slow cardiac repolarization as well as depolarization, and several important psychotropic drugs, including tricyclic antidepressants and phenothiazines. Histamine H_1-antagonists (**terfenadine**, **astemizole**) should be avoided for the same reason.

VERAPAMIL

Use

Verapamil is used as an anti-dysrhythmic:

- prophylactically to reduce the risk of recurrent SVT, by mouth;
- to reduce the ventricular rate in patients with atrial fibrillation who are not adequately controlled by **digoxin** alone (but beware interaction causing **digoxin** toxicity, see below);
- to terminate SVT in patients who are not haemodynamically compromised. In this setting it is given intravenously over five minutes. **Adenosine** is generally preferred, but **verapamil** may be useful in patients in whom adenosine is contraindicated (e.g. asthmatics).

Mechanism of action

Verapamil blocks L-type voltage-dependent Ca^{2+} channels. It is a class IV drug and has greater effects on cardiac conducting tissue than other Ca^{2+} antagonists. In common with other calcium antagonists, it relaxes the smooth muscle of peripheral arterioles and veins, and of coronary arteries. It is a negative inotrope, as cytoplasmic Ca^{2+} is crucial for cardiac contraction. As an anti-dysrhythmic drug, its major effect is to slow intracardiac conduction, particularly through the AV node. This reduces the ventricular response in atrial fibrillation and flutter, and abolishes most re-entry nodal tachycardias. Mild resting bradycardia is common, together with prolongation of the PR interval.

Adverse effects and contraindications

1. *Cardiovascular effects*: **Verapamil** is contraindicated in cardiac failure because of the negative inotropic effect. It is also contraindicated in sick sinus syndrome or intracardiac conduction block. It can cause hypotension, AV block or other bradydysrhythmias. It is contraindicated in WPW syndrome complicated by supraventricular tachycardia, atrial flutter or atrial fibrillation, as it can increase the rate of conduction through the accessory pathway. **Verapamil** is ineffective in ventricular dysrhythmias and its negative inotropic effect makes its inadvertent use in such dysrhythmias extremely hazardous.
2. *Gastrointestinal tract*: About one-third of patients experience constipation, although this can usually be prevented or managed successfully with advice about increased dietary intake of fibre and use of laxatives, if necessary.
3. *Other adverse effects*: Headache, dizziness and facial flushing are related to vasodilatation (compare with similar or worse symptoms caused by other calcium-channel blockers). Drug rashes, pain in the gums and a metallic taste in the mouth are uncommon.

Drug interactions

The important pharmacodynamic interaction of **verapamil** with β-adrenoceptor antagonists, which occurs especially when one or other member of the pair is administered intravenously, contraindicates their combined use by this route.

Verapamil reduces **digoxin** excretion and the dose of **digoxin** should therefore be halved when these drugs are combined. For the same reason, **verapamil** is contraindicated in patients with **digoxin** toxicity, especially as these drugs also have a potentially fatal additive effect on the AV node.

ADENOSINE

Use

Adenosine is used to terminate SVT. In addition to its use in regular narrow complex tachycardia, it is useful diagnostically in patients with regular broad complex tachycardia which is suspected of being SVT with aberrant conduction. If **adenosine** terminates the tachycardia, this implies that the AV node is indeed involved. However, if this diagnosis is wrong (as is not infrequently the case) and the patient actually has VT, little or no harm results, in contrast to the use of **verapamil** in VT.

Mechanism of action

Adenosine acts on specific adenosine receptors. A_1-receptors block AV nodal conduction. **Adenosine** also constricts bronchial smooth muscle by an A_1 effect, especially in asthmatics. It relaxes vascular smooth muscle, stimulates nociceptive afferent neurones in the heart and inhibits platelet aggregation via A_2-receptors.

Adverse effects and contraindications

Chest pain, flushing, shortness of breath, dizziness and nausea are common but short-lived. Chest pain can be alarming if the patient is not warned of its benign nature before the drug is administered. **Adenosine** is contraindicated in patients with asthma or heart block (unless already paced) and should be used with care in patients with WPW syndrome in whom the ventricular rate during atrial fibrillation may be accelerated as a result of blocking the normal AV nodal pathway and hence favouring conduction through the abnormal pathway. This theoretically increases the risk of ventricular fibrillation; however, this risk is probably small and should not discourage the use of **adenosine** in patients with broad complex tachycardias of uncertain origin.

Pharmacokinetics

Adenosine is rapidly cleared from the circulation by uptake into red blood cells and by enzymes on the luminal surface of endothelial cells. It is deaminated to inosine. The circulatory effects of a bolus therapeutic dose of adenosine last for 20–30 seconds, although effects on the airways in asthmatics persist for longer.

Drug interactions

Dipyridamole blocks cellular **adenosine** uptake and potentiates its action. **Theophylline** blocks **adenosine** receptors and inhibits its action.

DIGOXIN

For more information on **digoxin**, see also Chapter 31.

Use

The main use of **digoxin** is to control the ventricular rate (and hence improve cardiac output) in patients with atrial fibrillation. **Digoxin** is usually given orally, but if this is impossible, or if a rapid effect is needed, it can be given intravenously. Since the $t_{1/2}$ is approximately one to two days in patients with normal renal function, repeated administration of a maintenance dose results in a plateau concentration within about three to six days. This is acceptable in many settings, but if clinical circumstances are more urgent, a therapeutic plasma concentration can be achieved more rapidly by administering a loading dose.

The dose is adjusted according to the response, sometimes supplemented by plasma concentration measurement.

Mechanism of action

1. **Digoxin** inhibits membrane Na^+/K^+ adenosine triphosphatase (Na^+/K^+ ATPase), which is responsible for the active extrusion of Na^+ from myocardial, as well as other cells. This results in accumulation of intracellular Na^+, which indirectly increases the intracellular Ca^{2+} content via Na^+/Ca^{2+} exchange and intracellular Ca^{2+} storage. The rise in availability of intracellular Ca^{2+} accounts for the positive inotropic effect of **digoxin**.
2. Slowing of the ventricular rate results from several mechanisms, particularly increased vagal activity:
   - delayed conduction through the atrioventricular node and bundle of His;
   - increased cardiac output due to the positive inotropic effect of **digoxin** reduces reflex sympathetic tone;
   - small doses of digitalis sensitize the sinoatrial node to vagal impulses. The cellular mechanism of this effect is not known.

ATROPINE

Use

Atropine is administered intravenously to patients with haemodynamic compromise due to inappropriate sinus bradycardia. (It is also used for several other non-cardiological indications, including anaesthetic premedication, topical application to the eye to produce mydriasis and for patients who have been poisoned with organophosphorous anticholinesterase drugs; see Chapter 54).

Mechanism of action

Acetylcholine released by the vagus nerve acts on muscarinic receptors in atrial and cardiac conducting tissues. This increases K^+ permeability, thereby shortening the cardiac action potential and slowing the rate of increase of pacemaker potentials and cardiac rate. **Atropine** is a selective antagonist of acetylcholine at muscarinic receptors, and it thereby counters these actions of acetylcholine, accelerating the heart rate in patients with sinus bradycardia by inhibiting excessive vagal tone.

Adverse effects and contraindications

Parasympathetic blockade by **atropine** produces widespread effects, including reduced salivation, lachrymation and sweating, decreased secretions in the gut and respiratory tract, tachycardia, urinary retention in men, constipation, pupillary dilatation and ciliary paralysis. It is contraindicated in patients with narrow-angle glaucoma. **Atropine** can cause central nervous system effects, including hallucinations.

Pharmacokinetics

Although **atropine** is completely absorbed after oral administration, it is administered intravenously to obtain a rapid effect when treating sinus bradycardia, in the event of haemodynamic compromise, for example following myocardial infarction.

ADRENALINE

Use

Although not usually classed as an 'anti-dysrhythmic' drug (it is, of course, powerfully pro-dysrhythmogenic in healthy individuals), **adrenaline** (also called **epinephrine**) is used in the emergency treatment of patients with cardiac arrest (whether due to asystole or ventricular fibrillation). For these indications it is administered intravenously (or sometimes directly into the heart or down an endotracheal tube, as discussed in the above section on cardiac arrest). It has important uses other than in cardiac arrest, being essential for the treatment of anaphylactic shock (see Chapter 50) and useful in combination with local anaesthetics to reduce the rate of removal from the injection site (see Chapter 24).

Mechanism of action

Adrenaline is a potent and non-selective agonist at both α- and β-adrenoceptors. It causes an increased rate of depolarization of cardiac pacemaker potential, thereby increasing heart rate, in addition to increasing the force of contraction of the heart and intense α_1-mediated peripheral vasoconstriction (thereby producing a very marked pressor response), which is partly offset by β_2-mediated arterial vasodilation.

Adverse effects

Adrenaline is powerfully pro-dysrhythmogenic and increases the work of the heart (and hence its oxygen requirement). Its peripheral vasoconstrictor effect can reduce tissue perfusion. For these reasons, it is only used systemically in emergency situations.

Pharmacokinetics

Adrenaline is rapidly eliminated from the circulation by a high-affinity/low-capacity uptake process into sympathetic nerve terminals ('uptake 1') and by a lower-affinity/higher-capacity process into a variety of tissues ('uptake 2'). It is subsequently metabolized by monoamine oxidase and catechol-*O*-methyl transferase, and is excreted in the urine as inactive metabolites, including vanillyl mandelic acid (VMA).

Drug interactions

Tricyclic antidepressants block uptake 1 and so may potentiate the action of **adrenaline**. Adrenoceptor antagonists, both α and β, block its actions at these receptors.

CALCIUM CHLORIDE

Use

Calcium chloride is uniquely valuable when given (slowly) intravenously for treating the broad complex ('sine-wave') ventricular tachycardia that is a preterminal event in patients with severe hyperkalaemia (often secondary to renal failure; see Chapter 36). Its use may 'buy time' during which other measures to lower the plasma potassium concentration (e.g. glucose with insulin, ion-binding resins, dialysis) can take effect or be mobilized. In addition, **calcium chloride** is used in patients with hypocalcaemia, but these usually present with tetany rather than with cardiac dysrhythmia. It may be useful for treating patients who have received an overdose of Ca^{2+}-antagonists such as **verapamil** or **diltiazem**.

Mechanism of action

Ca^{2+} is a divalent cation. Divalent cations are involved in maintaining the stability of the membrane potential in excitable tissues, including the heart. The outer aspects of cell membranes contain fixed negative charges that influence the electric field in the membrane, and hence the state of activation of voltage-dependent ion channels (Na^+ and Ca^{2+}) in the membrane. Divalent cations bind to the outer membrane, neutralizing the negative charges and in effect hyperpolarizing the membrane. Conversely, if the extracellular concentration of Ca^{2+} falls, Ca^{2+} dissociates from the membrane, rendering it more unstable.

Adverse effects and contraindications

Calcium phosphate can precipitate in the kidneys of patients with hyperphosphataemia, worsening renal function. However, this consideration is irrelevant when one is faced with a hyperkalaemic patient with broad complex tachycardia.

Drug interactions

- Calcium carbonate precipitates if calcium chloride solution is mixed with sodium bicarbonate. Therefore, these should not be given through the same line, or consecutively without an intervening saline flush.
- Calcium increases **digoxin** toxicity and **calcium chloride** must not be administered if this is suspected.

MAGNESIUM

Use

Magnesium sulphate by intravenous infusion is used in broad complex tachycardia in the peri-arrest situation, in conjuction with other treatment (DC shock, **lidocaine** and correction of hypokalaemia). Intravenous **magnesium sulphate** is sometimes effective in treating dysrhythmias caused by **digoxin** and in drug-induced torsades de pointes. It is invaluable in eclampsia in prevention of further convulsions (see Chapter 28). **Magnesium chloride** may be particularly useful in settings where magnesium deficiency is common. These include prior chronic diuretic treatment, hypocalcaemia, hypokalaemia, alcoholism, diarrhoea, vomiting, drainage from a fistula, pancreatitis, hyperaldosteronism or prolonged infusion of intravenous fluid without magnesium supplementation. There is no simple test currently available to detect total body magnesium deficiency, since Mg^{2+} is predominantly an intracellular cation. However, serial plasma magnesium determinations may be useful in preventing excessive dosing with accumulation and toxicity.

Mechanism of action

Mg^{2+} is a divalent cation and at least some of its beneficial effects are probably due to the consequent neutralization of fixed negative charges on the outer aspect of the cardiac cell membranes (as for Ca^{2+}). In addition, Mg^{2+} is a vasodilator and releases prostacyclin from damaged vascular tissue in vitro.

Adverse effects and contraindications

- Excessively high extracellular concentrations of Mg^{2+} can cause neuromuscular blockade. **Magnesium chloride** should be used with great caution in patients with renal impairment or hypotension, and in patients receiving drugs with neuromuscular blocking activity, including aminoglycoside antibiotics.
- Mg^{2+} can cause AV block.

Pharmacokinetics

Magnesium salts are not well absorbed from the gastrointestinal tract, accounting for their efficacy as osmotic laxatives when given by mouth. Mg^{2+} is eliminated in the urine and therapy with magnesium salts should be avoided or the dose reduced (and frequency of determination of plasma Mg^{2+} concentration increased) in patients with glomerular filtration rates <20 mL/min.

Drug interactions

Magnesium salts form precipitates if they are mixed with sodium bicarbonate and, as with calcium chloride, magnesium salts should not be administered at the same time as sodium bicarbonate, or through the same line without an intervening saline flush. Hypermagnesaemia increases neuromuscular blockade caused by drugs with nicotinic-receptor-antagonist properties (e.g. **pancuronium**, aminoglycosides).

Case history

A 16-year-old girl is brought to the Accident and Emergency Department by her mother having collapsed at home. As a baby she had cardiac surgery and was followed up by a paediatric cardiologist until the age of 12 years, when she rebelled. She was always small for her age and did not play games, but went to a normal school and was studying for her GCSEs. On examination, she is ill and unable to give a history, and has a heart rate of 160 beats per minute (regular) and blood pressure of 80/60 mmHg. There are cardiac murmurs which are difficult to characterize. The ECG shows a broad complex regular tachycardia which the resident medical officer (RMO) is confident is an SVT with aberrant conduction.
Question

Decide whether initial management might reasonably include each of the following:

(a) i.v. verapamil.
(b) DC shock;
(c) i.v. adenosine;
(d) i.v. lidocaine.

Answer

(a) False
(b) True
(c) True
(d) False

Comment
This patient clearly has underlying heart disease and is acutely haemodynamically compromised by the dysrhythmia. It is difficult to distinguish SVT with aberrant conduction from ventricular tachycardia, but if the RMO is correct, then lidocaine will not be effective. Verapamil, while often effective in SVT, is potentially catastrophic in this setting, but a therapeutic trial of adenosine could be considered because of its short duration of action. Alternatively (or subsequently if adenosine is not effective, which would suggest that the rhythm is really ventricular), direct current (DC) shock is appropriate.

Case history

A 66-year-old man made a good recovery from a transmural (Q-wave) anterior myocardial infarction complicated by mild transient left ventricular dysfunction, and was sent home taking aspirin, atenolol, enalapril and simvastatin. Three months later, when he is seen in outpatients, he is feeling reasonably well, but is worried by palpitations. His pulse is irregular, but there are no other abnormal findings on examination and his ECG shows frequent multifocal ventricular ectopic beats.
Question
Decide whether management might appropriately include each of the following:

(a) consideration of cardiac catheterization;
(b) invasive electrophysiological studies, including provocation of dysrhythmia;
(c) adding flecainide;
(d) stopping atenolol;
(e) adding verapamil;
(f) adding amiodarone.

Answer

(a) True
(b) False
(c) False
(d) False
(e) False
(f) False

Comment
It is important to continue a beta-blocker, which will improve this patient's survival. It is appropriate to consider cardiac catheterization to define his coronary anatomy and to identify whether he would benefit from some revascularization procedure. Other classes of anti-dysrhythmic drugs have not been demonstrated to prolong life in this setting. If the symptom of palpitation is sufficiently troublesome, it would be reasonable to consider switching from atenolol to regular (i.e. racemic) sotalol.

Case history

A 24-year-old medical student arrives at the Accident and Emergency Department complaining of rapid regular palpitations coming on abruptly while he was studying in the library for his final examinations which start next week. There is no relevant past history. He looks pale but otherwise well, his pulse is 155 beats per minute and regular, his blood pressure is 110/60 mmHg and the examination is otherwise unremarkable. The cardiogram shows a supraventricular tachycardia.

Question

Decide whether initial management might reasonably include each of the following:

(a) i.v. amiodarone;
(b) vagal manoeuvres;
(c) i.v. digoxin;
(d) reassurance;
(e) DC shock;
(f) overnight observation;
(g) specialized tests for phaeochromocytoma.

Answer

(a) False
(b) True
(c) False
(d) True
(e) False
(f) True
(g) False

Comment

Students who are studying for examinations often consume excessive amounts of coffee and a history of caffeine intake should be sought. The rhythm is benign and the patient should be reassured. Vagal manoeuvres may terminate the dysrhythmia but, if not, overnight observation may see the rhythm revert spontaneously to sinus. Intravenous amiodarone or initial DC shock would be inappropriate, and i.v. digoxin (while increasing vagal tone) could render subsequent DC shock (if necessary) more hazardous.

FURTHER READING

Delacretaz E. Clinical practice: supraventricular tachycardia. *New England Journal of Medicine* 2006; **354**: 1039–51.

Goldberger Z, Lampert R. Implantable cardioverter-defibrillators: expanding indications and technologies. *Journal of the American Medical Association* 2006; **295**: 809–18.

Hall MC, Todd DM. Modern management of arrhythmias. *Postgraduate Medical Journal* 2006; **82**: 117–25.

Nattel S, Opie LH. Controversies in atrial fibrillation. *Lancet* 2006; **367**: 262–72.

PART V

THE RESPIRATORY SYSTEM

CHAPTER 33

THERAPY OF ASTHMA, CHRONIC OBSTRUCTIVE PULMONARY DISEASE (COPD) AND OTHER RESPIRATORY DISORDERS

PATHOPHYSIOLOGY OF ASTHMA

Asthma is characterized by fluctuating airways obstruction, with diurnal variation and nocturnal exacerbations. This manifests as the triad of wheeze, cough and breathlessness. These symptoms are due to a combination of constriction of bronchial smooth muscle, oedema of the mucosa lining the small bronchi, and plugging of the bronchial lumen with viscous mucus and inflammatory cells (Figure 33.1). Asthma is broadly categorized into non-allergic and allergic, but there is considerable overlap. In allergic asthma, which is usually of early onset, extrinsic allergens produce a type I allergic reaction in atopic subjects. Type I reactions are triggered via reaginic antibodies (IgE) on the surface of mast cells and other immune effector cells, especially activated Th2 lymphocytes, which release cytokines that recruit eosinophils and promote further IgE synthesis and sensitivity. Patients with non-allergic (late-onset) asthma do not appear to be sensitive to any single well-defined antigen, although infection (usually viral) often precipitates an attack. Inflammatory mediators implicated in asthma include histamine, several leukotrienes (LTC_4/D_4 and E_4) 5-hydroxytryptamine (serotonin), prostaglandin D_2, platelet-activating factor (PAF), neuropeptides and tachykinins. Increased parasympathetic tone due to local and centrally mediated stimuli also promotes bronchoconstriction.

MANAGEMENT OF ACUTE SEVERE ASTHMA

The proposed management is based on the British Thoracic Society guidelines and involves the following:

- assessment of asthma severity (e.g. unable to complete sentences in one breath, pulse rate and pulsus paradox, if measurable, respiratory rate, breath sounds peak expiratory flow rate, pulse oximetry and blood gases if arterial O_2 saturation <92%) to define the need for hospitalization. Life-threatening asthma (e.g. silent chest, exhaustion, cyanosis, peak flow <33% of predicted or best, saturation <92%) needs urgent treatment with:
- high flow oxygen (FiO_2 40–60% oxygen);
- glucocorticosteroids: hydrocortisone i.v., followed by prednisolone p.o.;
- nebulized β_2-agonist (e.g. **salbutamol**) plus **ipratropium**; via oxygen-driven nebulizer;
- if the response to the above bronchodilator treatment is inadequate or not sustained, consider intravenous bronchodilator: β_2-agonist (e.g. **salbutamol** by i.v. infusion), or aminophylline/theophylline (by slow i.v. injection);
- in refractory cases, consider magnesium sulphate (slow i.v. injection/short infusion);

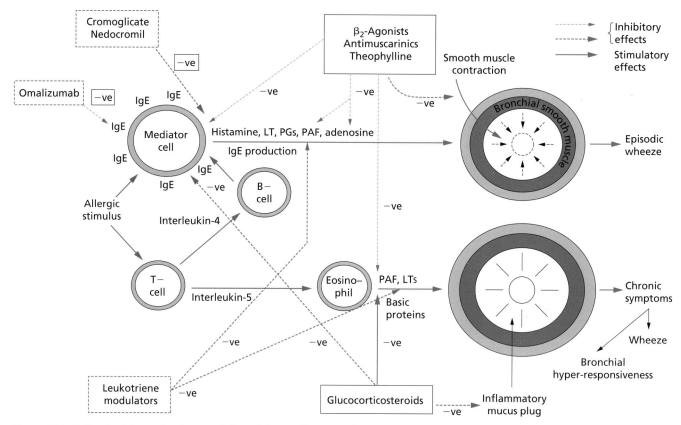

Figure 33.1: Pathophysiology of asthma and sites of drug action. PAF, platelet-activating factor; LTs, leukotrienes; PGs, prostaglandins.

- an antibiotic (e.g. **co-amoxiclav** or **clarithromycin**), if bacterial infection is strongly suspected – beware potential interactions with **theophylline**, see below;
- if the patient fails to respond and develops increasing tachycardia, with increasing respiratory rate and a fall in PaO_2 to <8 kPa or a rise in $PaCO_2$ to <6 kPa, assisted ventilation will probably be needed;
- sedation is absolutely contraindicated, except with assisted ventilation.
- general care: monitor fluid/electrolyte status (especially hypokalaemia) and correct if necessary.

CHRONIC ASTHMA

The primary objectives of the pharmacological management of chronic asthma are to obtain full symptom control, prevent exacerbations and achieve the best possible pulmonary function, with minimal side effects. The British Thoracic Society/Scottish Intercollegiate Guideline Network (BTS/SIGN) have proposed a five-step management plan, with initiation of therapy based on the assessed severity of the disease at that timepoint. Figure 33.2 details the treatment in the recommended steps in adult asthmatics. Step 1 is for mild asthmatics with intermittent symptoms occurring only once or twice a week; step 2 is for patients with more symptoms (more than three episodes of asthma symptoms per week or nocturnal symptoms). Step 3 is for patients who have continuing symptoms despite step 2 treatment and steps 4 and 5 are for more chronically symptomatic patients or patients with worsening symptoms, despite step 3 or 4 treatment.

PRINCIPLES OF DRUG USE IN TREATING CHRONIC ASTHMA

1. Metered dose inhalers (MDIs) of β_2-agonists are convenient and with correct usage little drug enters the systemic circulation. Aerosols are particularly useful for treating an acute episode of breathlessness. Long-acting β_2-agonist (e.g. **salmeterol**) should be taken regularly with top-ups of 'on-demand' shorter-acting agents. Oral preparations have a role in young children who cannot co-ordinate inhalation with activation of a metered-dose inhaler. Children over five years can use inhaled drugs with a 'spacer' device. There are several alternative approaches, including breath-activated devices and devices that administer the dose in the form of a dry powder that is sucked into the airways.
2. Patients should contact their physician promptly if their clinical state deteriorates or their β_2-agonist use is increasing.
3. Inhaled glucocorticosteroids (e.g. **beclometasone**, **fluticasone**, **budesonide**) are initiated when symptoms are not controlled or when:
   - regular (rather than occasional, as needed) doses of short-acting β_2-agonist bronchodilator are required;
   - repeated attacks interfere with work or school.

Adverse effects are minimized by using the inhaled route. Severely affected patients require oral glucocorticosteroids (e.g. **prednisolone**).

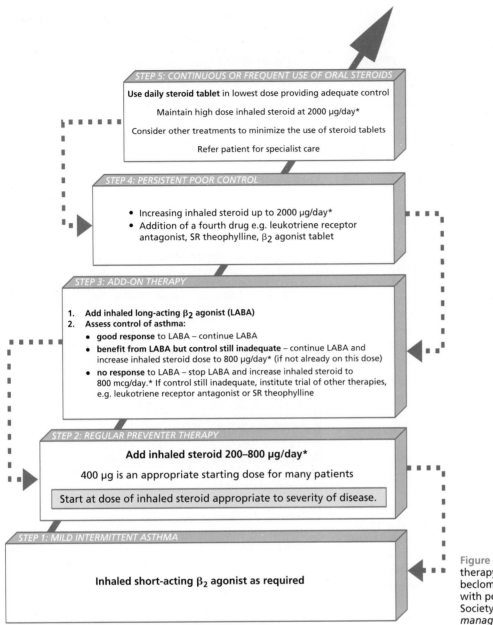

STEP 5: CONTINUOUS OR FREQUENT USE OF ORAL STEROIDS

Use daily steroid tablet in lowest dose providing adequate control

Maintain high dose inhaled steroid at 2000 μg/day*

Consider other treatments to minimize the use of steroid tablets

Refer patient for specialist care

STEP 4: PERSISTENT POOR CONTROL

- Increasing inhaled steroid up to 2000 μg/day*
- Addition of a fourth drug e.g. leukotriene receptor antagonist, SR theophylline, β₂ agonist tablet

STEP 3: ADD-ON THERAPY

1. **Add inhaled long-acting β₂ agonist (LABA)**
2. **Assess control of asthma:**
   - **good response** to LABA – continue LABA
   - **benefit from LABA but control still inadequate** – continue LABA and increase inhaled steroid dose to 800 μg/day* (if not already on this dose)
   - **no response** to LABA – stop LABA and increase inhaled steroid to 800 mcg/day.* If control still inadequate, institute trial of other therapies, e.g. leukotriene receptor antagonist or SR theophylline

STEP 2: REGULAR PREVENTER THERAPY

Add inhaled steroid 200–800 μg/day*

400 μg is an appropriate starting dose for many patients

Start at dose of inhaled steroid appropriate to severity of disease.

STEP 1: MILD INTERMITTENT ASTHMA

Inhaled short-acting β₂ agonist as required

* BDP or equivalent

Figure 33.2: Stepwise approach to asthma therapy in a non-acute situation. BDP, beclometasone dipropionate. (Redrawn with permission from the British Thoracic Society, *British guideline on the management of asthma*, p 26.)

4. Leukotriene receptor antagonists (e.g. **montelukast**) are used in adults and children for long-term maintenance therapy and can reduce glucocorticosteroid requirements.
5. In moderate to severe steroid-dependent chronic asthma, the anti-IgE monoclonal antibody **omalizumab** can improve asthmatic control and reduce the need for glucocorticosteroids.
6. Hypnotics and sedatives should be avoided, as for acute asthma.
7. Patients can perform home peak flow monitoring first thing in the morning and last thing at night, as soon as asthmatic symptoms develop or worsen. This allows adjustment of inhaled medication, or appropriate urgent medical assessment if the peak flow rate falls to less than 50% of normal, or diurnal variation (morning 'dipping') exceeds 20%.

ACUTE BRONCHITIS

Acute bronchitis is common. There is little convincing evidence that antibiotics confer benefit in otherwise fit patients presenting with cough and purulent sputum, and usually the most important step is to stop smoking. In the absence of fever or evidence of pneumonia, it seems appropriate to avoid antibiotics for this self-limiting condition.

CHRONIC BRONCHITIS AND EMPHYSEMA

Chronic bronchitis is associated with a chronic or recurrent increase in the volume of mucoid bronchial secretions sufficient to cause expectoration. At this stage, there need be no disability and measures such as giving up smoking (which may be aided by the use of nicotine replacment; see Chapter 53) and avoidance of air pollution improve the prognosis. Simple hypersecretion may be complicated by infection or the development of airways obstruction. Bacterial infection is usually due to mixed infections including organisms such as *Haemophilus influenzae*, although pneumococci, staphylococci or occasionally *Branhamella* may also be responsible. The commonly encountered acute bronchitic exacerbation is due to bacterial infection in only about one-third of cases. In the rest, other factors – such as increased air pollution, environmental temperature changes or viruses – are presumably responsible. *Mycoplasma pneumoniae* infections may be responsible for some cases and these respond to macrolides. Antibiotic therapy is considered when there is increased breathlessness, increased sputum volume and, in particular, increased sputum purulence. Rational antibiotic choice is based on adequate sputum penetration and the suspected organisms. The decision is seldom assisted by sputum culture or Gram stain, in contrast to the treatment of pneumonia. It is appropriate to vary the antibiotic used for different attacks, since effectiveness presumably reflects the sensitivity of organisms resident in the respiratory tract. Commonly used antibacterials include:

- **azithromycin** or **clarithromycin**;
- **amoxicillin** or **co-amoxiclav**;
- oral cephalosporin, e.g. **cefadroxil**;
- fluoroquinolone, e.g. **ciprofloxacin**.

Prevention of acute exacerbations is difficult. Stopping smoking is beneficial. Patients are often given a supply of antibiotic to take as soon as their sputum becomes purulent. Despite recovery from an acute attack, patients are at greatly increased risk of death or serious illness from intercurrent respiratory infections, and administration of influenza and pneumococcal vaccines is important. Airways obstruction is invariably present in chronic bronchitis, but is of variable severity. In some patients there is a reversible element, and a formal trial of bronchodilators, either β_2-adrenoceptor agonists or anticholinergics, e.g. **ipratropium**, is justified to assess benefit. Similarly, a short therapeutic trial of oral glucocorticosteroids, with objective monitoring of pulmonary function (FEV$_1$/FVC), is often appropriate. Many patients are not steroid responsive; approaches designed to reverse glucocorticosteroid resistance, including **theophylline**, are currently under investigation.

Long-term oxygen therapy (LTOT), usually at least 15 hours daily, in severely disabled bronchitis patients with pulmonary hypertension decreases mortality and morbidity. The mortality of such patients is related to pulmonary hypertension, which is increased by chronic hypoxia. Relief of hypoxia on a long-term basis by increasing the concentration of inspired oxygen reverses the vasoconstriction in the pulmonary arteries and decreases pulmonary hypertension. Long-term oxygen therapy cannot be safely offered to patients who continue to smoke because of the hazards of fire and explosion.

> **Key points**
>
> Therapy of chronic obstructive airways disease.
>
> Acute exacerbation
>
> - Controlled oxygen therapy (e.g. FiO$_2$ 24–28%);
> - Nebulized β_2-agonists (**salbutamol** every 2–4 hours, if needed) or intravenously if refractory;
> - Nebulized anticholinergics, such as **ipratropium bromide**;
> - Antibiotics (e.g. **clarithromycin, co-amoxiclav, levofloxacin**).
> - Short-term oral **prednisolone**.
>
> Chronic disease
>
> - Stop smoking cigarettes.
> - Optimize inhaled bronchodilators (**salbutamol/ipratropium bromide**) and their administration.
> - Consider oral **theophylline** and/or inhaled glucocorticosteroids.
> - Treat infection early and aggressively with antibiotics.
> - Offer long-term oxygen therapy (LTOT) for at least 15 hours per day for cor pulmonale.
> - Diuretics should be used for peripheral oedema.
> - Consider venesection for severe secondary polycythaemia.
> - Exercise, within limits of tolerance.

DRUGS USED TO TREAT ASTHMA AND CHRONIC OBSTRUCTIVE PULMONARY DISEASE

β_2-AGONISTS

Use

β_2-Agonists (e.g. **salbutamol** and the long-acting β_2-agonist **salmeterol**) are used to treat the symptoms of bronchospasm in asthma (both in an acute attack and as maintenance therapy) and chronic obstructive pulmonary disease (COPD). (Intravenous **salbutamol** is also used in obstetric practice to inhibit premature labour). For asthma, β_2-agonists are given via inhalation where possible, see also Table 33.1.

1. Inhalation formulations include:
   - metered-dose inhaler – aerosol. Some patients are unable to master this technique;
   - aerosol administered via a nebulizer;
   - as a dry powder – almost all patients can use a dry-powder inhaler correctly.
2. Oral formulations, including slow-release preparations.

Intravenous administration

The increase in FEV$_1$ after inhaling **salbutamol** begins within 5–15 minutes, peaks at 30–60 minutes and persists for 4–6 hours.

Pharmacological effects, mechanism of action and adverse effects

Agonists occupying β_2-adrenoceptors increase cyclic adenosine monophosphate (cAMP) by stimulating adenylyl cyclase via stimulatory G-proteins. Cyclic AMP phosphorylates a

Table 33.1: Comparative pharmacology of other β_2-agonists

Drug	Formulations available	Pharmacokinetics/ pharmacodynamics	Other comments
Terbutaline	Metered-dose inhaler Dry powder Nebulizer solution Tablets/syrup Slow-release tablets	Plasma $t_{1/2}$ is 3–4 h Gastro-intestinal and hepatic metabolism	Similar to salbutamol

Salmeterol	Metered-dose inhaler
	
	Dry powder
		Onset slow; 12 h duration
		  of action. Hepatic metabolism
			Prophylaxis and exercise-
			  induced asthma. Not
			  for treatment of acute
			  bronchospasm

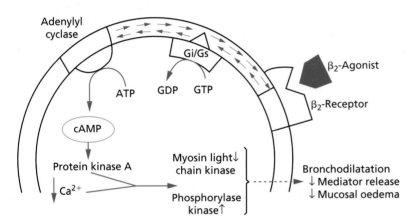

Figure 33.3: Membrane and intracellular events triggered when β_2-agonists stimulate β_2-receptors. Gi/Gs, inhibitory and stimulatory G-protein, GDP, guanosine diphosphate; GTP, guanosine triphosphate; cAMP, 3',5'-cyclic adenosine monophosphate.

cascade of enzymes (see Figure 33.3). This causes a wide variety of effects including:

1. relaxation of smooth muscle including bronchial, uterine and vascular;
2. inhibition of release of inflammatory mediators;
3. increased mucociliary clearance;
4. increase in heart rate, force of myocardial contraction, speed of impulse conduction and enhanced production of ectopic foci in the myocardium and automaticity in pacemaker tissue. This can cause dysrhythmias and symptoms of palpitations;
5. muscle tremor;
6. vasodilatation in muscle, part of this effect is indirect, via activation of endothelial NO biosynthesis;
7. metabolic effects:
   - hypokalaemia (via redistribution of K^+ into cells);
   - raised free fatty acid concentrations;
   - hyperglycaemia due to a greater increase in glycogenolysis than in insulin secretion.
8. desensitization.

Pharmacokinetics

Salbutamol undergoes considerable presystemic metabolism in the intestinal mucosa (sulphation) and hepatic conjugation

to form an inactive metabolite that is excreted in the urine. Most (approximately 90%) of the dose administered by aerosol is swallowed, but the 10–15% which is inhaled largely remains as free drug in the airways. The plasma elimination half-life ($t_{1/2}$) is two to four hours.

Salmeterol is long acting, with a duration of action of at least 12 hours, allowing twice daily administration. The lipophilic side-chain of **salmeterol** binds firmly to an exo-site that is adjacent to, but distinct from, the β_2-agonist binding site. Consequently, **salmeterol** functions as an almost irreversible agonist. The onset of bronchodilatation is slow (15–30 minutes). **Salmeterol** should not therefore be used to treat acute attacks of bronchospasm. It is now advised as first-line in prophylactic therapy, on a twice daily basis, with 'top ups' of short acting β_2-agonists. **Salmeterol** should be used in conjunction with inhaled glucocorticosteroids.

MUSCARINIC RECEPTOR ANTAGONISTS

Use

Osler recommended **stramonium** – which contains **atropine** – in the form of cigarettes for asthmatics! In comparison to **atropine**, modern agents, e.g. **ipratropium**, are quaternary ammonium analogues and have reduced systemic absorption due to their positive charge. **Ipratropium** is given three or four times daily from a metered-dose inhaler or nebulizer. Inhaled muscarinic receptor antagonists are most effective in older patients with COPD. The degree and rate of onset of bronchodilatation are less than those of **salbutamol**, but the duration of response is longer. **Ipratropium** has a place in maintenance therapy and the treatment of acute severe attacks of asthma and chronic bronchitis. It is compatible with β_2-agonists, and such combinations are additive. **Tiotropium** is a long-acting antimuscarinic bronchodilator administered by inhalation in the management of COPD patients. It is not used to treat acute bronchospasm.

Mechanism of action

There is increased parasympathetic activity in patients with reversible airways obstruction, resulting in bronchoconstriction through the effects of acetylcholine on the muscarinic (M_2, M_3) receptors in the bronchi. The final common pathway is via a membrane-bound G-protein which when stimulated leads to a fall in cAMP and increased intracellular calcium, with consequent bronchoconstriction. Antimuscarinic drugs block muscarinic receptors in the airways.

Adverse effects

These include:

- bitter taste (this may compromise compliance);
- acute urinary retention (in patients with prostatic hypertrophy);
- acute glaucoma has been precipitated when nebulized doses are given via a face mask;
- paradoxical bronchoconstriction due to sensitivity to benzalkonium chloride, which is the preservative in the nebulizer solution.

Pharmacokinetics

When administered by aerosol, it is poorly absorbed systemically. Plasma $t_{1/2}$ is three to four hours and inactive metabolites are excreted in the urine.

Several formulations of β_2-agonist combined with muscarinic antagonist bronchodilators are available to simplify treatment regimens.

Key points

Bronchodilator agents

- β_2-Agonists.
- Bronchodilate by increasing intracellular cAMP.
- Short-acting, rapid-onset agents (e.g. salbutamol) are used as needed to relieve bronchospasm in asthma.
- Long-acting, slower-onset agents (e.g. salmeterol) are used regularly twice daily.
- Common side effects include tremor, tachycardias, vasodilatation, hypokalaemia and hyperglycaemia.

Anticholinergics

- Antagonist at M_2 and M_3 muscarinic receptors in the bronchi, causing bronchodilatation.
- Slow onset of long-lasting bronchodilatation (given six- to eight-hourly), especially in older patients.
- Bitter taste.

- Little systemic absorption and side effects are rare (dry mouth, acute retention, exacerbation of glaucoma).

Theophylline

- Potent bronchodilator (also vasodilator).
- Aminophylline i.v. for acute severe episodes.
- Slow-release oral preparations for chronic therapy.
- Hepatic metabolism, multiple drug interactions (e.g. clarithromycin, ciprofloxacin).
- Therapeutic drug monitoring of plasma concentrations.
- Side effects include gastro-intestinal disturbances, vasodilatation, dysrhythmias, seizures and sleep disturbance.

METHYLXANTHINES

Use

Aminophylline (theophylline, 80%; ethylene diamine, 20%) is occasionally used intravenously in patients with severe refractory bronchospasm. Oral **theophylline** may be used for less severe symptoms or to reduce nocturnal asthma symptoms. Recently, the use of **theophylline** has markedly declined, but it is still sometimes used in refractory cases.

For intravenous **aminophylline**, a loading dose given slowly (20–30 minutes) is followed by a maintenance infusion. Oral **theophylline** sustained-release preparations can provide effective therapeutic concentrations for up to 12 hours following a single dose. Because of their slow release rate they have a reduced incidence of gastro-intestinal side effects.

Mechanism of action and pharmacological effects

It is not clear exactly how **theophylline** produces bronchodilation. Its pharmacological actions include the following:

- relaxation of airway smooth muscle and inhibition of mediator release (e.g. from mast cells). **Theophylline** raises intracellular cAMP by inhibiting phosphodiesterase. However, phosphodiesterase inhibition is modest at therapeutic concentrations of **theophylline**;
- antagonism of adenosine (a potent bronchoconstrictor) at A_2-receptors;
- anti-inflammatory activity on T-lymphocytes by reducing release of platelet-activating factor (PAF).

Adverse effects

The adverse effects of **theophylline** are:

- *Gastro-intestinal*: nausea, vomiting, anorexia.
- *Cardiovascular*: (1) dilatation of vascular smooth muscle – headache, flushing and hypotension; (2) tachycardia and cardiac dysrhythmias (atrial and ventricular).
- *Central nervous system*: insomnia, anxiety, agitation, hyperventilation, headache and fits.

Pharmacokinetics

Theophylline is well absorbed from the small intestine. It is 85–90% eliminated by hepatic metabolism (CYP1A2). The therapeutic concentration range is 5–20 mg/L, but it is preferable not to exceed 10 mg/L in children.

Drug interactions

Although synergism between β_2-adrenergic agonists and **theophylline** has been demonstrated in vitro, clinically the effect of this combination is at best additive. Many drugs inhibit CYP1A2-mediated **theophylline** metabolism, e.g. **erythromycin** (and other macrolides), fluoroquinolones (e.g. **ciprofloxacin**), **interferon** and **cimetidine**, thus precipitating **theophylline** toxicity. **Theophylline** metabolism is induced in the presence of hepatic CYP450-inducing agents, such as **rifampicin**.

GLUCOCORTICOSTEROIDS

Glucocorticosteroids are used in the treatment of asthma and in severe exacerbations of COPD because of their potent anti-inflammatory effect. This involves interaction with an intracellular glucocorticosteroid receptor that in turn interacts with nuclear DNA, altering the transcription of many genes and thus the synthesis of pro-inflammatory cytokines, β_2-adrenoceptors, tachykinin-degrading enzymes and lipocortin (an inhibitor of phospholipase A_2, reducing free arachidonic acid and thus leukotriene synthesis). They are used both in maintenance therapy (prophylaxis) and in the treatment of the acute severe attack.

SYSTEMIC GLUCOCORTICOSTEROIDS

For more information on the use of systemic glucocorticosteroids, see Chapter 40.

Hydrocortisone is given intravenously in urgent situations. Improvement (a rise in FEV_1 and forced vital capacity, FVC) does not begin until after six hours, and is usually maximal 10–12 hours following the start of treatment. This delay is due to the action of glucocorticosteroids via altered gene transcription and subsequent modified protein synthesis. Oral glucocorticosteroids (e.g. **prednisolone**) are usually started within 12–24 hours.

INHALED GLUCOCORTICOSTEROIDS (E.G. BECLOMETASONE, BUDESONIDE, FLUTICASONE, MOMETASONE)

Use

Modern inhalational devices deliver up to 20% of the administered dose to the lungs.

Glucocorticosteroids can be administered via nebulizers, 'spacer' devices, metered-dose inhalers or as dry powders. The fluorinated derivatives are extremely potent and mainly exert a local action because they are highly polar and hence only a small fraction of the dose is systemically absorbed. Approximately 15–20% enters the lungs, the rest being swallowed and then rapidly converted to inactive metabolites by intestinal and hepatic CYP3A enzymes.

The comparative pharmacology of the commonly used inhaled glucocorticosteroids is summarized in Table 33.2.

Adverse effects of inhaled steroids

- At the lowest recommended daily dose for adults, there is no prolonged suppression of the hypothalamic–pituitary–adrenal (HPA) axis. Higher doses can produce clinically important depression of adrenal function.
- Candidiasis of the pharynx or larynx occurs in 10–15% of patients. Using the minimum effective dose, or a 'spacer device', or gargling/using mouthwashes after dosing, minimizes this problem.
- A hoarse voice may develop due to a laryngeal myopathy at high doses. This is reversible and its occurrence is minimized by the use of a 'spacer'.
- Bruising and skin atrophy occur at high doses.
- Inhibition of long bone growth during prolonged high-dose treatment in children.
- Posterior subcapsular cataracts may develop following prolonged use.

CROMOGLICATE AND NEDOCROMIL

Use

Sodium cromoglicate may be used to prevent exercise-induced asthma and as prophylaxis for allergic asthma in children. Its use as a prophylactic in children has been largely superseded by inhaled glucocorticosteroids which are more effective. It is used as a nasal spray for perennial and allergic rhin-itis, and as eyedrops in allergic conjunctivitis. **Cromoglicate** produces no benefit during an acute asthmatic attack. **Nedocromil sodium** is an alternative to **cromoglicate**.

Mechanism of action

Cromoglicate and **nedocromil** inhibit mediator release from sensitized mast cells in vitro, and also reduce firing of sensory

---

Key points

Anti-inflammatory agents – cromoglicate and glucocorticosteroids

Sodium cromoglicate

- Its mechanism of action is unclear. It has an anti-inflammatory effect.
- Largely superseded in chronic prophylactic therapy of 'allergic asthma' by glucocorticosteroids.
- Prevents exercise-induced asthma.
- Inhaled therapy is administered via metered-dose inhaler or dry powder.
- Side-effects are minimal (headache, cough).
- Its use is very safe in children.

Glucocorticosteroids

- Mechanism is anti-inflammatory.
- They are administered systemically (i.v./p.o.) in severe acute and chronic asthma.
- They are inhaled topically or nebulized in chronic asthma.
- Glucocorticosteroids are well absorbed from the gastro-intestinal tract–hepatic (CYP3A) metabolism.
- Dosing is once daily for oral glucocorticosteroids and twice daily for inhaled agents.
- Side effects are minimal with topical therapy (oral thrush, hoarse voice, HPA suppression only at high dose).
- Side effects with systemic therapy are the features of Cushing's syndrome.

Table 33.2: Comparative pharmacology of some inhaled glucocorticosteroids

Drug	Relative binding affinity to receptors[a]	Relative blanching potency[a]	Comments
Beclometasone dipropionate	0.4	600	Equi-effective compared to budesonide. May be used in children
Budesonide	9.4	980	Nebulized formulation (0.5–1mg/2 mL) available. May be used in children to avoid systemic steroids
Fluticasone	18	1200	May cause fewer systemic side effects than others

[a]Relative to dexamethasone binding to glucocorticosteroid receptors in vitro and blanching of human skin in vitro.

C-fibres in response to tachykinins (e.g. bradykinin). However, the complete mechanism underlying their therapeutic efficacy is uncertain.

Adverse effects

- **Sodium cromoglicate** is virtually non-toxic. The powder can (very rarely) produce bronchospasm or hoarseness.
- Nausea and headache are rare adverse effects.
- Nedocromil has a bitter taste.

Pharmacokinetics

Sodium cromoglicate, an inhaled powder, undergoes little systemic absorption. Most of the powder is swallowed, about 10% reaching the alveoli. **Nedocromil sodium** has similarly low systemic bioavailability.

LEUKOTRIENE MODULATORS

These fall into two classes, namely leukotriene receptor antagonists and 5'-lipoxygenase inhibitors.

Leukotrienes (LT) are fatty acid-derived mediators containing a conjugated triene structure. They are formed when arachidonic acid (Chapter 26) is liberated from the cell membrane of cells, as a result of cell activation by allergic or other noxious stimuli. 5'-Lipoxygenase is the enzyme required for the synthesis of LTA_4, which is an unstable epoxide precursor of the two subgroups of biologically important leukotrienes. LTB_4 is a dihydroxy 20-carbon-atom fatty acid which is a potent pro-inflammatory chemo-attractant. The other group is the cysteinyl leukotrienes (LTC_4, LTD_4 and LTE_4). LTC_4 is a conjugate of LTA_4 plus glutathione, a tripeptide which combines with LTA_4 via its cysteine residue. LTC_4 is converted to an active metabolite (LTD_4) by the removal of the terminal amino acid in the peptide side-chain. Removal of a second amino acid results in a less active metabolite (LTE_4). LTC_4, LTD_4 and LTE_4, the 'sulphidopeptide leukotrienes' or 'cysteinyl leukotrienes', collectively account for the activity that used to be referred to as 'slow-reacting substance of anaphylaxis' (SRS-A). They all (but especially LTD_4) bind to the Cys-LT_1 receptor to cause bronchoconstriction, attraction of eosinophils and production of oedema.

LEUKOTRIENE C_4 AND D_4 ANTAGONISTS

Use

Leukotriene receptor antagonists are used to treat asthma and are given orally, usually in the evening. **Montelukast** was the first of these drugs to become available clinically. It reduced the requirement for glucocorticosteroid and improved symptoms in chronic asthma. It is also useful in the prophylaxis of exercise- or antigen-induced asthma. **Montelukast** is effective in aspirin-sensitive asthma, which is associated with diversion of arachidonic acid from the cyclo-oxygenase pathway (blocked by **aspirin**) to the formation of leukotrienes via 5'-lipoxygenase.

Mechanism of action

Montelukast is a competitive inhibitor of LTD_4 and LTC_4 at the Cys-LT_1 receptor.

Adverse effects

Montelukast is generally well tolerated, but side effects include:

- gastro-intestinal upsets;
- asthenia and drowsiness;
- rash, fever, arthralgias;
- elevation of serum transaminases.

Pharmacokinetics

This drug is rapidly absorbed from the gastro-intestinal tract. The mean plasma $t_{1/2}$ is 2.7–5.5 hours. It undergoes hepatic metabolism by CYP 3A and 2C9, and is mainly excreted in the bile.

Drug interactions

No clinically important drug–drug interactions are currently recognized.

5'-LIPOXYGENASE INHIBITORS

Zileuton (available in the USA) is a competitive inhibitor of the 5'-lipoxygenase enzyme. It is used in asthma therapy and administered orally and undergoes hepatic metabolism. Its use in asthma has declined considerably, with the efficacy of the leukotriene receptor antagonists.

ANTI-IGE MONOCLONAL Ab

Omalizumab is a recombinant humanized IgG1 monoclonal anti-IgE antibody. It is used as additional therapy in patients with severe persistent allergic asthma due to IgE-mediated sensitivity to inhaled allergens and inadequately controlled by glucocorticosteroids plus long-acting β_2-agonists. It binds to IgE at the same epitope on the Fc region that binds FcϵRI, this means it cannot react with IgE already bound to the mast cell or basophils and is not anaphylactogenic. It is administered subcutaneously every two to four weeks. It causes a 80–90% reduction in free IgE and it reduces FcϵRI expression on inflammatory cells. It has a $t_{1/2}$ of 20–30 days and is cleared via the reticuloendothelial system. Side effects include rashes, urticaria, pruritus, sinusitis, gastro-intestinal upsets, injection site reactions and possibly secondary haematologic malignancies. It can be used in children, but is a very expensive therapy.

Key points

Leukotriene modulation in asthma

- Leukotriene B$_4$ is a powerful chemo-attractant (eosinophils and neutrophils) and increases vascular permeability producing mucosal oedema.
- Leukotrienes C$_4$, D$_4$ and E$_4$ (cysteinyl leukotrienes) are potent spasmogens and pro-inflammatory substances ('SRS-A').
- Clinically used agents that modulate leukotrienes are leukotriene antagonists (which antagonize cysteinyl leukotrienes – LTD$_4$, LTC$_4$ at the Cys-LT$_1$ receptor)
- Leukotriene antagonists (e.g. montelukast) are effective as oral maintenance therapy in chronic persistent asthma. Montelukast has anti-inflammatory properties and is a mild, slow-onset bronchodilator.

ANTIHISTAMINES

H₁-BLOCKERS

See Chapter 50 for further information.

Antihistamines are not widely used in the treatment of asthma, but have an adjunctive role in asthmatics with severe hay fever. **Cetirizine** and **loratadine** are non-sedating H₁-antagonists with a plasma $t_{1/2}$ of 6.5–10 hours and 8–10 hours, respectively. **Cetirizine** and **loratidine** do not cause the potentially fatal drug–drug interaction (polymorphic VT) with macrolide antibiotics, as was the case with **astemizole** (or **terfenadine**).

ALTERNATIVE ANTI-INFLAMMATORY AGENTS

Other anti-inflammatory drugs, such as **methotrexate** or **ciclosporin**, reduce glucocorticosteroid requirements in

chronic asthmatics, but because of their long-term toxicities (Chapters 26 and 50), they are not used routinely.

RESPIRATORY FAILURE

Respiratory failure is the result of impaired gas exchange. It is defined by a low PaO_2 (less than 8 kPa (60 mmHg)). Causes include:

1. Type I (ventilation/perfusion inequality) is characterized by a low PaO_2 and a normal or low $PaCO_2$. Causes include:
   - acute asthma;
   - pneumonia;
   - left ventricular failure;
   - pulmonary fibrosis;
   - shock lung.

2. Type II (ventilatory failure) is characterized by a low PaO_2 and a raised $PaCO_2$ (>6.3 kPa). This occurs in:
   - severe acute asthma as the patient tires;
   - some patients with chronic bronchitis or emphysema;
   - reduced activity of the respiratory centre (e.g. from drug overdose or in association with morbid obesity and somnolence – Pickwickian syndrome);
   - peripheral neuromuscular disorders (e.g. Guillain–Barré syndrome or myasthenia gravis).

TREATMENT OF TYPE I RESPIRATORY FAILURE

The treatment of ventilation/perfusion inequality is that of the underlying lesion. Oxygen at high flow rate is given by nasal cannulae or face mask. Shock lung is treated by controlled ventilation, oxygenation and positive end expiratory pressure (PEEP).

TREATMENT OF TYPE II RESPIRATORY FAILURE

Sedatives (e.g. benzodiazepines) or respiratory depressants (e.g. opiates) must never be used unless the patient is being artifically ventilated.

SUPPORTIVE MEASURES
Physiotherapy

Physiotherapy is used to encourage coughing to remove tracheobronchial secretions and to encourage deep breathing to preserve airway patency.

Oxygen

Oxygen improves tissue oxygenation, but high concentrations may further depress respiration by removing the hypoxic respiratory drive. A small increase in the concentration of inspired oxygen to 24% using a Venturi-type mask should be tried. If the $PaCO_2$ does not increase, or increases by <0.66 kPa and the level of consciousness is unimpaired, the inspired oxygen concentration should be increased to 28% and after further assessment to 35%. If oxygen produces respiratory depression, assisted ventilation may be needed urgently.

Specific measures

Respiratory failure can be precipitated in chronic bronchitis by infection, fluid overload (e.g. as the pulmonary artery pressure increases and cor pulmonale supervenes) or bronchoconstriction. Antibacterial drugs are indicated if the sputum has become purulent. Bronchospasm may respond to **salbutamol** given frequently via nebulizer (often supplemented by nebulized **ipratropium**). **Hydrocortisone** is given intravenously for 72 hours. If the PaO_2 continues to fall and the $PaCO_2$ continues to rise, endotracheal intubation with suction and intermittent mandatory mechanical ventilation should be considered, especially if consciousness becomes impaired.

Key points
Respiratory failure
• Type I (hypocapnic hypoxaemia) and type II (hypercapnic hypoxaemia).
• Therapy for type I is supportive with high-percentage oxygen (FiO$_2$ 40–60%).
• Therapy for type II is low-percentage oxygen (FiO$_2$ 24–28%) and treatment of reversible factors – infection and bronchospasm (with antibiotics, bronchodilators and glucocorticosteroids).
• Type I or type II respiratory failure may necessitate mechanical ventilation.
• Central nervous system (CNS)-depressant drugs (e.g. opiates, benzodiazepines) may exacerbate or precipitate respiratory failure, usually type II.
• Sedatives are absolutely contraindicated (unless the patient is already undergoing mechanical ventilation).

COUGH

COUGH SUPPRESSANTS

Cough is a normal physiological reflex that frees the respiratory tract of accumulated secretions and removes particulate matter. The reflex is usually initiated by irritation of the mucous membrane of the respiratory tract and is co-ordinated by a centre in the medulla. Ideally, treatment should not impair elimination of bronchopulmonary secretions nor a thorough diagnostic search. A number of antitussive drugs are available, but critical evaluation of their efficacy is difficult. Patients with chronic cough are often poor judges of the antitussive effect of drugs. Objective recording methods have demonstrated dose-dependent antitussive effects for cough suppressants, such as **codeine** and **dextromethorphan**. However, cough should not be routinely suppressed, because of its protective function. Exceptions include intractable cough in carcinoma of the bronchus and cases in which an unproductive cough interferes with sleep or causes exhaustion. Bland demulcent syrups containing soothing substances (e.g. menthol or simple linctus BPC) provide adequate comfort for many patients. **Codeine** depresses the medullary cough centre and is effective as are **pholcodine** and **dextromethorphan**, other opioid analogues.

EXPECTORANTS

Difficulty in clearing viscous sputum is often associated with chronic cough. Various expectorants and mucolytic agents are available, but they are not very efficacious.

• Mixtures containing a demulcent and an antihistamine, a decongestant such as **pseudoephedrine** and sometimes a cough suppressant, such as **codeine**, are often prescribed. This combination is less harmful than anticipated, probably because the doses of most of its components are too low to exert much of an effect.

• Drugs which reduce the viscosity of sputum by altering the nature of its organic components are also available. They are sometimes called mucolytics, and the traditional agents are unhelpful because they reduce the efficacy of mucociliary clearance (which depends on beating cilia being mechanically coupled to viscous mucus). The increased viscosity of infected sputum is due to nucleic acids rather than mucopolysaccharides, and is not affected by drugs such as **bromhexine** or **acetyl cysteine**, which are therefore ineffective. **rhDNAase(Pulmozyme)** (phosphorylated glycosylated recombinant human deoxyribonuclease 1 enzyme), given by jet nebulizer, cleaves extracellular bacterial DNA, is proven effective in cystic fibrosis patients, decreasing sputum viscosity and reducing the rate of deterioration of lung function. Its major adverse effects are pharyngitis, voice changes, rashes and urticaria.

PULMONARY SURFACTANTS

Several pulmonary surfactants are available. **Colfosceril palmitate** (synthetic dipalmitoyl-phosphatidylcholine with hexadecanol and tyloxapol) is used in newborn infants undergoing mechanical ventilation for respiratory distress syndrome (RDS). It reduces complications, including pneumothorax and bronchopulmonary dysplasia, and improves survival. **Colfosceril** is given via the endotracheal tube, repeated after 12 hours if still intubated. Heart rate and arterial blood oxygenation/saturation must be monitored. The administered surfactant is rapidly dispersed and undergoes the same recycling as natural surfactant. Its principal adverse effects are obstruction of the endotracheal tubes by mucus, increased incidence of pulmonary haemorrhage and acute hyperoxaemia due to a rapid improvement in the condition.

α₁-ANTITRYPSIN DEFICIENCY

α_1-Antitrypsin is a serine protease produced by the liver. It inhibits neutrophil elastase in lungs. In patients with

α_1-antitrypsin deficiency, neutrophil elastase destroys the alveolar wall, leading to early-onset emphysema which is rapidly progressive. Such patients usually die of respiratory failure. Diagnosis is by measurement of α_1-antitrypsin concentrations in the blood. Replacement therapy with α_1-antitrypsin can be given. Replacement therapy with heat-treated (HIV- and hepatitis virus-negative) pooled plasma from donors is given intravenously weekly. The $t_{1/2}$ of α_1-antitrypsin is 5.2 days and its only adverse effect is post-infusion fever. Plasma concentrations rise into the normal range and several small longitudinal clinical studies with weekly dosing suggest reduction in the rate of decline in FEV_1 compared to historical controls. Aerosolized administration on a weekly basis appears safe and effective in children. The use of recombinant α_1-antitrypsin is being more widely investigated and α_1-antitrypsin gene therapy is now in early stage clinical investigation.

DRUG-INDUCED PULMONARY DISEASE

The lungs may be adversely affected by drugs in many important ways. Physical irritation by dry powder inhalers can precipitate cough/bronchospasm in asthmatics. Allergy to drugs of the immediate variety (type I) is particularly common in atopic individuals. Specific reaginic antibodies (IgE) to drugs can produce disturbances ranging from mild wheezing to laryngeal oedema or anaphylactic shock. Delayed bronchospasm may be due to drug interactions involving IgG antibodies (type III). Any drug may be responsible for allergic reactions, but several antibiotics are powerful allergens. β-Adrenoceptor antagonists can produce prolonged and sometimes fatal bronchospasm in asthmatics. **Aspirin** and other non-steroidal anti-inflammatory drugs (Chapters 25, 26 and 30) cause bronchoconstriction in sensitive asthmatic individuals (an estimated 2–7% of asthmatics have such sensitivity) who may also have nasal polyps and urticaria. Parasympathomimetic drugs (e.g. **bethanechol**, **methacholine**) and acetylcholinesterase inhibitors, such as **physostigmine**, can promote bronchial secretions and increase airways resistance. A dry cough can be caused by cytokines or more commonly (9–30% of patients) by angiotensin-converting enzyme (ACE) inhibitors (Chapters 28 and 29) and is dose dependent.

Pulmonary eosinophilia presents as dyspnoea, cough and fever. The chest x-ray shows widespread patchy changing shadows, and there is usually eosinophilia in the peripheral blood. The pathogenesis of the condition is not fully understood, but several drugs have been implicated, including **aspirin**, ACE inhibitors, **clarithromycin**, **imipramine**, **isoniazid**, **montelukast**, NSAIDs, **penicillin**, sulphonamides, **simvastatin**. The lungs can be involved by pleuritic reactions, pneumonia-like illness and impaired respiratory function due to small, stiff lungs in drug-induced systemic lupus erythematosus. Examples of drugs that cause this include **hydralazine**, **bromocriptine** and **procainamide**. Many drugs can produce interstitial pulmonary fibrosis, including **amiodarone, bepredil, bleomycin, cyclophosphamide, gemcitabine, gold salts, methotrexate** and **rituximab**.

Case history

A 35-year-old woman with a history of mild asthma in childhood (when she was diagnosed as being sensitive to aspirin) was seen in the Medical Outpatients Department because of sinus ache, some mild nasal stuffiness and itchy eyes. She had hay fever. For her asthma she was currently taking prn salbutamol (2 × 100 μg puffs) and beclomethasone 500 μg/day. She was given a prescription for an antihistamine, ketotifen 2 mg twice daily. She took the prescription to her local chemist rather than the hospital chemist, and started taking the tablets that day. She awoke in the early hours of the next morning very breathless and wheezy, and was rushed to hospital with acute severe bronchospasm requiring ventilation, but recovered. Fortunately, at the time of her admission her husband brought in all of the prescribed medications she was taking, and this led to her physicians establishing why she had deteriorated so suddenly.

Question
What led to this severe asthma attack? How could it have been avoided?

Answer
This patient was successfully treated with oxygen, IPPV, glucocorticosteroids and nebulized bronchodilators. Among her medications they found a bottle of ketoprofen (an NSAID) which she had started that morning (two 100 mg tablets twice a day). The pharmacist had not checked for NSAID sensitivity and the patient was not expecting an NSAID prescription after what the hospital doctor had told her about ketotifen. As the literature suggests, 2–7% of asthmatics are aspirin/NSAID sensitive, it is always important to check this with the patient.

On reviewing the prescription, the handwriting could have been thought to read 'ketoprofen', but the practitioner was adamant that she had written 'ketotifen'. The second issue in this case was a poorly written prescription for a drug with which the patient was unfamiliar, namely ketotifen, an antihistamine that may have additional cromoglicate-like properties, but whose anti-allergic effects have been disappointing in clinical practice. The importance of clearly written appropriate drug prescriptions cannot be over-emphasized. Computerized prescribing may minimize such errors in the future. Possible 'look-alike' drug pairs which have the potential for confusion include amiodarone and amlodipine, alprazolam and alprostadil, chlorpheniramine and chlorpromazine, digoxin and doxepin, esmolol and ethambutol, fexofenadine and fenfluramine, metoprolol and misoprostol, and omeprazole and omalizumab. Proprietary names further multiply the opportunities for 'sound-alike–look-alike' confusion.

FURTHER READING AND WEB MATERIAL

Barnes PJ. Drug therapy: inhaled glucocorticoids for asthma. *New England Journal of Medicine* 1995; **332**: 868–75.

British Thoracic Society; Scottish Intercollegiate Guidelines Network. British guideline on the management of asthma. *Thorax* 2003; **58** (Suppl. 1): s1–94 and www.sign.ac.uk/pdf/grg63.pdf

Currie GP, Srivastava P, Dempsey OJ, Lee DK. Therapeutic modulation of allergic airways disease with leukotriene receptor antagonists. *QJM: Monthly Journal of the Association of Physicians* 2005; **98**: 171–82.

O'Byrne PM, Parameswaran K. Pharmacological management of mild or moderate persistent asthma. *Lancet* 2006; **368**: 794–803.

Seddon P, Bara A, Ducharme FM, Lasserson TJ. Oral xanthines as maintenance treatment for asthma in children. *Cochrane Database of Systematic Reviews* 2006; (1):CD002885.

PART VI

THE ALIMENTARY SYSTEM

CHAPTER 34

ALIMENTARY SYSTEM AND LIVER

CONTRIBUTION BY DR DIPTI AMIN

PEPTIC ULCERATION

PATHOPHYSIOLOGY

Peptic ulcer disease affects approximately 10% of the population of western countries. The incidence of duodenal ulcer (DU) is four to five times higher than that of gastric ulcer (GU). Up to 1 million of the UK population suffer from peptic ulceration in a 12-month period. Its aetiology is not well understood, but there are four major factors of known importance:

1. acid–pepsin secretion;
2. mucosal resistance to attack by acid and pepsin;
3. non-steroidal anti-inflammatory drugs (NSAIDs);
4. the presence of *Helicobacter pylori*.

Key points

Peptic ulceration

- Affects 10% of the population.
- Duodenal ulcers are more common than gastric ulcers (4:1).
- Most gastric ulcers are related to *Helicobacter pylori* or NSAID therapy.
- Relapse is common.

ACID–PEPSIN SECRETION

Gastric parietal (oxyntic) cells secrete isotonic hydrochloric acid. Figure 34.1 illustrates the mechanisms that regulate gastric acid secretion. Acid secretion is stimulated by gastrin, acetylcholine and histamine. Gastrin is secreted by endocrine cells in the gastric antrum and duodenum. Zollinger–Ellison syndrome is an uncommon disorder caused by a gastrin-secreting adenoma associated with very severe peptic ulcer disease.

MUCOSAL RESISTANCE

Some endogenous mediators suppress acid secretion and protect the gastric mucosa. Prostaglandin E_2 (the principal prostaglandin synthesized in the stomach) is an important gastroprotective mediator. It inhibits secretion of acid, promotes secretion of protective mucus and causes vasodilatation of submucosal blood vessels. The gastric and duodenal mucosa is protected against acid–pepsin digestion by a mucus layer into which bicarbonate is secreted. Agents such as salicylate, ethanol and bile impair the protective function of this layer. Acid diffuses from the lumen into the stomach wall at sites of damage where the protective layer of mucus is defective. The presence of strong acid in the submucosa causes further damage, and persistence of H^+ ions in the interstitium initiates or perpetuates peptic ulceration. H^+ ions are cleared from the submucosa by diffusion into blood vessels and are then buffered in circulating blood. Local vasodilatation in the stomach wall is thus an important part of the protective mechanism against acid–pepsin damage.

NON-STEROIDAL ANTI-INFLAMMATORY DRUGS

Aspirin and other NSAIDs inhibit the biosynthesis of prostaglandin E_2, as well as causing direct irritation and damage to the gastric mucosa.

HELICOBACTER PYLORI

The presence of the bacterium *Helicobacter pylori* has now been established as a major causative factor in the aetiology of peptic ulcer disease. Although commonly found in the gastric antrum, it may also colonize other areas of the stomach, as well as patches of gastric metaplasia in the duodenum. *H. pylori* is present in all patients with active type B antral gastritis and in 90–95% of those with duodenal ulcers. After exclusion of gastric ulcers caused by non-steroidal anti-inflammatory drug therapy and Zollinger–Ellison syndrome, the incidence of *H. pylori* infection in patients with gastric ulcer approaches 100%. The strongest evidence of a causal relationship between *H. pylori* and peptic ulcer disease is the marked reduction in

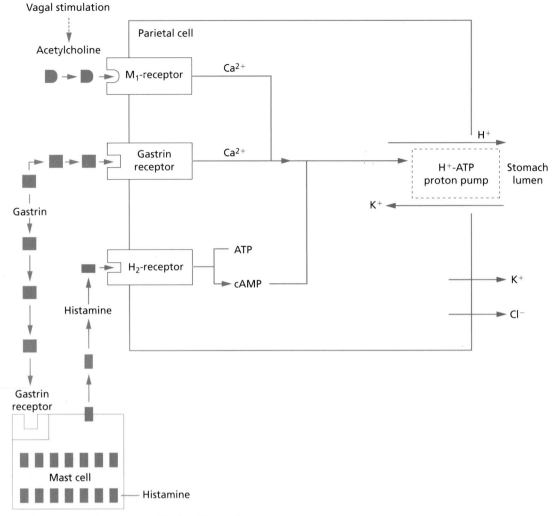

Figure 34.1: Mechanisms regulating hydrochloric acid secretion.

ulcer recurrence and complications following successful eradication of the organism. It has been shown that the speed of ulcer healing obtained with acid-suppressing agents is accelerated if *H. pylori* eradication is achieved concomitantly. Moreover, eradication of *H. pylori* infection prior to the commencement of NSAID therapy reduces the occurrence of gastro-duodenal ulcers in patients who have not had previous exposure to NSAIDs. *H. pylori* appears to be associated with increased risk of gastric cancer of the corpus and antrum.

Key points

Recommendations for eradication of *Helicobacter pylori*

- duodenal ulcer
- gastric ulcer
- mucosa-associated lymphoid tissue (MALT) lymphoma
- severe *H. pylori* gastritis.
- patients requiring long-term proton-pump inhibitor treatment (risk of accelerated gastric atrophy)
- blind treatment with eradication therapy is not recommended.

PRINCIPLES OF MANAGEMENT

The therapeutic objectives are as follows:

- symptomatic relief;
- promotion of ulcer healing;
- prevention of recurrence, once healing has occurred;
- prevention of complications.

GENERAL MANAGEMENT

- Stopping smoking increases the healing rate of gastric ulcers and is more effective in preventing the recurrence of duodenal ulcers than H_2-receptor antagonists.
- Diet is of symptomatic importance only. Patients usually discover for themselves which foods aggravate symptoms.
- Avoid 'ulcerogenic' drugs, including **caffeine** (as strong coffee or tea), alcohol, **aspirin** and other NSAIDs (**paracetamol** is a safe minor analgesic in these cases), and glucocorticosteroids.

- With regard to drug therapy, several drugs (see below) are effective. Documented duodenal or gastric ulcerations should be treated with an H_2-blocker or proton-pump inhibitor.
- Test for the presence of *H. pylori* by using the urease CLO test or antral biopsy at endoscopy.
- All suspected gastric ulcers should be endoscoped and biopsied to exclude malignancy, with repeat endoscopy following treatment, to confirm healing and for repeat biopsy.
- The current recommendation in relation to *H. pylori* is summarized above.

Key points
General management of peptic ulceration
• Stop smoking.
• Avoid ulcerogenic drugs (e.g. NSAIDs, alcohol, glucocorticosteroids).
• Reduce caffeine intake.
• Diet should be healthy (avoid obesity, and foods that give rise to symptoms).
• Test for the presence of *H. pylori*.

The choice of regimen used to eradicate *H. pylori* is based on achieving a balance between efficacy, adverse effects, compliance and cost. Most regimens include a combination of acid suppression and effective doses of two antibiotics. A typical regime for eradication of *H. pylori* is shown in Table 34.1.

Eradication should be confirmed, preferably by urea breath test at a minimum of four weeks post-treatment.

Non-steroidal anti-inflammatory drug-associated ulcer

NSAID-related ulcers will usually heal if the NSAID is withdrawn and a proton-pump inhibitor is prescribed for four weeks. If the NSAID has to be restarted (preferably after healing), H_2-receptor antagonists or proton-pump inhibitors or **misoprostol** (see below) should be co-prescribed. If *H. pylori* is present it should be eradicated.

Key points
Ulcer-healing drugs
Reduction of acidity:
• antacids;
• H_2-blockers;
• proton-pump inhibitors;
• muscarinic blockers (pirenzapine).
Mucosal protection:
• misoprostol (also reduces gastric acid secretion);
• bismuth chelate (also toxic to *H. pylori*);
• sucralfate;
• carbenoxolone (rarely prescribed).

Table 34.1: Typical triple therapy *Helicobacter pylori* eradication regime

Lansoprazole	30 mg bd	
Amoxicillin[a]	1 g bd	all for 1 week
Clarithromycin	500 mg bd	

[a] Metronidazole 400 mg bd if patient is allergic to penicillin.

DRUGS USED TO TREAT PEPTIC ULCERATION BY REDUCING ACIDITY

ANTACIDS

Use and adverse effects

Antacids have a number of actions which include neutralizing gastric acid and thus relieving associated pain and nausea, reducing delivery of acid into the duodenum following a meal, and inactivation of the proteolytic enzyme pepsin by raising the gastric pH above 4–5. In addition, it is thought that antacid may increase lower oesophageal sphincter tone and reduce oesophageal pressure.

A number of preparations are available and the choice will depend on the patient's preference, often determined by the effect on bowel habit (see Table 34.2).

In general terms, antacids should be taken approximately one hour before or after food, as this maximizes the contact time with stomach acid and allows the antacid to coat the stomach in the absence of food.

Drug interactions

Magnesium and aluminium salts can bind other drugs in the stomach, reducing the rate and extent of absorption of antibacterial agents such as **erythromycin, ciprofloxacin, isoniazid, norfloxacin, ofloxacin, pivampicillin, rifampicin** and most tetracyclines, as well as other drugs such as **phenytoin, itraconazole, ketoconazole, chloroquine, hydroxychloroquine**, phenothiazines, **iron** and **penicillamine**. They increase the excretion of **aspirin** (in alkaline urine).

H_2-RECEPTOR ANTAGONISTS

H_2-receptors stimulate gastric acid secretion and are also present in human heart, blood vessels and uterus (and probably brain). There are a number of competitive H_2-receptor antagonists in clinical use, which include **cimetidine** and **ranitidine**. The uses of these are similar and will be considered together in this section. Because each drug is so widely prescribed, separate sections on their individual adverse effects, pharmacokinetics and interactions are given below, followed by a brief consideration of the choice between them.

Use

1. H_2-receptor agonists are effective in healing both gastric and duodenal ulcers. A four-week course is usually

Table 34.2: Antacids

Antacid	Features	Adverse effects
Sodium bicarbonate	Rapid action	Produces carbon dioxide, causing belching and distension; excess can cause metabolic alkalosis; best avoided in renal and cardiovascular disease
Calcium carbonate	High acid–neutralizing capacity	Acid rebound; excess may cause hypercalcaemia and constipation
Magnesium salts (e.g. dihydroxide, carbonate, trisilicate)	Poor solubility, weak antacids; the trisilicates inactivate pepsin; increase lower oesophageal sphincter tone, and may be of use in reflux	Diarrhoea
Aluminium hydroxide	Forms an insoluble colloid in the presence of acid, and lines the gastric mucosa to provide a physical and chemical barrier; weak antacid, slow onset of action, inactivates pepsin	Constipation; absorption of dietary phosphate may lead to calcium depletion and negative calcium balance

adequate. Nearly all duodenal ulcers and most gastric ulcers that are not associated with NSAIDs are associated with *H. pylori*, which should be eradicated (see above). Most regimens include an H$_2$-receptor antagonist or a proton-pump inhibitor. It is essential to exclude carcinoma endoscopically, as H$_2$-blockers can improve symptoms caused by malignant ulcers. Without gastric acid, the functions of which include providing a barrier to infection, patients on H$_2$-antagonists and proton-pump inhibitors are predisposed to infection by enteric pathogens and the rate of bacterial diarrhoea is increased.

2. Oesophagitis may be treated with H$_2$-antagonists, but proton-pump inhibitors are more effective.
3. In cases of acute upper gastrointestinal haemorrhage and stress ulceration, the use of H$_2$-blockers is rational, although their efficacy has not been proven.
4. Replacement of pancreatic enzymes in steatorrhoea due to pancreatic insufficiency is often unsatisfactory due to destruction of the enzymes by acid and pepsin in the stomach. H$_2$-blockers improve the effectiveness of these enzymes in such cases.
5. In anaesthesia, H$_2$-receptor blockers can be given before emergency surgery to prevent aspiration of acid gastric contents, particularly in obstetric practice (Mendelson's syndrome).
6. The usual oral dose of **cimetidine** is 400 mg bd or 800 mg nocte, while for **ranitidine** it is 150 mg bd or 300 mg nocte to treat benign peptic ulceration.

CIMETIDINE

Cimetidine is well absorbed (70–80%) orally and is subject to a small hepatic first-pass effect. Intramuscular and intravenous injections produce equivalent blood levels. Diarrhoea,

rashes, dizziness, fatigue, constipation and muscular pain (usually mild and transient) have all been reported. Mental confusion can occur in the elderly. **Cimetidine** transiently increases serum prolactin levels, but the significance of this effect is unknown. Decreased libido and impotence have occasionally been reported during **cimetidine** treatment. Chronic cimetidine administration can cause gynaecomastia, which is reversible and appears with a frequency of 0.1–0.2%. Rapid intravenous injection of **cimetidine** has rarely been associated with bradycardia, tachycardia, asystole or hypotension. There have been rare reports of interstitial nephritis, urticaria and angioedema.

Drug interactions

1. Absorption of **ketoconazole** (which requires a low pH) and **itraconazole** is reduced by **cimetidine**.
2. Metabolism of several drugs is reduced by **cimetidine** due to inhibition of cytochrome P450, resulting in raised plasma drug concentrations. Interactions of potential clinical importance include those with **warfarin**, **theophylline**, **phenytoin**, **carbamazepine**, **pethidine** and other opioid analgesics, tricyclic antidepressants, **lidocaine** (**cimetidine**-induced reduction of hepatic blood flow is also a factor in this interaction), terfenadine, **amiodarone**, flecainide, **quinidine** and **fluorouracil**.
3. **Cimetidine** inhibits the renal excretion of **metformin** and **procainamide**, resulting in increased plasma concentrations of these drugs.

RANITIDINE

Ranitidine is well absorbed after oral administration, but its bioavailability is only 50%, suggesting that there is appreciable first-pass metabolism. Absorption is not affected by food.

Ranitidine has a similar profile of minor side effects to **cimetidine**. There have been some very rare reports of breast swelling and tenderness in men. However, unlike **cimetidine**, **ranitidine** does not bind to androgen receptors, and impotence and gynaecomastia in patients on high doses of **cimetidine** have been reported to resolve when they were switched to **ranitidine**. Cardiovascular effects have been even more infrequently reported than with **cimetidine**. Small amounts of **ranitidine** penetrate the central nervous system (CNS) and (like, but less commonly than, **cimetidine**) it can (rarely) cause mental confusion, mainly in the elderly and in patients with hepatic or renal impairment.

Drug interactions

Ranitidine has a lower affinity for cytochrome P450 than **cimetidine** and does not inhibit the metabolism of **warfarin**, **phenytoin** and **theophylline** to a clinically significant degree.

Choice of H₂-antagonist

All of the H_2-receptor antagonists currently available in the UK are effective in peptic ulceration and are well tolerated. **Cimetidine** and **ranitidine** are most commonly prescribed and have been available for the longest time. **Cimetidine** is the least expensive, but in young men who require prolonged treatment **ranitidine** may be preferable, due to a lower reported incidence of impotence and gynaecomastia. **Ranitidine** is also preferable in the elderly, where **cimetidine** occasionally causes confusion, and also when the patient is on drugs whose metabolism is inhibited by **cimetidine** (e.g. **warfarin**, **phenytoin** or **theophylline**).

Other H_2-receptor antagonists available for use in the UK include **famotidine** and **nizatidine**, but they offer no significant advantage over **ranitidine**.

PROTON-PUMP INHIBITORS

The proton-pump inhibitors inhibit gastric acid by blocking the H^+/K^+-adenosine triphosphatase enzyme system (the proton pump) of the gastric parietal cell. Examples are **omeprazole**, **esomeprazole**, **lansoprazole**, **pantoprazole** and **rabeprazole**. The main differences, if any, appear to be in relation to drug interactions. As yet there do not appear to be any clinically significant drug interactions with **pantoprazole**, whereas **omeprazole** inhibits cytochrome P450 and **lansoprazole** is a weak inducer of cytochrome P450. The indications for proton-pump inhibitors include the following:

* benign duodenal and gastric ulcers;
* NSAID-associated peptic ulcer and gastro-duodenal erosions;
* in combination with antibacterial drugs to eradicate *H. pylori*;
* Zollinger–Ellison syndrome;
* gastric acid reduction during general anaesthesia;
* gastro-oesophageal reflux disease (GORD);
* stricturing and erosive oesophagitis where they are the treatment of choice.

DRUGS THAT ENHANCE MUCOSAL RESISTANCE

PROSTAGLADIN ANALOGUES

Misoprostol is a synthetic analogue of prostaglandin E_1 which inhibits gastric acid secretion, causes vasodilatation in the submucosa and stimulates the production of protective mucus.

Uses

These include the following:

1. healing of duodenal ulcer and gastric ulcer, including those induced by NSAIDs;
2. prophylaxis of gastric and duodenal ulceration in patients on NSAID therapy.

Adverse effects

Diarrhoea, abdominal pain, nausea and vomiting, dyspepsia, flatulence, abnormal vaginal bleeding, rashes and dizziness may occur. The most frequent adverse effects are gastrointestinal and these are usually dose dependent.

Contraindications

Pregnancy (or desired pregnancy) is an absolute contraindication to the use of **misoprostol**, as the latter causes abortion.

BISMUTH CHELATE

Colloidal tripotassium dicitratobismuthate precipitates at acid pH to form a layer over the mucosal surface and ulcer base, where it combines with the proteins of the ulcer exudate. This coat is protective against acid and pepsin digestion. It also stimulates mucus production and may chelate with pepsin, thus speeding ulcer healing. Several studies have shown it to be as active as **cimetidine** in the healing of duodenal and gastric ulcers after four to eight weeks of treatment. It has a direct toxic effect on *H. pylori* and may be used as part of triple therapy.

Bismuth chelate elixir is given diluted with water 30 minutes before meals and two hours after the last meal of the day. This liquid has an ammoniacal, metallic taste and odour which is unacceptable to some patients, and chewable tablets can be used instead. Antacids or milk should not be taken concurrently.

Ranitidine bismuth citrate tablets are also available for the treatment of peptic ulcers and for use in *H. pylori* eradication regimes.

Adverse effects

Adverse effects include blackening of the tongue, teeth and stools (causing potential confusion with melaena) and nausea. The latter may limit dosing. Bismuth is potentially neurotoxic. Urine bismuth levels rise with increasing oral dosage, indicating some intestinal absorption. Although with normal doses the blood concentration remains well below the toxic threshold, bismuth should not be used in renal failure or for maintenance treatment.

SUCRALFATE

Use

Sucralfate is used in the management of benign gastric and duodenal ulceration and chronic gastritis. Its action is entirely local, with minimal if any systemic absorption. It is a basic aluminium salt of sucrose octasulphate which, in the presence of acid, becomes a sticky adherent paste that retains antacid efficacy. This material coats the floor of ulcer craters, exerting its acid-neutralizing properties locally, unlike conventional antacid gels which form a diffusely distributed antacid dispersion. In addition it binds to pepsin and bile salts and prevents their contact with the ulcer base. **Sucralfate** compares favourably with **cimetidine** for healing both gastric and duodenal ulcers, and is equally effective in symptom relief. The dose is 1 g (one tablet) four times daily for four to six weeks. Antacids may be given concurrently.

Adverse effects

Sucralfate is well tolerated but, because it contains aluminium, constipation can occur and in severe renal failure accumulation is a potential hazard.

Case history

A 75-year-old retired greengrocer who presented to the Accident and Emergency Department with shortness of breath and a history of melaena is found on endoscopy to have a bleeding gastric erosion. His drug therapy leading up to his admission consisted of digoxin, warfarin and piroxicam for a painful hip, and over-the-counter cimetidine self-initiated by the patient for recent onset indigestion.
Question
How may this patient's drug therapy have precipitated or aggravated his bleeding gastric erosion?
Answer
NSAIDs inhibit the biosynthesis of prostaglandin E_2, as well as causing direct damage to the gastric mucosa. Warfarin is an anticoagulant and will increase bleeding. Cimetidine inhibits CYP450 enzymes and therefore inhibits the metabolism of warfarin, resulting in higher blood concentrations and an increased anticoagulant effect.

OESOPHAGEAL DISORDERS

REFLUX OESOPHAGITIS

Reflux oesophagitis is a common problem. It causes heartburn and acid regurgitation and predisposes to stricture formation.

NON-DRUG MEASURES

Non-drug measures which may be useful include the following:

1. sleeping with the head of the bed raised. Most damage to the oesophagus occurs at night when swallowing is much reduced and acid can remain in contact with the mucosa for long periods;

2. avoiding:
   - large meals;
   - alcohol and/or food before bed;
   - smoking, which lowers the lower oesophageal sphincter pressure, and coffee;
   - **aspirin** and NSAIDs;
   - constricting clothing around the abdomen;
3. weight reduction;
4. bending from the knees and not the spine;
5. regular exercise.

DRUG THERAPY

Drugs that may be useful include the following:

1. **metoclopramide**, which increases oesophageal motility as well as being anti-emetic. It may also improve gastro-oesophageal sphincter function and accelerate gastric emptying;
2. a mixture of alginate and antacids is symptomatically useful – the alginate forms a viscous layer floating on the gastric contents;
3. symptomatic relief may be obtained with antacids, but there is a risk of chronic aspiration of poorly soluble particles of magnesium or aluminium salts if these are taken at night;
4. H_2-antagonists;
5. proton-pump inhibitors are the most effective agents currently available for reflux oesophagitis and are the drugs of choice for erosive reflux oesophagitis.

Case history

A 25-year-old male estate agent complains of intermittent heartburn, belching and sub-xiphisternal pain which has been present on most nights for two weeks. It was particularly severe the previous Saturday night after he had consumed a large curry and several pints of beer. The symptoms were not improved by sleeping on two extra pillows or by taking ibuprofen. He smokes ten cigarettes daily. Examination revealed him to be overweight, but was otherwise unremarkable.
Question
Outline your management of this patient.
Answer
Life-style advice – stop smoking, lose weight and exercise, adopt a low-fat diet, avoid tight clothing, avoid large meals or eating within three hours of going to bed. Raise the head of the bed (do not add pillows). Avoid NSAIDs and excessive alcohol.
Prescribe alginate/antacids.
If there is an inadequate response or early relapse, prescribe an H_2-blocker or proton-pump inhibitor for six weeks. If symptoms have still not completely resolved, refer the patient for endoscopy.

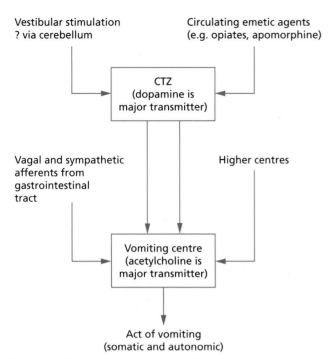

Vestibular stimulation
? via cerebellum

Circulating emetic agents
(e.g. opiates, apomorphine)

CTZ
(dopamine is
major transmitter)

Vagal and sympathetic
afferents from
gastrointestinal
tract

Higher centres

Vomiting centre
(acetylcholine is
major transmitter)

Act of vomiting
(somatic and autonomic)

Figure 34.2: The central mechanisms of vomiting.

ANTI-EMETICS

Complex processes underlie nausea and vomiting. Nausea is associated with autonomic effects (sweating, bradycardia, pallor and profuse salivary secretion). Vomiting is preceded by rhythmic muscular contractions of the 'respiratory' muscles of the abdomen (retching) and is a somatic rather than an autonomic function. Central co-ordination of these processes occurs in a group of cells in the dorsolateral reticular formation in the floor of the fourth ventricle of the medulla oblongata in close proximity to the cardiovascular and respiratory centres with which it has synaptic connections. This vomiting centre (Figure 34.2) is not directly responsive to chemical emetic stimuli, but is activated by one or more inputs. The major efferent pathways from the vomiting centre are the phrenic nerve, the visceral efferent of the vagus to the stomach and oesophagus, and the spinal nerves to the abdominal musculature.

An important receptor area for emetic stimuli, namely the chemoreceptor trigger zone (CTZ), is a group of neurones in the area postrema of the fourth ventricle which is sensitive to emetic stimuli such as radiation, bacterial toxins and uraemia. **Dopamine** excites CTZ neurones, which in turn activate the vomiting centre and cause emesis. Emetic stimuli originating in the pharynx, oesophagus and gut are transmitted directly to the vomiting centre via the vagus and glossopharyngeal nerves. Those from the vestibular organs (in travel sickness and Ménière's disease) act indirectly via the CTZ. A histamine pathway is apparently involved in labyrinthine vomiting.

Anti-emetic drugs can be classified pharmacologically as shown in Table 34.3. They should only be used when the cause of nausea or vomiting is known, otherwise the symptomatic relief produced could delay diagnosis of a remediable and

Table 34.3: Classification of anti-emetics

Anticholinergics (e.g. hyoscine)

Antihistamines (H_1-blockers) (e.g. promethazine)

Dopamine antagonists (e.g. metoclopramide)

Phenothiazines (e.g. prochlorperazine)

5-Hydroxytryptamine ($5HT_3$)-receptor antagonists (e.g. ondansetron)

Neurokinin antagonists (e.g. aprepitant)

Cannabinoids (e.g. nabilone)

Miscellaneous:

Glucocorticosteroids

Benzodiazepines

serious cause. Nausea and sickness during the first trimester of pregnancy will respond to most anti-emetics, but are rarely treated with drugs because of the possible dangers (currently unquantifiable) of teratogenesis.

Key points

Use of anti-emetics

- The cause of vomiting should be diagnosed.
- Symptomatic relief may delay investigation of the underlying cause.
- Treatment of the cause (e.g. diabetic ketoacidosis, intestinal obstruction, intracerebral space-occupying lesion) usually cures the vomiting.
- The choice of drug depends on the aetiology.

MUSCARINIC RECEPTOR ANTAGONISTS

These act partly by their antimuscarinic action on the gut, as well as by some central action. **Hyoscine** (0.3 mg) is effective in preventing motion sickness and is useful in single doses for short journeys, as the anticholinergic side effects make it unsuitable for chronic use. **Hyoscine** is an alternative to antihistamines and phenothiazines for the treatment of vertigo and nausea associated with Ménière's disease and middle ear surgery. Drowsiness, blurred vision, dry mouth and urinary retention are more common at therapeutic doses than is the case with antihistamines.

ANTIHISTAMINES (H_1-BLOCKERS)

These are most effective in preventing motion sickness and treating vertigo and vomiting caused by labyrinthine disorders. They have additional anticholinergic actions, and these contribute to their anti-emetic effect. They include **cyclizine**, **promethazine**, **betahistine** and **cinnarizine**. The main limitations of these drugs are their modest efficacy and common dose-related adverse effects, in addition to antimuscarinic effects.

- **Cyclizine** given either orally or by injection is effective in opiate-induced vomiting and has been given widely in pregnancy without any untoward effects on the fetus. The main side effects are drowsiness and a dry mouth.
- **Promethazine** is also an effective anti-emetic. It is more sedative than **cyclizine**.
- **Betahistine** is used in vertigo, tinnitus and hearing loss associated with Ménière's disease.
- **Cinnarizine** is an antihistamine and calcium antagonist. It has an action on the labyrinth and is effective in the treatment of motion sickness and vertigo.

DOPAMINE ANTAGONISTS

METOCLOPRAMIDE

Use

Metoclopramide is effective for:

- post-operative vomiting;
- radiation sickness;
- drug-induced nausea;
- migraine (see Chapter 23);
- diagnostic radiology of the small intestine is facilitated by **metoclopramide**, which reduces the time required for barium to reach the caecum and decreases the number of films required;
- facilitation of duodenal intubation and endoscopy;
- emergency anaesthesia (including that required in pregnancy) to clear gastric contents;
- symptoms of reflux oesophagitis may be improved, as it prevents nausea, regurgitation and reflux.

Adverse effects

Adverse effects are usually mild but can be severe. Extra-pyramidal effects (which occur in about 1% of patients) consist of dystonic effects including akathisia, oculogyric crises, trismus, torticollis and opisthotonos, but parkinsonian features are absent. These effects are more common in females and in the young. They are treated by stopping **metoclopramide** and giving **benztropine** or **diazepam** acutely if necessary (see also Chapter 21). Overdosage in infants has produced convulsions, hypertonia and irritability. Milder effects include dizziness, drowsiness, lassitude and bowel disturbances.

Mechanism of action

Metoclopramide increases the amount of acetylcholine released at post-ganglionic terminals.

It is a central dopamine antagonist and raises the threshold of the CTZ. It also decreases the sensitivity of the visceral nerves that carry impulses from the gut to the emetic centre. It is relatively ineffective in motion sickness and other forms of centrally mediated vomiting.

High doses of **metoclopramide** block $5HT_3$ receptors.

Pharmacokinetics

Metoclopramide is well absorbed orally and is also given by intravenous or intramuscular injection. It undergoes metabolism by dealkylation and amide hydrolysis, about 75% being excreted as metabolites in the urine. The mean plasma $t_{1/2}$ is four hours.

Drug interactions

Metoclopramide potentiates the extrapyramidal effects of phenothiazines and butyrophenones. Its effects on intestinal motility result in numerous alterations in drug absorption, including increased rates of absorption of several drugs such as **aspirin**, **tetracycline** and **paracetamol**.

DOMPERIDONE

Domperidone is a dopamine-receptor antagonist similar to **metoclopramide**. It does not penetrate the blood–brain barrier, however, and therefore seldom causes sedation or extrapyramidal effects. However, the CTZ lies functionally outside the barrier and thus **domperidone** is an effective anti-emetic which can logically be given with centrally acting dopamine agonists or **levodopa** or **apomorphine** to counter their emetogenic effect (see Chapter 21).

PHENOTHIAZINES

Use

Phenothiazines (see Chapter 20) act on the CTZ and larger doses depress the vomiting centre as well. Phenothiazines used as anti-emetics include **prochlorperazine**, **trifluoperazine**, **perphenazine** and **chlorpromazine**.

These are effective against opioid- and radiation-induced vomiting and are sometimes helpful in vestibular disturbances. They are least effective in the treatment of motion sickness. All of them carry a risk of extrapyramidal disturbances, dyskinesia and restlessness. **Perphenazine** is probably the most soporific of this group.

5-HYDROXYTRYPTAMINE ($5HT_3$)-RECEPTOR ANTAGONISTS

The serotonin ($5HT_3$)-receptor antagonists are highly effective in the management of acute nausea and vomiting due to cytotoxic chemotheraphy, although they offer little advantage for delayed emesis, occurring secondary to cytotoxic chemotherapy and radiotherapy. They are also effective in the treatment of post-operative nausea and vomiting.

Their exact site of action is uncertain. It may be peripheral at abdominal visceral afferent neurones, or central within the area postrema of the brain, or a combination of both.

Examples include **ondansetron**, **granisetron**, **dolasetron** and **tropisetron**.

CANNABINOIDS

Cannabis and its major constituent, D-9-tetrahydrocannabinol (THC), have anti-emetic properties and have been used to prevent vomiting caused by cytotoxic therapy. In an attempt to reduce side effects and increase efficacy, a number of analogues, including **nabilone**, have been synthesized. The site of action of **nabilone** is not known, but an action on cortical centres affecting vomiting via descending pathways seems probable. There is some evidence that opioid pathways are involved in these actions. They are only moderately effective.

Adverse effects

Adverse effects include sedation, confusion, loss of coordination, dry mouth and hypotension. These effects are more prominent in older patients.

MISCELLANEOUS AGENTS

Large doses of glucocorticosteroids exert some anti-emetic action when used with cytotoxic drugs and the efficacy of the $5HT_3$-antagonists has been shown to be improved when concomitant **dexamethasone** is given. Their mode of action is not known. Benzodiazepines given before treatment with cytotoxics reduce vomiting, although whether this is a specific anti-emetic action or a reduction in anxiety is unknown.

INFLAMMATORY BOWEL DISEASE

Mediators of the inflammatory response in ulcerative colitis and Crohn's disease include kinins and prostaglandins. The latter stimulate adenylyl cyclase, which induces active ion secretion and thus diarrhoea. Synthesis of prostaglandin E_2, thromboxane A_2 and prostacyclin by the gut increases during disease activity, but not during remission. The aminosalicylates influence the synthesis and metabolism of these eicosanoids, and influence the course of disease activity.

Apart from correction of dehydration, nutritional and electrolyte imbalance (which in an acute exacerbation is potentially life-saving) and other non-specific treatment, glucocorticosteroids, aminosalicylates and immunosuppressive drugs are valuable.

GLUCOCORTICOSTEROIDS

Steroids modify every part of the inflammatory response and glucocorticosteroids (see Chapter 40) remain the standard by which other drugs are judged. **Prednisolone** and **hydrocortisone** given orally or intravenously are of proven value in the treatment of acute colitis or exacerbation of Crohn's disease. Topical therapy in the form of a rectal drip, foam or enema of **hydrocortisone** or **prednisolone** is very effective in milder attacks of ulcerative colitis and Crohn's colitis; some systemic absorption may occur.

Diffuse inflammatory bowel disease or disease that does not respond to local therapy may require oral glucocorticosteroid treatment, e.g. **prednisolone** for four to eight weeks. **Prednisolone** is preferred to **hydrocortisone** as it has less mineralocorticoid effect at equipotent anti-inflammatory doses. Modified-release **budesonide** is licensed for Crohn's disease affecting the ileum and the ascending colon; it causes fewer systemic side effects than oral **prednisolone**, due to extensive hepatic first-pass metabolism, but may be less effective. Glucocorticosteroids are not suitable for maintenance treatment because of side effects.

AMINOSALICYLATES

5-Aminosalicylic acid (5ASA) acts at many points in the inflammatory process and has a local effect on the colonic mucosa. However, as it is very readily absorbed from the small intestine, it has to be attached to another compound or coated in resin to ensure that it is released in the large bowel. Although these drugs are only effective for controlling mild to moderate ulcerative colitis when given orally, they are very effective for reducing the incidence of relapse per year from about 70 to 20%. The aminosalicylates are not effective in small-bowel Crohn's disease. For rectosigmoid disease, suppository or enema preparations are as effective as systemic steroids.

Drugs currently available in this group are **sulfasalazine**, **mesalazine**, **balsalazide** and **olsalazine**. **Sulfasalazine** remains the standard agent, but **mesalazine**, **balsalazide** and **olsalazine** avoid the unwanted effects of the sulphonamide carrier molecule (sulphapyridine) of **sulfasalazine**, while delivering 5ASA to the colon. Although usually well tolerated, the adverse effects of **sulfasalazine** are nausea, vomiting, epigastric discomfort, headache and rashes (including toxic dermal necrolysis). All of the adverse effects associated with sulphonamides can occur with **sulfasalazine**, and they are more pronounced in slow acetylators. Toxic effects on red cells are common (70% of cases) and in some cases lead to haemolysis, anisocytosis and methaemoglobinaemia. **Sulfasalazine** should be avoided in patients with glucose-6-phosphate dehydrogenase (G6PD) deficiency. Temporary oligospermia with decreased sperm motility and infertility occurs in up to 70% of males who are treated for over three years. Uncommon adverse effects include pancreatitis, hepatitis, fever, thrombocytopenia, agranulocytosis, Stevens–Johnson syndrome, neurotoxicity, photosensitization, a systemic lupus erythematosus (SLE)-like syndrome, myocarditis, pulmonary fibrosis, and renal effects including proteinuria, haematuria, orange urine and nephrotic syndrome.

The newer agents are useful in patients who cannot tolerate **sulfasalazine** and in men who wish to remain fertile.

Key points

Aminosalicylates and blood dyscrasias

- Any patient who is receiving aminosalicylates must be advised to report unexplained bleeding, bruising, purpura, sore throat, fever or malaise.
- If the above symptoms occur, a blood count should be performed.
- If there is suspicion of blood dyscrasia, stop aminosalicylates.
- Aminosalicylates are associated with agranulocytosis, aplastic anaemia, leukopenia, neutropenia and thrombocytopenia.

IMMUNOSUPPRESSIVE DRUGS

Although the exact pathogenetic mechanisms involved in inflammatory bowel disease remain unclear, there is abundant evidence that the immune system (both cellular and humoral) is activated in the intestine of patients with inflammatory bowel disease. This forms the rationale for the use of immuno-suppressive agents in the group of patients who do not respond to therapy with aminosalicylates or glucocorticosteroids. General indications for their use include patients who have been on steroids for more than six months despite efforts to taper them off, those who have frequent relapses, those with chronic continuous disease activity and those with Crohn's disease with recurrent fistulas. Patients with ulcerative colitis may benefit from a short course of **ciclosporin** (unlicensed indication). Patients with unresponsive or chronically active inflammatory bowel disease may benefit from **azathioprine** or **mercaptopurine**, or (in the case of Crohn's disease) once-weekly **methotrexate** (these are all unlicensed indications).

Infliximab, a monoclonal antibody that inhibits tumour nerosis factor α (see Chapters 16 and 26) is licensed for the management of severe active Crohn's disease and moderate to severe ulcerative colitis in patients whose condition has not responded adequately to treatment with a glucocorticosteroid and a conventional immunosuppressant or who are intolerant of them. **Infliximab** is also licensed for the management of refractory fistulating Crohn's disease. Maintenance therapy with **infliximab** should be considered for patients who respond to the initial induction course.

OTHER THERAPIES

Metronidazole may be beneficial for the treatment of active Crohn's disease with perianal involvement, possibly through its antibacterial activity. It is usually given for a month, but no longer than three months because of concerns about develop-ing peripheral neuropathy. Other antibacterials should be given if specifically indicated (e.g. sepsis associated with fis-tulas and perianal disease) and for managing bacterial over-growth in the small bowel.

Antimotility drugs such as **codeine** and **loperamide** (see below) and antispasmodic drugs may precipitate paralytic ileus and megacolon in active ulcerative colitis; treatment of the inflammation is more logical. Laxatives may be required in proctitis. Diarrhoea resulting from the loss of bile-salt absorp-tion (e.g. in terminal ileal disease or bowel resection) may improve with **colestyramine**, which binds bile salts.

> **Key points**
>
> Inflammatory bowel disease
> The cause is unknown.
> There is local and sometimes systemic inflammation.
>
> - Correct dehydration, nutritional and electrolyte imbalance.
> - Drug therapy: aminosalicylates; glucocorticosteroids; other immunosuppressive agents.

CONSTIPATION

When constipation occurs, it is important first to exclude both local and systemic disease which may be responsible for the symptoms. Also, it is important to remember that many drugs can cause constipation (Table 34.4).

In general, patients with constipation present in two ways:

1. Long-standing constipation in otherwise healthy people may be due to decreased colon motility or to dyschezia, or to a combination of both. It is usually sufficient to reassure the patient and to instruct them in the importance of re-establishing a regular bowel habit. This should be combined with an increased fluid intake and increased bulk in the diet. Bran is cheap and often satisfactory. As an alternative, non-absorbed bulk substances such as **methylcellulose**, **ispaghula** or **sterculia** are helpful. The other laxatives described below should only be tried if these more 'natural' treatments fail.

2. Loaded colon or faecal impaction – sometimes it is necessary to evacuate the bowel before it is possible to start re-education, particularly in the elderly or those who are ill. In these cases, a laxative such as **senna** combined with **glycerol suppositories** is appropriate.

Table 34.4: Drugs that can cause constipation

Aluminium hydroxide
Amiodarone
Anticholinergics (older antihistamines)
Diltiazem
Disopyramide
Diuretics
Iron preparations
Opioids
Tricyclic antidepressants
Verapamil

LAXATIVES

Laxatives are still widely although often inappropriately used by the public and in hospital. There is now a greater know-ledge of intestinal pathophysiology, and of outstanding import-ance is the finding that the fibre content of the diet has a marked regulatory action on gut transit time and motility and on defecation performance.

As a general rule, laxatives should be avoided. They are employed:

- if straining at stool will cause damage (e.g. post-operatively, in patients with haemorrhoids or after myocardial infarction);

- in hepatocellular failure to reduce formation and/or absorption of neurotoxins produced in the bowel;
- occasionally in drug-induced constipation.

BULK LAXATIVES

Plant fibre

Plant fibre is the portion of the walls of plant cells that resists digestion in the intestine. The main effect of increasing the amount of fibre in the diet is to increase the bulk of the stools and decrease the bowel transit time; this is probably due to the ability of fibre to take up water and swell. Fibre also binds organic molecules, including bile salts. It does not increase the effective caloric content of the diet, as it is not digested or absorbed.

The main uses of plain fibre (e.g. bran) are as follows:

- in constipation, particularly if combined with a spastic colon. By increasing the bulk of the intestinal contents, fibre slowly distends the wall of the colon, and this causes an increase in useful propulsive contraction. The main result is a return of the large bowel function towards normal. Similar results are obtained in diverticular disease in which there is colon overactivity associated with a high intraluminal pressure.
- the proposed effects of fibre in preventing large-bowel carcinoma, piles, appendicitis, coronary artery disease and varicose veins are still speculative.

The starting 'dose' of bran is a dessertspoonful daily and this can be increased at weekly intervals until a satisfactory result is obtained. It may be mixed with food, as it is difficult to swallow if taken 'neat'.

Adverse effects and contraindications

Bran usually causes some flatulence which is dose related. Phytates in bran could theoretically bind calcium and zinc ions. Bran should be avoided in gluten enteropathy and is contraindicated in bowel obstruction.

Other bulk laxatives

Methylcellulose takes up water in the bowel and swells, thus stimulating peristalsis. It is a reasonable substitute if bran is not satisfactory.

OSMOTIC AGENTS

For many years, these have been thought to act by retaining fluid in the bowel by virtue of the osmotic activity of their unabsorbed ions. The increased bulk in the lumen would then stimulate peristalsis. However, 5 g of **magnesium sulphate** would be isotonic in only 130 mL and acts within one to two hours, well before it could have reached the colon, so mechanisms other than osmotic effects must account for its laxative properties. It has been postulated that, because magnesium ions can also contract the gall-bladder, relax the sphincter of Oddi and increase gastric, intestinal and pancreatic enzyme secretion, they may act indirectly via cholecystokinin.

Magnesium ions themselves may also have direct pharmacological effects on intestinal function.

Magnesium sulphate (Epsom salts) and other magnesium salts are useful where rapid bowel evacuation is required. It should be remembered that a certain amount of magnesium may be absorbed, and accumulation can occur in renal failure.

Macrogols are inert polymers of ethylene glycol which sequester fluid in the bowel; giving fluid with macrogols may reduce the dehydrating effect sometimes seen with osmotic laxatives.

Phosphate enemas are useful in bowel clearance before radiology, endoscopy and surgery.

Lactulose is a disaccharide which passes through the small intestine unchanged, but in the colon is broken down by carbohydrate-fermenting bacteria to unabsorbed organic anions (largely acetic and lactic acids) which retain fluid in the gut lumen and also make the colonic contents more acid. This produces a laxative effect after two to three days. It is effective and well tolerated, but relatively expensive. It is of particular value in the treatment of hepatic encephalopathy, as it discourages the proliferation of ammonia-producing organisms and the absorption of ammonia.

LUBRICANTS AND STOOL SOFTENERS

These agents were formerly believed to act by softening or lubricating the faeces, but they act at least in part in a similar manner to stimulant purgatives by inhibiting intestinal electrolyte transport.

DIOCTYL SODIUM SULPHOSUCCINATE

Dioctyl sodium sulphosuccinate is a surface-active agent that acts on hard faecal masses and allows more water to penetrate the mass and thus soften it. Its use should be confined to patients with faecal impaction, and it should not be given over long periods.

ARACHIS OIL

Enemas containing **arachis oil** lubricate and soften impacted faeces and promote a bowel movement.

CHEMICAL STIMULANTS

Many of the agents in this class (e.g. **castor oil, phenolphthalein**) are now obsolete because of their toxicity, but **senna, co-danthramer** and **bisacodyl** are still useful if bulk laxatives are ineffective. **Glycerol** suppositories act as a rectal stimulant due to the local irritant action of **glycerol** and are useful if a rapid effect is required. Phosphate enemas are similarly useful.

LAXATIVE ABUSE

Persistent use of laxatives, particularly in increasing doses, causes ill health.

After prolonged use of stimulant laxatives, the colon becomes dilated and atonic with diminished activity. The cause is not clear, but this effect is perhaps due to damage to the intrinsic nerve plexus of the colon. The disorder of bowel motility may improve after withdrawing the laxative and using a high-residue diet.

Some people, mainly women, take purgatives secretly. This probably bears some relationship to disorders such as anorexia nervosa that are concerned with weight loss, and is also associated with self-induced vomiting and with diuretic abuse. The clinical and biochemical features can closely mimic Bartter's syndrome and this possibility should always be investigated in patients in whom the diagnosis of this rare disorder is entertained, especially adults in whom true Bartter's syndrome almost never arises de novo. Features include:

- sodium depletion – hypotension, cramps, secondary hyperaldosteronism;
- potassium depletion – weakness, polyuria and nocturia and renal damage.

In addition, there may be features suggestive of enteropathy and osteomalacia.

Diagnosis and treatment are difficult; melanosis coli may provide a diagnostic clue. Urinary electrolyte determinations may help, but can be confounded if the patient is also surreptitiously taking diuretics.

Case history

A 70-year-old woman who was previously very active but whose mobility has recently been limited by osteoarthritis of the knees and hips sees her general practitioner because of a recent change in bowel habit from once daily to once every three days. Her current medication includes regular co-codamol for her osteoarthritis, oxybutynin for urinary frequency, aluminium hydroxide prn for dyspepsia, and bendroflumethiazide and verapamil for hypertension. Following bowel evacuation with a phosphate enema, proctoscopy and colonoscopy are reported as normal.
Question
Which of this patient's medications may have contributed to her constipation?
Answer

- Co-codamol, which contains an opioid–codeine phosphate.
- Aluminium hydroxide.
- Bendroflumethiazide.
- Verapamil.
- Oxybutynin (an anticholinergic).

DIARRHOEA

The most important aspect of the treatment of acute diarrhoea is the maintenance of fluid and electrolyte balance, particularly in children and in the elderly. In non-pathogenic diarrhoea or viral gastroenteritis, antibiotics and antidiarrhoeal drugs are best avoided. Initial therapy should be with oral rehydration preparations (such as Dioralyte® or Electrolade®), which contain electrolytes and glucose. Antibiotic treatment is indicated for patients with systemic illness and evidence of bacterial infection.

Adjunctive symptomatic treatment is sometimes indicated. Two main types of drug may be employed, that either decrease intestinal transit time or increase the bulk and viscosity of the gut contents.

DRUGS THAT DECREASE INTESTINAL TRANSIT TIME

OPIOIDS

For more information on opioid use, see Chapter 25.

Codeine is widely used for this purpose in doses of 15–60 mg. **Morphine** is also given, usually as a **kaolin** and **morphine** mixture. **Diphenoxylate** is related to **pethidine** and also has structural similarities to anticholinergic drugs. It may cause drug dependence and euphoria and is usually prescribed as 'Lomotil' (diphenoxylate plus atropine). Overdose with this drug in children causes features of both opioid and atropine intoxication and may be fatal.

LOPERAMIDE

Loperamide is an effective, well-tolerated antidiarrhoeal agent. It antagonizes peristalsis, possibly by antagonizing acetylcholine release in the intramural nerve plexus of the gut, although non-cholinergic effects may also be involved. It is poorly absorbed and probably acts directly on the bowel. The dose is 4 mg initially, followed by 2 mg after each loose stool up to a total dose of 16 mg/day. Adverse effects are unusual, but include dry mouth, dizziness, skin rashes and gastric disturbances. Excessive use (especially in children) is to be strongly discouraged.

DRUGS THAT INCREASE BULK AND VISCOSITY OF GUT CONTENTS

Adsorbents, such as **kaolin**, are not recommended for diarrhoea. Bulk-forming drugs, such as **ispaghula**, **methylcellulose** and **sterculia** are useful in controlling faecal consistency in ileostomy and colostomy, and in controlling diarrhoea associated with diverticular disease.

TRAVELLERS' DIARRHOEA

This is a syndrome of acute watery diarrhoea lasting for one to three days and associated with vomiting, abdominal cramps and other non-specific symptoms, resulting from infection by one of a number of enteropathogens, the most common being enterotoxigenic *Escherichia coli*. It probably reflects colonization of the bowel by 'unfamiliar' organisms. Because of the variable nature of the pathogen, there is no specific treatment.

Ciprofloxacin is occasionally used for prophylaxis against travellers' diarrhoea, but routine use is not recommended due to consequent encouragement of bacterial resistance. Lactobacillus preparations have not been shown to be effective. Early treatment of diarrhoea with **ciprofloxacin** will control the great majority of cases and this, together with oral replacement of salts and water, is the currently preferred approach.

PSEUDOMEMBRANOUS COLITIS

Broad-spectrum antibacterial drug therapy is sometimes associated with superinfection of the intestine with toxin-producing *Clostridium difficile*. Debilitated and immunosuppressed patients are at particular risk. The infection can be transmitted from person to person. Withdrawal of the antibacterial drug and the introduction of oral **metronidazole** or **vancomycin** should be instituted.

IRRITABLE BOWEL SYNDROME

This motility disorder of the gut affects approximately 10% of the population. Although the symptoms are mostly colonic, patients with the syndrome have abnormal motility throughout the gut and this may be precipitated by dietary items, such as alcohol or wheat flour. The important management principles are first to exclude a serious cause for the symptoms and then to determine whether exclusion of certain foods or alcohol would be worthwhile. An increase in dietary fibre over the course of several weeks may also reduce the symptoms. Psychological factors may be important precipitants and counselling may be helpful. Drug treatment is symptomatic and often disappointing.

- Anticholinergic drugs, such as **hyoscine**, have been used for many years, although evidence of their efficacy is lacking. The oral use of better absorbed anticholinergics, such as **atropine**, is limited by their side effects.
- **Mebeverine** (135 mg before meals three times daily) directly relaxes intestinal smooth muscle without anticholinergic effects. Its efficacy is marginal.
- **Peppermint** oil relaxes intestinal smooth muscle and is given in an enteric-coated capsule which releases its contents in the distal small bowel. It is given before meals three times daily.
- Antidiarrhoeal drugs, such as **loperamide**, reduce associated diarrhoea.
- Psychotropic drugs, such as antipsychotics and antidepressants with anticholinergic properties, have also been effective in some patients. In general, however, they should be avoided for such a chronic and benign condition because of their serious adverse effects (see Chapters 19 and 20).

PANCREATIC INSUFFICIENCY

It is important to remember that, amongst the many causes of pancreatitis, certain drugs can very occasionally be an aetiological factor (Table 34.5).

Exocrine pancreatic insufficiency is an important cause of steatorrhoea. The pancreas has a large functional reserve and malabsorption does not usually occur until enzyme output is reduced to 10% or less of normal. This type of malabsorption is usually treated by replacement therapy with pancreatic extracts (usually of porcine origin). Unfortunately, although useful, these preparations rarely abolish steatorrhoea. A number of preparations are available, but the enzyme activity varies between preparations – one with a high lipase activity is most likely to reduce steatorrhoea. Unfortunately, less than 10% of the lipase activity and 25% of the tryptic activity is recoverable from the duodenum regardless of the dose schedule. This limited effectiveness of oral enzymes is partly due to acid–peptic inactivation in the stomach and duodenum. H$_2$-antagonists decrease both acidity and volume of secretion and retard the inactivation of exogenous pancreatic enzymes. They are given as an adjunct to these preparations.

Supplements of **pancreatin** are given to compensate for reduced or absent exocrine secretion in cystic fibrosis, pancreatectomy, total gastrectomy and chronic pancreatitis. **Pancreatin** is inactivated by gastric acid and therefore preparations are best taken with or immediately before or after food. Gastric acid secretion can be reduced by giving an H$_2$-blocker about one hour beforehand, or antacids may be given concurrently to reduce acidity.

Pancreatin is inactivated by heat and, if mixed with liquids or food, excessive heat should be avoided. The dose is adjusted according to size, number and consistency of stools such that the patient thrives.

Pancreatin can irritate the perioral skin and buccal mucosa if it is retained in the mouth and excessive doses can cause perianal irritation. The most frequent side effects are gastrointestinal ones including nausea, vomiting and abdominal discomfort. Hyperuricaemia and hyperuricuria have been associated with very high doses of the drug.

Table 34.5: Drugs that are associated with pancreatitis (this is uncommon)

Asparaginase	Oestrogens
Azathioprine	Pentamidine
Corticosteroids	Sodium valporate
Dideoxyinosine (DDI)	Sulphonamides and
Ethanol	sulfasalazine
	Tetracycline
	Thiazides

LIVER DISEASE

PRINCIPLES UNDERLYING DRUG TREATMENT OF HEPATIC ENCEPHALOPATHY AND LIVER FAILURE

In severe liver dysfunction, neuropsychiatric changes occur and can progress to coma. The mechanism which produces these changes is not established, but it is known that in hepatic coma and pre-coma, the blood ammonia concentration increases. In many patients, the time-course of encephalopathy parallels the rise in blood ammonia concentrations. Orally administered nitrogenous compounds (e.g. protein, amino acids, ammonium chloride) yield ammonia in the gut, raise blood ammonia concentrations and provoke encephalopathy. The liver is the only organ that extracts ammonia from the blood and converts it to urea. Bacterial degradation products of nitrogenous material within the gut enter the systemic circulation because of a failure of first-pass hepatic extraction (due to hepatocellular damage), or due to bypass of the hepatocytes by collateral circulation or intrahepatic shunting. Another source is urea, which undergoes enterohepatic circulation and yields approximately 3.5 g/day of ammonia (see Figure 34.3).

Ammonia diffuses into the blood across the large intestine epithelium, where it is trapped by becoming ionized due to the lower pH of blood compared to colonic contents. Ammonia is not the only toxin involved, as perhaps 20% of patients with encephalopathy have normal blood ammonia concentrations, and methionine can provoke encephalopathy without causing a significant rise in blood ammonia concentration. Furthermore, ammonia toxicity affects the cortex but not the brainstem, which is also involved in encephalopathy.

Other toxins of potential relevance include the following:

- Intestinal bacterial decarboxylation produces hydroxyphenyl amines, such as octopamine (from tyramine), which could replace normal transmitters at nerve endings in the central and peripheral nervous systems, thus acting as 'false transmitters' and changing the balance of inhibition and excitation at central synapses.

- Changes in fatty acid metabolism increase plasma free fatty acids, some of which have anaesthetic properties. In addition, these determine the availability of tryptophan to the brain and hence have an effect on 5-hydroxytryptamine synthesis.

Glutathione synthesis is impaired in severe liver disease. Cellular damage due to free radical excess can produce multi-organ dysfunction. Intravenous administration of **acetylcysteine** is used prophylactically in some centres to enhance glutathione synthesis and thereby reduce oxidant (free radical) stresses by scavenging these reactive entities.

Treatment of hepatic encephalopathy includes the following measures:

- dietary protein restriction to as little as 20 g/day, while ensuring an adequate intake of essential amino acids;
- emptying the lower bowel by means of enemas and purgatives to reduce the bacterial production of ammonia;
- oral or rectal administration of non-absorbable antibiotics, such as **neomycin**, to reduce the bacterial population of the large bowel. **Neomycin**, 1–2 g four times daily, is often used. It should be remembered, if the patient also has renal impairment, that **neomycin** may accumulate and produce toxicity;
- oral lactulose improves encephalopathy. This disaccharide is not a normal dietary constituent and humans do not possess a lactulase enzyme, so lactulose is neither digested nor absorbed but reaches the colon unchanged, where the bacterial flora breaks it down to form lactate, acetate and other acid products. These trap ammonia and other toxins within the intestinal lumen by reducing its pH, and in addition they act as a cathartic and reduce ammonia absorption by reducing the colonic transit time;
- bleeding may occur due to interference with clotting factor synthesis or thrombocytopenia. Vitamin K is given and fresh frozen plasma or platelets are used as required. H_2 antagonists (e.g. **ranitidine**) or proton-pump inhibitors (e.g. **omeprazole**) are often used to prevent gastric erosions and bleeding;
- sedatives should be avoided as patients with liver disease are extremely sensitive to such drugs. If sedation is essential (e.g. because of agitation due to alcohol

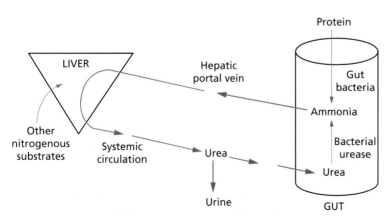

Figure 34.3: Enterohepatic circulation of urea and ammonia.

withdrawal), small doses of benzodiazepines that are metabolized to inactive glucuronide conjugates, e.g. **oxazepam** are preferred to those with longer-lived metabolites. The hazards of narcotic analgesics to the patient with acute or chronic liver disease cannot be over-emphasized;

- prophylactic broad-spectrum intravenous antibiotics, especially if there is evidence of infection (e.g. spontaneous peritonitis);
- intravenous **acetylcysteine** (the precise value of this has not yet been fully confirmed).

Key points

Treatment of hepatic encephalopathy

- Supportive.
- Measures to reduce absorption of ammonia from the gut (e.g. low-protein diet, lactulose ± neomycin).
- Prophylactic broad spectrum antibiotics, prompt treatment of infection.
- Prophylactic vitamin K.
- Fresh frozen plasma/platelets as indicated.
- H_2 antagonist (e.g. ranitidine) or proton-pump inhibitor (e.g. omeprazole) to prevent gastric erosions and bleeding.
- i.v. acetylcysteine (unproven).
- Avoidance of sedatives, potassium-losing diuretics, opioids, drugs that cause constipation and hepatotoxic drugs whenever possible.

DRUG THERAPY OF PORTAL HYPERTENSION AND OESOPHAGEAL VARICES

Oesophageal varices form a collateral circulation in response to raised blood pressure in the portal system and are of clinical importance because of their tendency to bleed. Two-thirds of patients with varices die as a result and of these, one-third die of the first bleed, one-third rebleed within six weeks and only one-third survive for one year. Sclerotherapy and surgical shunt procedures are the mainstay of treatment, and drug therapy must be judged against these gloomy survival figures. In addition to resuscitation, volume replacement and, when necessary, balloon tamponade using a Sengstaken–Blakemore tube, the emergency treatment of bleeding varices may include vasoconstrictor drugs, e.g **vasopressin** analogues. These reduce portal blood flow through splanchnic arterial constriction.

Drugs currently used for the management of acute variceal haemorrhage include **octreotide** (the long-acting analogue of **somatostatin**), **vasopressin** and **terlipressin** (a derivative of **vasopressin**). **Terlipressin** and **octreotide** are used to reduce portal pressure urgently, to control bleeding before more definitive treatment, such as sclerotherapy or variceal banding. Beta-blockers and vasodilators, such as nitrates, are used for long-term therapy to reduce portal pressure. **Somatostatin** and its long-acting analogue **octreotide** reduce blood flow and cause a significant reduction in variceal pressure without effects on the systemic vasculature. To date, a clear-cut response in variceal bleeding has not been demonstrated. Side effects include vomiting, anorexia, abdominal pain, diarrhoea, headache and dizziness. Newer vasoactive drugs, such as **terlipressin**, appear to have a better therapeutic index and fewer side effects, although **terlipressin** has a short half-life and needs to be administered frequently or as an infusion.

A number of trials have demonstrated efficacy of non-cardioselective beta-adrenergic antagonists (**propranolol**, **nadolol**) in reducing the incidence of gastro-intestinal bleeding in patients with portal hypertension, especially in combination with endoscopic sclerotherapy.

MANAGEMENT OF CHRONIC VIRAL HEPATITIS

Chronic viral hepatitis is associated with chronic liver disease, cirrhosis and hepatocellular carcinoma. The carrier rate for hepatitis B in the UK is 0.1–1% (it is particularly prevalent in socially deprived areas of inner cities) and the seroprevalence for hepatitis C is 0.1–0.7%. Chronic viral hepatitis is diagnosed when there is evidence of continuing hepatic damage and infection for at least six months after initial viral infection. In hepatitis C, the liver function may remain normal for months to years, while the patient's blood remains infectious (confirmed by hepatitis C virus RNA detection). The course of the liver damage often fluctuates. While up to 90% of patients with acute hepatitis B clear the virus spontaneously, up to 60% of those with hepatitis C virus do not do so. About 20% of those with chronic active hepatitis progress insidiously to cirrhosis, and about 2–3% go on to develop hepatocellular carcinoma.

Hepatitis B virus is a DNA virus that is not directly cytopathic and hepatic damage occurs as a result of the host immune response. Hepatocytes infected with hepatitis B virus produce a variety of viral proteins, of which the 'e' antigen (HBeAg) is clinically the most important. HBeAg is a marker for continued viral replication and therefore for infectivity. Hepatitis C virus is a single-stranded RNA virus. Controlled trials have shown that **interferon-alfa**, **lamivudine** (a nucleoside analogue inhibitor of viral DNA polymerase) and **adefovir dipivoxil** (a phosphorylated nucleotide analogue inhibitor of viral DNA polymerases) are beneficial in reducing the viral load in patients with chronic hepatitis B virus infection. Pegylated interferon alfa-2a (**peginterferon alfa-2a**) may be preferred to interferon alfa. Pegylation (polyethylene glycol-conjugation) prolongs the interferon half-life in the blood, allowing subcutaneous once weekly dosing. The National Institute of Health and Clinical Excellence (NICE) has recommended **adefovir** as an option in chronic hepatitis B if **interferon** is unsuccessful, if relapse occurs following successful initial interferon treatment, or if interferon is poorly tolerated or contraindicated (see Chapters 45 and 46).

In chronic hepatitis C, the combination of **peginterferon alfa** and **ribavarin** (see Chapter 45) is recommended. Details on the regimens can be found at www.nice.org.uk/TA075.

Table 34.6: Dose-dependent hepatotoxicity

Drug	Mechanism	Comment/predisposing factors
Paracetamol	Hepatitis	See Chapter 54
Salicylates	Focal hepatocellular necrosis	Autoimmune disease (especially systemic lupus erythematosus)
	Reye's sydrome	In children with viral infection (contraindicated in children <16 years)
Tetracycline	Central and mid-zonal necrosis with fat droplets	–
Azathioprine	Cholestasis and hepatitis	Underlying liver disease
Methotrexate	Hepatic fibrosis	–
Fusidic acid	Cholestasis, conjugated hyperbilirubinaemia	Rare
Rifampicin	Cholestasis, conjugated and unconjugated hyperbilirubinaemia	Transient
Synthetic oestrogens	Cholestasis, may precipitate gallstone disease	Underlying liver disease, rare now that low-dose oestrogens are generally given
HMG CoA reductase inhibitors	Unknown	Usually mild and asymptomatic (statins)

DRUG-INDUCED LIVER DISEASE

After oral administration, the entire absorbed dose of a drug is exposed to the liver during the first pass through the body. The drug itself or its metabolites may affect liver function. Metabolic pathways may become saturated at high concentrations and drug or metabolites may accumulate, leading to toxicity. The drugs shown in Table 34.6 predictably cause hepatotoxicity at excessive doses. Although hepatotoxicity is traditionally divided into dose-dependent and dose-independent hepatotoxicity, the relationship is not always clear-cut. For example, even with predictable hepatotoxins, there is considerable inter-individual variation in susceptibility to hepatic damage. This can sometimes be attributed to genetic polymorphism or to environmental stimuli affecting hepatic microsomal enzymes, or to previous liver disease. Although dose-independent hepatotoxicity is used to classify those reactions that are 'idiosyncratic' and usually unpredictable (Table 34.7), the severity of the resulting liver disease may be related to dose or to duration of therapy. Particular drugs tend to produce distinctive patterns of liver injury, but this is not invariable (see also Chapter 12).

INVESTIGATION AND MANAGEMENT OF HEPATIC DRUG REACTIONS

Depending on the clinical presentation the most important differential diagnoses are hepatic dysfunction due to viral infection (which may be asymptomatic), malignant disease, alcohol and congestive cardiac failure. The aetiology of a minor elevation of transaminases is often undetermined. If the patient is being treated for a disease associated with hepatic dysfunction, particularly with multiple drugs, identification of the responsible agent is particularly difficult. Minor elevations of transaminase

activity are often picked up on routine biochemical profiles. If they are considered to be drug related, but further treatment is indicated, it is reasonable to continue the drug with regular monitoring of liver enzymes if a better alternative therapy is not available. If the transaminases reach more than twice, and/or the bilirubin rises to >1.5 × the upper limit of the normal range, it is prudent to stop the drug if the clinical situation permits.

DRUGS THAT MODIFY APPETITE

APPETITE-SUPPRESSING (ANORECTIC) DRUGS

The most common form of malnutrition in the UK is obesity. Obesity is a major risk factor for cardiovascular disease, stroke and type 2 diabetes mellitus. It is preventable, since obese patients are fat because they eat too many calories for their energy needs. Naturally, a calorie-controlled diet and adequate but sensible amounts of exercise are the essentials of treatment. Unfortunately, the results of treating patients at weight-reduction clinics are disappointing and only a few individuals achieve permanent weight loss. There has accordingly been a great deal of interest in the possibility of altering appetite pharmacologically in order to help the patient to reduce his or her calorie intake. Unfortunately, the causes of obesity are only currently being more comprehensively studied.

In 1994, the gene for obesity (OB) in the mouse was identified. The OB gene encodes the protein leptin, which is produced only in fat cells and is secreted into the blood. The human homologue of the OB gene has now been identified. Leptin is thought to be a blood-borne signal from the adipose tissue that informs the brain about the size of an individual's fat mass. Much more research is required to determine its exact role in neuroendocrine, reproductive, haematopoietic

Table 34.7: Dose-independent hepatotoxicity

Drug	Mechanism	Comment/predisposing factors
Captopril	Cholestatic jaundice	
Chlorpromazine	Cholestatic hepatitis	Estimated incidence 0.5% associated with fever, abdominal pain, pruritus; subclinical hepatic dysfunction is more common
Flucloxacillin	Cholestatic jaundice and hepatitis	Very rare, may occur up to several weeks after treatment. Elderly are at particular risk
Tolbutamide	Cholestatic jaundice	
Telithromycin	Hepatocellular damage	
Isoniazid	Hepatitis	Mild and self-limiting in 20% and severe hepatitis in 0.1% of cases. Possibly more common in rapid acetylators
Pyrazinamide	Hepatitis	Similar to isoniazid, but more clearly related to dose
Methyldopa	Hepatitis	About 5% of cases have subclinical, raised transaminases; clinical hepatitis is rare
Phenytoin	Hypersensitivity reaction	Resembles infectious mononucleosis; pharmacogenetic predisposition; cross-reaction with carbamazepine
Isoniazid	Chronic active hepatitis	Associated with prolonged treatment, usually regresses when drug is discontinued
Nitrofurantoin Dantrolene Halothane Ketoconazole	Hepatitis/hepatic necrosis	See Chapter 24

and metabolic control pathways, as well as its exact effects on body weight and energy expenditure. In the future, modulation of leptin activity may provide a target for treating obesity.

One hypothesis is that lean people do not become obese when they overeat because their tissues preferentially liberate heat (particularly from brown fat). Despite this uncertainty, there is no doubt that starvation leads to weight loss. Therefore, research into drugs for the treatment of obesity has concentrated on finding substances that inhibit appetite.

Learned behaviour is probably important in determining the frequency of eating and whether food is taken between major meals. Stretch receptors in the stomach are stimulated by distention, but the main factors that terminate eating are humoral. Bombesin and somatostatin are two candidates for humoral satiety factors released by the stomach. The most important satiety factor released from the gastro-intestinal tract beyond the stomach is cholecystokinin (CCK). A small peptide fragment of this (CCK-8) has been synthesized and has been found to cause humans to reduce their food intake, possibly by acting on the appetite/satiety centre in the hypothalamus, but this agent is not in clinical use.

Amphetamines and related drugs suppress appetite but are toxic and have considerable abuse potential. The site of action of amphetamines appears to be in the hypothalamus, where they increase noradrenaline and dopamine concentrations by causing transmitter release and blocking re-uptake. Cardiovascular effects are frequently observed with amphetamines, a dose-related increase in heart rate and blood pressure being the most

common effect. **Dexfenfluramine, fenfluramine** and **phentermine** were associated with less abuse potential, but have been withdrawn from use in the UK, because they were associated with valvular heart disease and rarely pulmonary hypertension.

Sibutramine inhibits the re-uptake of noradrenaline and serotonin. It reduces appetite and is used as an adjunct to diet for up to one year. Blood pressure and pulse should be monitored. Contraindications include major psychiatric illness, ischaemic heart disease, dysrrythmias, hyperthyroidism and pregnancy. Side effects include dry mouth, nausea, abnormal taste, constipation, myalgia, palpitations, alopecia, seizures and bleeding disorders.

In 2006, **rimonabant** was approved in Europe. It is an oral selective cannabinoid CB1 receptor antagonist which is used as an adjunct to diet to achieve weight loss. **Rimonabant** is contraindicated in (and may cause) depression. Adverse effects include nausea, vomiting, diarrhoea, mood changes, anxiety, impaired memory, dizziness and sleep disorders. It is highly protein bound and metabolized by hepatic CYP3A4. The half-life is six to nine days in those with normal BMI, but approximately 16 days in obese patients.

Orlistat, is an inhibitor of gastro-intestinal lipases, reduces fat absorption and is licensed for use to treat obesity in combination with a weight management programme, including a mildly hypocaloric diet. NICE has recommended that if weight reduction is less than 10% after six months, treatment should be stopped. Systemic absorption is minimal. The main adverse effects are oily spotting from the rectum, flatus with discharge, faecal urgency and oily faeces. Although there is less absorption of the fat-soluble vitamins (vitamins A, D, E and K) and of β-carotene, this does not appear to cause pathological vitamin deficiency, and vitamin supplementation is not routinely indicated.

BULK AGENTS

Substances such as methylcellulose and guar gum act as bulking agents in the diet and are ineffective at producing weight loss. A high-fibre diet may help weight loss, provided that total caloric intake is reduced, and is desirable for other reasons as well.

MISCELLANEOUS

Diuretics cause a transient loss of weight through fluid loss, and their use for such an effect is to be deplored. Myxoedema is associated with weight gain. Thyroxine has been used to increase the basal metabolic rate and reduce weight in euthyroid obese patients. This is both dangerous and irrational.

APPETITE STIMULATION

This is often difficult, as patients with a poor appetite may have a debilitating systemic illness or an underlying psychiatric disorder. Drugs that inhibit serotonin (5HT) receptors, (e.g. **cyproheptadine**, **pizotifen**) increase appetite and cause weight gain. Weight gain occurs during treatment with various other drugs, including atypical neuroleptics, e.g. **risperidone**, **amitriptyline**, **lithium**, glucocorticosteroids and ACTH, as well as the oral contraceptive pill. Glucocorticosteroids may help to improve appetite in terminally ill patients.

FURTHER READING

Bateson MC. Advances in gastroenterology and hepatology. *Postgraduate Medical Journal* 2000; **76**: 328–32.

Reidenburg M. Drugs and the liver. *British Journal of Clinical Pharmacology* 1998; **46**: 351–9.

Zaman A, Chalasani N. Bleeding caused by portal hypertension. *Gastroenterology Clinics of North America* 2005; **34**: 623–42.

VITAMINS AND TRACE ELEMENTS

INTRODUCTION

Vitamins were discovered during investigations of clinical syndromes that proved to be a consequence of deficiency states (e.g. scurvy, beriberi). They are nutrients that are essential for normal cellular function, but are required in much smaller quantities than the aliments (carbohydrates, fats and proteins). Vitamins are essential cofactors to or components of enzymes that are integral in intermediary metabolism and many other biochemical processes.

GENERAL PHYSIOLOGY OF VITAMINS

Humans are unable to synthesize adequate amounts of vitamins. Vitamin deficiency usually results from either inadequate dietary intake, increased demand (e.g pregnancy or growth) or impaired absorption (e.g coeliac disease, cystic fibrosis, pancreatic insufficiency or as a result of certain drugs, notably **orlistat** which causes fat malabsorption). Vitamin deficiencies are rarely diagnosed in the UK, but their true incidence may be under-recognized, particularly in the elderly, alcoholics, poor people and certain ethnic groups.

The concept that various vitamin supplements might decrease the incidence of a variety of diseases, including cancer and atheroma, has been under investigation. Several large prospective placebo-controlled intervention trials have investigated these hypotheses, but to date evidence of clear clinical benefit is lacking. Not all vitamins are harmless when taken in excess (especially vitamins A and D). In general vitamins should only be prescribed for the prevention or treatment of vitamin deficiency.

Vitamins are divided into two categories:

1. *water soluble* – vitamin B complex (including vitamin B$_{12}$, folate, thiamine, nicotinic acid, pantothenic acid and biotin), vitamin C;
2. *fat soluble* – vitamins A, D, E and K.

Vitamin B$_{12}$ and folate are discussed in Chapter 49, vitamin D in Chapter 39, and vitamin K in Chapter 30.

Key points

Major categories of vitamins

- Originally identified by characteristic deficiency states (now uncommon in most developed countries).
- Water-soluble vitamins include the vitamin B complex and vitamin C.
- Fat-soluble vitamins include vitamins A, D, E and K.
- The vitamin B complex includes vitamins B$_1$ (thiamine), B$_6$ (pyridoxine), B$_{12}$, folate, plus B$_2$ (riboflavin), B$_3$ (nicotinic acid).

VITAMIN A (RETINOIC ACID) AND ITS DERIVATIVES

Physiology

This vitamin exists in several forms that are interconverted. Retinol (vitamin A$_1$) is a primary alcohol and is present in the tissues of animals and marine fishes; 3-dehydroretinol (vitamin A$_2$) is present in freshwater fish; retinoic acid shares some but not all of the actions of retinol. Carotene is provitamin A and is readily converted into retinol in the body. Vitamin A has many physiological functions (Figure 35.1). Its deficiency retards growth and development, and causes night blindness, keratomalacia, dry eyes and keratinization of the skin. Dietary sources of vitamin A include eggs, fish liver oil, liver, milk and vegetables.

Use

Vitamin A is used to prevent and treat deficiency states. Dietary supplementation with halibut liver oil capsules BP (containing the daily requirement of vitamin A and vitamin D) is used to

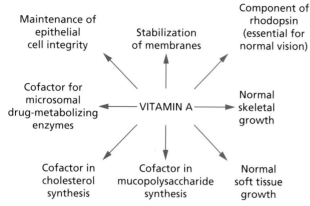

Figure 35.1: Functions of vitamin A.

prevent vitamin A deficiency. Regular dietary or parenteral supplementation of vitamin A may be necessary in patients with steatorrhoea.

Adverse effects

Long-term ingestion of more than double the recommended daily intake of vitamin A can lead to toxicity and chronic hyper-vitaminosis A.

Chronic toxicity includes:

1. anorexia and vomiting;
2. itching and dry skin;
3. raised intracranial pressure (benign intracranial hypertension), irritability and headache;
4. tender hyperostoses in the skull and long bones;
5. hepatotoxicity;
6. congenital abnormalities.

Acute poisoning causes:

1. headache, vomiting and papilloedema;
2. desquamation.

Pharmacokinetics

Gastro-intestinal absorption of retinol via a saturable active transport mechanism is very efficient, but is impaired in patients with steatorrhoea. Carotene is metabolized to vitamin A in the intestine. Esterified retinol reaches peak plasma concentrations four hours after ingestion. Retinol is partly conjugated to a glucuronide and undergoes enterohepatic circulation. Clinical evidence of vitamin A deficiency usually appears only months after reduced intake, when hepatic stores have been depleted.

Contraindications

Excess vitamin A during pregnancy causes birth defects (closely related compounds are involved in controlling morphogenesis in the fetus). Therefore pregnant women should not take vitamin A supplements, and should also avoid liver in their diet.

DERIVATIVES OF VITAMIN A (RETINOIDS)

RETINOIDS AND THE SKIN

Vitamin A derivatives, e.g. **etretinate**, are discussed in Chapter 51.

RETINOIDS AND CANCER

This is discussed in Chapter 48.

VITAMIN B₁ (THIAMINE)

Physiology

All plant and animal cells require thiamine (in the form of thiamine pyrophosphate) for carbohydrate metabolism, as it is a coenzyme for decarboxylases and transketolases. Thiamine deficiency leads to the various manifestations of beriberi, including peripheral neuropathy and cardiac failure. Increased carbohydrate utilization requires increased intake because thiamine is consumed during carbohydrate metabolism. It is therefore useful to express thiamine needs in relation to the calorie intake. Diets associated with beriberi contain less than 0.3 mg thiamine per 1000 kcal. If the diet provides more than this, the excess is excreted in the urine. Thus the recommended daily intake of 0.4 mg/1000 kcal provides a considerable safety margin. The body possesses little ability to store thiamine and with absolutely deficient intake, beriberi develops within weeks.

Acute thiamine deficiency may be precipitated by a carbohydrate load in patients who have a marginally deficient diet. This is especially important in alcoholics and thiamine replacement should precede intravenous dextrose in alcoholic patients with a depressed conscious level. Failure to do this has historically been associated with worsening encephalopathy and permanent sequelae (e.g. Korsakoff's psychosis). Thiamine is found in many plant and animal foods (e.g. yeast and pork).

Use

Thiamine is used in the treatment of beriberi and other states of thiamine deficiency, or in their prevention. Such conditions include alcoholic neuritis, Wernicke's encephalopathy and the neuritis of pregnancy, as well as chronic diarrhoeal states and after intestinal resection. The parenteral route of administration is used in confused patients. Once the deficiency state has been corrected, the oral route is preferred, unless gastrointestinal disease interferes with ingestion or absorption of the vitamin.

Adverse effects

Anaphylactoid reactions following parenteral thiamine dosing have been reported, so parenteral administration should be restricted to situations where it is essential.

Pharmacokinetics

Absorption of thiamine following intramuscular injection is rapid and complete. Thiamine is also well absorbed through the mucosa of the upper part of the small intestine by both active and passive mechanisms, and surplus intake is excreted unchanged in the urine.

VITAMIN B₃ (NIACIN AND NICOTINIC ACID)

Physiology

Niacin is found in yeast, rice, liver and other meats. Its vital metabolic role is as a component of nicotinamide adenine dinucleotide (NAD) and nicotinamide adenine dinucleotide phosphate (NADP). Niacin can be generated in the body in small amounts from tryptophan. Deficiency of niacin causes pellagra, that can manifest clinically as a syndrome complex which includes dementia, dermatitis and diarrhoea.

Uses

1. Niacin is used to treat and prevent pellagra. If oral treatment is not possible, intravenous injections are available.
2. Nicotinic acid (or nicotinic acid analogues, e.g. **acipomox**) may be used to treat dyslipidaemia (Chapter 27), but hypolipidaemic dosing is limited by vasodilatation/flushing.

Adverse effects

In replacement therapy for pellagra, adverse effects are uncommon. High doses (as used for hyperlipidaemia) cause the following:

1. vasodilatation due to prostaglandin D_2 – this can be reduced by premedication with **aspirin**;
2. nausea, vomiting and itching;
3. hyperglycaemia;
4. exacerbation of hyperuricaemia.

Pharmacokinetics

Both niacin and nicotinamide are well absorbed via the intestine and are widely distributed to tissues. When the usual dietary amounts are administered, a high proportion is excreted as *N*-methyl nicotinamide and other metabolites. When increased doses are administered, a higher proportion is excreted unchanged in the urine.

VITAMIN B₆ (PYRIDOXINE)

Physiology

Vitamin B_6 occurs naturally in three forms, namely pyridoxine, pyridoxal and pyridoxamine. All three forms are converted in the body into pyridoxal phosphate, which is an essential cofactor in several metabolic reactions, including decarboxylation, transamination and other steps in amino acid metabolism. Pyridoxine is present in wheatgerm, yeast, bran, rice and liver. Deficiency causes glossitis, seborrhoea, fits, peripheral neuropathy and sideroblastic anaemia. **Isoniazid** prevents the activation of pyridoxal to pyridoxal phosphate by inhibiting the enzyme pyridoxal kinase, and slow acetylators of **isoniazid** are at increased risk of developing peripheral neuropathy for this reason (Chapters 14 and 44).

Use

Pyridoxine hydrochloride is given to patients at risk (e.g. alcoholics) during long-term therapy with **isoniazid** to prevent peripheral neuropathy, and in deficiency states. Large doses

are used in sideroblastic anaemia. **Pyridoxine** is also used to treat certain uncommon inborn errors of metabolism, including primary hyperoxaluria. Large doses are sometimes used to treat premenstrual syndrome, and there is a lobby of enthusiasts for this, despite a paucity of evidence.

Adverse effects

There have been reports of ataxia and sensory neuropathy following administration of large doses (2 g/day) of pyridoxine for more than two months.

VITAMIN C (ASCORBIC ACID)

Physiology

Ascorbic acid is present in large quantities in citrus fruits, tomatoes and green vegetables. Vitamin C is essential to humans, monkeys and guinea pigs which, unlike other mammals, cannot synthesize it from glucose. Dietary lack of vitamin C causes scurvy, which is characterized by bleeding gums and perifollicular purpura. Ascorbic acid is involved in several metabolic processes (Figure 35.2). It is a potent water-soluble anti-oxidant. The nutritional status of vitamin C can be assessed by measuring the intracellular leukocyte concentration, but this is not routinely performed or available.

Uses

1. **Ascorbic acid** is used in the prophylaxis and treatment of scurvy. (Perhaps the first recorded clinical trial involved the distribution of citrus fruit to some, but not all, British naval vessels and observation of the incidence of scurvy. The Admiralty were (after some prevarication) convinced and British sailors were subsequently provided with limes – whence the term 'limeys'.)
2. **Ascorbic acid** increases the absorption of orally administered iron.
3. The reducing properties of ascorbate may be used in the treatment of methaemoglobinaemia.
4. In scorbutic patients, wound healing is delayed and this is restored to normal by administration of **ascorbic acid**.

Adverse effects

Ascorbic acid is non-toxic in low doses. However, administration of ≥4 g daily raises the urinary excretion of oxalate. Large

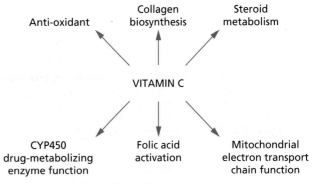

Figure 35.2: Functions of vitamin C.

doses of vitamin C taken chronically have resulted in calcium oxalate urolithiasis. There is theoretical concern that high doses of vitamin C (in common with other anti-oxidants) can have pro-oxidant actions.

Pharmacokinetics

Ascorbic acid is well absorbed following oral administration and its sodium salt may be given by intramuscular or intravenous injection. **Ascorbic acid** is mainly metabolized by oxidation to oxalic acid. Normally about 40% of urinary oxalate is derived from **ascorbic acid**. When the body stores of **ascorbic acid** are saturated, some ingested **ascorbic acid** is excreted in the urine unchanged.

VITAMIN E (TOCOPHEROL)

Vitamin E is found in many foods, including nuts, wheatgerm and bananas. Deficiency in animals causes abortion and degeneration of the germinal epithelium of the testes. No defined deficiency syndrome exists in humans, but low vitamin E intake is associated with anaemia in premature and malnourished infants. Vitamin E protects erythrocytes against haemolysis, and is a fat-soluble anti-oxidant and detoxifies free radicals. Free radicals cause membrane and epithelial injury and have been implicated in the pathophysiology of numerous diseases, including cancer and atheroma. Epidemiological studies suggested that reduced vitamin E intake is associated with increased atherogenesis (Chapter 27). Large studies of vitamin E supplementation for a number of cardiovascular disorders and cancers have not shown clear benefit, and there is a theoretical risk that prolonged ingestion of high doses could be harmful.

Key points

Vitamin deficiency and disease

- In general, vitamin deficiencies are due to inadequate dietary intake or malabsorption.
- Vitamin B deficiencies do not often occur in isolation.
- Vitamin A deficiency causes night blindness.
- Vitamin B_1 (thiamine) deficiency causes beriberi (neuropathy, paralysis, muscle wasting and cardiac failure).
- Vitamin B_3 (nicotinic acid) deficiency causes pellagra (photosensitive dermatitis, diarrhoea, dementia and death (the 4 Ds)).
- Vitamin B_{12} deficiency causes megaloblastic anaemia, dementia and neuropathy.
- Vitamin C deficiency causes scurvy (perifollicular petechiae, gingivitis and swollen joints).
- Vitamin D deficiency causes rickets (in young) and osteomalacia (adults).
- Folate deficiency causes megaloblastic anaemia and neural tube defects (in the developing fetus).

Key points

Population groups at high risk for vitamin deficiency

- Infants
- Pregnant women
- Elderly people, especially the elderly with chronic disease
- Alcoholics and drug abusers
- Vegans and undernourished populations
- Patients taking long-term anticonvulsants
- Patients with malabsorption syndromes.

Key points

Vitamin toxicities

- Vitamin A – gastro-intestinal upsets, headache (raised intracranial pressure), desquamation, hepatotoxicity and teratogenicity.
- Nicotinic acid – flushing, vasodilatation and hepatotoxicity.
- Vitamin C – hyperoxaluria and oxalate stones.
- Vitamin D – hypercalcaemia.

ESSENTIAL FATTY ACIDS

Several naturally occurring unsaturated fatty acids are essential dietary components. Linoleic and linolenic acids occur in vegetable oils and nuts, arachidonic acid occurs in meat, and longer-chain fatty acids (eicosapentanoic acid and docosahexanoic acid) are found in cold-water oily fish. Humans synthesize arachidonic acid (C20:4) from shorter-chain (C18:2) essential fatty acids by chain elongation and desaturation. Arachidonic acid is present in the lipid component of cell membranes throughout the body. It is esterified on the 2′-position of glycerol in membrane phospholipids and is liberated by phospholipases when cells are injured or stimulated. Free arachidonic acid is the precursor of the 2-series of prostaglandins, thromboxanes, the 4-series of leukotrienes and epoxyeicosatetraenoic acids which are important in many physiologic and pathologic states, including control of inflammation, haemostasis and vascular tone. Deficiency states have been described in patients receiving long-term parenteral nutrition and are prevented by the use of lipid emulsions.

TRACE ELEMENTS

A total of 13 nutritionally essential trace elements are recognized, namely fluorine, silicon, vanadium, chromium, manganese, iron, cobalt, nickel, copper, zinc, selenium, tin and iodine. These are required in the human body at <0.01% of body weight. Most of them are highly reactive chemically and one or more of these elements is present at the active site of many enzymes. They are present in small but adequate amounts in a normal diet, but evidence is accumulating that in addition to iron, cobalt (Chapter 49) and iodine (Chapter 38), zinc,

Table 35.1: Common trace element deficiencies

Element	Clinical features of deficiency	Biochemical activity	Normal serum/tissue concentration	Other comments
Copper	Osteoporosis, costochondral cartilage cupping and anaemia/leukopenia. Menke's syndrome in children	Major enzyme dysfunction (e.g. cytochrome oxidase)	Plasma copper (12–26 μmol/L) does not reflect tissue copper status well Reduced red cell superoxide dismutase activity is a better indicator	Premature babies are predisposed to copper deficiency, as copper stores are built up in late pregnancy
Zinc	Skin rash, hair thinning, diarrhoea, (acrodermatitis enteropathica); mental apathy and impaired T-cell function	At the active site of glutathione peroxidase and protects against oxidant stresses	Serum zinc 5.6–25 μmol/L	Adverse effects of zinc include dyspepsia and abdominal pain

copper, selenium and molybdenum deficiencies can contribute to disease. Trace element deficiencies are most commonly due to inadequate intake or to intestinal disease reducing absorption; treatment is with adequate replacement.

The features of copper and zinc deficiencies are summarized in Table 35.1.

Case history

A 24-year-old woman with epilepsy is well controlled on phenytoin. Months after starting treatment, she complained of fatigue. Her haemoglobin was 8.0 g/dL and mean corpuscular volume (MCV) was 103 fL.
Question
What additional investigations would you undertake? What is the most likely diagnosis and how should you treat this patient?
Answer
This patient has a macrocytic anaemia. Your investigations show her serum folate to be low, with a normal B_{12}. This confirms your suspicion of phenytoin-induced folate deficiency. A dietary assessment reveals an adequate folate intake; there is no evidence of other causes of malabsorption. Phenytoin commonly causes folate deficiency, impairing the absorption of dietary folate by inducing gastro-intestinal enzymes involved in its catabolism. Treatment should consist of daily oral folate supplementation, keeping her on the phenytoin (as this has controlled her epilepsy), and further monitoring of her haematological status for response. During follow up, she should also be monitored for possible development of osteomalacia (suggested by proximal myopathy with low serum phosphate and calcium and raised alkaline phosphatase), as phenytoin also induces the metabolic inactivation of vitamin D.

FURTHER READING AND WEB MATERIAL

Ahmed FE. Effect of diet, life style, and other environmental/chemopreventive factors on colorectal cancer development, and assessment of the risks. *Journal of Environmental Science and Health. Part C, Environmental Carcinogenesis and Ecotoxicology Reviews* 2004; **22**: 91–147.

van Poppel G, van den Berg H. Vitamins and cancer. *Cancer Letters* 1997; **114**: 195–202.

Bender DA. *Nutritional biochemistry of the vitamins*. Cambridge: Cambridge University Press, 1992.

Fitzgerald FT, Tierney LM. Trace metals and human disease. *Advances in Internal Medicine* 1984; **30**: 337–58.

Useful websites: www.nlm.nih.gov/medlineplus/vitamins, www.indstate.edu/thcme/mwking/vitamins

PART VII

FLUIDS AND ELECTROLYTES

CHAPTER **36**

NEPHROLOGICAL AND RELATED ASPECTS

INTRODUCTION

The 'internal environment' is tightly controlled so that plasma concentrations of electrolytes remain within narrow limits despite substantial variations in dietary intake, as a result of renal processes that ensure that the amounts excreted balance those taken in. Fluid and electrolyte disturbances are important in many diseases (e.g. heart failure, see Chapter 31). In the present chapter, we consider general aspects of their management. This usually involves dietary restriction and the use of drugs that act on the kidney – especially various diuretics. Additionally, we consider briefly drugs that act on the bladder and other components of the genito-urinary system.

VOLUME OVERLOAD (SALT AND WATER EXCESS)

Volume overload is usually caused by an excess of sodium chloride with accompanying water. Effective treatment is directed at the underlying cause (e.g. heart failure or renal failure), in addition to improving volume status per se by reducing salt intake and increasing its elimination by the use of diuretics. Limiting water intake is seldom useful in patients with volume overload, although modest limitation is of value in patients with ascites due to advanced liver disease and in other patients with hyponatraemia.

Diuretics increase urine production and Na^+ excretion. They are of central importance in managing hypertension (Chapter 28), as well as the many diseases associated with oedema and volume overload, including heart failure, cirrhosis, renal failure and nephrotic syndrome, where it is important to assess the distribution of salt and water excess in different body compartments. Glomerular filtrate derives from plasma, so diuretic treatment acutely reduces plasma

volume. It takes time for tissue fluid to re-equilibrate after an acute change in blood volume. Consequently, attempts to produce a vigorous diuresis are inappropriate in some oedematous states and may lead to cardiovascular collapse and 'prerenal' renal failure – i.e. caused by poor renal perfusion, often signalled by an increase in serum urea disproportionate to the creatinine concentration. The principles of using diuretics in the management of hypertension (Chapter 28) and heart failure (Chapter 31) are described elsewhere. Here, we describe briefly the management of hypoalbuminaemic states: nephrotic syndrome and cirrhosis. Hypoalbuminaemia affects the kinetics of several drugs through its effects on protein binding (Chapter 7) and causes an apparently inadequate intravascular volume in the face of fluid overload in the body as a whole. This results in an increased risk of nephrotoxicity from several common drugs, particularly non-steroidal anti-inflammatory drugs (NSAIDs, Chapter 26). Particular caution is needed when prescribing and monitoring the effects of therapy for intercurrent problems in such patients.

NEPHROTIC SYNDROME

The primary problem in nephrotic syndrome is impairment of the barrier function of glomerular membranes with leakage of plasma albumin into the urine. Plasma albumin concentration falls together with its oncotic pressure and water passes from the circulation into the tissue spaces, producing oedema. The fall in effective blood volume stimulates the renin–angiotensin–aldosterone system, causing sodium retention. Depending on the nature of the glomerular pathology, it may be possible to reduce albumin loss with glucocorticosteroid or other immunosuppressive drugs (Chapter 50). However, treatment is often only symptomatic. Diuretics are of limited value, but diet is important. Adequate protein intake is needed to support hepatic synthesis of albumin. Salt intake should be restricted.

CIRRHOSIS

Fluid retention in cirrhosis usually takes the form of ascites, portal hypertension leading to loss of fluid into the peritoneal cavity, although dependent oedema also occurs. Other important factors are hypoalbuminaemia (caused by failure of synthesis by the diseased liver) and hyperaldosteronism (due to activation of volume receptors and reduced hepatic aldosterone catabolism). Transplantation may be appropriate in cases where the underlying pathology (e.g. alcoholism) is judged to have been cured or (as in some rare inherited metabolic disorders) will not recur in a donor liver. Nevertheless, symptomatic treatment is all that is available for most patients.

Diet is important. Protein is restricted in the presence of hepatic encephalopathy, and should be of high quality to provide an adequate supply of essential amino acids. High energy intake from carbohydrate minimizes catabolism of body protein. Salt restriction is combined with moderate water restriction monitored by daily weighing. Excessive diuresis may precipitate renal failure: loss of approximately 0.5 kg body weight (as fluid) daily is ideal.

Thiazides or loop diuretics exacerbate potassium depletion and alkalosis and can precipitate hepatic encephalopathy. **Amiloride** or **spironolactone** are used in this setting (see below), combined subsequently with loop diuretics if necessary.

DIURETICS

Many diuretics block sodium ion reabsorption from renal tubular fluid (Figure 36.1). This causes natriuresis (i.e. increased excretion of sodium ions), so diuretics are used to treat patients with volume overload. Some diuretics have additional distinct therapeutic roles because of additional effects on the kidney (e.g. the use of **furosemide** to treat hypercalcaemia or the use of

thiazide diuretics to treat nephrogenic diabetes insipidus) or elsewhere in the body (e.g. **mannitol** for cerebral oedema).

CARBONIC ANHYDRASE INHIBITORS

Acetazolamide, a sulphonamide, is a non-competitive inhibitor of carbonic anhydrase. Carbonic anhydrase plays an important part in bicarbonate reabsorption from the proximal tubule (Figure 36.1). Consequently, **acetazolamide** inhibits reabsorption of sodium bicarbonate, resulting in an alkaline diuresis with loss of sodium and bicarbonate in the urine. Since chloride (rather than bicarbonate) is the preponderant anion in the plasma (and hence in glomerular filtrate), carbonic anhydrase inhibitors influence only a small fraction of sodium reabsorption and are thus weak diuretics.

Uses

More importantly than its diuretic effect, **acetazolamide** inhibits carbonic anhydrase in the eye and thereby decreases the rate of secretion of the aqueous humour and lowers intraocular pressure. Treatment of glaucoma is currently the major use of **acetazolamide**. **Dorzolamide** is a topical carbonic anhydrase inhibitor for use in glaucoma (Chapter 52). Carbonic anhydrase in the choroid plexus participates in the formation of cerebrospinal fluid and **acetazolamide** has been used in the management of benign intracranial hypertension. **Acetazolamide** is used in the prevention of mountain sickness, since it permits rapid acclimatization to altitude (which entails renal compensation for respiratory alkalosis caused by hyperventilation) by facilitating bicarbonate excretion. Urinary alkalinization with **acetazolamide** has been used in the treatment of children with cysteine stones due to cysteinuria, as cysteine is more soluble at alkaline than at acid pH. (Many of these uses are unlicensed.)

Unwanted effects

As a consequence of increased urinary elimination of bicarbonate during **acetazolamide** treatment, the plasma bicarbonate

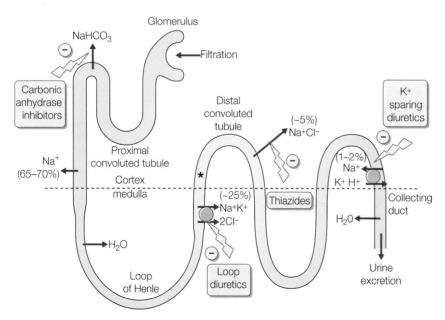

★ thick ascending limb of Loop of Henle

Figure 36.1: Sites of action of different diuretics in the nephron.

concentration falls without accumulation of any unmeasured anions, giving a non-anion gap metabolic acidosis, as in renal tubular acidosis. The reduction in plasma bicarbonate leads to a reduced filtered load of this ion, so less bicarbonate is available for reabsorption from proximal tubular fluid. The diuretic effect of **acetazolamide** is therefore self-limiting. Large doses cause paraesthesiae, fatigue and dyspepsia. Prolonged use predisposes to renal stone formation due to reduced urinary citrate (citrate increases the solubility of calcium in the urine). Hypersensitivity reactions and blood dyscrasias are a problem, as with other sulphonamides.

LOOP DIURETICS

Uses

The main clinical use of loop diuretics (e.g. **furosemide**) is for heart failure (Chapter 31). **Furosemide** is also useful in patients with chronic renal failure who are suffering from fluid overload and/or hypertension. Large doses may be needed to produce diuresis in patients with severe renal impairment. In patients with incipient acute renal failure, intravenous infusion sometimes produces diuresis, and may prevent the development of established failure, although this is difficult to prove.

Loop diuretics increase urinary calcium excretion (in contrast to thiazides). This is exploited in the treatment of hypercalcaemia when **furosemide** is given after volume replacement with 0.9% sodium chloride.

Mechanism of action

Loop diuretics have steep dose–response curves and much higher maximum effects than thiazide or other diuretics,

being capable of increasing fractional sodium excretion to as much as 35%. They act from within the tubular fluid to inhibit a co-transporter in the thick ascending limb of the loop of Henle which transports Na^+ and K^+ together with $2Cl^-$ ions from the lumen ('$Na^+ K^+ 2Cl^-$ cotransport'), see Figure 36.1.

Pharmacokinetics

Furosemide is rapidly and extensively absorbed from the gut. It is 95% bound to plasma protein and elimination is mainly via the kidneys, by filtration and proximal tubular secretion. Approximately two-thirds of water reabsorption occurs iso-osmotically in the proximal convoluted tubule, so **furosemide** is substantially concentrated before reaching its site of action in the thick ascending limb. This accounts for its selectivity for the renal $Na^+ K^+ 2Cl^-$ cotransport mechanism, as opposed to $Na^+ K^+ 2Cl^-$ cotransport at other sites, such as the inner ear. The luminal site of action of **furosemide** also contributes to diuretic insensitivity in nephrotic syndrome, where heavy albuminuria results in binding of **furosemide** to albumin within the lumen.

Adverse effects

1. Acute renal failure – loop diuretics in high dose cause massive diuresis. This can abruptly reduce blood volume. Acute hypovolaemia can precipitate prerenal renal failure.
2. Hypokalaemia – inhibition of K^+ reabsorption in the loop of Henle and increased delivery of Na^+ to the distal nephron (where it can be exchanged for K^+) results in increased urinary potassium loss and hypokalaemia.
3. Hypomagnesaemia.
4. Hyperuricaemia and gout.
5. Otoxicity with hearing loss is associated with excessive peak plasma concentrations caused by too rapid intravenous injection. It may be related to inhibition of $Na^+ K^+ 2Cl^-$ cotransporter in the ear, which is involved in the formation of endolymph.
7. Metabolic alkalosis – the increased water and chloride excretion caused by loop diuretics results in contraction alkalosis.
8. Idiosyncratic blood dyscrasias occur rarely.

Drug interactions

Loop diuretics increase the nephrotoxicity of first-generation cephalosporins, e.g. **cephaloridine**, and increase aminoglycoside toxicity. **Lithium** reabsorption is reduced by loop diuretics and the dose of lithium carbonate often needs to be reduced.

THIAZIDE DIURETICS

The mechanism, adverse effects, contraindications and interactions of thiazide diuretics are covered in Chapter 28, together with their first-line use in hypertension.

Uses

Thiazides are used in:

1. hypertension (Chapter 28)
2. mild cardiac failure (Chapter 31);
3. resistant oedema – thiazides or related drugs (e.g. **metolazone**) are extremely potent when combined with a loop diuretic;
4. prevention of stones – thiazides reduce urinary calcium excretion and thus help to prevent urinary stone formation in patients with idiopathic hypercalciuria;
5. diabetes insipidus – paradoxically, thiazides reduce urinary volume in diabetes insipidus by preventing the formation of hypotonic fluid in the distal tubule; they are therefore sometimes used to treat nephrogenic diabetes insipidus.

POTASSIUM-SPARING DIURETICS

Some diuretics inhibit distal Na^+/K^+ tubular exchange (Figure 36.1), causing potassium retention at the same time as natriuresis. They fall into two categories:

1. competitive antagonists, structurally related to aldosterone: **spironolactone**, **eplerenone**;
2. Na^+/K^+ exchange antagonists that do not compete with aldosterone: **amiloride**, **triamterene**.

These are not potent diuretics, since only a small fraction of the filtered Na^+ is reabsorbed by this mechanism, but **spironolactone** prolongs survival in heart failure (Chapter 31) and is useful when there is hyperaldosteronism, whether primary (Conn's syndrome, resistant hypertension) or secondary (e.g. in cirrhosis with ascites). High doses of **spironolactone** causes gynaecomastia and breast tenderness in men and menstrual irregularity in women – oestrogenic side effects. **Eplerenone** is more selective and lacks these oestrogenic effects. It is much more expensive but has been shown to improve survival following myocardial infarction (Chapter 29).

Amiloride and **triamterene** also inhibit Na^+/K^+ exchange, but not by competition with **aldosterone**. They are marketed as combination tablets with loop or thiazide diuretics as a means of avoiding hypokalaemia. Hypokalaemia is important if drugs such as **digoxin** (Chapters 31 and 32) or **sotalol** (Chapter 32) are co-prescribed, because their toxicity is increased by hypokalaemia. Conversely K^+-retaining diuretics predispose to hyperkalaemia if used with ACEI or sartans in patients with renal impairment.

OSMOTIC DIURETICS

Use and mechanism of action

Osmotic diuretics undergo glomerular filtration but are poorly reabsorbed from the renal tubular fluid. Their main diuretic action is exerted on the proximal tubule. This section of the tubule is freely permeable to water, and under normal circumstances sodium is actively reabsorbed accompanied by an

> **Key points**
>
> Salt overload and diuretics
>
> - Several diseases are associated with retention of excess salt and water, including:
>   - heart failure;
>   - renal failure;
>   - nephrotic syndrome;
>   - cirrhosis.
> - Treatment involves restriction of dietary salt and administration of diuretics to increase salt excretion.
> - The main classes of diuretics for these indications are:
>   - thiazides;
>   - loop diuretics;
>   - K^+-sparing diuretics.
> - In addition to treating salt/water overload, diuretics are also used in:
>   - systemic hypertension;
>   - glaucoma (carbonic anhydrase inhibitors);
>   - acute reduction of intracranial or intra-ocular pressure (osmotic diuretics);
>   - hypercalcaemia (furosemide);
>   - nephrogenic diabetes insipidus (thiazides).

isoosmotic quantity of water. The presence of a substantial quantity of a poorly absorbable solute opposes this, because as water is reabsorbed the concentration and hence the osmotic activity of the solute increases. Osmotic diuretics (e.g. **mannitol**) also interfere with the establishment of the medullary osmotic gradient which is necessary for the formation of concentrated urine. **Mannitol** is poorly absorbed from the intestine and is given intravenously in gram quantities.

Unlike other diuretics, osmotic diuretics increase the plasma volume (by increasing the entry of water to the circulation as a result of increasing intravascular osmolarity), so they are unsuitable for the treatment of most causes of oedema, especially cardiac failure. It is possible that, if used early in the course of incipient acute renal failure, osmotic diuretics may stave off the occurrence of acute tubular necrosis by increasing tubular fluid flow and washing away material that would otherwise plug the tubules. Osmotic diuretics are mainly used for reasons unconnected with their ability to cause diuresis. Because they do not enter cells or some anatomical areas, such as the eye and brain, they cause water to leave cells down the osmotic gradient. This 'dehydrating' action is used in two circumstances:

1. reduction of intra-ocular pressure: pre-operatively for urgent reduction of intra-ocular pressure and in closed-angle glaucoma;
2. emergency reduction of intracranial pressure.

SIADH: OVERHYDRATION

Overhydration without excess salt is much less common than salt and water overload, but occurs when antidiuretic hormone (ADH) is secreted inappropriately (e.g. by a neoplasm or following head injury or neurosurgery), giving rise to the syndrome of inappropriate secretion of ADH (SIADH). This is sometimes caused by drugs, notably the anticonvulsant **carbamazepine**, which stimulates ADH release from the posterior pituitary, and sulphonylureas, which potentiate its action on the renal collecting ducts. Antidiuretic hormone secretion results in a concentrated urine, while continued drinking (as a result of dietary habit) leads to progressive dilution of the plasma, which becomes hypo-osmolar and hyponatraemic. The plasma volume is slightly increased and urinary sodium loss continues. Some causes of SIADH resolve spontaneously (e.g. some cases of head injury), whereas others may improve after specific treatment of the underlying cause (e.g. following chemotherapy for small-cell carcinoma of the bronchus). Hyponatraemia that has arisen gradually can be corrected gradually by restricting fluid intake. This does not cause thirst (because the plasma is hypo-osmolar), but may not be well tolerated because of habit. Rapid correction of hyponatraemia to levels greater than 125 mmol/L is potentially harmful and is associated with central pontine myelinolysis, with resultant devastating loss of brainstem function.

Demeclocycline inhibits adenylyl cyclase and renders the collecting ducts insensitive to ADH (thereby producing a form of nephrogenic diabetes insipidus). It has been used to treat SIADH. In common with other tetracyclines, it increases plasma urea levels and can produce deterioration of renal function and increased loss of sodium in the urine. Electrolytes and renal function must be monitored during treatment.

VOLUME DEPLETION

PRINCIPLES OF FLUID REPLACEMENT

Volume depletion is seldom treated with drugs. Even in Addisonian crisis, where the definitive treatment is replacement with glucocorticoid and mineralocorticoid hormones, emergency treatment pivots on replacement of what is depleted, i.e. salt and water, usually in the form of adequate volumes of isotonic 0.9% sodium chloride solution (Chapter 40). The same is true of diabetic ketoacidosis, where the critical life-saving intervention is the rapid infusion of large volumes of isotonic saline, as well as insulin (Chapter 37). In patients with hypovolaemia due to acute and rapid blood loss, the appropriate fluid with which to replace is blood. In some situations, particularly when hypoalbuminaemia and oedema coexist with acute blood volume depletion, infusion of solutions of high-molecular-weight colloid (e.g. gelatin) may be preferable to isotonic saline. Anaphylactoid reactions are an unusual but severe adverse effect of such treatment. Lactate is metabolized aerobically with the production of bicarbonate and Ringer's lactate solution is used to avoid hyperchloraemic acidosis. Bicarbonate-containing solutions for i.v. use are being developed.

DIABETES INSIPIDUS AND VASOPRESSIN

'Pure' water deprivation (i.e. true dehydration) is much less common than loss of salt and water (i.e. desalination). Plasma osmolality rapidly increases if fluid intake is inadequate. This causes thirst, which leads to drinking and restoration of plasma osmolality, and to secretion of antidiuretic hormone (ADH, arginine vasopressin) by the posterior pituitary, which results in the formation of a small volume of concentrated urine. ADH combines with receptors coupled to G-proteins. The most physiologically important actions of vasopressin, including its antidiuretic effect, are mediated by V_2-receptors which are coupled to adenylyl cyclase. V_1-receptors activate the phosphatidyl inositol signalling system in vascular smooth muscle, mobilizing cytoplasmic calcium and causing vasoconstriction.

Vasopressin renders the collecting ducts permeable to water. Consequently, water leaves the collecting ducts passively down its osmotic gradient from tubular fluid (which is hypotonic at the beginning of the distal tubule) into the highly concentrated papillary interstitium. This process results in the formation of a small volume of highly concentrated urine under the influence of vasopressin.

Control of plasma osmolarity via thirst fails when a patient is denied oral fluid, usually because of surgery ('nil by mouth'). Fluid must then be administered parenterally if dehydration with increased plasma sodium ion concentration is to be prevented. An isotonic (5%) solution of glucose is used in these circumstances, as the glucose is rapidly metabolized to carbon dioxide, leaving water unaccompanied by solute. Surgical patients also lose salt, but unless they have been vomiting or losing electrolyte-rich fluid from the gastro-intestinal tract via a drain or fistula, salt is lost at a lower rate than water. Consequently, post-operative patients are often given two or three volumes of 5% glucose for every volume of isotonic saline, adjusted in the light of serial serum electrolyte determinations.

Diabetes insipidus is an uncommon disorder in which either the secretion of ADH is deficient ('central' diabetes insipidus which can follow neurosurgery or head injury or complicate diseases such as sarcoid that can infiltrate the posterior pituitary), or in which the sensitivity of the collecting ducts to ADH is deficient ('nephrogenic' diabetes insipidus). Nephrogenic diabetes insipidus is sometimes drug induced, **lithium** being a common cause. Severe nephrogenic diabetes insipidus is a rare X-linked disease caused by a mutation in the V_2-receptor gene. In such cases, exogenous **vasopressin** or **desmopressin** (see below) is ineffective. Paradoxically, thiazide diuretics (see above) reduce polyuria in nephrogenic diabetes insipidus by reducing the hypotonicity of fluid entering the distal tubule, and are combined with mild salt restriction.

Dehydration is not a problem in diabetes insipidus provided the patient has access to water, because increasing plasma osmolality stimulates thirst. The consequent polydipsia prevents dehydration and hypernatraemia. However, patients with diabetes insipidus are at greatly increased risk of dehydration if they become unconscious for any reason (e.g. anaesthesia for an intercurrent surgical problem).

Polydipsia and polyuria in central diabetes insipidus can be prevented by **vasopressin**. Treatment with ADH necessitates repeated injections. Currently, the usual treatment is therefore with a stable analogue, namely desamino-D-arginine vasopressin (DDAVP, **desmopressin**). This is sufficiently well absorbed through the nasal mucosa for it to be administered intranasally. It is selective for V_2-receptors and lacks the pressor effect of ADH.

Desmopressin is also used for nocturnal enuresis in children over seven years old, and intravenously in patients with von Willebrand's disease before undergoing elective surgery, because it increases circulating von Willebrand factor. It also increases factor VIII in patients with mild/moderate haemophilia.

Key points

Volume depletion

- Volume depletion can be caused by loss of blood or other body fluids (e.g. vomiting, diarrhoea, surgical fistulas).
- Replacement should be with appropriate volumes of crystalloid or blood in the case of haemorrhage.
- Excessive renal loss of salt (e.g. Addison's disease) or water (e.g. diabetes insipidus) can be due to renal or endocrine disorders and requires appropriate treatment (e.g. fludrocortisone in Addison's disease, desmopressin in central diabetes insipidus).

DISORDERED POTASSIUM ION BALANCE

HYPOKALAEMIA

Hypokalaemia commonly accompanies loss of fluid from the gastro-intestinal tract (e.g. vomiting or diarrhoea), or loss of potassium ions into the urine due to diuretic therapy (see above). Hypokalaemia in untreated patients with hypertension is suggestive of mineralocorticoid excess (e.g. Conn's syndrome, liquorice abuse). Bartter's syndrome is a rare cause of severe hypokalaemia that should be considered in normotensive children who are not vomiting. Severe hypokalaemia causes symptoms of fatigue and nocturia (because of loss of renal concentrating ability), and can cause dysrhythmias. Mild degrees of hypokalaemia (often associated with diuretic use) are generally well tolerated and of little clinical importance. Risk factors for more serious hypokalaemia include:

1. high-dose diuretics, especially combinations of loop diuretic and thiazide;
2. other drugs that cause potassium loss/redistribution (e.g. systemic steroids, chronic laxative treatment, high dose β_2-agonists);
3. low potassium intake;
4. primary or secondary hyperaldosteronism.

POTASSIUM REPLACEMENT

There are two ways to increase plasma potassium concentrations: potassium supplements, or potassium-sparing diuretics.

POTASSIUM SUPPLEMENTS

Potassium salts may be given orally as either an effervescent or slow-release preparation. Diet can be supplemented by foods with a high potassium content, such as fruit and vegetables (bananas and tomatoes are rich in potassium ions). Intravenous potassium salts are usually given as potassium chloride. This is used either to maintain body potassium levels in patients receiving intravenous feeding, or to restore potassium levels in severely depleted patients (e.g. those with diabetic ketoacidosis). The main danger associated with intravenous potassium is hyperkalaemia, which can cause cardiac arrest. Potassium chloride has the dubious distinction of causing the highest frequency of fatal adverse reactions. Potassium chloride solution is infused at a maximum rate of 10 mmol/hour unless there is severe depletion, when 20 mmol/hour can be given with electrocardiographic monitoring. Particular care is needed if there is impaired renal function. Potassium chloride for intravenous replacement should be dilute whenever possible (e.g. mini-bags of prediluted fluid); strong potassium solutions (the most dangerous) should be restricted to areas such as intensive care units where patients may need i.v. potassium while also severely restricting fluid intake.

POTASSIUM-SPARING DIURETICS

An alternative to potassium supplementation is to combine a thiazide or loop diuretic with a potassium-retaining diuretic (see above). Potassium-retaining diuretics are better tolerated than oral potassium supplements.

Key points

Disordered K^+ metabolism

- Hypokalaemia is caused by urinary or gastro-intestinal K^+ loss in excess of dietary intake, or by a shift of K^+ into cells. Diuretics are often the cause. Endocrine causes include Conn's syndrome. β_2-Agonists shift K^+ into cells.
- Mild hypokalaemia is often unimportant, but severe hypokalaemia can cause dysrhythmias. Hypokalaemia increases digoxin toxicity.
- Emergency treatment (e.g. in diabetic ketoacidosis) involves intravenous replacement, which requires close monitoring (including ECG).
- Foods rich in K^+ include fruit and vegetables. Oral K^+ preparations are unpalatable and not very effective.
- K^+-retaining diuretics are used to prevent hypokalaemia. They predispose to hyperkalaemia, especially in patients with impaired renal function or with concomitant use of K^+ supplements, ACEI or NSAIDs.

HYPERKALAEMIA

Hyperkalaemia in untreated patients suggests the possibility of renal failure or of mineralocorticoid deficiency (e.g. Addison's disease). Most commonly, however, it is caused by drugs. Hyperkalaemia can develop either with potassium supplements or with potassium-sparing diuretics (see above). Hyperkalaemia is particularly likely to occur in patients with impaired renal function, in the elderly (in whom renal impairment may be unrecognized because the plasma creatinine concentration is normal) and in patients receiving ACE inhibitors, K^+ supplements or NSAID.

Treatment

1. Calcium gluconate is a potentially life-saving emergency treatment in patients with dysrhythmias caused by hyperkalaemia (Chapter 32). It is given intravenously with ECG monitoring.
2. Glucose and insulin shift extracellular K^+ into cells.
3. Sodium bicarbonate, given intravenously, also shifts K^+ into cells.
4. High-dose nebulized β_2-agonists shift K^+ into cells.
5. Ion-exchange resin made of sodium or calcium polystyrene sulphonate removes potassium from the body in stool. The main adverse effect when resins are given chronically for patients with chronic renal failure is constipation, which can be avoided if the resins are suspended in a solution of **sorbitol**.
6. Emergency haemofiltration or dialysis.

Key points

Drugs and plasma potassium

- Hypokalaemia (and hypomagnesaemia) predisposes to digoxin toxicity and to torsades de pointes caused by drugs that prolong the QT interval (e.g. amiodarone, sotalol). Mild hypokalaemia associated with thiazide or loop diuretics is common and seldom harmful per se.
- Where hypokalaemia is clinically important it can be corrected and/or prevented with K^+ supplements or more conveniently with K^+-retaining diuretics. However, these predispose to hyperkalaemia.
- Hyperkalaemia can cause dysrhythmias that can be fatal. ACEI predispose to hyperkalaemia, especially when there is renal impairment.
- Emergency treatment of broad complex tachycardia caused by hyperkalaemia includes i.v. calcium gluconate.
- Glucose and insulin i.v. cause redistribution of potassium into cells.
- Sodium bicarbonate i.v. can cause redistribution of potassium into cells in exchange for hydrogen ions.
- β_2-Agonists i.v./high-dose nebulized cause intracellular shift of K^+.
- Haemodialysis or haemofiltration is frequently indicated in acute hyperkalaemic emergencies.
- Ion-exchange resins administered by mouth are useful.

DRUGS THAT ALTER URINE pH

ACIDIFICATION

Ammonium chloride given orally results in urinary acidification and is used in specialized diagnostic tests of renal tubular acidosis. It is a gastric irritant and is given as enteric-coated tablets. The elimination of some basic drugs (e.g. **amfetamine**) is enhanced by acidification of the urine, though this is rarely used in clinical practice.

ALKALINIZATION

Sodium bicarbonate causes urinary alkalinization; intravenously it is used to alkalinize the urine in salicylate overdose (see Chapter 54). However, if given by mouth it reacts with hydrochloric acid in the stomach to produce carbon dioxide, so it is poorly tolerated and not very effective. Instead, a citric acid/potassium citrate mixture can be used orally, as citrate is absorbed from the gut and metabolized via the tricarboxylic acid cycle with generation of bicarbonate. Potassium must be avoided in renal failure, as retention of potassium ions may cause hyperkalaemia.

Use

Alkalinization of the urine is used to give symptomatic relief for the dysuria of cystitis and to prevent the formation of uric acid stones, especially in patients who are about to undergo cancer chemotherapy. The use of alkaline diuresis to increase urinary excretion of salicylate following overdose is discussed in Chapter 54.

DRUGS THAT AFFECT THE BLADDER AND GENITO-URINARY SYSTEM

DRUGS TO INCREASE BLADDER ACTIVITY

Drugs that increase bladder activity (e.g. muscarinic agonists, such as **bethanechol**, or anticholinesterases, such as **distigmine**) have been used to treat patients with chronic retention of urine, but catheterization is usually preferable.

DRUGS FOR URINARY INCONTINENCE

Stress incontinence is usually managed without drugs, often surgically, although **duloxetine** (an amine uptake inhibitor) is licensed for use in women with moderately severe stress incontinence in conjunction with pelvic floor exercises. Alpha blockers (e.g. **doxazosin**, see Chapter 28) can worsen incontinence in women with pelvic floor pathology and should be discontinued if possible.

Urge incontinence is common. Infection should be excluded. When unstable detrusor contraction is responsible, drug treatment to reduce bladder activity is of limited use, combined with pelvic floor exercises and bladder training. Antimuscarinic drugs, such as **oxybutynin**, have a high incidence of antimuscarinic side effects (e.g. dry mouth, dry eyes, blurred vision, constipation, confusion). These may be minimized by starting with a low dose and by slow release formulation. **Solifenacin** is a newer and more expensive drug.

DRUGS FOR PROSTATIC OBSTRUCTION

Prostatic obstruction is often managed surgically. Symptoms of benign prostatic hypertrophy may be improved by a 5α-reductase inhibitor (e.g. **finasteride**, Chapters 41 and 48) or by an α_1-adrenoceptor antagonist (e.g. **doxazosin**, Chapter 28). **Tamsulosin**, an α_1-adrenoceptor antagonist selective for the α_{1A}-adrenoceptor subtype, produces less postural hypotension than non-selective α_1-adrenoceptor antagonists. Hormonal manipulation with anti-androgens and analogues of luteinizing hormone-releasing hormone (LHRH) is valuable in patients with prostatic cancer (Chapter 48).

ERECTILE DYSFUNCTION

Erectile failure has several organic, as well as numerous psychological, causes. Replacement therapy with testosterone, given by skin patch, is effective in cases caused by proven androgen deficiency. Nitric oxide is involved in erectile function both as a vascular endothelium-derived mediator and as a non-adrenergic non-cholinergic neurotransmitter. This has led to the development of type V phosphodiesterase inhibitors as oral agents to treat erectile dysfunction. **Sildenafil** (Viagra™) was the first of these to be introduced, there are several other longer-acting agents in this class currently. These drugs are discussed in Chapter 41.

Case history

A 35-year-old woman has proteinuria (3 g/24 hours) and progressive renal impairment (current serum creatinine 220 μmol/L) in the setting of insulin-dependent diabetes mellitus. In addition to insulin, she takes captopril regularly and buys ibuprofen over the counter to take as needed for migraine. She develops progressive oedema which does not respond to oral furosemide in increasing doses of up to 250 mg/day. Amiloride (10 mg daily) is added without benefit and metolazone (5 mg daily) is started. She loses 3 kg over the next three days. One week later, she is admitted to hospital having collapsed at home. She is conscious but severely ill. Her blood pressure is 90/60 mmHg, heart rate is 86 beats/minute and regular, and she has residual peripheral oedema, but the jugular venous pressure is not raised. Serum urea is 55 mmol/L, creatinine is 350 μmol/L, K+ is 6.8 mmol/L, glucose is 5.6 mmol/L and albumin is 3.0 g/dL. Urinalysis shows 4+ protein. An ECG shows tall peaked T-waves and broad QRS complexes.

Question

Decide whether each of the following statements is true or false.

(a) Insulin should be withheld until the patient's metabolic state has improved.
(b) Metolazone should be stopped.
(c) The furosemide dose should be increased in view of the persistent oedema.

(d) Ibuprofen could have contributed to the hyperkalaemia.
(e) Captopril should be withheld.

Answer

(a) False
(b) True
(c) False
(d) True
(e) True

Comment

Although highly effective in causing diuresis in patients with resistant oedema, combination diuretic treatment with loop, K+-sparing and thiazide diuretics can cause acute prerenal renal failure with a disproportionate increase in serum urea compared to creatinine. Resistance to furosemide may be related to the combination of reduced GFR plus albuminuria. The combination of an NSAID, captopril and amiloride is extremely dangerous, especially in diabetics, and will have contributed to the severe hyperkalaemia. The NSAID may also have led to reduced glomerular filtration. Glucose with insulin would be appropriate to lower the plasma K+.

Case history

A 73-year-old man has a long history of hypertension and of osteoarthritis. Three months ago he had a myocardial infarction, since when he has been progressively oedematous and dyspnoeic, initially only on exertion but more recently also on lying flat. He continues to take co-amilozide for his hypertension and naproxen for his osteoarthritis. The blood pressure is 164/94 mmHg and there are signs of fluid overload with generalized oedema and markedly elevated jugular venous pressure. Serum creatinine is 138 μmol/L and K+ is 5.0 mmol/L. Why would it be hazardous to commence furosemide in addition to his present treatment? What alternative strategy could be considered?

Comment

The patient may go into prerenal renal failure with the addition of the loop diuretic to the two more distal diuretics he is already taking in the co-amilozide combination. The NSAID he is taking makes this more likely, and also makes it more probable that his serum potassium level (which is already high) will become dangerously elevated. It would be appropriate to consider hospital admission, stopping naproxen (perhaps substituting paracetamol for pain if necessary), stopping the co-amilozide and cautiously instituting an ACE inhibitor (which could improve his prognosis from his heart failure as described in Chapter 31) followed by introduction of furosemide with close monitoring of blood pressure, signs of fluid overload and serum creatinine and potassium levels over the next few days.

FURTHER READING

Brater DC. Pharmacology of diuretics. *American Journal of Medical Science* 2000; **319**: 38–50.

Clark BA, Brown RS. Potassium homeostasis and hyperkalemic syndromes. *Endocrinology and Metabolism Clinics of North America* 1995; **24**: 573–91.

Greger R, Lang F, Sebekova, Heidland A. Action and clinical use of diuretics. In: Davison AMA, Cameron JS, Grunfeld J-P et al (eds). *Oxford textbook of clinical nephrology*, 3rd edn. Oxford: Oxford University Press, 2005: 2619–48.

Reid IR, Ames RW, Orr-Walker BJ et al. Hydrochlorothiazide reduces loss of cortical bone in normal postmenopausal women: a randomized controlled trial. *American Journal of Medicine* 2000; **109**: 362–70.

Saggar-Malik AK, Cappuccio FP. Potassium supplements and potassium-sparing diuretics. A review and guide to appropriate use. *Drugs* 1993; **46**: 986–1008.

Shankar SS, Brater DC. Loop diuretics: from the Na-K-2Cl transporter to clinical use. *American Journal of Physiology. Renal Physiology* 2003; **284**: F11–21.

Weinberger MH. Eplerenone – a new selective aldosterone receptor antagonist. *Drugs of Today* 2004; **40**: 481–5.

PART VIII

THE ENDOCRINE SYSTEM

DIABETES MELLITUS

INTRODUCTION

Before the discovery of **insulin**, type 1 diabetes – where insulin deficiency can lead to ketoacidosis – was invariably fatal. Since the introduction of insulin, the therapeutic focus has broadened from treating and preventing diabetic ketoacidosis to preventing long-term vascular complications. Type 2 diabetes – where insulin resistance and a relative lack of insulin lead to hyperglycaemia – not only causes symptoms related directly to hyperglycaemia (polyuria, polydipsia and blurred vision – see below), but is also a very powerful risk factor for atheromatous disease. Glucose intolerance and diabetes mellitus are increasingly prevalent in affluent and developing countries, and represent a major public health challenge. Addressing risk factors distinct from blood glucose, especially hypertension, is of paramount importance and is covered elsewhere (Chapters 27 and 28). In this chapter, we focus mainly on the types of insulin and oral hypoglycaemic agents.

PATHOPHYSIOLOGY

Insulin is secreted by β-cells (also called B-cells) of the islets of Langerhans. It lowers blood glucose, but also modulates the metabolic disposition of fats and amino acids, as well as carbohydrate. It is secreted together with inactive C-peptide, which provides a useful index of insulin secretion: its plasma concentration is low or absent in patients with type 1 diabetes, but very high in patients with insulinoma (an uncommon tumour which causes hypoglycaemia by secreting insulin). This should not be confused with 'C-reactive peptide' (CRP) which is an acute phase protein synthesized by the liver and used as a non-specific index of inflammation. C-peptide concentration is not elevated in patients with hypoglycaemia caused by injection of insulin.

Diabetes mellitus (fasting blood glucose concentration of $\geqslant 7\,\text{mmol/L}$) is caused by an absolute or relative lack of insulin. In type 1 diabetes there is an absolute deficiency of insulin. Such patients are usually young and non-obese at presentation. There is an inherited predisposition. However, concordance in identical twins is somewhat less than 50%, so it is believed that genetically predisposed individuals must also be exposed to an environmental factor. Viruses (including Coxsackie and Echo viruses) are one such factor and may initiate an autoimmune process that then destroys the islet cells.

In type 2 diabetes there is a relative lack of insulin secretion, coupled with marked resistance to its action. The circulating concentration of immunoreactive insulin measured by standard assays (which do not discriminate well between insulin and pro-insulin) may be normal or even increased, but more discriminating assays indicate that there is an increase in pro-insulin, and that the true insulin concentration is reduced. Such patients are usually middle-aged or older at presentation, and obese. Concordance of this form of diabetes in identical twins is nearly 100%. Type 2 diabetes is rarely if ever associated with diabetic ketoacidosis, although it can be complicated by non-ketotic hyperosmolar coma or, rarely (in association with treatment with a biguanide drug such as metformin, see below), with lactic acidosis.

An increased concentration of glucose in the circulating blood gives rise to osmotic effects:

1. diuresis (polyuria) with consequent circulating volume reduction, causing thirst and polydipsia;
2. the refractive index of a high glucose concentration solution in the eye differs from healthy aqueous humour, causing blurred vision.

In addition, glycosuria predisposes to *Candida* infection, especially in women. The loss of calories in the urine is coupled with inability to store energy as glycogen or fat, or to lay down protein in muscle, and weight loss with loss of fat and muscle ('amyotrophy') is common in uncontrolled diabetics.

Both types of diabetes mellitus are complicated by vascular complications. Microvascular complications include retinopathy, which consists of background retinopathy (dot and blot haemorrhages and hard exudates which do not of themselves threaten vision), and proliferative retinopathy which can cause retinal haemorrhage and blindness. Cataracts are common. Diabetic neuropathy causes a glove and stocking distribution of loss of sensation with associated painful paraesthesiae. Approximately one-third of diabetic patients develop diabetic nephropathy, which leads to renal failure. Microalbuminuria is a forerunner of overt diabetic nephropathy.

Macrovascular disease is the result of accelerated atheroma and results in an increased incidence of myocardial infarction, peripheral vascular disease and stroke. There is a strong association (pointed out by Reaven in his 1988 Banting Lecture at the annual meeting of the American Diabetes Association) between diabetes and obesity, hypertension and dyslipidaemia (especially hypertriglyceridaemia), and type 2 diabetes is strongly associated with endothelial dysfunction, an early event in atherogenesis (Chapter 27).

PRINCIPLES OF MANAGEMENT

It is important to define ambitious but achievable goals for each patient. In young type 1 patients there is good evidence that improved diabetic control reduces microvascular complications. It is well worth trying hard to minimize the metabolic derangement associated with diabetes mellitus in order to reduce the development of such complications. Education and support are essential to motivate the patient to learn how to adjust their insulin dose to optimize glycaemic control. This can only be achieved by the patient performing blood glucose monitoring at home and learning to adjust their insulin dose accordingly. The treatment regimen must be individualized. A common strategy is to combine injections of a short-acting insulin before each meal with a once daily injection of a long-acting insulin to provide a low steady background level during the night. Follow up must include structured care with assessment of chronic glycaemic control using HbA1c and regular screening for evidence of microvascular disease. This is especially important in the case of proliferative retinopathy and maculopathy, because prophylactic laser therapy can prevent blindness.

By contrast, striving for tight control of blood sugar in type 2 patients is only appropriate in selected cases. Tight control reduces macrovascular complications, but at the expense of increased hypoglycaemic attacks, and the number of patients that needs to be treated in this way to prevent one cardiovascular event is large. In contrast, aggressive treatment of hypertension is of substantial benefit, and the target blood pressure should be lower than in non-diabetic patients (<130 mmHg systolic and <80 mmHg diastolic, see Chapter 28). In older type 2 patients, hypoglycaemic treatment aims to minimize symptoms of polyuria, polydipsia or recurrent *Candida* infection, and to prevent hyperosmolar coma.

DIET IN DIABETES MELLITUS

It is important to achieve and maintain ideal body weight on a non-atherogenic diet. Caloric intake must be matched with insulin injections. Patients who rely on injected insulin must time their food intake accordingly. Simple sugars should be restricted because they are rapidly absorbed, causing postprandial hyperglycaemia, and should be replaced by foods that give rise to delayed and reduced glucose absorption, analogous to slow release drugs (quantified by nutritionists as 'glycaemic index'). (Artificial sweeteners are useful for those with a 'sweet tooth'.) A fibre-rich diet reduces peak glucose levels after meals and reduces the insulin requirement. Beans and lentils flatten the glucose absorption curve. Saturated fat and cholesterol intake should be minimized. Low fat sources of protein are favoured. There is no place for commercially promoted 'special diabetic foods', which are expensive and also often high in fat and calories at the expense of complex carbohydrate.

DRUGS USED TO TREAT DIABETES MELLITUS

INSULINS

Insulin is a polypeptide. Animal insulins have been almost entirely replaced by recombinant human insulin and related analogues. These are of consistent quality and cause fewer allergic effects. Insulin is available in several formulations (e.g. with protamine and/or with zinc) which differ in pharmacokinetic properties, especially their rates of absorption and durations of action. So-called 'designer' insulins are synthetic polypeptides closely related to insulin, but with small changes in amino acid composition which change their properties. For example, a lysine and a proline residue are switched in **insulin lispro**, which consequently has a very rapid absorption and onset (and can therefore be injected immediately before a meal), whereas **insulin glargine** is very slow acting and is used to provide a low level of insulin activity during the 24-hour period.

Use

Insulin is indicated in all patients with type 1 diabetes mellitus (although it is not strictly necessary during the early 'honeymoon' period before islet cell destruction is complete) and in about one-third of patients with type 2 disease. **Insulin** is usually administered by subcutaneous injection, although recently an inhaled preparation has been licensed for use in type 2 diabetics. (Note: This was not commercially successful, and has been withdrawn in the UK for this reason.) The effective dose of human insulin is usually rather less than that of animal insulins because of the lack of production of blocking antibodies. Consequently, the dose is reduced when switching from animal to human insulin.

Soluble insulin is the only preparation suitable for intravenous use. It is administered intravenously in diabetic emergencies and given subcutaneously before meals in chronic management. Formulations of human insulins are available in various ratios of short-acting and longer-lasting forms (e.g. 30:70, commonly used twice daily). Some of these are marketed in prefilled injection devices ('pens') which are convenient for patients. The small dose of soluble insulin controls hyperglycaemia just after the injection. The main danger is of hypoglycaemia in the early hours of the morning. When starting a diabetic on a two dose per day regime, it is therefore helpful to divide the daily dose into two-thirds to be given before breakfast and one-third to be given before the evening meal. If the patient engages in strenuous physical work, the morning dose of **insulin** is reduced somewhat to prevent exercise-induced hypoglycaemia.

Insulin is also required for symptomatic type 2 diabetics in whom diet and/or oral hypoglycaemic drugs fail. Unfortunately, **insulin** makes weight loss considerably more difficult because it stimulates appetite, but its anabolic effects are valuable in wasted patients with diabetic amyotrophy. **Insulin** is needed in acute diabetic emergencies such as ketoacidosis, during pregnancy, peri-operatively and in severe intercurrent disease (infections, myocardial infarction, burns, etc.).

Insulin requirements are increased by up to one-third by intercurrent infection and patients must be instructed to intensify home blood glucose monitoring when they have a cold or other infection (even if they are eating less than usual) and increase the **insulin** dose if necessary. The dose will subsequently need to be reduced when the infection has cleared. Vomiting often causes patients incorrectly to stop injecting **insulin** (for fear of hypoglycaemia) and this may result in ketoacidosis.

Patients for elective surgery should be changed to soluble **insulin** preoperatively. During surgery, soluble **insulin** can be infused i.v. with glucose to produce a blood glucose concentration of 6–8 mmol/L. This is continued post-operatively until oral feeding and intermittent subcutaneous injections

of **insulin** can be resumed. A similar regime is suitable for emergency operations, but more frequent measurements of blood glucose are required. Patients with type 2 diabetes can sometimes be managed without **insulin**, but the blood glucose must be regularly checked during the post-operative period.

Ketoacidosis

The metabolic changes in diabetic ketoacidosis (DKA) resemble those of starvation since, despite increased plasma glucose concentrations, glucose is not available intracellularly ('starving amidst plenty'). Hyperglycaemia leads to osmotic diuresis and electrolyte depletion. Conservation of K^+ is even less efficient than that of Na^+ in the face of acidosis and an osmotic diuresis, and large amounts of intravenous K^+ are often needed to replace the large deficit in total body K^+. However, plasma K^+ concentration in DKA can be increased due to a shift from the intracellular to the extracellular compartment, so large amounts of potassium chloride should not be administered until plasma electrolyte concentrations are available and high urine output established. Fat is mobilized from adipose tissue, releasing free fatty acids that are metabolized by β-oxidation to acetyl coenzyme A (CoA). In the absence of glucose breakdown, acetyl CoA is converted to acetoacetate, acetone and β-hydroxybutyrate (ketones). These are buffered by plasma bicarbonate, leading to a fall in bicarbonate concentration (metabolic acidosis – with an increased 'anion gap' since anionic ketone bodies are not measured routinely) and compensatory hyperventilation ('Küssmaul' breathing). There are therefore a number of metabolic abnormalities:

- *Sodium and potassium deficit* A generous volume of physiological saline (0.9% sodium chloride), given intravenously, is crucial in order to restore extracellular fluid volume. Monitoring urine output is necessary. When blood glucose levels fall below 17 mmol/L, 5% glucose is given in place of N-saline. Potassium must be replaced and if the urinary output is satisfactory and the plasma potassium concentration is <4.5 mEq/L, up to 20 mmol/hour KCl can be given, the rate of replacement being judged by frequent measurements of plasma potassium concentration and ECG monitoring.
- *Hyperglycaemia* Intravenous insulin is infused at a rate of up to 0.1 unit/kg/hour with a syringe pump until ketosis resolves (judged by blood pH, serum bicarbonate and blood or urinary ketones).
- *Metabolic acidosis* This usually resolves with adequate treatment with physiological sodium chloride and insulin. Bicarbonate treatment to reverse the extracellular metabolic acidosis is controversial, and may paradoxically worsen intracellular and cerebrospinal fluid acidosis. If arterial pH is <7.0, the patient is often given bicarbonate, should be managed on an intensive care unit if possible and may need inotropic support.
- *Other measures* include aspiration of the stomach, as gastric stasis is common and aspiration can be severe and may be fatal, and treatment of the precipitating cause of coma (e.g. antibiotics for bacterial infection).

Key points

Type 1 diabetes mellitus and insulin

- Type 1 (insulin-dependent) diabetes mellitus is caused by degeneration of β-cells in the islets of Langerhans leading to an absolute deficiency of insulin.
- Without insulin treatment, such patients are prone to diabetic ketoacidosis (DKA).
- Even with insulin treatment, such patients are susceptible to microvascular complications of retinopathy, nephropathy and neuropathy, and also to accelerated atherosclerotic (macrovascular) disease leading to myocardial infarction, stroke and gangrene.
- Management includes a healthy diet low in saturated fat (Chapter 27), high in complex carbohydrates and with the energy spread throughout the day.
- Regular subcutaneous injections of recombinant human insulin are required indefinitely. Mixtures of soluble and longer-acting insulins are used and are given using special insulin 'pens' at least twice daily. Regular self-monitoring of blood glucose levels throughout the day with individual adjustment of the insulin dose is essential to achieve good metabolic control, which reduces the risk of complications.
- DKA is treated with large volumes of intravenous physiological saline, intravenous soluble insulin and replacement of potassium and, if necessary, magnesium.

Hyperosmolar non-ketotic coma

Less **insulin** is required in this situation, as the blood pH is normal and **insulin** sensitivity is retained. Fluid loss is restored using physiological saline (there is sometimes a place for half-strength, 0.45% saline) and large amounts of intravenous potassium are often required. Magnesium deficiency is common, contributes to the difficulty of correcting the potassium deficit, and should be treated provided renal function is normal. In this hyperosmolar state, the viscosity of the blood is increased and a **heparin** preparation (Chapter 30) should be considered as prophylaxis against venous thrombosis.

Mechanism of action

Insulin acts by binding to transmembrane glycoprotein receptors. Receptor occupancy results in:

1. activation of insulin-dependent glucose transport processes (in adipose tissue and muscle) via a transporter known as 'Glut-4';
2. inhibition of adenylyl cyclase-dependent metabolism (lipolysis, proteolysis, glycogenolysis);
3. intracellular accumulation of potassium and phosphate, which is linked to glucose transport in some tissues.

Secondary effects include increased cellular amino acid uptake, increased DNA and RNA synthesis and increased oxidative phosphorylation.

Adverse reactions

1. Hypoglycaemia is the most important and severe complication of **insulin** treatment. It is treated with an intravenous injection of glucose in unconscious patients, but sugar is given as a sweet drink in those with milder symptoms. **Glucagon** (1 mg intramuscularly, repeated after a few minutes if necessary) is useful if the patient is unconscious and intravenous access is not achievable (e.g. to ambulance personnel or a family member).
2. **Insulin**-induced post-hypoglycaemic hyperglycaemia (Somogyi effect) occurs when hypoglycaemia (e.g. in the early hours of the morning) induces an overshoot of hormones (adrenaline, growth hormone, glucocorticosteroids, glucagon) that elevate blood glucose (raised blood glucose on awakening). The situation can be misinterpreted as requiring increased **insulin**, thus producing further hypoglycaemia.
3. Local or systemic allergic reactions to **insulin**, with itching, redness and swelling at the injection site.
4. Lipodystrophy: the disappearance of subcutaneous fat at or near injection sites. Atrophy is minimized by rotation of injection sites. Fatty tumours occur if repeated injections are made at the same site.
5. **Insulin** resistance, defined arbitrarily as a daily requirement of more than 200 units, due to antibodies, is unusual. Changing to a highly purified **insulin** preparation is often successful, a small starting dose being used to avoid hypoglycaemia.

Pharmacokinetics

Insulin is broken down in the gut and by the liver and kidney, and is given by injection. The $t_{1/2}$ is three to five minutes. It is metabolized to inactive α and β peptide chains largely by hepatic/renal insulinases (insulin glutathione transhydrogenase). **Insulin** from the pancreas is mainly released into the portal circulation and passes to the liver, where up to 60% is degraded before reaching the systemic circulation (presystemic metabolism). The kidney is also important in the metabolism of **insulin** and patients with progressive renal impairment often have a reduced requirement for **insulin**. There is no evidence that diabetes ever results from increased hepatic destruction of **insulin**, but in cirrhosis the liver fails to inactivate **insulin**, thus predisposing to hypoglycaemia.

ORAL HYPOGLYCAEMIC DRUGS AND TYPE 2 DIABETES

Oral hypoglycaemic drugs are useful in type 2 diabetes as adjuncts to continued dietary restraint. They fall into four groups:

1. biguanides (**metformin**);
2. sulphonylureas and related drugs;
3. thiazolidinediones (glitazones);
4. α-glucosidase inhibitors (**acarbose**).

Most type 2 diabetic patients initially achieve satisfactory control with diet either alone or combined with one of these agents. The small proportion who cannot be controlled with drugs at this stage (primary failure) require **insulin**. Subsequent failure after initially adequate control (secondary failure) occurs in about one-third of patients, and is treated with **insulin**. Inhaled **insulin** is effective but expensive. Its bioavailability is affected by smoking and by respiratory infections, and currently should only be used with great caution in patients with asthma/COPD.

BIGUANIDES: METFORMIN

Uses

Metformin is the only biguanide available in the UK. It is used in type 2 diabetic patients inadequately controlled by diet. Its anorectic effect aids weight reduction, so it is a first choice drug for obese type 2 patients, provided there are no contraindications. It must not be used in patients at risk of lactic acidosis and is contraindicated in:

- renal failure (it is eliminated in the urine, see below);
- alcoholics;
- cirrhosis;
- chronic lung disease (because of hypoxia);
- cardiac failure (because of poor tissue perfusion);
- congenital mitochondrial myopathy (which is often accompanied by diabetes);
- acute myocardial infarction and other serious intercurrent illness (**insulin** should be substituted).

Metformin should be withdrawn and **insulin** substituted before major elective surgery. Plasma creatinine and liver function tests should be monitored before and during its use.

Mechanism of action

This remains uncertain. Biguanides do not produce hypoglycaemia and are effective in pancreatectomized animals. Effects of **metformin** include:

- reduced glucose absorption from the gut;
- facilitation of glucose entry into muscle by a non-insulin-responsive mechanism;
- inhibition of gluconeogenesis in the liver;
- suppression of oxidative glucose metabolism and enhanced anaerobic glycolysis.

Adverse effects

Metformin causes nausea, a metallic taste, anorexia, vomiting and diarrhoea. The symptoms are worst when treatment is initiated and a few patients cannot tolerate even small doses. Lactic acidosis, which has a reported mortality in excess of 60%, is uncommon provided that the above contraindications are respected. Treatment is by reversal of hypoxia and circulatory collapse and peritoneal or haemodialysis to alleviate sodium overloading and removing the drug. **Phenformin** (withdrawn in the UK and USA) was more frequently associated with this problem than **metformin**. Absorption of vitamin B_{12} is reduced by **metformin**, but this is seldom clinically important.

Pharmacokinetics

Oral absorption of **metformin** is 50–60%; it is eliminated unchanged by renal excretion, clearance being greater than the glomerular filtration rate because of active secretion into the tubular fluid. **Metformin** accumulates in patients with renal impairment. The plasma $t_{1/2}$ ranges from 1.5 to 4.5 hours, but its duration of action is considerably longer, permitting twice daily dosing.

Drug interactions

Other oral hypoglycaemic drugs are additive with **metformin**. **Ethanol** predisposes to **metformin**-related lactic acidosis.

SULPHONYLUREAS AND RELATED DRUGS
Use

Sulphonylureas (e.g. **tolbutamide**, **glibenclamide**, **gliclazide**) are used for type 2 diabetics who have not responded adequately to diet alone or diet and **metformin** with which they are additive. They improve symptoms of polyuria and polydipsia, but (in contrast to **metformin**) stimulate appetite. **Chlorpropamide**, the longest-acting agent in this group, has a higher incidence of adverse effects (especially hypoglycaemia) than other drugs of this class and should be avoided. This is because of a protracted effect and reduced renal clearance in patients with renal dysfunction and the elderly; thus it is hardly ever used. **Tolbutamide** and **gliclazide** are shorter acting than **glibenclamide**, so there is less risk of hypoglycaemia, and for this reason they are preferred in the elderly. Related

drugs (e.g. **repaglinide**, **nateglinide**) are chemically distinct, but act at the same receptor. They are shorter acting even than **tolbutamide**, but more expensive. They are given before meals.

Mechanism of action

The hypoglycaemic effect of these drugs depends on the presence of functioning B cells. Sulphonylureas, like glucose, depolarize B cells and release **insulin**. They do this by binding to sulphonylurea receptors (SUR) and blocking ATP-dependent potassium channels (KATP); the resulting depolarization activates voltage-sensitive Ca^{2+} channels, in turn causing entry of Ca^{2+} ions and **insulin** secretion.

Adverse effects

Sulphonylureas can cause hypoglycaemia. **Chlorpropamide**, the longest-acting agent, was responsible for many cases. It also causes flushing in susceptible individuals when **ethanol** is consumed, and can cause dilutional hyponatraemia (by potentiating ADH, see Chapter 42). Allergic reactions to sulphonylureas include rashes, drug fever, gastrointestinal upsets, transient jaundice (usually cholestatic) and haematopoietic changes, including thrombocytopenia, neutropenia and pancytopenia. Serious effects other than hypoglycaemia are uncommon.

Pharmacokinetics

Sulphonylureas are well absorbed from the gastrointestinal tract and the major differences between them lie in their relative potencies and rates of elimination. **Glibenclamide** is almost completely metabolized by the liver to weakly active metabolites that are excreted in the bile and urine. The activity of these metabolites is only clinically important in patients with renal failure, in whom they accumulate and can cause hypoglycaemia. **Tolbutamide** is converted in the liver to inactive metabolites which are excreted in the urine. The $t_{1/2}$ shows considerable inter-individual variability, but is usually four to eight hours. **Gliclazide** is extensively metabolized, although up to 20% is excreted unchanged in the urine. The plasma $t_{1/2}$ ranges from 6 to 14 hours. **Repaglinide** and **nateglinide** exhibit rapid onset and offset kinetics, rapid absorption (time to maximal plasma concentration approximately 55 minutes after an oral dose) and elimination (half-life approximately three hours). These features lead to short duration of action and a low risk of hypoglycaemia. They are administered shortly before a meal to reduce the postprandial glucose rise in type 2 diabetic patients.

Drug interactions

Monoamine oxidase inhibitors potentiate the activity of sulphonylureas by an unknown mechanism. Several drugs (e.g. glucocorticosteroids, growth hormone) antagonize the hypoglycaemic effects of sulphonylureas by virtue of their actions on **insulin** release or sensitivity.

THIAZOLIDINEDIONES (GLITAZONES)

Glitazones (e.g. **piolitazone**, **rosiglitazone**) were developed from the chance finding that a fibrate drug (Chapter 27) increased **insulin** sensitivity.

Use

Glitazones lower blood glucose and haemoglobin A1c (HbA1c) in type 2 diabetes mellitus patients who are inadequately controlled on diet alone or diet and other oral hypoglycaemic drugs. An effect on mortality or diabetic complications has yet to be established, but they have rapidly become very widely used.

Mechanism of action

Glitazones bind to the peroxisome-proliferating activator receptor γ (PPARγ), a nuclear receptor found mainly in adipocytes and also in hepatocytes and myocytes. It works slowly, increasing the sensitivity to **insulin** possibly via effects of circulating fatty acids on glucose metabolism.

Adverse effects

The first two glitazones caused severe hepatotoxicity and are not used. Hepatotoxicity has not proved problematic with **rosiglitazone** or **pioglitazone**, although they are contraindicated in patients with hepatic impairment and liver function should be monitored during their use. The most common adverse effects are weight gain (possibly partly directly related to their effect on adipocytes) and fluid retention due to an effect of PPARγ receptors on renal tubular sodium ion absorption. They can also exacerbate cardiac dysfunction and are therefore contraindicated in heart failure. Recently, an association with increased bone fractures and osteoporosis has been noted. They are contraindicated during pregnancy. A possible increase in myocardial infarction with **rosiglitazone** has been noted, but the data are controversial.

Pharmacokinetics

Both **rosiglitazone** and **pioglitazone** are well absorbed, highly protein bound and subject to hepatic metabolism.

Drug interactions

Glitazones are additive with other oral hypoglycaemic drugs. They potentiate **insulin**, but this combination is contraindicated in Europe because of concerns that it might increase the risk of heart failure, although the combination is widely used in the USA. **Pioglitazone** is an inducer of CYP3A and may cause treatment failure with concomitantly administered drugs which are CYP3A substrates (e.g. reproductive steroids).

ACARBOSE

Acarbose is used in type 2 diabetes mellitus in patients who are inadequately controlled on diet alone or diet and other oral hypoglycaemic agents. **Acarbose** is a reversible competitive inhibitor of intestinal α-glucoside hydrolases and delays the absorption of starch and sucrose, but does not affect the absorption of ingested glucose. The postprandial glycaemic rise after a meal containing complex carbohydrates is reduced and its peak is delayed. Fermentation of unabsorbed carbohydrate in the intestine leads to increased gas formation which results in flatulence, abdominal distension and occasionally diarrhoea. As with any change in a diabetic patient's medication, diet or activities, the blood glucose must be monitored.

Key points

Type 2 diabetes mellitus and oral hypoglycaemic agents

- Type 2 (non-insulin-dependent) diabetes mellitus is caused by relative deficiency of insulin in the face of impaired insulin sensitivity. Such patients are usually obese.
- About one-third of such patients finally require insulin treatment. This is especially important when they are losing muscle mass.
- The dietary goal is to achieve ideal body weight by consuming an energy-restricted healthy diet low in saturated fat (Chapter 27).
- Oral hypoglycaemic drugs are useful in some patients as an adjunct to diet.
- Metformin, a biguanide, lowers blood glucose levels and encourages weight loss by causing anorexia. Diarrhoea is a common adverse effect. It is contraindicated in patients with renal impairment, heart failure, obstructive pulmonary disease or congenital mitochondrial myopathies because of the risk of lactic acidosis, a rare but life-threatening complication.
- Acarbose, an α-glucosidase inhibitor, delays the absorption of starch and sucrose. It flattens the rise in plasma glucose following a meal and may improve control when added to diet with or without other drugs. However, it can cause bloating, flatulence and diarrhoea associated with carbohydrate malabsorption.
- Sulphonylureas (e.g. tolbutamide) and related drugs (e.g. nateglinide) release insulin from β-cells by closing ATP-sensitive K$^+$ channels, thereby depolarizing the cell membrane. They are well tolerated and improve blood glucose at least initially, but stimulate appetite, promoting weight gain. They differ from one another in their kinetics, the longer-acting drugs being particularly likely to cause hypoglycaemia which can be severe, especially in the elderly and should not be used in these patients.
- Thiazolidinediones (e.g. pioglitazone, rosiglitazone) activate PPARγ receptors and increase insulin sensitivity. They lower blood sugar but cause weight gain and fluid retention. They are contraindicated in heart failure. Effects on longevity or complications are unknown.

Case history

A 56-year-old woman with a positive family history of diabetes presents with polyuria, polydipsia, blurred vision and recurrent attacks of vaginal thrush. She is overweight at 92 kg, her fasting blood sugar is 12 mmol/L and haemoglobin A1C is elevated at 10.6%. She is treated with glibenclamide once daily in addition to topical antifungal treatment for the thrush. Initially, her symptoms improve considerably and she feels generally much better, but after nine months the polyuria and polydipsia recur and her weight has increased to 102 kg.
Comment
Treatment with a sulphonylurea without attention to diet is doomed to failure. This patient needs to be motivated to take dietary advice, restricting her energy intake and reducing her risk of atherosclerosis. If hyperglycaemia is still not improved, metformin (which reduces appetite) would be appropriate.

FURTHER READING

American Diabetes Association. Implications of the diabetes control and complications trial. *Diabetes* 1993; **42**: 1555–8.

Bolli GB, Owens DR. Insulin glargine. *Lancet* 2000; **356**: 443–5.

deFronzo RA, Goodman AM. Efficacy of metformin in patients with non-insulin-dependent diabetes mellitus. *New England Journal of Medicine* 1995; **333**: 541–9 (see also accompanying editorial on metformin by OB Crofford, pp. 588–9).

Dornhorst A. Insulinotropic meglitinide analogues. *Lancet* 2001; **358**: 1709–16.

Gale EAM. Lessons from the glitazones: a story of drug development. *Lancet* 2001; **357**: 1870–5.

Gerich JE. Oral hypoglycemic agents. *New England Journal of Medicine* 1989; **321**: 1231–45.

Hirsch IB. Drug therapy: Insulin analogues. *New England Journal of Medicine* 2005; **352**: 174–83.

Owens DR, Zinman B, Bolli GB. Insulins today and beyond. *Lancet* 2001; **358**: 739–46.

Perfetti R, D'Amico E. Rational drug design and PPAR agonists. *Current Diabetes Report* 2005; **5**: 340–5.

Pickup JC, Williams J (eds). *Handbook of diabetes*, 3rd edn. Oxford: Blackwell Science, 2004.

Skyler JS, Cefalu WT, Kourides IA et al. Efficacy of inhaled human insulin in type 1 diabetes mellitus: a randomized proof-of-concept study. *Lancet* 2001; **357**: 324–5.

Yki-Jarvinen H. Drug therapy: thiazolidinediones. *New England Journal of Medicine* 2004; **351**: 1106–18.

THYROID

INTRODUCTION

The thyroid secretes thyroxine (T_4) and tri-iodothyronine (T_3), as well as calcitonin, which is discussed in Chapter 39. The release of T_3 and T_4 is controlled by the pituitary hormone thyrotrophin (thyroid-stimulating hormone, TSH). This binds to receptors on thyroid follicular cells and activates adenylyl cyclase, which stimulates iodine trapping, iodothyronine synthesis and release of thyroid hormones. TSH is secreted by basophil cells in the adenohypophysis. Secretion of TSH by the anterior pituitary is stimulated by the hypothalamic peptide thyrotrophin-releasing hormone (TRH). Circulating T_4 and T_3 produce negative-feedback inhibition of TSH at the pituitary and hypothalamus.

Drug treatment is highly effective in correcting under- or over-activity of the thyroid gland. The diagnosis of abnormal thyroid function and monitoring of therapy have been greatly facilitated by accurate and sensitive assays measuring TSH, because the serum TSH level accurately reflects thyroid state, whereas the interpretation of serum concentrations of T_3 and T_4 is complicated by very extensive and somewhat variable protein binding. Negative feedback of biologically active thyroid hormones ensures that when there is primary failure of the thyroid gland, serum TSH is elevated, whereas when there is overactivity of the gland, serum TSH is depressed. Hypothyroidism caused by hypopituitarism is relatively uncommon and is associated with depressed sex hormone and adrenal cortical function. Hyperthyroidism secondary to excessive TSH is extremely rare.

PATHOPHYSIOLOGY AND PRINCIPLES OF TREATMENT

Thyroid disease is more common in women than in men, and is manifested either as goitre or as under- or over-activity of the gland. Hypothyroidism is common, especially in the elderly. It is usually caused by autoimmune destruction of the gland and, if untreated, leads to the clinical picture of myxoedema. Treatment is by lifelong replacement with thyroxine.

Hyperthyroidism is also common and again autoimmune processes are implicated. Treatment options comprise:

- antithyroid drugs;
- radioactive iodine;
- surgery.

Antithyroid drugs enable a euthyroid state to be maintained until the disease remits or definitive treatment with radio-iodine or surgery is undertaken. Radioactive iodine is well tolerated and free of surgical complications (e.g. laryngeal nerve damage), whereas surgery is most appropriate when there are local mechanical problems, such as tracheal compression.

In older patients, the most common cause of hyperthyroidism is multinodular toxic goitre. In young women it is usually caused by Graves' disease, in which an immunoglobulin binds to and stimulates the TSH receptor, thereby promoting synthesis and release of T_3 and T_4 independent of TSH. In addition to a smooth vascular goitre, there is often deposition of mucopolysaccharide, most notably in the extrinsic eye muscles which become thickened and cause proptosis. Graves' disease has a remitting/relapsing course and often finally leads to hypothyroidism. Other aetiologies of hyperthyroidism include acute viral or autoimmune thyroiditis (which usually resolve spontaneously), iatrogenic iodine excess (e.g. thyroid storm following iodine-containing contrast media and hyperthyroidism in patients treated with drugs, such as **amiodarone**; see below and Chapter 32), and acute postpartum hyperthyroidism.

IODINE

The thyroid gland concentrates iodine. Dietary iodide normally amounts to 100–200 mg per day and is absorbed from the stomach and small intestine by an active process. Following systemic absorption and uptake into the thyroid gland, iodide is oxidized to iodine, which is the precursor to various iodinated tyrosine compounds including T_3 and T_4. Iodine is used to treat simple non-toxic goitre due to iodine deficiency. Potassium iodide (3 mg daily p.o.) prevents further enlargement of the gland, but seldom actually shrinks it. Iodized salt is used to prevent this type of endemic goitre in areas where the diet is iodine deficient, according to a defined World Health Organization (WHO) policy.

Preoperative treatment with Lugol's iodine solution (an aqueous solution of iodine and potassium iodide) in combination with **carbimazole** or **propylthiouracil** (see below) is used to reduce the vascularity of the gland and inhibit thyroid hormone release. This action of iodine in inhibiting thyroid hormone release is only maintained for one to two weeks, after which thyroid hormone release is markedly increased if the cause of the hyperthyroidism has not been dealt with.

THYROXINE AND TRI-IODOTHYRONINE

Use

L-Thyroxine is used in the treatment of uncomplicated hypothyroidism, the dose being individualized according to serum TSH. The dose is titrated every four weeks until the patient has responded clinically and the TSH level has fallen to within the normal range. Excessive dosage may precipitate cardiac complications, particularly in patients with ischaemic heart disease in whom the starting dose should be reduced. If angina pectoris limits the dose of thyroxine, the addition of a beta-blocker (e.g. **atenolol**) will allow further increments in thyroxine dosage. Long-term overdosage is undesirable and causes osteoporosis, as well as predisposing to cardiac dysrhythmias.

Congenital hypothyroidism is treated similarly and thyroxine must be given as early as possible. In the UK, the adoption of the Guthrie test has greatly facilitated the early detection of neonatal hypothyroidism.

The rapid action of T_3 is useful in treating myxoedema coma. It is given intramuscularly while starting maintenance therapy with thyroxine. Hypothyroidism sometimes coexists with Addison's disease (also autoimmune in aetiology) and hydrocortisone is given empirically to patients with myxoedema coma.

Hypothyroidism may result from hypopituitarism. This is also treated with oral thyroxine in the usual doses. Glucocorticosteroid replacement must be started first, otherwise acute adrenal insufficiency will be precipitated.

Mechanism of action

Thyroxine is a prohormone. After entering cells it is converted to T_3, which binds to the thyroid hormone nuclear receptor and the ligand–receptor complex increases transcription of genes involved in the following cellular functions:

- stimulation of metabolism – raised basal metabolic rate;
- promotion of normal growth and maturation, particularly of the central nervous system and skeleton;
- sensitization to the effects of catecholamines.

Adverse effects

The adverse effects of the thyroid hormones relate to their physiological functions and include cardiac dysrhythmia, angina, myocardial infarction and congestive cardiac failure.

Tremor, restlessness, heat intolerance, diarrhoea and other features of hyperthyroidism are dose-dependent toxic effects of these hormones. Chronic **thyroxine** excess is an insidious cause of osteoporosis.

Pharmacokinetics

Thyroid hormones are absorbed from the gut. The effects of T_4 are not usually detectable before 24 hours and maximum activity is not attained for many days during regular daily dosing. T_3 produces effects within six hours and peak activity is reached within 24 hours. The $t_{1/2}$ of T_4 is six to seven days in euthyroid individuals, but may be much longer than this in hypothyroidism, and that for T_3 is two days or less. It is unnecessary to administer thyroid hormone more frequently than once a day. The liver conjugates thyroid hormones, which undergo enterohepatic recirculation.

Key points

Iodine and thyroid hormones

- Iodized salt is used to prevent endemic goitre in regions where the diet is iodine-deficient. Lugol's iodine (a solution of iodine in aqueous potassium iodide) is also used pre-operatively to reduce the vascularity of the thyroid.
- Thyroxine (T_4) is used as a physiological replacement in patients who are hypothyroid. It is converted in the tissues to the more active tri-iodothyronine (T_3).
- T_3 has a shorter elimination half-life than T_4 and is therefore used for emergency treatment of myxoedema coma (often with glucocorticoids because of the possibility of coexisting hypoadrenalism).

ANTITHYROID DRUGS

CARBIMAZOLE

Use

Carbimazole is used to treat hyperthyroidism. The patient is usually rendered euthyroid within four to six weeks, and the dose is then reduced. Treatment is maintained for one to two years and the drug is then gradually withdrawn. If relapse occurs, the dose is raised until clinical improvement is restored. If dosage adjustment proves difficult, smoother control may be obtained by giving a replacement dose of **thyroxine** together with a blocking dose of **carbimazole**.

Mechanism of action

The action of **carbimazole** is via its active metabolite **methimazole**, which is a substrate-inhibitor of peroxidase and is itself iodinated and degraded within the thyroid, diverting oxidized iodine away from thyroglobulin and decreasing thyroid hormone biosynthesis. **Methimazole** is concentrated by cells with a peroxidase system (salivary gland, neutrophils and macrophage/monocytes, in addition to thyroid follicular cells). It has an immunosuppressive action within the thyroid and interferes with the generation of oxygen radicals by macrophages, thereby interfering with the presentation of antigen to lymphocytes. **Methimazole** does not affect hormone secretion directly. Thus hormone release decreases after a latent period, during which time the thyroid becomes depleted of hormone.

Adverse effects

Carbimazole is usually well tolerated, although pruritus and rashes are fairly common. These usually respond to switching to **propylthiouracil** (see below). Neutropenia is a rare but potentially fatal adverse effect. Patients must be warned to report sore throat or other evidence of infection immediately, an urgent white cell count must be obtained and the drug should be stopped if there is neutropenia. Nausea, hair loss, drug fever, leukopenia and arthralgia are rare, but recognized adverse effects. Use of **carbimazole** during pregnancy has rarely been associated with aplasia cutis in the newborn.

Pharmacokinetics

Carbimazole is rapidly absorbed after oral administration and hydrolysed to **methimazole**, which is concentrated in the thyroid within minutes of administration. **Methimazole** has an apparent volume of distribution equivalent to body water and the $t_{1/2}$ varies according to thyroid status, being approximately seven, nine and 14 hours in hyperthyroid, euthyroid and hypothyroid patients, respectively. It is metabolized in the liver and thyroid.

PROPYLTHIOURACIL

Use

Propylthiouracil has similar actions, uses and toxic effects to **carbimazole**, but in addition inhibits the peripheral conversion of T_4 to active T_3. As with **carbimazole**, dangerous leukopenia may develop, but is very rare. The scheme of attaining a euthyroid state with a large initial dose which is then reduced is as for **carbimazole**. **Propylthiouracil** is rapidly absorbed from the intestine. The plasma $t_{1/2}$ is short, but the duration of action within the thyroid is prolonged and, as with **carbimazole**, **propylthiouracil** can be given once daily. It is used (by specialists) in pregnancy (see below) and has some advantages over **carbimazole** in this setting.

β-ADRENOCEPTOR ANTAGONISTS

Beta-blockers improve symptoms of hyperthyroidism, including anxiety, tachycardia and tremor. They inhibit the conversion of T_4 to T_3 in the tissues. They are useful:

- while awaiting laboratory confirmation, if the diagnosis is in doubt;
- during initiation of therapy with antithyroid drugs;
- before treatment with radio-iodine, because they do not interfere with the uptake of iodine by the gland;
- in thyroid crisis;
- with iodine, as a rapid preparation for surgery on a hyperactive thyroid goitre;

- in neonatal hyperthyroidism due to thyroid-stimulating immunoglobulin from the mother – this remits within about six weeks as maternal-derived immunoglobulin is cleared by the infant.

Hyperthyroid patients treated with beta-blockers are not biochemically euthyroid, even if they appear clinically euthyroid, and thyroid crisis ('storm') can supervene if treatment is discontinued.

RADIOACTIVE IODINE

Radioactive iodine is an effective oral treatment for thyrotoxicosis caused by Graves' disease or by toxic nodular goitre. It is safe, causes no discomfort to the patient and has largely replaced surgery, except when there are local mechanical problems, such as tracheal compression. It is contraindicated in pregnancy. Dosing has been the subject of controversy. It is now standard practice in many units to give an ablative dose followed by replacement therapy with **thyroxine**, so late-onset undiagnosed hypothyroidism is avoided. The isotope usually employed is ^{131}I with a $t_{1/2}$ of eight days. **Thyroxine** replacement is started after four to six weeks and continued for life. There is no increased incidence of leukemia, thyroid or other malignancy after therapeutic use of ^{131}I, but concern remains regarding its use in children or young women. However, the dose of radiation to the gonads is less than that in many radiological procedures and there is no evidence that therapeutic doses of radioactive iodine damage the germ cells or reduce

> **Key points**
>
> Antithyroid drugs
>
> - Carbimazole works via its active metabolite, methimazole. This is concentrated in cells that contain peroxidase, including neutrophils as well as thyroid epithelium. It is iodinated in the thyroid, diverting iodine from the synthesis of T_3 and T_4 and depleting the gland of hormone. It does not inhibit secretion of preformed thyroid hormones, so there is a latent period before its effect is evident after starting treatment.
> - Neutropenia is an uncommon but potentially fatal adverse effect. Patients who develop sore throat or other symptoms of infection need to report for an urgent white blood count. Pruritus and rash are more common but less severe.
> - Propylthiouracil is similar in its effects and adverse effects to carbimazole/methimazole, but in addition it inhibits peripheral conversion of T_4 to the more active T_3, and is therefore preferred in thyroid storm.
> - β-Adrenoceptor antagonists suppress manifestations of hyperthyroidism and are used when starting treatment with specific antithyroid drugs, and in treating thyroid storm (together with propylthiouracil and glucocorticoids, which also suppress the conversion of T_4 to T_3).
> - Radioactive iodine (^{131}I) is safe in non-pregnant adults and has largely replaced surgery in the treatment of hyperthyroidism, except when there are local mechanical complications, such as tracheal obstruction. Replacement therapy with T_4 is required after functional ablation.

fertility. It is contraindicated during pregnancy because it damages the fetus, causing congenital hypothyroidism and consequent mental retardation. Patients are usually treated as outpatients during the first ten days of the menstrual cycle and after a negative pregnancy test. Pregnancy should be avoided for at least four months and a woman should not breast-feed for at least two months after treatment. High-dose ^{131}I is used to treat patients with well-differentiated thyroid carcinoma to ablate residual tumour after surgery. **Thyroxine** is stopped at least one month before treatment to allow TSH levels to increase, thereby stimulating uptake of the isotope by the gland. Patients are isolated in hospital for several days initially after dosing, to protect potential contacts.

SPECIAL SITUATIONS

GRAVES' OPHTHALMOPATHY

Eye signs usually occur within 18 months of the onset of Graves' disease and commonly resolve over one to two years, irrespective of the state of the thyroid. Over-aggressive treatment of hyperthyroidism in patients with eye signs must be avoided because of a strong clinical impression that iatrogenic hypothyroidism can exacerbate eye disease. Peri-orbital oedema can be reduced by sleeping with the head of the bed elevated. Simple moisturizing eye drops (e.g. **hypromellose**) may be useful. Tarsoroplasty is indicated to prevent corneal abrasion in severe cases. Radiotherapy is used in moderate Graves' ophthalmopathy, provided that this is not threatening vision. Severe and distressing exophthalmos warrants a trial of **prednisolone**. Urgent surgical decompression of the orbit is required if medical treatment is not successful and visual acuity deteriorates due to optic nerve compression.

THYROID CRISIS

Thyroid crisis is a severe, abrupt exacerbation of hyperthyroidism with hyperpyrexia, tachycardia, vomiting, dehydration and shock. It can arise post-operatively, following radioiodine therapy or with intercurrent infection. Rarely, it arises spontaneously in a previously undiagnosed or untreated patient. Mortality is high. Urgent treatment comprises:

- β-adrenoceptor antagonists;
- intravenous saline;
- cooling;
- propylthiouracil;
- Lugol's iodine;
- glucocorticoids;
- fast atrial fibrillation can be especially difficult to treat: DC cardioversion may be needed.

Aspirin must be avoided, because salicylate displaces bound T_4 and T_3 and also because of its uncoupling effect on oxidative phosphorylation, which renders the metabolic state even more severe.

PREGNANCY AND BREAST-FEEDING

Radioactive iodine is absolutely contraindicated in pregnancy and surgery should be avoided if possible. T_4 and T_3 do not cross the placenta adequately and, if a fetus is hypothyroid, this results in congenital hypothyroidism with mental retardation caused by maldevelopment of the central nervous system. Antithyroid drugs (**carbimazole** and **propylthiouracil**) cross the placenta and enter breast milk, and management of hyperthyroidism during pregnancy requires specialist expertise. Overtreatment with antithyroid drugs must be avoided. Blocking doses of antithyroid drugs with added T_4 must never be used in pregnancy, as the antithyroid drugs cross the placenta but T_4 does not, leading inevitably to a severely hypothyroid infant. **Propylthiouracil** may be somewhat less likely than **carbimazole** to produce effects in the infant, since it is more highly protein bound and is ionized at pH 7.4. This reduces its passage across the placenta and into milk. Minimal effective doses of **propylthiouracil** should be used during pregnancy and breast-feeding.

DRUG-INDUCED THYROID DYSFUNCTION

Other drugs are known to cause thyroid hypofunction. Iodinated radio-contrast dyes can cause transient hyperthyroidism. **Amiodarone**, interferons and interleukins can cause hypo- or hyperthyroidism. **Lithium** and several of the novel kinase inhibitors (**imatinib**, **sorafenib**, **sunitinib**, see Chapter 48) can cause hypothyroidism and/or goitre. The patient should be assessed for the need for continuing the implicated drug and the degree of thyroid dysfunction evaluated. If drug therapy has to be continued, antithyroid or replacement thyroxine therapy with careful monitoring of the thyroid axis is the standard treatment.

Case history

A 19-year-old Chinese woman develops secondary amenorrhoea followed by symptoms of palpitations, nervousness, heat intolerance and sweating. There is a strong family history of autoimmune disease. On examination, she appears anxious and sweaty, her pulse is 120 beats per minute regular and there is a smooth goitre with a soft bruit. There is tremor of the outstretched fingers and lid lag is present. A pregnancy test is positive and you send blood to the laboratory for standard investigations, including T_3 and T_4.
Comment
This young woman has the clinical picture of Graves' disease, which is common in this ethnic group. Management is complicated by the fact that she is probably pregnant, and specialist input will be essential. Treatment with a β-adrenoreceptor antagonist and a low dose of an antithyroid drug (propylthiouracil is preferred as it crosses the placenta poorly) should be considered. Radioactive iodine is absolutely contraindicated in pregnancy and a high dose of antithyroid drug should be avoided because of the risk of causing congenital hypothyroidism, and consequent mental retardation, in the baby.

FURTHER READING

Cooper DS. Drug therapy: antithyroid drugs. *New England Journal of Medicine* 2005; **352**: 905–17.

Franklin JA. The management of hyperthyroidism. *New England Journal of Medicine* 1995; **330**: 1731–8.

Franklin JF, Sheppard M. Radioiodine for hyperthyroidism: perhaps the best option. *British Medical Journal* 1992; **305**: 728–9.

Klein I, Ojamaa K. Mechanisms of disease: thyroid hormone and the cardiovascular system. *New England Journal of Medicine* 2001; **344**: 501–9.

Larkins R. Treatment of Graves' ophthalmology. *Lancet* 1993; **342**: 941–2.

Lazarus JH. Hyperthyroidism. *Lancet* 1997; **349**: 339–43.

Lindsay RS. Hypothyroidism. *Lancet* 1997; **349**: 413–17.

Nayak B, Burman K. Thyrotoxicosis and thyroid storm. *Endocrinology and Metabolism Clinics of North America* 2006; **35**: 663–86.

Weetman AP. Medical progress: Graves' disease. *New England Journal of Medicine* 2000; **343**: 1236–48.

CALCIUM METABOLISM

INTRODUCTION

Plasma calcium is sensed by a calcium-sensitive receptor (CaSR) in parathyroid and renal tubular cells, and maintained within a narrow physiological range by parathyroid hormone (PTH), vitamin D and calcitonin. The plasma calcium concentration is the major factor controlling PTH secretion and a reduction in calcium concentration stimulates PTH release. PTH raises plasma calcium and lowers phosphate concentration. It acts on kidney and bone. PTH causes phosphaturia and increases renal tubular reabsorption of calcium, which in association with mobilization of calcium from bone, increases the plasma calcium concentration. Effects of PTH on bone include stimulation of osteoclast activity, formation of new osteoclasts from progenitor cells and transient depression of osteoblast activity. PTH also plays a role in the regulation of vitamin D metabolism, indirectly increasing gut absorption of calcium by stimulating production of the active metabolite 1,25-dihydroxycholecalciferol (1,25-DHCC or calcitriol, see below).

Several important metabolic diseases affect the bones, notably hyperparathyroidism, osteomalacia and rickets, Paget's disease and osteoporosis. Some of these diseases (e.g. osteomalacia) are associated with normal or low plasma calcium concentrations, some (e.g. hyperparathyroidism) are associated with hypercalcaemia and some (e.g. osteoporosis) are associated with normal plasma calcium concentrations. Post-menopausal osteoporosis is the most common of these disorders; iatrogenic glucocorticoid or thyroid hormone excess are important contributory causes. Those at risk should take adequate dietary calcium and vitamin D (see below) and contributory factors corrected if possible. Hormone replacement therapy (HRT) with oestrogen (Chapter 41) is no longer first line as a prophylaxis against osteoporosis in women over 50 because of an excess of thrombotic events, although it is at least temporarily effective if started soon after menopause. **Raloxifene** is an alternative (Chapter 41). Bisphosphonates and **teriparatide** (see below) are effective in treating post-menopausal osteoporosis.

Key points

Pathophysiology of common metabolic bone disease

- Osteoporosis is characterized by reduced bone quantity (density).
- Paget's disease is characterized by excessive new bone formation and bone resorption.
- Osteomalacia is characterized by lack of bone mineralization.

VITAMIN D

The term 'vitamin D' covers several related compounds that share the ability to prevent or cure rickets. These include ergo-calciferol (vitamin D_2), cholecalciferol (vitamin D_3), α-calcidol (1-α-hydroxycholecalciferol) and calcitriol (1,25-DHCC). The metabolic pathway of vitamin D is summarized in Figure 39.1. Vitamin D_3 is synthesized in skin in response to ultraviolet light or absorbed in the upper small intestine. It is fat soluble, so bile is necessary for its absorption. Renal 1-α-hydroxylase is activated by PTH and inhibited by phosphate, which thus influence the amount of active 1,25-DHCC produced. 1,25-DHCC is, in effect, a hormone synthesized in the kidney. It augments intestinal calcium absorption, mobilizes calcium from bone and stimulates calcium reabsorption in the kidney (a minor effect). Storage of vitamin D occurs in the body, so a single large dose may be effective for several weeks. Enzyme induction (Chapter 5), e.g. by anti-epileptic drugs, increases metabolic inactivation of vitamin D and can lead to osteomalacia.

Uses

Dietary deficiency of vitamin D occurs where there is poverty and poor diet, accentuated by lack of sunlight. Asian communities living in northern regions of the UK are at risk (chapatis and other unleavened breads also reduce the absorption of vitamin D), as are elderly people living alone. Pregnant and lactating women have increased requirements. Several vitamin D preparations are available, with different potencies and uses.

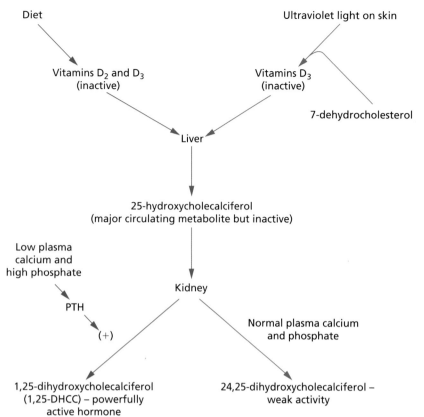

Figure 39.1: Metabolic pathway of vitamin D. PTH, parathormone.

1. Calcium and **ergocalciferol** tablets provide a physiological dose of vitamin D. They are used in the prophylaxis of rickets and osteomalacia. The small dose of calcium is unnecessary, but a preparation of vitamin D alone is not available.
2. **Calciferol** tablets provide a pharmacological dose of vitamin D and are used for treatment of hypo-parathyroidism and in cases of vitamin D-resistant rickets due to intestinal malabsorption or chronic liver disease.
3. α-Calcidol rapidly undergoes hydroxylation to 1,25-DHCC. It is used in:
   - renal rickets, together with a phosphate-binding agent;
   - hypoparathyroidism and (paradoxically) secondary hyperparathyroidism;
   - vitamin D-resistant rickets;
   - nutritional and malabsorptive rickets can be treated with small doses of α-calcidol instead of conventional vitamin D.
4. **Calcitriol** (1,25-DHCC) is also available for the treatment of vitamin D-resistant rickets and is the treatment of choice for pseudohypoparathyroidism (an uncommon metabolic disorder where low plasma calcium is caused by resistance to the biochemical action of PTH).

Adverse effects

Hypercalcaemia, which can accelerate renal dysfunction, is the main problem. Regular plasma calcium and creatinine measurements (weekly initially) are essential.

CALCIUM

Calcium salts (lactate or gluconate) are used in conjunction with **calciferol** in the treatment of rickets and osteomalacia, and in hypocalcaemic tetany. Calcium chloride (i.v.) is uniquely

Key points

Vitamin D and calcium metabolism

- Plasma calcium concentrations are tightly controlled by the balance of hypocalcaemic effects of calcitonin and hypercalcaemic effects of PTH and vitamin D and Ca^{2+} intake.
- Vitamin D is available in a number of forms, many of which are derived from each other by sequential metabolism in the skin, liver and kidney, and each of which has specific indications.
- The most potent and rapid-acting orally available vitamin D preparations are 1,25 dihydroxy-cholecalciferol, and 1-α-hydroxycholecalciferol. They are used in renal rickets or vitamin D-resistant rickets.
- When patients are hypocalcaemic, calcium can be supplemented orally as calcium carbonate with or without various preparations of vitamin D. If urgent calcium replacement is required, a 10% solution of calcium lactate or gluconate (the former yielding more calcium) may be administered intravenously.
- Patients who are receiving vitamin D plus calcium should have periodic checks of their serum Ca^{2+} and creatinine concentrations, as the major adverse effect is hypercalcaemia.

effective in life-threatening hyperkalaemia-induced cardiac dysrhythmias (Chapter 32). Calcium and vitamin D supplements are used in patients at risk of osteoporosis if intake is below 1 g of elemental calcium daily. Effervescent or chewable preparations are available and easy to take.

TREATMENT OF HYPERCALCAEMIA

Hypercalcaemia may be a life-threatening emergency. Causes include hyperparathyroidism, malignancy with bone metastases or ectopic PTH synthesis, sarcoidosis and vitamin D intoxication. Treating the underlying cause is crucial. Management of hypercalcaemia per se buys time for this and can be divided into general and specific measures.

GENERAL MEASURES

The following general measures apply:

1. rehydration;
2. avoid thiazide diuretics (cause Ca^{2+} retention, see Chapter 36);
3. avoid excessive vitamin D;
4. avoid immobilization if possible.

Specific measures to:

1. increase calcium excretion:
   - intravenous saline increases calcium excretion;
   - once extravascular volume has been restored, **furosemide** further increases urinary calcium excretion.
2. decrease bone resorption:
   - bisphosphonates (see below);
   - calcitonin (see below);
3. glucocorticosteroids:
   - glucocorticosteroids are useful for treating the hypercalcaemia associated with sarcoidosis.

Key points

Management of acute hypercalcaemia

- Avoid thiazides, vitamin D (milk), any calcium preparations and, if possible, immobilization.
- Vigorously replace fluid losses with intravenous 0.9% sodium chloride. Once replete, furosemide administration further increases urinary calcium loss.
- Give parenteral bisphosphonates (e.g. disodium etidronate or disodium pamidronate).
- Calcitonin lowers calcium levels more rapidly than bisphosphonates, and may be used concomitantly in severe cases.
- Glucocorticosteroids are used for the hypercalcaemia of sarcoidosis.

BISPHOSPHONATES

Bisphosphonates resemble pyrophosphate structurally, except that the two phosphorus atoms are linked by carbon rather than by oxygen. The P-C-P backbone structure renders such compounds very stable – no enzyme is known that degrades them.

Uses

Alendronic acid or **risedronate** (by mouth) are first-choice bisphosphonates for the prevention and treatment of osteoporosis; **etidronate** is an alternative if these are not tolerated. Bisphosphonates are also used to treat Paget's disease of bone, in the treatment of hypercalcaemia of malignancy (e.g. **pamidronate** i.v.) and to reduce skeletal complications in breast cancer metastatic to bone and multiple myeloma (e.g. **clodronate** p.o. or i.v.). They are effective for glucocorticoid-associated and post-menopausal osteoporosis. In Paget's disease, **risedronate** is given for two months and this can be repeated after at least two months off treatment. **Etidronate** is started at low dosage up to six months when many patients achieve remission; a further course may be given following relapse. Use for longer than six months at a time does not prolong remission. High doses should be used only if lower doses fail or if rapid control of disease is needed. Serum alkaline phosphatase, phosphate and if possible urinary hydroxyproline are monitored during treatment of Paget's disease.

Mechanism of action

Bisphosphonates modify the crystal growth of calcium hydroxyapatite by chemical adsorption to the crystal surface, reducing bone remodelling and turnover by osteoclasts.

Adverse effects

Renal impairment is a caution or contraindication for all bisphosphonates. Oesophagitis and ulceration can be severe. This is minimized by taking **alendronic acid** or **risedronate** when sitting upright or standing, on an empty stomach before breakfast, and remaining standing for half an hour before eating. Other adverse effects include the gamut of gastrointestinal symptoms. **Etidronate** increases the risk of fracture in patients with Paget's disease.

Key points

Bisphosphonates and bone disease

- Used to treat malignant hypercalcaemia, bone pain from metastatic cancer (breast, prostate) and Paget's disease, and to prevent and reduce the progression of osteoporosis.
- Inhibit bone resorption by osteoclasts; etidronate also inhibits mineralization with chronic use.
- Oral absorption is poor; short $t_{1/2}$ in plasma and long $t_{1/2}$ in bone; renal clearance.
- Food and/or calcium-containing antacids further reduce gastrointestinal absorption of bisphosphonates.
- The most common side effects are gastro-intestinal disturbances (*Note*: with regard to oesophagitis and ulceration with alendronic acid, this drug must be taken with water and the patient must be able to stand for 30 minutes post-ingestion).

Pharmacokinetics

Bisphosphonates are incompletely absorbed (<10%) and food and antacids further reduce absorption. They disappear rapidly from the blood, distributing to bone, where their effects are long lived. Within 24 hours, approximately 50% of the absorbed dose is excreted unchanged in the urine, but the remainder is excreted over many weeks.

CALCITONIN

This is a 32-amino-acid polypeptide hormone secreted by thyroid parafollicular C-cells. Secretion is determined mainly by the plasma Ca^{2+} concentration.

Uses

Synthetic or recombinant salmon calcitonin (**salcatonin**) is used to lower the plasma calcium concentration in hypercalcaemia, especially from malignancy, and in the treatment of pain and some of the neurological complications (e.g. deafness due to VIII nerve compression) of severe Paget's disease and for post-menopausal osteoporosis (together with calcium and vitamin D supplements, if diet is inadequate). **Calcitonin** is given by subcutaneous or intramuscular injection, or as a nasal spray. Plasma calcium, phosphate, alkaline phosphatase and if possible urine hydroxyproline excretion are monitored.

Mechanism of action

The main action of **calcitonin** is on bone; it inhibits bone resorption by binding to a specific receptor on osteoclasts inhibiting their action. In the kidney, it decreases the reabsorption of both Ca^{2+} and phosphate in the proximal tubules.

Adverse effects

Adverse effects include the following:

1. pain at the injection site;
2. nausea and diarrhoea;
3. flushing.

STRONTIUM RANELATE

Strontium is a bone-seeking element; it was widely used for osteoporosis in the 1950s, but there were concerns that it inhibited calcitriol synthesis and might cause defective bone mineralization. These adverse effects may have reflected a calcium-deficient diet and incorrect dosing. Recent evidence indicates that **strontium ranelate** reduces bone reabsorption and increases bone formation, and reduces vertebral and hip fractures in women with post-menopausal osteoporosis. It is given by mouth at night to older women with osteoporosis and a history of bone fracture when bisphosphonates are contraindicated or not tolerated. It causes gastro-intestinal adverse effects.

TERIPARATIDE

Teriparatide is a PTH agonist. It is a recombinant fragment of PTH, used by experts in metabolic bone disease for the treatment of post-menopausal osteoporosis. It is contraindicated in patients with other metabolic bone diseases, including hyperparathyroidism, Paget's disease or previous radiation therapy to the skeleton and used with caution if there is renal impairment or cardiac disease. It is given daily by subcutaneous injection for periods up to 18 months, monitoring serum calcium, phosphate, alkaline phosphatase, creatinine and electrolytes.

CINACALCET

Cinacalcet is a calcimimetic drug which enhances signalling through the calcium sensing receptor (CaSR). It is an allosteric activator of CaSR and reduces secretion of PTH. This is accompanied by a modest reduction in plasma calcium and phosphate. It also reduces expression of the PTH gene (and hence the synthesis of PTH) and diminishes parathyroid hyperplasia. It is given by mouth for secondary hyperparathyroidism in patients on dialysis for end-stage renal disease and for hypercalcaemia caused by parathyroid carcinoma, with monitoring of serum calcium and PTH.

Case history

A 52-year-old woman has had epilepsy since childhood, treated with phenytoin 300 mg/day and her fits have been well controlled. Since the loss of her job and the death of her husband she has become an alcoholic. At the age of 54 years, she is seen by her local GP because of weakness in her legs, difficulty in climbing stairs and getting out of her chair. She has no sensory symptoms in her limbs and no sphincter problems. Neurological examination of her legs is normal apart from signs of thigh and hip muscle weakness and slight wasting. Clinical investigations reveal that haemoglobin, white blood and platelets are normal, but her erythrocyte sedimentation rate is 30 mm per hour, her blood glucose level is 5.4 mM, sodium is 136 mM, K is 4.6 mM, urea is 10 mM and creatinine is 80 μM. Liver function tests are all normal, except for an elevated alkaline phosphatase of 600 IU/L, and bilirubin is normal. A chest x-ray is normal. Further biochemical investigation reveals a plasma calcium concentration of 1.8 mM and a phosphate concentration of 0.6 mM.
Question
What is the likely cause of her metabolic disturbance and leg weakness, and how would you treat it ?
Answer
This patient has hypocalcaemia with hypophosphataemia and a raised alkaline phosphatase, but no evidence of renal dysfunction. This is the clinical picture of a patient with osteomalacia. The aetiology is secondary to her chronic phenytoin therapy. The mechanism of these effects is complex and relates to several actions of the drug. Phenytoin is a potent inducer of hepatic drug metabolizing enzyme systems, including the enzymes involved in vitamin D metabolism, specifically metabolism of calciferol to 25'-hydroxycholecalciferol by the liver, and its further metabolism to inactive products. It also impairs the absorption of vitamin D from the gut. Treatment of this form of drug-induced osteomalacia consists of giving the patient oral Ca^{2+} supplements together with low-dose 1-α-hydroxy vitamin D (0.5 μg per day), and continuing the phenytoin if necessary.

Further reading

Block GA, Martin KJ, de Francisco ALM et al. Cinacalcet for secondary hyperparathyroidism in patients receiving hemodialysis. *New England Journal of Medicine* 2004; **350**: 1516–25.

Delmas P. Treatment of postmenopausal osteoporosis. *Lancet* 2002; **359**; 2018–26.

Jackson RD, LaCroix AZ, Gass M et al. Calcium plus vitamin D supplementation and the risk of fractures. *New England Journal of Medicine* 2006; **354**: 669–83.

Kleerekoper M, Schein JR. Comparative safety of bone remodeling agents with a focus on osteoporosis therapies. *Journal of Clinical Pharmacology* 2001; **41**: 239–50.

Lopez FJ. New approaches to the treatment of osteoporosis. *Current Opinion in Chemical Biology* 2000; **4**: 383–93.

Marx SJ. Medical progress – Hyperparathyroid and hypoparathyroid disorders. *New England Journal of Medicine* 2000; **343**: 1863–75.

Meunier PJ, Roux C, Seeman E et al. The effects of strontium ranelate on the risk of vertebral fracture in women with postmenopausal osteoporosis. *New England Journal of Medicine* 2004; **350**: 459–68.

Reeve J. Recombinant human parathyroid hormone: osteoporosis is proving amenable to treatment. *British Medical Journal* 2002; **324**: 435–6.

Reichel H, Koeftler HP, Norman AW. The role of the vitamin D endocrine system in health and disease. *New England Journal of Medicine* 1989; **320**: 980–91.

Rosen CJ, Bilezekian JP. Anabolic therapy for osteoporosis. *Journal of Clinical Endocrinology and Metabolism* 2001; **86**: 957–64.

ADRENAL HORMONES

ADRENAL CORTEX

The adrenal cortex secretes:

1. glucocorticosteroids, principally cortisol (hydrocortisone);
2. mineralocorticoids – principally aldosterone;
3. androgens (relatively small amounts).

GLUCOCORTICOSTEROIDS

The actions of glucocorticosteroids and the effects of their over-secretion (Cushing's syndrome) and under-secretion (Addison's disease) are summarized in Table 40.1. Glucocorticosteroids influence carbohydrate and protein metabolism, and play a vital role in the response to stress. Glucocorticosteroids stimulate the mobilization of amino acids from skeletal muscle, bone and skin, promoting their transport to the liver where they are converted into glucose (gluconeogenesis) and stored as glycogen. Fat mobilization by catecholamines is potentiated by glucocorticosteroids. The major therapeutic uses of the glucocorticosteroids exploit their powerful anti-inflammatory and immunosuppressive properties. They reduce circulating eosinophils, basophils and T-lymphocytes, while increasing neutrophils. Applied topically to skin or mucous membranes, potent steroids can cause local vasoconstriction and massive doses administered systemically can cause hypertension due to generalized vasoconstriction.

Mechanism of action

Glucocorticosteroids combine with a cytoplasmic glucocorticosteroid receptor causing its dissociation from a phosphorylated heat shock protein complex. The receptor–glucocorticosteroid complex translocates to the nucleus, where it binds to glucocorticosteroid response elements (GREs) in DNA and acts as a transcription factor. This increases the transcription of various signal transduction proteins. In addition, the glucocorticosteroid receptor interacts with both NFκB and AP-1 and inhibits them from enhancing transcription of many pro-inflammatory proteins. Thus glucocorticosteroids produce a delayed but profound anti-inflammatory effect.

Adverse effects

Adverse effects of glucocorticosteroids are common to all members of the group, and will be discussed before considering the uses of individual drugs.

Chronic administration causes iatrogenic Cushing's syndrome (see Table 40.1). Features include:

- Cushingoid physical appearance;
- impaired resistance to infection;
- salt and water retention; hypokalaemia;
- hypertension;
- hyperglycaemia;
- osteoporosis;
- glucocorticosteroid therapy is weakly linked with peptic ulceration, and can mask the symptoms and signs of gastrointestinal perforation;
- mental changes: anxiety, elation, insomnia, depression and psychosis;
- posterior cataracts;
- proximal myopathy;
- growth retardation in children;
- aseptic necrosis of bone.

Acute adrenal insufficiency can result from rapid withdrawal after prolonged glucocorticosteroid administration. Gradual tapered withdrawal is less hazardous. However, even in patients who have been successfully weaned from chronic treatment with glucocorticosteroids, for one to two years afterwards a stressful situation (such as trauma, surgery or infection) may precipitate an acute adrenal crisis and necessitate the administration of large amounts of sodium chloride, glucocorticosteroids, glucose and water. Suppression of the adrenal cortex is unusual if the daily glucocorticosteroid dose is lower than the amount usually secreted physiologically. The rate at which patients can be weaned off glucocorticosteroids depends on their underlying condition and also on the dose and duration of therapy. After long-term glucocorticosteroid therapy has been discontinued the patient should continue to carry a steroid card for at least one year.

Table 40.1: Actions of cortisol and consequences of under- and over-secretion

	Actions	Deficiency	Excess
Carbohydrate, protein and fat metabolism	Enhances gluconeogenesis; antagonizes insulin; hyperglycaemia with or without diabetes mellitus; centripetal fat deposition; hypertriglyceridaemia; hypercholesterolaemia; decreased protein synthesis (e.g. diminished skin collagen)	Hypoglycaemia, loss of weight	Cushing's syndrome: weight gain, increase in trunk fat, moon face, skin striae, bruising, atrophy, wasting of limb muscles
Water and salt metabolism	Inhibits fluid shift from extracellular to intracellular compartment; antagonizes vasopressin action on kidney; increases vasopressin destruction and decreases its production. Sodium and water retention, potassium loss	Loss of weight, hypovolaemia, hyponatraemia	Oedema, thirst, polyuria; hypertension; muscular weakness
Haematological	Lowers lymphocyte and eosinophil counts; increases neutrophils, platelets and clotting tendency		Florid complexion and polycythaemia
Alimentary	Increases production of gastric acid and pepsin	Anorexia and nausea	Dyspepsia; aggravation of peptic ulcer
Cardiovascular system	Sensitizes arterioles to catecholamines; enhances production of angiotensinogen. Fall in high-density lipoprotein with increased total cholesterol	Hypotension, fainting	Hypertension, atherosclerosis
Skeletal	Decrease production of cartilage and osteoporosis; antivitamin D; increased renal loss of calcium; renal calculus formation		Backache due to osteoporosis, renal calculi, dwarfing in children (also anti-GH effect)
Nervous system	Altered neuronal excitability; inhibition of uptake of catecholamines		Depression and other psychiatric changes
Anti-inflammatory	Reduces formation of fluid and cellular exudate; fibrous tissue repair		Increased spread of and proneness to infections
Immunological	Large dose lysis lymphocytes and plasma cells (transient release of immunoglobulin)		Reduced lymphocyte mass, diminished immunoglobulin production
Feedback	Inhibits release of ACTH and MSH		Pigmentation of skin and mucosa

ACTH, adrenocorticotropic hormone; MSH, melanocyte-stimulating hormone; GH, growth hormone.

HYDROCORTISONE (CORTISOL)

Uses

Hydrocortisone has predominantly glucocorticoid effects, but also has significant mineralocorticoid activity (Table 40.2). At physiological concentrations, it plays little if any part in controlling blood glucose, but it does cause hyperglycaemia (and can precipitate frank diabetes mellitus) when administered in pharmacological doses. This is caused by enhanced gluconeogenesis combined with reduced sensitivity to insulin. **Hydrocortisone** is given (usually with **fludrocortisone** to replace mineralocorticoid) as replacement therapy in patients with adrenocortical insufficiency.

High-dose intravenous **hydrocortisone** is used short term to treat acute severe asthma (usually followed by oral **prednisolone**) or autoimmune inflammatory diseases (e.g. acute inflammatory bowel disease). **Hydrocortisone acetate** is an insoluble suspension which can be injected into joints or

Table 40.2: Relative potencies of glucocorticosteroids and mineralocorticosteroids

Compound	Relative potency	
	Anti-inflammatory	**Mineralocorticoid**
Glucocorticosteroids		
Cortisol (hydrocortisone)	1	1
Cortisone	0.8	1
Prednisolone and prednisone	4	0.8
Methylprednisolone	5	0.5
Triamcinolone	5	0
Dexamethasone	25–30	0
Betamethasone	25–30	0
Mineralocorticosteroids		
Aldosterone	0	1000[a]
Fludrocortisone	10	500

[a]Injected (other preparations administered as oral doses).

inflamed bursae to provide a localized anti-inflammatory effect. **Hydrocortisone** cream is relatively low in potency and is of particular use on the face where more potent steroids are contraindicated.

Pharmacokinetics

Hydrocortisone is rapidly absorbed from the gastro-intestinal tract, but there is considerable inter-individual variation in bioavailability due to variable presystemic metabolism. It is metabolized in the liver (by CYP3A) and other tissues to tetrahydrometabolites that are conjugated with glucuronide before being excreted in the urine. The plasma $t_{1/2}$ is approximately 90 minutes, but the biological $t_{1/2}$ is longer (six to eight hours).

Key points

Glucocorticosteroids – pharmacodynamics and pharmacokinetics

- They have a potent anti-inflammatory action which takes six to eight hours to manifest after dosing.
- They act as positive transcription factors for proteins involved in inhibition of the production of inflammatory mediators (e.g. lipocortin) and they inhibit the action of transcription factors for pro-inflammatory cytokines.
- Mineralocorticoid effects decrease as the anti-inflammatory potency of synthetic glucocorticoids increases.
- Glucocorticosteroids have relatively short half-lives and are metabolized to inactive metabolites.
- Used in a wide range of inflammatory disorders of lung, gut, liver, blood, nervous system, skin and musculoskeletal systems, and for immunosuppression in transplant patients.

Key points

Glucocorticosteroids – major side effects

- Adrenal suppression, reduced by once daily morning or alternate-day administration.
- After chronic therapy – slow-dose tapering is needed, otherwise an adrenal crisis is likely to be precipitated.
- Metabolic effects including hyperglycaemia and hypokalaemia occur rapidly, as does insomnia and mood disturbances.
- Chronic side effects include Cushingoid appearance, hypertension, osteoporosis and proximal myopathy.
- Immunosuppression – susceptibility to infections.
- Mask acute inflammation (e.g. perforated intra-abdominal viscus).
- Patients on chronic steroid treatment require an increased dose for stresses, such as infection or surgery.

PREDNISOLONE

Uses

Prednisolone is an analogue of **hydrocortisone** that is approximately four times more potent than the natural hormone with regard to anti-inflammatory metabolic actions, and involution of lymphoid tissue, but slightly less active as a mineralocorticoid.

The anti-inflammatory effect of **prednisolone** can improve inflammatory symptoms of connective tissue and vasculitic diseases (see Chapter 26), but whether this benefits the underlying course of the disease is often unclear. Treatment must therefore be re-evaluated regularly and if long-term use is deemed essential, the dose reduced to the lowest effective maintenance dose. Alternate-day dosing produces less suppression of the pituitary–adrenal axis, but not all diseases are adequately treated in this way (e.g. giant cell arteritis). **Prednisolone** is considered in progressive rheumatoid arthritis when other forms of treatment have failed, or as an interim measure while a disease-modifying drug, such as **methotrexate**, has time to act. Intra-articular injection may be useful, but if done repeatedly carries a substantial risk of damage to the joint. Low doses of **prednisolone** may be symptomatically useful in the short-term management of patients with severe articular symptoms from systemic lupus erythematosus and larger doses may be appropriate for limited periods in such patients with steroid-responsive forms of glomerulonephritis or with progressive central nervous system involvement.

Other diseases where **prednisolone** may be indicated include severe asthma and some interstitial lung diseases, e.g. fibrosing alveolitis and some patients with sarcoidosis (Chapter 33), some forms of acute hepatitis and chronic active hepatitis, acute and chronic inflammatory bowel disease (where suppositories or enemas are used), and minimal-change nephrotic syndrome. The immunosuppressant effect of **prednisolone** is further utilized in transplantation, usually in combination with **ciclosporin** or **azathioprine**, in order to prevent rejection (Chapter 50). Benign haematological disorders for which **prednisolone** is indicated include autoimmune haemolytic anaemia and idiopathic thrombocytopenic purpura and is an essential component of chemotherapeutic regimens for lymphoma and Hodgkin's disease (Chapters 48 and 49).

DEXAMETHASONE

Uses

Dexamethasone is powerfully anti-inflammatory, but is virtually devoid of mineralocorticoid activity. It is generally reserved for a few distinct indications, including:

- as a diagnostic agent in the investigation of suspected Cushing's syndrome (low- and high-dose **dexamethasone** suppression tests) as it does not cross-react with endogenous cortisol in conventional radioimmunoassays;
- in the symptomatic treatment of cerebral oedema associated with brain tumours;
- to prevent respiratory distress syndrome in premature babies by administration to pregnant mothers;
- in combination with other anti-emetics to prevent cytotoxic chemotherapy-induced nausea and vomiting;
- when a corticosteroid is indicated, but fluid retention is problematic.

MINERALOCORTICOIDS

ALDOSTERONE

Aldosterone is the main mineralocorticoid secreted by the zona glomerulosa of the adrenal cortex. It has no glucocorticoid activity, but is about 1000 times more active than **hydrocortisone** as a mineralocorticoid. The main factors that control its release are plasma sodium, plasma potassium and angiotensin II. Pituitary failure, which results in a total absence of ACTH and of cortisol secretion, allows **aldosterone** production to continue.

Aldosterone acts on the distal nephron, promoting Na^+/K^+ exchange, causing sodium retention and urinary loss of potassium

and hydrogen ions. Primary hyperaldosteronism (Conn's syndrome) is due to either a tumour or hyperplasia of the zona glomerulosa of the adrenal cortex. Clinical features include nocturia, hypokalaemia, hypomagnesaemia, weakness, tetany, hypertension and sodium retention. **Spironolactone** and **eplerenone** are mineralocorticoid antagonists (see Chapters 31 and 36) that compete with **aldosterone** and other mineralocorticoids for the cytoplasmic mineralocorticosteroid receptor. They are used as potassium-sparing diuretics and to treat primary or secondary hyperaldosteronism in the contexts of hypertension and/or heart failure (Chapters 28 and 36).

FLUDROCORTISONE

Fludrocortisone (9-α-fluorohydrocortisone) is a potent synthetic mineralocorticoid, being approximately 500 times more powerful than hydrocortisone. It binds to the mineralocorticoid steroid receptor and mimics the action of **aldosterone**. It undergoes significant presystemic metabolism, but unlike **aldosterone** is active by mouth. It is used as replacement therapy in patients with adrenocortical insufficiency. It is sometimes used to treat patients with symptomatic postural hypotension, but at the cost of causing features of Conn's syndrome.

Key points

Mineralocorticoids

- Mineralocorticoids mimic aldosterone's effects on the distal nephron, causing sodium retention and potassium excretion.
- The synthetic mineralocorticoid fludrocortisone, is effective orally.
- Fludrocortisone is used when mineralocorticoid replacement is needed in patients with adrenal insufficiency.
- Occasionally, fludrocortisone is used to treat severe postural hypotension.
- Mineralocorticoid antagonists (e.g. spironolactone, Chapter 36) are used to treat mineralocorticoid excess (e.g. Conn's syndrome).

ADRENAL MEDULLA

Adrenaline (**epinephrine**) is the main hormone produced by the adrenal medulla. It is used in emergency situations, such as cardiac arrest (Chapter 32), anaphylactic shock (Chapter 50) and other life-threatening disorders that require combined potent α- and β-agonist activity (e.g. shock, beta-blocker overdose). It is used to prolong the action of local anaesthetics (via its vasoconstrictor action). **Dipivefrine** is a prodrug eye-drop formulation of **adrenaline** used to treat chronic open angle glaucoma (Chapter 52). Tumours of the adrenal medulla that secrete adrenaline and other pharmacologically active catecholamines (phaeochromocytoma) are treated surgically; in these patients preoperative blockade with **phenoxybenzamine**, a long-acting α-blocker, followed by β-blockade is essential.

Case history

A 32-year-old man presents after collapsing in the street complaining of severe lower abdominal pain.

His relevant past medical history is that for 10 years he has had chronic asthma, which is normally controlled with β_2-agonists and inhaled beclometasone 2000 μg/day. Initial assessment shows that he has peritonitis, and emergency laparotomy reveals a perforated appendix and associated peritonitis. His immediate post-operative state is stable, but approximately 12 hours post-operatively he becomes hypotensive and oliguric. The hypotension does not respond well to intravenous dobutamine and dopamine and extending the spectrum of his antibiotics. By 16 hours post-operatively, he remains hypotensive on pressor agents (blood pressure 85/50 mmHg) and he becomes hypoglycaemic (blood glucose 2.5 mM). His other blood biochemistry shows Na^+ 124 mM, K^+ 5.2 mM and urea 15 mM.

Question

What is the diagnosis here and how could you confirm it? What is the correct acute and further management of this patient?

Answer

In a chronic asthmatic patient who is receiving high-dose inhaled steroids (and may have received oral glucocorticosteroids periodically), any severe stress (e.g. infection or surgery) could precipitate acute adrenal insufficiency. In this case, the development of refractory hypotension in a patient who is on antibiotics and pressors, and the subsequent hypoglycaemia, should alert one to the probability of adrenal insufficiency. This possibility is further supported by the low sodium, slightly increased potassium and elevated urea levels. This could be confirmed by sending plasma immediately for ACTH and cortisol estimation, although the results would not be available in the short term.

The treatment consists of immediate administration of intravenous hydrocortisone and intravenous glucose. Hydrocortisone should then be given eight hourly for 24–48 hours, together with intravenous 0.9% sodium chloride, 1 L every three to six hours initially (to correct hypotension and sodium losses). Glucose should be carefully monitored further. With improvement, the patient could then be given twice his normal dose of prednisolone or its parenteral equivalent for five to seven days. This unfortunate clinical scenario could have been avoided if parenteral hydrocortisone was given preoperatively and every eight hours for the first 24 hours post-operatively. Glucocorticosteroids should be continued at approximately twice their normal dose for the next two to three days post-operatively, before reverting to his usual dose (clinical state permitting).

FURTHER READING

Arlt W, Allolio B. Adrenal insufficiency. Lancet 2003; **361**: 1881–93.

Cooper MS, Stewart PM. Current concepts – corticosteroid insufficiency in acutely ill patients. *New England Journal of Medicine* 2003; **348**: 727–34.

Falkenstein E, Tillmann HC, Christ M et al. Multiple actions of steroid hormones – a focus on rapid, nongenomic effects. *Pharmacology Reviews* 2000; **52**: 513–56.

Ganguly A. Current concepts – primary aldosteronism. *New England Journal of Medicine* 1998; **339**: 1828–34.

Goulding NJ, Flower RJ (eds). *Glucocorticoids*. In: Parnham MJ, Bruinvels J (series eds). Milestones in drug therapy. Berlin: Birkhauser, 2001.

Hayashi R, Wada H, Ito K, Adcock IM. Effects of glucocorticoids on gene transcription. *European Journal of Pharmacology* 2004; **500**: 51–62.

Lamberts SWJ, Bruining HA, de Jong FS. Corticosteroid therapy in severe illness. *New England Journal of Medicine* 1997; **337**: 1285–92.

Rhen T, Cidlowski JA. Antiinflammatory action of glucocorticoids – new mechanisms for old drugs. *New England Journal of Medicine* 2005; **353**: 1711–23.

Schacke H, Docke WD, Asadullah K. Mechanisms involved in the side effects of glucocorticoids. *Pharmacology and Therapeutics* 2002; **96**: 23–43.

Tak PP, Firestein GS. NF-kappaB: a key role in inflammatory diseases. *Journal of Clinical Investigation* 2001; **107**: 7–11.

White PC. Mechanisms of disease – disorders of aldosterone biosynthesis and action. *New England Journal of Medicine* 1994; **331**: 250–8.

CHAPTER 41

REPRODUCTIVE ENDOCRINOLOGY

CONTRIBUTION BY DR DIPTI AMIN

FEMALE REPRODUCTIVE ENDOCRINOLOGY

INTRODUCTION

Appropriate sexual development at puberty and the cyclical processes of ovulation and menstruation involve a complex interaction of endocrine and target organs. Gonadotrophin-releasing hormones (GnRH) regulate the release of the gonadotrophins luteinizing hormone (LH) and follicle-stimulating hormone (FSH) from the anterior pituitary gland. LH and FSH promote maturation of ova and secretion of oestrogen and progesterone from the ovaries.

Oestrogen and progesterone are derived from cholesterol. They stimulate the breast, uterus and vagina and exert both negative and positive feedback on the central nervous system (CNS)–hypothalamic–pituitary unit resulting in inhibition and stimulation of gonadotrophin secretion.

The main hormones secreted by the ovary are oestradiol-17β, oestrone, progesterone and androgens. Oestrogens influence the development of secondary sexual characteristics, including breast development and the female distribution of fat, as well as ovulation during the reproductive years.

From the start of menses until the menopause, the primary oestrogen is oestradiol-17β, whereas in post-menopausal women oestrone predominates. Oestriol is only present in significant amounts during pregnancy and is made by the placenta which converts dehydroisoepiandrosterone (DHEA) from the adrenal cortex of the fetus to oestriol.

OESTROGENS

Properties

The properties of oestrogens include the following:

- stimulation of endometrial growth;
- maintenance of blood vessels and skin;
- reduction of bone resorption and increase of bone formation;
- increase uterine growth;
- increase the hepatic production of binding proteins;
- increase circulating clotting factors II, VII, IX, X and plasminogen;
- increase high-density lipoprotein (HDL);
- increase biliary cholesterol;
- control salt and water retention.

Uses

Oestrogens are used in:

- oral contraception;
- the treatment of symptoms of menopause;
- the prevention of osteoporosis. Fractures of the spine, wrist and hips are reduced by 50–70% and there is about a 5% increase in spinal bone density in those women treated with oestrogen within three years of the onset of menopause and for five to ten years thereafter.
- the treatment of vaginal atrophy;
- the treatment of hypo-oestrogenism (as a result of hypogonadism, castration or primary ovarian failure);
- treatment of primary amenorrhoea;
- treatment of dysmenorrhoea;
- treatment of oligomenorrhoea;
- treatment of certain neoplastic diseases;
- treatment of hereditary haemorrhagic telangiectasia (Osler–Weber–Rendu syndrome);
- palliative treatment of prostate cancer.

Ethinylestradiol, a synthetic oestrogen, is an alternative for many of the above indications.

Oestrogens are no longer used to suppress lactation because of the risk of thromboembolism. **Bromocriptine** is used instead.

> **Key points**
>
> Main uses of oestrogen
>
> - oral contraception;
> - replacement therapy.

Adverse effects

Common symptoms include nausea and vomiting, abdominal cramps and bloating, breast enlargement and tenderness, premenstrual symptoms, sodium and fluid retention. Salt and water retention with oedema, hypertension and exacerbation of heart failure can occur with pharmacological doses. In men, gynaecomastia and impotence are predictable dose-dependent effects. There is an increased risk of thromboembolism. Oestrogens are carcinogenic in some animals and there is an increased incidence of endometrial carcinoma in women who have uninterrupted treatment with exogenous oestrogen unopposed by progestogens.

Pharmacokinetics

Oestrogens are absorbed by mouth and via the skin and mucous membranes. The most potent natural oestrogen is oestradiol-17β which is largely oxidized to oestrone and then hydrated to produce oestriol. All three oestrogens are metabolized in the liver and excreted as glucuronide and sulphate conjugates in the bile and urine. Estimation of urinary oestrogen excretion provides a measure of ovarian function. **Ethinylestradiol** has a prolonged action because of slow hepatic metabolism with a half-life of about 25 hours.

PROGESTOGENS

Progesterone is a steroid hormone involved in the female menstrual cycle, pregnancy (it supports gestation) and embryogenesis. Progesterone is the precursor of 17-hydroxyprogesterone which is converted to androstenedione which subsequently is converted to testosterone, oestrone and oestradiol. Progesterone is produced in the adrenal glands, by the corpus luteum, the brain and by the placenta.

Progestogens act on tissues primed by oestrogens whose effects they modify. There are two main groups of progestogens, namely the naturally occurring hormone progesterone and its analogues, and the testosterone analogues, such as **norethisterone** and **norgestrel**. All progestogens have anti-oestrogenic and anti-gonadotrophic properties, and differ in their potency and their side effects.

Uses of progesterone

The uses of progesterone are:

- to control anovulatory bleeding;
- to prepare the uterine lining in infertility therapy and to support early pregnancy;
- for recurrent pregnancy loss due to inadequate progesterone production;
- in the treatment of intersex disorders, to promote breast development.

Uses of progestogens

The uses of progestogens are:

- as part of the combined oral contraceptive and in the progestogen-only pill. **Medroxyprogesterone acetate** administered by depot injection is used when parenteral contraception is indicated.
- as an anti-androgen in androgen-sensitive tumours, such as prostate cancer, e.g. **cyproterone acetate**;
- as part of hormone replacement therapy in women with an intact uterus to counteract the effects of unopposed oestrogen on the endometrium which can result in endometrial carcinoma;

- endometriosis;
- in menstrual disorders, such as premenstrual tension, dysmenorrhoea and menorrhagia;
- progestogens in common use include **norethisterone**, **levonorgestrel**, **desogestrel**, **norgestimate** and **gestodene**, which are all derivatives of **norgestrel**. These differ considerably in potency. The newer progestogens, **desogestrel**, **gestodene** and **norgestimate** produce good cycle control and have a less marked adverse effect on plasma lipids; however, studies have shown that oral contraceptives containing **desogestrel** and **gestodene** are associated with an increase of around two-fold in the risk of venous thromboembolism compared to those containing other progestogens and should be avoided in women with risk factors for thromboembolic disease. **Desogestrel**, **drospirenone** (a derivative of spironolactone with anti-androgenic and anti-mineralocorticoid properties) and **gestodene** should be considered for women who have side effects, such as acne, headache, depression, weight gain, breast symptoms and breakthrough bleeding with other progestogens. The progestogen **norelgestromin** is combined with **ethinylestradiol** in a transdermal contraceptive patch.

Mechanism of action

Progestogens act on intracellular cytoplasmic receptors and initiate new protein formation. Their main contraceptive effect is via an action on cervical mucus which renders it impenetrable to sperm. **Nortestosterone** derivatives are partially metabolized oestrogenic metabolites which may account for some additional anti-ovulatory effect. A pseudodecidual change in the endometrium further discourages implantation of the zygote.

Pharmacokinetics

Progesterone is subject to presystemic hepatic metabolism and is most effective when injected intramuscularly or administered sublingually. It is excreted in the urine as pregnanediol and pregnanelone. It has prolonged absorption and an elimination half-life of 25–50 hours. It is highly protein bound. **Norethisterone**, a synthetic progestogen used in many oral contraceptives, is rapidly absorbed orally, is subject to little presystemic hepatic metabolism and has a half-life of 7.5–8 hours.

THE COMBINED ORAL CONTRACEPTIVE

Since the original pilot trials in Puerto Rico proved that steroid oral contraception was feasible, this method has become the leading method of contraception world-wide. Nearly 50% of all women in their twenties in the UK use this form of contraception. It is the most consistently effective contraceptive method and allows sexual relations to proceed without interruption, but it lacks the advantage of protection against sexually transmitted disease that is afforded by condoms. The most commonly used oestrogen is ethinylestradiol. The main contraceptive action of the combined oral contraceptive (COC) is to suppress ovulation by interfering with gonadotrophin release by the pituitary via negative feedback on the hypothalamus. This prevents the mid-cycle rise in LH which triggers ovulation.

Progestogens currently used in combined oral contraceptives include **desogestrel**, **gestodene** and **norgestimate**. These 'third-generation' progestogens are only weak anti-oestrogens, have less androgenic activity than their predecessors (**norethisterone**, **levonorgestrel** and **ethynodiol**) and are associated with less disturbance of lipoprotein metabolism. However, **desogestrel** and **gestadene** have been associated with an increased risk of venous thrombo-embolism.

Endocrine effects of the combined oral contraceptive include:

1. prevention of the normal premenstrual rise and mid-cycle peaks of LH and FSH and of the rise in progesterone during the luteal phase;
2. increased hepatic synthesis of proteins, including thyroid-binding globulin, ceruloplasmin, transferrin, coagulation factors and renin substrate, while increased fibrinogen synthesis can raise the erythrocyte sedimentation rate;
3. reduced carbohydrate tolerance;
4. decreased albumin and haptoglobulin synthesis.

Adverse effects of the COC

The overall acceptability of the combined pill is around 80% and minor side effects can often be controlled by a change in preparation. Users have an increased risk of venous thrombo-embolic disease, this risk being greatest in women over 35 years of age, especially if they smoke cigarettes, are obese and have used oral contraceptives for five years or more continuously. The increased risk of venous thrombo-embolism (VTE) has made it desirable to reduce the oestrogen dose as much as possible. Progestogen-only pills may be appropriate in women at higher risk of thrombotic disease.

In healthy non-pregnant women not taking an oral contraceptive, the incidence of VTE is about five cases per 100 000 women per year. For those using the COC containing a second-generation progestogen such as **levonorgestrel**, the incidence is 15 per 100 000 women per year of use. Some studies have shown a greater risk of VTE in women who are using COC preparations that contain third-generation progestogens, such as **desogestrel** and **gestodene**, reporting incidences of about 25 per 100 000 women per year of use. However, as the overall risk is still very small and well below the risk associated with pregnancy, provided that women are well informed about the relative risks and accept them, the choice of a COC should be made jointly by the prescriber and the woman concerned in light of individual medical history and any contraindications.

Increased blood pressure is common with the pill, and is clinically significant in about 5% of patients. When medication is stopped, the blood pressure usually falls to the pretreatment value. In normotensive non-smoking women without other risk factors for vascular disease, there is no upper age limit on using the combined oral contraceptive, but it is prudent to use the lowest effective dose of oestrogen, especially in women aged 35 years or over. Mesenteric artery thrombosis and small bowel ischaemia, and hepatic vein thrombosis and Budd–Chiari

syndrome are rare but serious adverse events linked to the use of combined oral contraception. These cardiovascular adverse effects are related to oestrogen. Jaundice similar to that of pregnancy cholestasis can occur, usually in the first few cycles. Recovery is rapid on drug withdrawal.

Oral contraceptives may affect migraine in the following ways:

1. precipitation of attacks in the previously unaffected;
2. exacerbation of previously existing migraine;
3. alteration of the pattern of attacks – in particular, focal neurological features may appear;
4. occasionally the incidence of attacks may decrease or they may even be abolished while the patient is on the pill.

Other important adverse effects include an increased incidence of gallstones. There is a small increased risk of liver cancer. There is a decreased incidence of benign breast lesions and functional ovarian cysts. Diabetes mellitus may be precipitated by the COC. Amenorrhoea after stopping combined oral contraception is not unusual (about 5% of cases) but is rarely prolonged, and although there may be temporary impairment of fertility, permanent sterility is very uncommon.

> **Key points**
>
> Combined oral contraception (COC) – adverse effects
>
> - thrombo-embolic disease;
> - increased blood pressure;
> - jaundice;
> - migraine – precipitates attacks or aggravates previously existing migraine;
> - increased incidence of gallstones;
> - associated with increased risk of liver cancer.

Risk–benefit profile

COCs cause no increased incidence of coronary artery disease, but there is a two-fold increase in ischaemic stroke. The data with regard to breast cancer suggest that there may be a small increased risk, but this is reduced to zero ten years after stopping the COC. With regards to cervical cancer, there is a small increase after five years and a two-fold increase after ten years of treatment. The risk of ovarian cancer and endometrial cancer is halved and this benefit persists for ten years or more.

> **Key point**
>
> The main mechanism of action of the combined oral contraceptive is suppression of ovulation.

Contraindications of the COC

- *Absolute contraindications*: pregnancy, thrombo-embolism, multiple risk factors for arterial disease, ischaemic heart disease, severe hypertension, migraine with focal neurological symptoms, severe liver disease, porphyria, otosclerosis, breast or genital tract carcinoma, undiagnosed vaginal bleeding and breast-feeding.

- *Relative contraindications*: uncomplicated migraine, cholelithiasis, hypertension, dyslipidaemia, diabetes mellitus, varicose veins, severe depression, long-term immobilization, sickle-cell disease, inflammatory bowel disease.

Key points

Combined oral contraceptive (COC) – absolute contraindications

- pregnancy;
- thrombo-embolism;
- multiple risk factors for arterial disease;
- ischaemic heart disease;
- severe hypertension;
- otosclerosis;
- breast or genital carcinoma;
- undiagnosed vaginal bleeding;
- breast-feeding;
- porphyria.

Drug interactions with the COC

Oestrogens increase clotting factors and reduce the efficacy of oral anticoagulants. This is not a contraindication to their continued use in patients to be started on **warfarin** (in whom pregnancy is highly undesirable), but it is a reason for increased frequency of monitoring of the international normalized ratio (INR).

Antihypertensive therapy may be adversely affected by oral contraceptives, at least partly because of increased circulating renin substrate.

Enzyme inducers (e.g. **rifampicin**, **carbamazepine**, **phenytoin**, **nelfinavir**, **nevirapine**, **ritonavir**, **St John's wort**) decrease the plasma levels of contraceptive oestrogen, thus decreasing the effectiveness of the combined contraceptive pill. Breakthrough bleeding and/or unwanted pregnancy have been described.

Oral contraceptive steroids undergo enterohepatic circulation, and conjugated steroid in the bile is broken down by bacteria in the gut to the parent steroid and subsequently reabsorbed. Broad-spectrum antibiotics (e.g. **amoxicillin**, **tetracycline**) alter colonic bacteria, increase faecal excretion of contraceptive oestrogen and decrease plasma concentrations, resulting in possible contraceptive failure. This does not appear to be a problem with progestogen-only pills.

POST-COITAL CONTRACEPTION

Post-coital contraception (the 'morning-after' pill) consists of 1.5 mg **levonorgestrel**, given as soon as possible, preferably within 12 hours and no later than 72 hours after unprotected intercourse. This prevents approximately 84% of expected pregnancies. If vomiting occurs within three hours of ingestion,

the dose should be repeated. A single dose of **mifepristone** (a progesterone antagonist) is highly effective. The abortion statistics suggest that post-coital contraception is under-utilized in the UK.

Key point

Post-coital contraception

Levonorgestrel 1.5 g as a single dose as soon as possible, preferably within 12 hours of, and no later than 72 hours after, unprotected sexual intercourse.

PROGESTOGEN-ONLY CONTRACEPTIVES

Progestogen-only contraception is available as an oral pill, a depot injection administered every 12 weeks, a single flexible rod implanted subdermally into the lower surface of the upper arm which lasts up to three years and as an intra-uterine device. The single flexible rod implant releases **etonogestrel**. The intra-uterine device (IUD) releases **levonorgestrel** directly into the uterine cavity and is licensed for use as a contraceptive and for the treatment of primary menorrhagia, as well as prevention of endometrial hypoplasia during oestroegen replacement therapy. This IUD can be effective for up to five years.

Uses

Progestogen-only contraceptive pills (e.g. **norethisterone**, **norgestrel**) are associated with a high incidence of menstrual disturbances, but are useful if oestrogen-containing pills are poorly tolerated or contraindicated (e.g. in women with risk factors for vascular disease such as older smokers, diabetics or those with valvular heart disease or migraine) or during breast-feeding. Contraceptive effectiveness is less than with the combined pill, as ovulation is suppressed in only approximately 40% of women and the major contraceptive effect is on the cervical mucus and endometrium. This effect is maximal three to four hours after ingestion and declines over the next 16–20 hours, so the pill should be taken at the same time each day, preferably three to four hours before the usual time of intercourse. Pregnancy rates are of the same order as those with the intra-uterine contraceptive device or barrier methods (approximately 1.5–2 per 100 women per year, compared to 0.3 per 100 women per year for the COCs). Progestogen-only pills are taken continuously throughout the menstrual cycle, which is convenient for some patients.

Depot **progesterone** injections are more effective than oral preparations. A single intramuscular injection of **medroxyprogesterone acetate** provides contraception for ten weeks with a failure rate of 0.25 per 100 women per year. It is mainly used as a temporary method (e.g. while waiting for vasectomy to become effective), but is occasionally indicated for long-term use in women for whom other methods are unacceptable. The side effects are essentially similar to those of oral progestogen-only preparations. After two years of treatment up to 40% of women develop amenorrhoea and infertility, so that pregnancy is unlikely for 9–12 months after the last injection.

Treatment with depot **progestogen** injections should not be undertaken without full counselling of the patient.

Adverse effects

The main problems are irregular menstrual bleeding (which can be heavy, but usually settles down after a few cycles), occasionally breast tenderness and uncommonly nausea, headache, appetite disturbance, weight changes and altered libido.

Contraindications

These include pregnancy, undiagnosed vaginal bleeding, severe arterial disease, liver adenoma and porphyria.

ANTI-PROGESTOGENS

Mifepristone is a competitive antagonist of progesterone. It is used as a medical alternative to surgical termination of early pregnancy (currently up to 63 days' gestation, although it is also effective during the second trimester). A single oral dose of **mifepristone** is followed by **gemeprost** (a prostaglandin that ripens and softens the cervix), as a vaginal pessary unless abortion is already complete. **Gemeprost** can cause hypotension, so the blood pressure must be monitored for six hours after the drug has been administered. The patient is followed up at 8–12 days and surgical termination is essential if complete abortion has not occurred. Contraindications include ectopic pregnancy.

HORMONE REPLACEMENT THERAPY

Uses and risk–benefit profile

Small doses of **oestrogen** have been shown to alleviate the vasomotor symptoms of the menopause, such as flushing, as well as menopausal vaginitis caused by oestrogen deficiency. There is now reliable evidence that giving doses of **oestrogen** for several years, starting at around the time of the menopause, reduces the degree of post-menopausal osteoporosis, but increases the risk of VTE and stroke. There is an increased risk of endometrial carcinoma after several years of use which can be countered by **progestogen**. In the main, the minimum effective dose should be used for the shortest duration.

For vaginal atrophy, **oestrogen** can be given as a local topical preparation for a few weeks at a time, repeated as necessary. However, the periods of treatment need to be limited, as again there is a risk of endometrial carcinoma. Vasomotor

symptoms require systemic therapy and this usually needs to be given for at least one year. In women with an intact uterus, **progestogen** needs to be added. Women undergoing an early natural or surgical menopause, i.e. before the age of 45 years, have a high risk of osteoporosis and have been shown to benefit from hormone replacement therapy (HRT) given until at least the age of 50 years.

There is a small increased risk of breast cancer associated with the duration of HRT. The risk of breast cancer with combined HRT does not appear to start to increase until four years after commencing HRT.

HRT users have a slightly increased risk of stroke and possibly also of myocardial infarction. A woman's baseline risk of stroke increases with age and using HRT further increases this risk.

Taking HRT increases the risk of venous thrombo-embolism (VTE) particularly in the first year of use, although the single biggest risk factor for a future episode is a personal history of VTE. The number of cases of VTE per 1000 non-HRT users over five years is three, compared to seven in those using combined HRT over five years in the 50–59 age group and the same figures are 8 and 17, respectively for the 60–69 year age group.

In women with a uterus, **oestrogen** is given daily with additional **progestogen** for the last 12–14 days of each 28-day cycle. Oestrogen is subject to first-pass metabolism via the oral route. Subcutaneous and transdermal routes of administration are available and may be suitable for certain women. Subcutaneous implants can cause rebound vasomotor symptoms, as abnormally high plasma concentrations may occur.

Hormone replacement therapy does not provide contraception and a woman is considered potentially fertile for two years after her last menstrual period if she is under 50 years of age, and for one year if she is over 50 years.

Women under 50 years without any of the risk factors for venous or arterial disease may use a low-oestrogen combined oral contraceptive pill to gain both relief of menopausal symptoms and contraception.

Contraindications

Pregnancy, oestrogen-dependent cancers, active thrombo-embolic disease, liver disease, undiagnosed vaginal bleeding and breast-feeding.

The relative contraindications include migraine, history of breast nodules and fibrocystic disease, pre-existing uterine fibroids, endometriosis, risk factors for thrombo-embolic disease.

Although caution is recommended in certain other conditions, such as hypertension, cardiac or renal disease, diabetes, asthma, epilepsy, melanoma, otosclerosis and multiple sclerosis, there is unsatisfactory evidence to support this, and many women with these conditions may benefit from HRT.

Side effects of HRT

These include nausea and vomiting, weight changes, breast enlargement and tenderness, premenstrual-like syndrome, fluid retention, changes in liver function, depression and headache, altered blood lipids, venous thrombo-embolism.

Oestrogens used in HRT include conjugated **oestrogens**, **mestranol**, **estradiol**, **estriol** and **oestropipate**. Progester-ones used in HRT include **medroxyprogesterone**, **norgestrel**, **norethisterone**, **levonorgestrel** and **dydrogesterone**. **Tibolone** has oestrogenic, progestogenic and weak androgenic activity.

Key points

HRT is much less used now because of worries about increased cardiovascular events and hormone-sensitive cancers (especially breast). Absolute contraindications:

- pregnancy;
- oestrogen-dependent cancers;
- active thrombo-embolic disease;
- liver disease;
- undiagnosed vaginal bleeding;
- breast-feeding.

REPRODUCTIVE HORMONE ANTAGONISTS

Uses

There are a number of agents now available that are used in early and advanced breast cancer due to their antagonistic or inhibitory effect on oestrogen, breast cancer commonly being an oestrogen-sensitive tumour.

Oestrogen receptor antagonists include **tamoxifen** which is licensed for breast cancer and anovulatory infertility, **fulvestrant** which is licensed for the treatment of oestrogen receptor-positive metastatic or locally advanced breast cancer in post-menopausal women, and **toremifene** which is licensed for hormone-dependent metastatic breast cancer in post-menopausal women.

The aromatase inhibitors block the conversion of androgens to oestrogens in the peripheral tissues. They do not inhibit ovarian oestrogen synthesis and are not suitable for use in premenopausal women who will continue to secrete ovarian oestrogens. Currently licensed agents include **anastrozole**, **letrozole** and **exemestane**.

The gonadorelin analogue **goserelin** is licensed for the management of advanced breast cancer in premenopausal women. It acts by initially stimulating and then depressing luteinizing hormone released by the pituitary, which in turn reduces oestrogen production.

Clomifene and **tamoxifen** are used in the treatment of female infertility due to oligomenorrhoea or secondary amenorrhoea (for example, that associated with polycystic ovarian disease). Both drugs can induce gonadotrophin release by occupying oestrogen receptors in the hypothalamus, thereby interfering with feedback mechanisms. As an adjunct, chorionic gonadotrophin is sometimes used.

Clomifene is used primarily for anovulatory infertility. Patients should be warned about the risks of multiple births. It is contraindicated in those with liver disease, ovarian cysts, hormone-dependent tumours and abnormal uterine bleeding of undetermined cause.

Side effects of **clomifene** include visual disturbances, ovarian hyperstimulation, hot flushes, abdominal discomfort, occasionally nausea, vomiting, depression, insomnia, breast tenderness, headache, intermenstrual spotting, menorrhagia, endometriosis, convulsions, weight gain, rashes, dizziness and hair loss.

GONADOTROPHINS

Follicle-stimulating hormone (FSH) and luteinizing hormone (LH) together, or follicle-stimulating hormone alone, and chorionic gonadotrophin, are used in the treatment of infertility in women with proven hypopituitarism or who have not responded to **clomifene**, or in superovulation treatment for assisted conception, for example in vitro fertilization (IVF).

DRUGS FOR SUPPRESSION OF LACTATION

Bromocriptine is a dopamine agonist and inhibits the release of prolactin by the pituitary. It is used for the treatment of galactorrhoea and cyclical benign breast disease, as well as the treatment of prolactinomas.

Cabergoline has actions and uses similar to those of **bromocriptine**, but its duration of action is longer. It has a different side-effect profile from **bromocriptine** and patients who may not tolerate the latter may be able to tolerate **cabergoline** and vice versa.

Although **bromocriptine** and **cabergoline** are licensed to suppress lactation, they are not recommended for routine suppression or for the relief of symptoms of postpartum pain and breast engorgement that can be adequately treated with simple analgesics and support.

PROSTAGLANDINS AND OXYTOCIC DRUGS

Prostaglandins and oxytocics are used to induce abortion, or induce or augment labour, and to minimize blood loss from the placental site. The commonly used drugs include **oxytocin**, **ergometrine** and the prostaglandins. All work by inducing uterine contractions with varying degrees of pain according to the strength of the contractions induced.

Synthetic prostaglandin E_2 (**dinoprostone**) is used for the induction of late (second-trimester) therapeutic abortion, because the uterus is sensitive to its actions at this stage, whereas oxytocin only reliably causes uterine contraction later in pregnancy.

Dinoprostone is preferred to **oxytocin** for the induction of labour in women with intact membranes regardless of parity or cervical favourability. Both are equally effective in inducing labour in women with ruptured membranes. However, **oxytocin** is preferred for this, because it lacks the many side effects of prostaglandin E_2 that relate to its actions on extra-uterine tissues. These include nausea, vomiting, diarrhoea, flushing, headache, hypotension and fever.

Dinoprostone is available as vaginal tablets, pessaries and vaginal gels. **Oxytocin** is administered by slow intravenous infusion using an infusion pump to induce or augment labour, usually in conjunction with rupture of membranes. Uterine activity must be monitored carefully and hyperstimulation avoided. Large doses of **oxytocin** can cause excessive fluid retention. **Oxytocin** should not be started within six hours of administration of vaginal prostaglandins.

A combination formulation of **ergometrine** and **oxytocin** (**syntometrine**) is used for bleeding due to incomplete abortion and in the routine management of the third stage of labour. This is administered by intramuscular injection with the delivery of the anterior shoulder. A useful alternative in severe postpartum haemorrhage in patients with an atonic uterus unresponsive to **ergometrine** and **oxytocin** is **carboprost**.

OXYTOCIN

Oxytocin produces contractions of the smooth muscle of the fundus of the pregnant uterus at term, and of the mammary gland ducts. It is released from the pituitary by suckling and also by emotional stimuli. Any role in the initiation of labour is not established. There is no known disease state of over- or under-production of **oxytocin**. Synthetic **oxytocin** is effective when administered by any parenteral route, and is usually given as a constant-rate intravenous infusion to initiate or augment labour, often following artificial rupture of the membranes. A low dose is used to initiate treatment titrated upwards if necessary.

The side effects of **oxytocin** include uterine spasm, tetanic contractions, water intoxication and hyponatraemia, and uterine hyperstimulation.

ERGOMETRINE

Ergometrine (an alkaloid derived from ergot, a fungus that infects rye) is a powerful oxytocic. The uterus is sensitive at all times, but especially so in late pregnancy. It is given intramuscularly, or intravenously in emergency. **Oxytocin** produces slow contractions with full relaxations between, whilst **ergometrine** produces faster contractions superimposed on a tonic persistent contraction (it is for this reason that **ergometrine** is unsuitable for induction of labour). If given intramuscularly, **oxytocin** acts within one to two minutes, although the contraction is brief, but **ergometrine** takes five minutes to act.

Ergometrine can cause hypertension, particularly in pre-eclamptic patients, in whom it should be used with care, if at all.

PROSTAGLANDINS

Prostaglandins are naturally occurring lipid-derived mediators. Prostaglandins are involved in a wide range of physiological and pathological processes, including inflammation (see Chapter 26) and haemostasis and thrombosis (see Chapter 30). Prostaglandin E_2 has a potent contractile action on the human uterus, and also softens and ripens the cervix. In addition, it has many other actions, including inhibition of acid secretion by the stomach, increased mucus secretion within the gastro-intestinal tract, contraction of gastro-intestinal smooth muscle, relaxation of vascular smooth muscle and increase in body temperature.

Specialized uses of prostaglandins in the perinatal period include the use of prostaglandin E_1 (**alprostadil**) in neonates with congenital heart defects that are 'ductus-dependent'. It preserves the patency of the ductus arteriosus until surgical correction is feasible. Conversely, in infants with inappropriately patent ductus arteriosus, **indometacin** given intravenously can cause closure of the ductus by inhibiting the endogenous biosynthesis of prostaglandins involved in the preservation of ductal patency.

MALE REPRODUCTIVE ENDOCRINOLOGY

INTRODUCTION

The principal hormone of the testis is testosterone, which is secreted by the interstitial (Leydig) cells. Testosterone circulates in the blood, bound to a plasma globulin. The plasma concentration is variable, but should exceed 10 nmol/L in adult males. Cells in target tissues convert testosterone into the more active androgen dihydrotestosterone by a 5-α-reductase enzyme. Both testosterone and dihydrotestosterone are inactivated in the liver. Androgens have a wide range of activities, the most important of which include actions on:

- development of male secondary sex characteristics (including male distribution of body hair, breaking of the voice, enlargement of the penis, sebum secretion and male-pattern balding);
- protein anabolic effects influencing growth, maturation of bone and muscle development;
- spermatogenesis and seminal fluid formation.

Testicular function is controlled by the anterior pituitary.

- Follicle-stimulating hormone acts on the seminiferous tubules and promotes spermatogenesis.
- Luteinizing hormone stimulates testosterone production.

The release of FSH and LH by the pituitary is in turn mediated by the hypothalamus via gonadotrophin-releasing hormone.

ANDROGENS AND ANABOLIC STEROIDS

Uses

Many cases of impotence are psychogenic in origin and treatment with androgens is inappropriate. In impotent patients with low concentrations of circulating testosterone, replacement therapy improves secondary sex characteristics and may restore erectile function and libido, but it does not restore fertility. (Treatment of patients with hypogonadism secondary to hypothalamic or pituitary dysfunction who wish to become fertile includes gonadotrophins or pulsatile gonadotrophin-releasing hormone.) Replacement therapy is most reliably achieved by intramuscular injection of testosterone esters in oil, of which various preparations are available. They should usually be given at two- to three-week intervals to control symptoms. Alternatively, **testosterone undecanoate** or **mesterolone** can be taken by mouth; these drugs are formulated in oil, favouring lymphatic absorption from the gastro-intestinal tract.

Delayed puberty due to gonadal deficiency (primary or secondary) or severe constitutional delay can be treated by testosterone esters or gonadotrophins. Care is needed because premature fusion of epiphyses may occur, resulting in short stature and such treatment is best supervised by specialist clinics.

Occasional patients with disseminated breast cancer derive considerable symptomatic benefit from androgen treatment.

Anabolic steroids (e.g. **nandrolone, stanozolol, danazol**) have proportionately greater anabolic and less virilizing effects than other androgens. They have generally been disappointing in therapeutics and have been widely abused by athletes and body builders. Their legitimate uses are few, but include the treatment of some aplastic anaemias, the vascular manifestations of Behçet's disease and the prophylaxis of recurrent attacks of hereditary angioneurotic oedema.

Mechanism of action

Testosterone and dihydrotestosterone interact with intracellular receptors in responsive cells, leading to new protein synthesis.

Adverse effects

Virilization in women and increased libido in men are predictable effects. In women, acne, growth of facial hair and deepening of the voice are common undesirable features produced by androgens. Other masculinizing effects and menstrual irregularities can also develop. In the male, excessive masculinization can result in frequent erections or priapism and aggressive behaviour. Children may undergo premature fusion of epiphyses. Other adverse effects include jaundice, particularly of the cholestatic type, and because of this complication **methyltestosterone** is no longer prescribed. Azospermia occurs due to inhibition of gonadotrophin secretion. In patients treated for malignant disease with androgens, hypercalcaemia (which may be severe) is produced by an unknown mechanism. Oral **testosterone** preparations in oil cause various gastro-intestinal symptoms including anorexia, vomiting, flatus, diarrhoea and oily stools.

Pharmacokinetics

Although **testosterone** is readily absorbed following oral administration, considerable presystemic metabolism occurs in the liver. It can be administered sublingually, although this route is seldom used. Testosterone in oil is well absorbed from intramuscular injection sites, but is also rapidly metabolized. Esters of testosterone are much less polar and are more slowly released from oily depot injections and are used for their prolonged effect. Inactivation of testosterone takes place in the liver. The chief metabolites are androsterone and etiocholanolone, which are mainly excreted in the urine. About 6% of administered testosterone appears in the faeces having undergone enterohepatic circulation.

ANTI-ANDROGENS

CYPROTERONE

Uses

Cyproterone acetate is used in men with inoperable prostatic carcinoma, before initiating treatment with gonadotrophin-releasing hormone analogues to prevent the flare of disease activity induced by the initial increase in sex hormone release. It has also been used to reduce sexual drive in cases of sexual deviation and in children with precocious puberty. In women, it has been used to treat hyperandrogenic effects (often seen in polycystic ovary disease), including acne, hirsutism and male-pattern baldness. The potentially adverse effects of **cyproterone** on HDL and LDL caution against long-term use, and the risk–benefit ratio should be considered carefully before embarking on treatment for relatively minor indications.

Mechanism of action

Cyproterone acts by competing with testosterone for its high-affinity receptors, thereby inhibiting prostatic growth, spermatogenesis and masculinization. It also has strong progestational activity and a very weak glucocorticoid effect.

Adverse effects

Side effects include gynaecomastia in approximately 20% of patients (occasionally with benign nodules and galactorrhoea), inhibition of spermatogenesis (which usually returns to normal six months after cessation of treatment) and tiredness and lassitude (which can be so marked as to make driving dangerous).

DUTASTERIDE AND FINASTERIDE

Use

Dutasteride and **finasteride** inhibit 5α-reductase and reduce prostate size with improvement in urinary flow rate and symptoms of obstruction. They are useful alternatives to alpha blockers (e.g. **doxazosin**) for benign prostatic hypertrophy, particularly in men with a significantly enlarged prostate.

Prostate-specific antigen should be measured as treatment must not delay the diagnosis of prostate cancer.

Adverse effects include impotence, decreased libido, ejaculation disorders, breast tenderness and enlargement. Women of child-bearing potential should avoid handling crushed or broken tablets of **finasteride** or leaking capsules of **dutasteride**.

A low strength of **finasteride** is licensed for treating male-pattern baldness in men.

DRUGS THAT AFFECT MALE SEXUAL PERFORMANCE

The complex interplay between physiological and psychological factors that determines sexual desire and performance makes it difficult to assess the influence of drugs on sexual function. In randomized placebo-controlled blinded studies, a small but significant proportion of men who receive placebo discontinue their participation because of the occurrence of impotence which they attribute to therapy. Drugs that affect the autonomic supply to the sex organs are not alone in interfering with sexual function. Indeed, **bendroflumethiazide**, a thiazide diuretic, caused significantly more impotence in the Medical Research Council (MRC) trial of mild hypertension than did **propranolol**, a β-adrenoceptor antagonist. Drugs that do interfere with autonomic function and can also cause erectile dysfunction include phenothiazines, butyrophenones and tricyclic antidepressants. Pelvic non-adrenergic, non-cholinergic nerves are involved in erectile function and utilize nitric oxide as their neurotransmitter. Nitric oxide release from endothelium in the corpus cavernosum is abnormal in some cases of organic impotence, e.g. in diabetes mellitus.

Phosphodiesterase type 5 inhibitors licensed for the treatment of erectile dysfunction include **sildenafil**, **tadalafil** and **vardenafil**. They have revolutionized the treatment of erectile dysfunction. Caution is needed in patients with cardiovascular disease, anatomical deformation of the penis, e.g. Peyronie's disease, and in those with a predisposition to prolonged erection, e.g. in sickle-cell disease. They are contraindicated in patients who are on nitrates and in patients with a previous history of non-arteritic anterior ischaemic optic neuropathy.

The side effects include dyspepsia, vomiting, headache, flushing, dizziness, myalgia, visual disturbances, raised intraocular pressure and nasal congestion.

Other therapeutic options for erectile dysfunction include intracavernosal injection or urethral application of **alprostadil** (prostaglandin E_1). Priapism and hypotension are side effects. Any treatment for erectile dysfunction should only be initiated after treatable medical causes have been excluded.

A few cases of reduced libido and impotence in males and females are associated with idiopathic hyperprolactinaemia, and in such cases **bromocriptine** may restore potency. Androgens play a role in both male and female arousal, but their use is not appropriate except in patients with reduced circulating concentrations of testosterone.

Case history

A 26-year-old woman consults you in your GP surgery regarding advice about starting the combined oral contraceptive pill.
Question
Outline your management of this patient.
Answer
It is very important to take a careful history in order to exclude any risk factors which would contraindicate the combined oral contraceptive, such as a past history of thrombo-embolic disease or risk factors for thrombo-embolic disease. In addition, it is important to ascertain whether the patient is a smoker and when she last had a cervical smear. It is important to exclude a history of migraine and to check her blood pressure.

The combined oral contraceptive is probably an appropriate form of contraception in a woman of this age, who would possibly be highly fertile, as it is the most reliable form of contraception available, provided that there are no risk factors to contraindicate the combined oral contraceptive. There are many COCs on the market and selection for this individual would be dependent on a balance of achieving good cycle

control and weighing the beneficial effects on plasma lipids offered by the newer progestogens, such as desogestrel, gestadine and norgestimate, against the recently reported two-fold increased risk of venous thrombo-embolism noted with desogestrel and gestadine. In a woman of this age, the beneficial effects on plasma lipids are probably of minor importance and in view of the increased risk of venous thrombo-embolism it would probably be appropriate to choose a pill containing norethisterone, levonorgestrel or norgestimate. The majority of women achieve good cycle control with combined oral contraceptives containing oestrogen at a dose of about 30–35 µg; pills containing the higher dose of oestrogen would only be required if the individual was on long-term enzyme-inducing therapy (e.g. rifampicin) or anticonvulsant medication.

Case history

A 50-year-old woman consults you about her symptoms of flushing and vaginal discomfort. She is thin and is a smoker.
Question
Outline the therapy most likely to be of benefit, including the reasons for this.
Answer
This woman is probably menopausal and is suffering the consequences of the vasomotor effects of the menopause, as well as vaginal dryness. The vaginal dryness could be treated locally with short periods of treatment with topical oestrogens. However, in view of her other symptoms, a better option would be to start her on hormone replacement therapy. If she still has an intact uterus then it is important to give both oestrogen and cyclical progestogen to protect the endometrium from hyperplasia. Depending on preference, life-style and the likelihood of compliance, either oral therapy or patches may be appropriate. In this woman, who has risk factors for osteoporosis, such as smoking and thinness, it may be of benefit to continue the hormone replacement therapy for a period of at least five years and possibly longer, although it is important to exercise caution with regard to her risk for breast cancer and cardiovascular disease.

FURTHER READING

Baird DT, Glasier AF. Science, medicine, and the future: Contraception. *British Medical Journal* 1999; **319**: 969–72.

Nelson HD. Assessing benefits and harms of hormone replacement therapy: clinical applications. *Journal of the American Medical Association* 2002; **288**: 882–4.

Nelson HD, Humphrey LL, Nygren P et al. Postmenopausal hormone replacement therapy: scientific review. *Journal of the American Medical Association* 2002; **288**: 872–81.

US Preventive Services Task Force. Hormone therapy for the prevention of chronic conditions in postmenopausal women: recommendations from the US Preventive Services Task Force. *Annals of Internal Medicine* 2005; **142**: 855–60.

Wathen CN, Feig DS, Feightner JW et al. and The Canadian Task Force on Preventive Health Care. Hormone replacement therapy for the primary prevention of chronic diseases: recommendation statement from the Canadian Task Force on Preventive Health Care. *Canadian Medical Association Journal* 2004; **170**: 1535–7.

CHAPTER 42

THE PITUITARY HORMONES AND RELATED DRUGS

ANTERIOR PITUITARY HORMONES AND RELATED DRUGS

GROWTH HORMONE: PHYSIOLOGY AND PATHOPHYSIOLOGY

Growth hormone (GH) is a 191-amino-acid protein secreted by the acidophil cells in the anterior pituitary. Secretion occurs in brief pulses, with a slower underlying diurnal variability, and is greatest during sleep. Secretion is much greater during growth than in older individuals. Secretion is stimulated by hypogly-caemia, fasting and stress, and by agonists at dopamine, serotonin and at α- and β-adrenoceptors. The serotoninergic pathway is involved in the stimulation of somatotropin release during slow-wave sleep. Secretion is inhibited by eating, by glucocorticos-teroids and by oestrogens. The hypothalamus controls GH secretion from the pituitary by secreting a GH-releasing hormone (GHRH), somatorelin and a GH-release-inhibiting hormone, somatostatin, which is also synthesized in D cells of the islets of Langerhans in the pancreas. GH-secreting pituitary adenomas cause acromegaly in adults (gigantism in children), whereas GH deficiency in children causes growth retardation and short stature.

GROWTH HORMONE (SOMATROPIN): THERAPEUTIC USE

Somatropin is the synthetic recombinant form of human growth hormone used therapeutically. It promotes protein synthesis and is synergistic with insulin. Its effect on skeletal growth is mediated by somatomedin (a small peptide synthe-sized in the liver, secretion of which depends on somatotropin).

Somatropin is used to treat children with dwarfism due to isolated growth hormone deficiency or deficiency due to hypo-thalamic or pituitary disease. This is often difficult to diagnose, and requires accurate sequential measurements of height together with biochemical measurements of endogenous GH during pharmacological (e.g. **insulin**, **clonidine**, **glucagon**, **argi-nine** or **L-dopa**) or physiological (e.g. sleep, exercise) stimula-tion. **Somatropin** treatment also increases height in children with Turner's syndrome. Injections should start well before

puberty in order to optimize linear growth, and should continue until growth ceases. Replacement therapy with gonadotrophin or sex hormones is delayed until max-imum growth has been achieved. Other indications are to increase growth in children with chronic renal failure, with Prader–Willi syndrome and in short children born short for gestational age. It is used in adults with severe GH deficiency accompanying deficiency of another pituitary hormone and associated with impaired quality of life. In this setting it should be discontinued if the quality of life does not improve after nine months of treatment. In adults aged less than 25 years in whom growth is complete, severe GH defi-ciency (e.g. following neurosurgery) should be treated with **somatropin** until adult peak bone mass has been achieved.

GROWTH HORMONE EXCESS

Over-secretion of GH is usually associated with a functional ade-noma of the acidophil cells of the adenohypophysis, and treat-ment is by neurosurgery and radiotherapy. The place of medical treatment is as an adjunct to this when surgery has not effected a cure, and while awaiting the effect of radiotherapy, which can be delayed by up to ten years. The visual fields and size of the pitu-itary fossa must be assessed repeatedly in order to detect further growth of the tumour during such treatment. Somatostatin low-ers GH levels in acromegalics, but has to be given by continuous intravenous infusion and also inhibits many gastro-intestinal hormones. **Octreotide** and **lanreotide** are long-acting analogues of somatostatin which lower somatotropin levels. They are given by intermittent injection. **Pegvisomant** is a selective antagonist of the GH receptor. It is a genetically modified GH analogue and is injected subcutaneously once daily. It is used for acromegaly with an inadequate response to surgery, radiotherapy and somatostatin analogues. It has a range of gastro-intestinal, meta-bolic, neurological and other adverse effects and should be used only by physicians experienced in treating acromegaly.

OCTREOTIDE

Uses

Octreotide is a synthetic octapeptide analogue of somatostatin which inhibits peptide release from endocrine-secreting tumours of the pituitary or gastro-intestinal tract. It is used to treat patients with symptoms caused by the release of pharmacologically active substances from gastro-enteropancreatic tumours, including patients with carcinoid syndrome, insulinoma, VIPoma or glucagonoma. It reduces symptoms of flushing, diarrhoea or skin rash, but does not reduce the size of the tumour. It is more effective than **bromocriptine** (now mainly used in Parkinson's disease, see Chapter 21) in lowering somatotropin levels in patients with acromegaly, but it is not generally an acceptable alternative to surgery, and must be administered parenterally (usually subcutaneously three times daily). It is also effective in patients with TSH-secreting basophil tumours of the adenohypophysis causing thyrotoxicosis (an extremely rare cause of hyperthyroidism). It reduces portal pressure in portal hypertension, and is effective in the acute therapy of bleeding oesophageal varices. It is also used to reduce ileostomy diarrhoea and the diarrhoea associated with cryptosporidiosis in AIDS patients. Gastro-intestinal side effects are minimized if **octreotide** is given between meals. A long-acting microsphere **octreotide** formulation in poly (alkyl cyanoacrylate) nanocapsules is administered intramuscularly once a month.

Adverse effects

These include:

- gastro-intestinal upset, including anorexia, nausea, vomiting, abdominal pain, diarrhoea and steatorrhoea;
- impaired glucose tolerance, by reducing insulin secretion;
- increased incidence of gallstones and/or biliary sludge after only a few months of treatment, especially at higher doses. Ultrasound evaluation of the gall bladder is recommended before starting therapy and if biliary symptoms occur during therapy.

Key points

Growth hormone (GH, somatropin)

- Somatropin (recombinant GH) is used to treat short stature due to:
  - GH deficiency;
  - Turner's syndrome;
  - Prader–Willi syndrome;
  - chronic renal impairment;
  - children who were born small for gestational age.
- Somatropin is also used for adults with severe symptomatic GH deficiency.
- GH secretion is controlled physiologically by:
  - somatorelin (stimulates GH secretion);
  - somatostatin (inhibits GH secretion).
- Somatostatin is secreted by D cells in the islets of Langerhans, as well as centrally, and inhibits the secretion of many gut hormones in addition to GH.
- Octreotide is a somatostatin analogue used:
  - in acromegalics with persistent raised GH despite surgery/radiotherapy;
  - in functional neuroendocrine tumours (e.g. carcinoid, VIPomas, glucagonomas);
  - to reduce portal pressure in variceal bleeding (unlicensed indication).
- Pegvisomant is a specific GH receptor antagonist: it is used for acromegaly when conventional treatment has failed.

GONADOTROPHINS

The human pituitary gland secretes follicle-stimulating hormone (FSH) and luteinizing hormone (LH). FSH is a glycoprotein which in females controls development of the primary ovarian follicle, stimulates granulosa cell proliferation and increases oestrogen production, while in males it increases spermatogenesis. LH is also a glycoprotein. It induces ovulation, stimulates thecal oestrogen production and initiates and maintains the corpus luteum in females. In males, LH stimulates androgen synthesis by Leydig cells, and thus has a role in the maturation of spermatocytes and the development of secondary sex characteristics.

Human menopausal urinary gonadotrophin (**HMG**), human chorionic gonadotrophin (**HCG**) and synthetic LH and recombinant FSH (**follitropin alfa** and **beta**) are all commercially available. They are used to induce ovulation in anovulatory women with secondary ovarian failure in whom treatment with **clomifene** (see Chapter 41) has failed. Treatment must be supervised by specialists experienced in the use of gonadotrophins and be carefully monitored with repeated pelvic ultrasound scans to avoid ovarian hyperstimulation and multiple pregnancies. Gonadotrophins are also effective in the treatment of oligospermia due to secondary testicular failure. They are, of course, ineffective in primary gonadal failure.

GONADORELIN ANALOGUES

Gonadorelin (gonadotrophin-releasing hormone, GnRH) is the FSH/LH-releasing factor produced in the hypothalamus. It may be used in a single intravenous dose to assess anterior pituitary reserve. Analogues of GnRH (Table 42.1) such as **goserelin**, **buserelin** and **leuprorelin** are also used to treat endometriosis, female infertility (see Chapter 41), prostate cancer and advanced breast cancer (see Chapter 48). **Buserelin** is given intranasally, and **goserelin** is usually given by subcutaneous injection/implant into the anterior abdominal. In benign conditions use should be limited to a maximum of six months because reduced oestrogen levels lead to reduced bone density, in addition to menopausal-type symptoms (see below). For indications such as endometriosis, it is possible to combine a GnRH analogue with low-dose **oestrogen** replacement to avoid this.

Mechanism of action

GnRH analogues initially stimulate the release of FSH/LH, but then downregulate this response (usually after two weeks)

Table 42.1: GnRH analogues

Drug	Use and additional comments
Goserelin	Used to treat endometriosis, prostate cancer and advanced breast cancer
Leuprorelin	Used to treat endometriosis and prostate cancer
Buserelin	Used to treat endometriosis. Prostate cancer. Induction of ovulation prior to IVF

and thereby reduce pituitary stimulation of male or female gonads, effectively leading to medical orchidectomy/ovariectomy (a state of hypopituitary hypogonadism).

Adverse effects

Menopausal symptoms are common in addition to decreased trabecular bone density, and local symptoms caused by irritation of the nasal mucosa with **buserelin**.

Pharmacokinetics

Gonadorelin analogues are peptides and are given parenterally. **Goserelin** may be given as intravenous pulses to mimic the physiological release of GnRH. Depot preparations are available to suppress FSH/LH release (see above). GnRH analogues are cleared by a combination of hepatic metabolism and renal excretion.

Key points

Gonadotrophins and GnRH analogues

- FSH and LH are secreted in pulses and stimulate gonadal steroid synthesis.
- GnRH analogues initially stimulate, but then downregulate the release of FSH and LH.
- GnRH analogues (e.g. goserelin, buserelin) are used in the treatment of :
  - endometriosis;
  - female infertility;
  - prostate cancer;
  - advanced breast cancer.
- Side-effects of GnRH analogues include:
  - menopausal symptoms;
  - reduced bone density (by reducing oestrogen secretion).

ADRENOCORTICOTROPHIC HORMONE

Adrenocorticotrophic hormone (ACTH, corticotropin) is no longer commercially available in the UK. A synthetic analogue of ACTH, containing only the first 24 amino acids, is available as **tetracosactide**. This possesses full biological activity, the remaining 15 amino acids of ACTH being species specific and associated with antigenic activity. The $t_{1/2}$ of **tetracosactide** (15 minutes) is slightly longer than that of ACTH, but otherwise its properties are identical. **Tetracosactide** is used as a diagnostic test in the evaluation of patients in whom Addison's disease (adrenal insufficiency) is suspected. A single intravenous or intramuscular dose is administered, followed by venous blood sampling for plasma cortisol determination. There is a small risk of anaphylaxis.

POSTERIOR PITUITARY HORMONES

Vasopressin (antidiuretic hormone, ADH) and **oxytocin** are related octapeptide hormones synthesized in the supra-optic and paraventricular hypothalamic nuclei and transported along nerve fibres to the posterior lobe of the pituitary gland for storage and subsequent release (neurosecretion). **Vasopressin** and **desmopressin** (DDAVP) are discussed in Chapter 36, in relation to the treatment of diabetes insipidus. **Demeclocycline** is an antagonist of ADH and has been used in patients with hyponatraemia caused by the syndrome of inappropriate ADH secretion (SIADH). More specific antagonists of ADH are in development. The use of **oxytocin** for induction of labour is described in Chapter 41.

Key points

Physiology of the pituitary

Anterior pituitary
secretes:

- growth hormone (GH);
- follicle-stimulating hormone (FSH);
- luteinizing hormone (LH);
- adrenocorticotrophic hormone (ACTH);
- prolactin;
- thyroid-stimulating hormone (TSH).

is controlled by:

- hypothalamic hormones (stimulatory/inhibitory);
- feedback inhibition.

Posterior pituitary
Related octapeptides, synthesized in the hypothalamus and released by neurosecretion:

1. Vasopressin (ADH):
   - increases blood pressure;
   - causes renal water retention.

2. Oxytocin:
   - stimulates uterine contractions;
   - used in obstretrics (for induction of labour).

Case history

A 64-year-old man was investigated for worsening chronic back pain and was found to have osteosclerotic bony metastases from prostate carcinoma. Analgesia with adequate doses of NSAIDs successfully controlled his bone pain, and he was started on GnRH analogue therapy with goserelin given subcutaneously, 3.6 mg per month. After one week his pain was worse, especially at night, without evidence of spinal compression.
Question
What is the likely cause of the deterioration in his symptoms and how would you treat him?
Answer
The most likely cause of his symptoms worsening in the first week of GnRH analogue therapy is the 'tumour flare reaction'. GnRH analogues increase secretion of FSH/LH for one to two weeks, causing an initial increase in testosterone. They subsequently produce downregulation, leading to decreased secretion of FSH/LH and hence decreased testosterone levels. In patients with metastatic prostate cancer it is essential to initiate GnRH analogue therapy only after several weeks of treatment with an androgen receptor antagonist such as cyproterone acetate, flutamide or bicalutamide. The use of anti-androgens prevents the 'tumour flare'. Thus this patient should be given adequate analgesia and an androgen receptor antagonist (e.g. oral flutamide) started at once. Goserelin can then be restarted in several weeks time.

FURTHER READING

Birnbaumer M. Vasopressin receptors. *Trends in Endocrinology and Metabolism* 2000; **11**: 406–10.

Drolet G, Rivest S. Corticotropin-releasing hormone and its receptors; an evaluation at the transcription level in vivo. *Peptides* 2001; **22**: 761–7.

Feenstra J, de Herder WW, ten Have SM et al. Combined therapy with somatostatin analogues and weekly pegvisomant in active acromegaly. *Lancet* 2005; **365**: 1644–6.

Freeman ME, Kanyicska B, Lerant A, Nagy G. Prolactin: structure, function and regulation of secretion. *Physiological Research* 2000; **80**: 1524–85.

Hays RM. Vasopressin antagonists – progress and promise. *New England Journal of Medicine* 2006; **355**: 2146–8.

Lamberts SWJ, van der Lely A-J, de Herder WW, Hofland LJ. 1996 Octreotide. *New England Journal of Medicine* 1996; **334**: 246–54.

Melmed S. Medical progress: acromegaly. *New England Journal of Medicine* 2006; **355**: 2558–73.

Okada S, Kopchick JJ. Biological effects of growth hormone and its antagonist. *Trends in Molecular Medicine* 2001; **7**: 126–32.

Thibonnier M, Coles P, Thibonnier A et al. 2001 The basic and clinical pharmacology of nonpeptide vasopressin receptor antagonists. *Annual Review of Pharmacology* 2001; **41**: 175–202.

Trainer PJ, Drake WM, Katznelson L et al. Treatment of acromegaly with the growth hormone-receptor antagonist pegvisomant. *New England Journal of Medicine* 2000; **342**: 1171–7.

Vance ML, Mauras N. Growth hormone therapy in adults and children. *New England Journal of Medicine* 1999; **341**: 1206–16.

Wenzel V, Krismer AC, Arntz HR et al. A comparison of vasopressin and epinephrine for out-of-hospital cardiopulmonary resuscitation. *New England Journal of Medicine* 2004; **350**: 105–13.

PART IX

SELECTIVE TOXICITY

CHAPTER 43

ANTIBACTERIAL DRUGS

PRINCIPLES OF ANTIBACTERIAL CHEMOTHERAPY

Bacteria are a common cause of disease, but have beneficial as well as harmful effects. For example, the gastrointestinal bacterial flora of the healthy human assists in preventing colonization by pathogens. The widespread use of antibacterial drugs has led to the appearance of multiresistant bacteria which are now a significant cause of morbidity and mortality in the UK. Consequently, antibacterial therapy should not be used indiscriminately.

A distinction is conventionally drawn between bactericidal drugs that kill bacteria and bacteriostatic drugs that prevent their reproduction, elimination depending on host defence (Table 43.1A). This difference is relative, as bacteriostatic drugs are often bactericidal at high concentrations and in the presence of host defence mechanisms. In clinical practice, the distinction is seldom important unless the body's defence mechanisms are depressed. Antibacterial drugs can be further classified into five main groups according to their mechanism of action (Table 43.1B).

The choice of antibacterial drug, together with its dose and route of administration, depend on the infection (in particular the responsible pathogen(s), but also anatomical site and severity), absorption characteristics of the drug, and patient factors (in particular age, weight, renal function). In addition, the dose may be guided by plasma concentration measurements of drugs with a narrow therapeutic index (e.g. aminoglycosides). The duration of therapy depends on the nature of the infection and response to treatment.

The *British National Formulary* provides a good guide to initial treatments for common bacterial infections. In view of regional variations in patterns of bacterial resistance, these may be modified according to local guidelines.

Close liaison with the local microbiology laboratory provides information on local prevalence of organisms and sensitivities.

The minimum inhibitory concentration (MIC) is often quoted by laboratories and in promotional literature. It is the minimal concentration of a particular agent below which bacterial growth is not prevented. Although the MIC provides useful information for comparing the susceptibility of organisms to antibacterial drugs, it is an in vitro test in a homogenous culture system, whilst in vivo the concentration at the

Table 43.1A: Classification of antibacterial agents into bactericidal and bacteriostatic

Bactericidal	Bacteriostatic
Penicillins	Erythromycin
Cephalosporins	Tetracyclines
Aminoglycosides	Chloramphenicol
Co-trimoxazole	Sulphonamides
	Trimethoprim

Table 43.1B: Classification of antibacterial agents according to mechanism of action

Mechanism of action	Antibacterial agent
Inhibition of cell wall synthesis	Penicillins
	Cephalosporins
	Monobactams
	Vancomycin
Inhibition of DNA gyrase	Quinolones
Inhibition of RNA polymerase	Rifampicin
Inhibition of protein synthesis	Aminoglycosides
	Tetracyclines
	Erythromycin
	Chloramphenicol
Inhibition of folic acid metabolism	Trimethoprim
	Sulphonamides

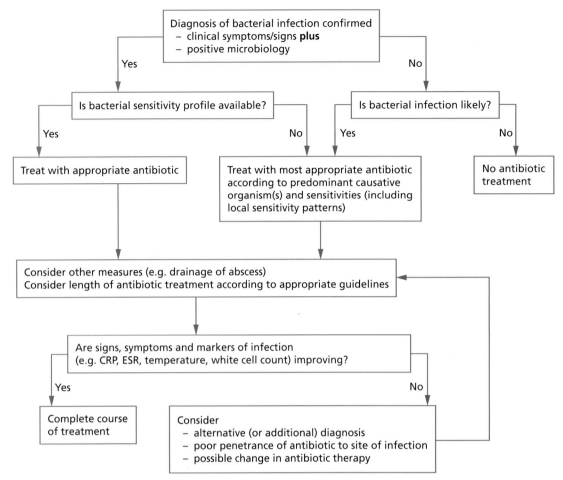

Figure 43.1: General algorithm for the treatment of bacterial infections.

site of infection may be considerably lower than the plasma concentration which one might predict to be bactericidal (e.g. drug penetration and concentration in an abscess cavity are very low).

Figure 43.1 gives a general algorithm for the treatment of bacterial infections.

BACTERIAL RESISTANCE

The resistance of bacterial populations to antimicrobial agents is constantly changing and can become a serious clinical problem, rendering previously useful drugs inactive. Overuse of antibiotics will lead to a future where infectious disease has the same impact as in in the pre-antibiotic era. The dates on tombstones in Victorian cemeteries should be required reading for over-enthusiastic prescribers and medical students! (Whole families of infants died in infancy, followed by their mother from puerperal sepsis.) Although most multiresistant bacteria have developed in hospitalized patients, the majority of antimicrobial prescribing in the UK takes place in primary care. Current guidelines therefore emphasize the following points:

1. no prescribing of antibiotics for coughs and colds or viral sore throats;
2. limit prescribing for uncomplicated cystitis to three days for otherwise fit women; and
3. limit prescribing of antibiotics over the telephone to exceptional cases.

Antimicrobial resistance is particularly common in intensive care units and transplant units, where the use of antimicrobial agents is frequent and the patients may be immunocompromised.

The evolution of drug resistance involves:

1. selection of naturally resistant strains (which have arisen by spontaneous mutation) that exist within the bacterial population by elimination of the sensitive strain by therapy. Thus the incidence of drug resistance is related to the prescription of that drug. The hospital environment with intensive and widespread use of broad-spectrum antibacterials is particularly likely to promote the selection of resistant organisms;

2. transfer of resistance between organisms can occur by transfer of naked DNA (transformation), by conjugation with direct cell-to-cell transfer of extrachromosomal DNA (plasmids), or by passage of the information by bacteriophage (transduction). In this way, transfer of genetic information concerning drug resistance (frequently to a group of several antibiotics simultaneously) may occur between species.

Mechanisms of drug resistance can be broadly divided into three groups:

1. inactivation of the antimicrobial agent either by disruption of its chemical structure (e.g. penicillinase) or by addition of a modifying group that inactivates the drug (e.g. chloramphenicol, inactivated by acetylation);
2. restriction of entry of the drug into the bacterium by altered permeability or efflux pump (e.g. sulphonamides, tetracycline);
3. modification of the bacterial target – this may take the form of an enzyme with reduced affinity for an inhibitor, or an altered organelle with reduced drug-binding properties (e.g. **erythromycin** and bacterial ribosomes).

DRUG COMBINATIONS

Most infections can be treated with a single agent. However, there are situations in which more than one antibacterial drug is prescribed concurrently:

- to achieve broad antimicrobial activity in critically ill patients with an undefined infection (e.g. **aminoglycoside** plus a **penicillin** to treat septicaemia);
- to treat mixed bacterial infections (e.g. following perforation of the bowel) in cases where no single agent would affect all of the bacteria present;
- to prevent the emergence of resistance (e.g. in treating tuberculosis; see Chapter 44);
- to achieve an additive or synergistic effect (e.g. use of **co-trimoxazole** in the treatment of *Pneumocystis carinii* pneumonia).

PROPHYLACTIC USE OF ANTIBACTERIAL DRUGS

On a few occasions it is appropriate to use antibacterial drugs prophylactically. Wherever possible a suitably specific narrow-spectrum drug should be used.

ANTIBIOTIC PROPHYLAXIS OF INFECTIVE ENDOCARDITIS

An important recent change is that fewer patients are deemed to require antibiotic prophylaxis against infective endocarditis; it should be restricted to patients who have previously had

endocarditis, cardiac valve replacement surgery (mechanical or biological prosthetic valves), or surgically constructed systemic or pulmonary shunts or conduits. In such patients, all dental procedures involving dento-gingival manipulation will require antibiotic prophylaxis, as will certain genito-urinary, gastro-intestinal, respiratory or obstetric/gynaecological procedures. Intravenous antibiotics are no longer recommended unless the patient cannot take oral antibiotics. The latest guidelines (2006) by the Working Party of the British Society for Antimicrobial Chemotherapy can be found at http://jac.oxfordjournals.org/cgi/reprint/dkl121v1. These are updated periodically.

For dental procedures, in addition to prophylactic antibiotics, the use of **chlorhexidine** 0.2% mouthwash five minutes before the procedure may be a useful supplementary measure.

PROPHYLACTIC PREOPERATIVE ANTIBIOTICS

GENERAL PRINCIPLES

1. Prophylaxis should be restricted to cases where the procedure commonly leads to infection, or where infection, although rare, would have devastating results.
2. The antimicrobial agent should preferably be bactericidal and directed against the likely pathogen.
3. The aim is to provide high plasma and tissue concentrations of an appropriate drug at the time of bacterial contamination. Intramuscular injections can usually be given with the premedication or intravenous injections at the time of induction. Drug administration should seldom exceed 48 hours. Many problems in this area arise because of failure to discontinue 'prophylactic' antibiotics, a mistake that is easily made by a busy junior house-surgeon who does not want to take responsibility for changing a prescription for a patient who is apparently doing well post-operatively. Local hospital drug and therapeutics committees can help considerably by instituting sensible guidelines on the duration of prophylactic antibiotics.
4. If continued administration is necessary, change to oral therapy post-operatively wherever possible.

The British National Formulary provides a good summary of the use of antibacterial drugs preoperatively, which may be varied according to local guidelines based on regional patterns of bacterial susceptibility/resistance.

COMMONLY PRESCRIBED ANTIBACTERIAL DRUGS

β-LACTAM ANTIBIOTICS

These drugs each contain a β-lactam ring. This can be broken down by β-lactamase enzymes produced by bacteria, notably by many strains of *Staphylococcus* and *Haemophilus influenzae*, which are thereby resistant. β-Lactam antibiotics kill bacteria by inhibiting bacterial cell wall synthesis. Penicillins are excreted in the urine. **Probenecid** blocks the renal tubular secretion of **penicillin**. This interaction may be used therapeutically to produce higher and more prolonged blood concentrations of **penicillin**. Antibiotics in this group include the penicillins, monobactams, carbapenems and cephalosporins.

PENICILLINS

Use

Benzylpenicillin (penicillin G) is the drug of choice for streptococcal, pneumococcal, gonococcal and meningococcal infections, and is also useful for treatment of anthrax, diphtheria, gas gangrene, leptospirosis, syphilis, tetanus, yaws and Lyme disease in children.

Adverse effects

The adverse effects include:

1. anaphylaxis (in approximately 1 in 100 000 injections);
2. rashes (3–5% of patients) can, rarely, be severe (e.g. Stevens–Johnson syndrome – see Chapter 12);
3. serum sickness – type III hypersensitivity;
4. other idiosyncratic reactions including haemolytic anaemia and thrombocytopenia;
5. in renal failure, high-dose **penicillin** causes encephalopathy and seizures.

Limitations of **benzylpenicillin** include:

1. It is acid labile and so must be given parenterally (inactivated in gastric acid).
2. It has a short half-life, so frequent injections are required.
3. Development of resistant β-lactamase-producing strains can occur.
4. It has a narrow antibacterial spectrum.

Two preparations with similar antibacterial spectra are used to overcome the problems of acid lability/frequent injection:

1. **Procaine benzylpenicillin** – this complex releases **penicillin** slowly from an intramuscular site, so a twice daily dosage only is required.
2. **Phenoxymethylpenicillin** ('penicillin V') – this is acid stable and so is effective when given orally (40–60% absorption). Although it is useful for mild infections, blood concentrations are variable, so it is not used in serious infections or with poorly sensitive bacteria. Tablets are given on an empty stomach to improve absorption.

β-LACTAMASE-RESISTANT PENICILLIN

Flucloxacillin was developed to overcome β-lactamase-producing strains. Otherwise, it has a similar antibacterial spectrum to **benzylpenicillin**. It is effective against β-lactamase-producing organisms. It is used for the treatment of staphylococcal infections (90% of hospital staphylococci are resistant to **benzylpenicillin** and 5–10% are resistant to **flucloxacillin**).

EXTENDED-RANGE PENICILLINS

AMPICILLIN/AMOXICILLIN

Uses

In addition to streptococcal (including pneumococcal) strains, **ampicillin** and **amoxicillin** are also effective against many strains of *Haemophilus influenzae*, *E. coli*, *Streptococcus faecalis* and *Salmonella*. They are used for a variety of chest infections (e.g. bronchitis, pneumonia), otitis media, urinary tract infections, biliary infections and the prevention of bacterial endocarditis (**amoxicillin**). **Amoxicillin** is somewhat more potent than **ampicillin**, penetrates tissues better and is given three rather than four times daily. Both are susceptible to β-lactamases.

Adverse effects

Rashes are common and may appear after dosing has stopped. There is an especially high incidence in patients with infectious mononucleosis or lymphatic leukaemia.

Pharmacokinetics

The half-life of each drug is about 1.5 hours and they are predominantly renally excreted.

CO-AMOXICLAV

Co-amoxiclav is a combination of **amoxicillin** and **clavulanic acid**, a β-lactamase inhibitor. In addition to those bacteria that are susceptible to **amoxicillin**, most *Staphylococcus aureus*, 50% of *E. coli*, some *Haemophilus influenzae* strains and many *Bacteroides* and *Klebsiella* species are susceptible to **co-amoxiclav**. Adverse effects are similar to those of **amoxicillin**, but abdominal discomfort is more common.

ANTIPSEUDOMONAL PENICILLINS

Standard penicillins are not effective against *Pseudomonas*. This is not usually a problem, as these organisms seldom cause disease in otherwise healthy people. However, *Pseudomonas* infection is important in neutropenic patients (e.g. those undergoing cancer chemotherapy) and in patients with cystic fibrosis. Penicillins with activity against *Pseudomonas* have been developed and are particularly useful in these circumstances. These include **piperacillin**, **azlocillin** and **ticarcillin**.

Uses

These expensive intravenous penicillins are not used routinely. Their efficacy against Gram-positive organisms is variable and poor. They are useful against Gram-negative infections, particularly with *Pseudomonas* and they are also effective against many anaerobes. These drugs have a synergistic effect when combined with aminoglycosides in *Pseudomonas* septicaemias. Combinations of **ticarcillin** or of **piperacillin** with β-lactamase inhibitors designed to overcome the problem of β-lactamase formation by *Pseudomonas* are commercially available.

Adverse effects

These drugs predispose to superinfection. Rashes, sodium overload, thrombocytopenia and platelet dysfunction can occur.

Pharmacokinetics

Absorption of these drugs from the gut is inadequate in the life-threatening infections for which they are mainly indicated. They are given intravenously every 4–6 hours. Their half-lives range from 1 to 1.5 hours and they are renally excreted.

CEPHALOSPORINS

FIRST-GENERATION CEPHALOSPORINS

So-called first-generation cephalosporins (e.g. **cephalexin, cefaclor, cefadroxil**) are effective against *Streptococcus pyogenes* and *Streptococcus pneumoniae*, *E. coli* and some staphylococci. They have few absolute (i.e. uniquely advantageous) indications. Their pharmacology is similar to that of the penicillins and they are principally renally eliminated.

SECOND- AND THIRD-GENERATION CEPHALOSPORINS

Second- and third-generation cephalosporins are active against *H. influenzae* and in some instances *Pseudomonas* and anaerobes, at the expense of reduced efficacy against Gram-positive organisms. β-Lactamase stability has been increased. Arguably the most generally useful member of the group is **cefuroxime**, which combines lactamase stability with activity against streptococci, staphylococci, *H. influenzae* and *E. coli*. It is given by injection eight-hourly (an oral preparation is also available, as **cefuroxime axetil**). It is expensive, although when used against Gram-negative organisms that would otherwise necessitate use of an aminoglycoside, this cost is partly offset by savings from the lack of need for plasma concentration determinations.

Of the third-generation cephalosporins, **ceftazidime, ceftriaxone** and **cefotaxime** are useful in severe sepsis, especially because (unlike earlier cephalosporins) they penetrate the blood–brain barrier well and are effective in meningitis.

Adverse effects

About 10% of patients who are allergic to penicillins are also allergic to cephalosporins. Some first-generation cephalosporins are nephrotoxic, particularly if used with **furosemide**, aminoglycosides or other nephrotoxic agents. Some of the third-generation drugs are associated with bleeding due to increased prothrombin times, which is reversible with vitamin K.

MONOBACTAMS

Monobactams (e.g. **aztreonam**) contain a 5-monobactam ring and are resistant to β-lactamase degradation.

AZTREONAM
Uses

Aztreonam is primarily active against aerobic Gram-negative organisms and is an alternative to an aminoglycoside. It is used in severe sepsis, often hospital acquired, especially infections of the respiratory, urinary, biliary, gastro-intestinal and female genital tracts. It has a narrow spectrum of activity and cannot be used alone unless the organism's sensitivity to **aztreonam** is known.

Mechanism of action

The 5-monobactam ring binds to bacterial wall transpeptidases and inhibits bacterial cell wall synthesis in a similar way to the penicillins.

Adverse effects

Rashes occur, but there appears to be no cross-allergenicity with penicillins.

Pharmacokinetics

Aztreonam is poorly absorbed after oral administration, so it is given parenterally. It is widely distributed to all body compartments, including the cerebrospinal fluid. Excretion is renal and the usual half-life (one to two hours) is increased in renal failure.

IMIPENEM–CILASTATIN AND MEROPENEM
Uses

Imipenem, a carbapenem, is combined with **cilastatin**, which is an inhibitor of the enzyme dehydropeptidase I found in the brush border of the proximal renal tubule. This enzyme breaks down **imipenem** in the kidney. **Imipenem** has a very broad spectrum of activity against Gram-positive, Gram-negative and anaerobic organisms. It is β-lactamase stable and is used for treating severe infections of the lung and abdomen, and in patients with septicaemia, where the source of the organism is unknown. **Meropenem** is similar to **imipenem**, but is stable to renal dehydropeptidase I and therefore can be given without **cilastatin**.

Adverse effects

Imipenem is generally well tolerated, but seizures, myoclonus, confusion, nausea and vomiting, hypersensitivity, positive Coombs' test, taste disturbances and thrombophlebitis have all been reported. **Meropenem** has less seizure-inducing potential and can be used to treat central nervous system infection.

Pharmacokinetics

Imipenem is filtered and metabolized in the kidney by dehydropeptidase I. This is inhibited by **cilastatin** in the combination. **Imipenem** is given intravenously as an infusion in three or four divided daily doses.

AMINOGLYCOSIDES

Uses

Aminoglycosides are highly polar, sugar-containing derivatives. They are powerful bactericidal agents that are active against many Gram-negative organisms and some Gram-positive organisms, with activity against staphylococci and

Enterococcus faecalis, but not (when used alone) against other streptococci. They synergize with penicillins in killing *Streptococcus faecalis* in endocarditis. Aminoglycosides are used in serious infections including septicaemia, sometimes alone but usually in combination with other antibiotics (penicillins or cephalosporins). **Gentamicin** is widely used and has a broad spectrum, but is ineffective against anaerobes, many streptococci and pneumococci.

Tobramycin is probably somewhat less nephrotoxic than **gentamicin**. **Amikacin** is more effective than **gentamicin** for pseudomonal infections and is occasionally effective against organisms resistant to **gentamicin**. It is principally indicated in serious infections caused by Gram-negative bacilli that are resistant to **gentamicin**. Topical **gentamicin** or **tobramycin** eye drops are used to treat eye infections.

Mechanism of action

These drugs are transported into cells and block bacterial protein synthesis by binding to the 30S ribosome.

Adverse effects

These are important and are related to duration of therapy and trough plasma concentrations. They are more frequent in the elderly and in renal impairment. Therapeutic monitoring is performed by measuring plasma concentrations before dosing (trough) and at 'peak' levels (usually at an arbitrary one hour after dosing). Eighth nerve damage is potentially catastrophic and is often irreversible. Acute tubular necrosis and renal failure are usually reversible if diagnosed promptly and the drug stopped or the dose reduced. Hypersensitivity rashes are uncommon. Bone marrow suppression is rare. Exacerbation of myasthenia gravis is predictable in patients with this disease.

Pharmacokinetics

Aminoglycosides are poorly absorbed from the gut and are given by intramuscular or intravenous injection. They are poorly protein bound (30%) and are excreted renally. The half-life is short, usually two hours, but once daily administration is usually adequate. This presumably reflects a post-antibiotic effect whereby bacterial growth is inhibited following clearance of the drug. In patients with renal dysfunction, dose reduction and/or an increased dose interval is required. Cerebrospinal fluid (CSF) penetration is poor.

Drug interactions

Aminoglycosides enhance neuromuscular blockade of non-depolarizing neuromuscular antagonists. Loop diuretics potentiate their nephrotoxicity and ototoxicity.

CHLORAMPHENICOL

Uses

Chloramphenicol has a broad spectrum of activity and penetrates tissues exceptionally well. It is bacteriostatic, but is extremely effective against streptococci, staphylococci, *H. influenzae*, salmonellae and others. Uncommonly it causes aplastic anaemia, so its use is largely confined to life-threatening disease (e.g. *H. influenzae* epiglottitis, meningitis, typhoid fever) and to topical use as eyedrops.

Mechanism of action

Chloramphenicol inhibits bacterial ribosome function by inhibiting the 50S ribosomal peptidyl transferase, thereby preventing peptide elongation.

Adverse effects

These include:

1. *haematological effects* – dose-related erythroid suppression is common and predictable, but in addition aplastic anaemia occurs unpredictably with an incidence of approximately 1:40 000. This is irreversible in 50% of cases. It is rarely, if ever, related to the use of eyedrops.
2. *grey baby syndrome* – the grey colour is due to shock (hypotension and tissue hypoperfusion). **Chloramphenicol** accumulates in neonates (especially if premature) due to reduced glucuronidation in the immature liver (see Chapter 10).
3. *other* – sore mouth, diarrhoea, encephalopathy and optic neuritis.

Pharmacokinetics

Chloramphenicol is well absorbed following oral administration and can also be given by the intramuscular and intravenous routes. It is widely distributed and CSF penetration is excellent. It mainly undergoes hepatic glucuronidation, but in neonates this is impaired.

Drug interactions

Chloramphenicol inhibits the metabolism of **warfarin**, **phenytoin** and **theophylline**.

MACROLIDES

Macrolide antibiotics (e.g. **erythromycin**, **clarithromycin**, **azithromycin**) have an antibacterial spectrum similar, but not identical to that of **penicillin**. Distinctively, they are effective against several unusual organisms, including *Chlamydia*, *Legionella* and *Mycoplasma*.

ERYTHROMYCIN

Uses

Uses include respiratory infections (including *Mycoplasma pneumoniae*, psittacosis and Legionnaires' disease), whooping cough, *Campylobacter enteritis* and non-specific urethritis. **Erythromycin** is a useful alternative to **penicillin** in penicillin-allergic patients (except meningitis: it does not penetrate the CSF adequately). It is useful for skin infections, such as low-grade cellulitis and infected acne, and is acceptable for patients with an infective exacerbation of chronic bronchitis. It is most commonly administered by mouth four times daily, although when necessary it may be given by intravenous infusion.

Mechanism of action

Macrolides bind to bacterial 50S ribosomes and inhibit protein synthesis.

Pharmacokinetics

Well absorbed orally and distributed adequately to most sites except the brain, macrolides are inactivated by hepatic N-demethylation, <15% being eliminated unchanged in the urine. Food delays absorption but may reduce gastro-intestinal side effects.

Adverse effects

Erythromycin is remarkably safe and may be used in pregnancy and in children. Nausea, vomiting, diarrhoea and abdominal cramps are the most common adverse effects reported, related to direct pharmacological actions rather than allergy. Cholestatic jaundice has been reported following prolonged use. Intravenous administration frequently causes local pain and phlebitis.

Drug interactions

Erythromycin inhibits cytochrome P450 and causes accumulation of **theophylline**, **warfarin** and **terfenadine**. This can result in clinically important adverse effects.

AZITHROMYCIN AND CLARITHROMYCIN

Each of these has greater activity than **erythromycin** against *H. influenzae*. **Azithromycin** is less effective against Gram-positive bacteria than **erythromycin**, but has a wider spectrum of activity against Gram-negative organisms. **Clarithromycin** is an **erythromycin** derivative with slightly greater activity than the parent compound; tissue concentrations are higher than with **erythromycin**. It is given twice daily.

Azithromycin and **clarithromycin** are more expensive than **erythromycin**, but cause fewer gastro-intestinal side effects.

TETRACYCLINES

Uses

Tetracyclines (e.g. **tetracycline, oxytetracycline, doxycycline**) have a broad range of antibacterial activity covering both Gram-positive and Gram-negative organisms and, in addition organisms such as *Rickettsia*, *Chlamydia* and *Mycoplasma*. They are used in atypical pneumonias and chlamydial and rickettsial infections, and remain useful in treating exacerbations of chronic bronchitis or community-acquired pneumonia. They are not used routinely for staphylococcal or streptococcal infections because of the development of resistance. Tetracyclines are used in the long-term treatment of acne (Chapter 51).

Mechanism of action

Tetracyclines bind to the 30S subunit of bacterial ribosomes and prevent binding of the aminoacyl-tRNA to the ribosome acceptor site, thereby inhibiting protein synthesis.

Adverse effects

These include:

1. nausea, vomiting and diarrhoea (pseudomembranous colitis due to *Clostridium difficile* reported occasionally);
2. hypersensitivity reactions (including rash, exfoliative dermatitis, Stevens–Johnson syndrome, urticaria, angioedema, anaphylaxis, pericarditis);
3. worsening of renal failure;
4. hepatotoxicity (rare);
5. discoloration and damage of the teeth and bones of the fetus if the mother takes tetracyclines after the fifth month of pregnancy, and of children; they should therefore be avoided in pregnancy and children under 12 years.

Pharmacokinetics

Tetracyclines are well absorbed orally when fasting, but their absorption is reduced by food and antacids. They undergo elimination by both the liver and the kidney. The half-life varies between different members of the group, ranging from six to 12 hours. The shorter-acting drugs are given four times daily and the longer-acting ones once daily. **Doxycycline** is given once daily, can be taken with food and is not contraindicated in renal impairment.

Drug interactions

Tetracyclines chelate calcium and iron in the stomach, and their absorption is reduced by the presence of antacids or food.

SODIUM FUSIDATE

Uses

Fusidic acid is combined with other drugs to treat staphylococcal infections, including **penicillin**-resistant strains. It penetrates tissues (including bone) well. It is normally used in conjunction with **flucloxacillin** for serious staphylococcal infections. It is also available as eyedrops for the treatment of bacterial conjunctivitis.

Mechanism of action

It inhibits bacterial protein synthesis.

Adverse effects

Adverse effects are rare, but include cholestatic jaundice.

Pharmacokinetics

When administered either orally or intravenously, its half-life is four to six hours and it is excreted primarily via the liver.

VANCOMYCIN

Uses and antibacterial spectrum

Vancomycin is valuable in the treatment of resistant infections due to *Staphylococcus pyogenes*. It is also rarely used to treat other infections, for example *Staphylococcus epidermidis* endocarditis, and is given orally for pseudomembranous colitis caused by *Clostridium difficile*.

Mechanism of action

Vancomycin inhibits bacterial cell wall synthesis.

Adverse effects

These include:

- hearing loss;
- venous thrombosis at infusion site;
- 'red man' syndrome due to cytokine/histamine release following excessively rapid intravenous administration;
- hypersensitivity (rashes, etc.);
- nephrotoxicity.

Pharmacokinetics

Vancomycin is not absorbed from the gut and is usually given as an intravenous infusion (except for the treatment of pseudomembranous colitis). It is eliminated by the kidneys. Because of its concentration-related toxicity, the dose is adjusted according to the results of plasma concentration monitoring.

TEICOPLANIN

Teicoplanin has a longer duration of action, but is otherwise similar to **vancomycin**.

METRONIDAZOLE

Uses

Metronidazole is a synthetic drug with high activity against anaerobic bacteria. It is also active against several medically important protozoa and parasites (see Chapter 47). It is used to treat trichomonal infections, amoebic dysentery, giardiasis, gas gangrene, pseudomembranous colitis and various abdominal infections, lung abscesses and dental sepsis. It is used prophylactically before abdominal surgery.

Mechanism of action

Metronidazole binds to DNA and causes strand breakage. In addition, it acts as an electron acceptor for flavoproteins and ferredoxins.

Adverse effects

These include:

1. nausea and vomiting;
2. peripheral neuropathy;
3. convulsions, headaches;
4. hepatitis.

Pharmacokinetics

Metronidazole is well absorbed after oral or rectal administration, but is often administered by the relatively expensive intravenous route. The half-life is approximately six hours. It is eliminated by a combination of hepatic metabolism and renal excretion. Dose reduction is required in renal impairment.

Drug interactions

Metronidazole interacts with alcohol because it inhibits aldehyde dehydrogenase and consequently causes a disulfiram-like reaction. It is a weak inhibitor of cytochrome P450.

SULPHONAMIDES AND TRIMETHOPRIM

Sulphonamides and **trimethoprim** inhibit the production of folic acid at different sites of its synthetic pathway and are synergistic in vitro. There is now widespread resistance to sulphonamides, and they have been largely replaced by more active and less toxic antibacterial agents. The sulfamethoxazole–trimethoprim combination (**co-trimoxazole**) is effective in urinary tract infections, prostatitis, exacerbations of chronic bronchitis and invasive *Salmonella* infections, but with the exception of *Pneumocystis carinii* infections (when high doses are used), **trimethoprim** alone is generally preferred as it avoids sulphonamide side effects, whilst having similar efficacy in vivo.

Sulphonamides are generally well absorbed after oral administration and are widely distributed. Acetylation and glucuronidation are the most important metabolic pathways. They may precipitate in acid urine. They frequently cause unwanted side effects, including hypersensitivity reactions such as rashes, fever and serum sickness-like syndrome and Stevens–Johnson syndrome (see Chapter 12). Rarely, agranulocytosis, megaloblastic, aplastic or haemolytic anaemia and thrombocytopenia occur. Sulphonamides are oxidants and can precipitate haemolytic anaemia in glucose-6-phosphate dehydrogenase (G6PD)-deficient individuals.

Sulphonamides potentiate the action of sulphonylureas, oral anticoagulants, **phenytoin** and **methotrexate** due to inhibition of their metabolism.

Trimethoprim is well absorbed, highly lipid soluble and widely distributed. At least 65% is eliminated unchanged in the urine. **Trimethoprim** competes for the same renal clearance pathway as creatinine. It is generally well tolerated, but occasionally causes gastro-intestinal disturbances, skin reactions and (rarely) bone marrow depression. Additionally, the high doses used in the management of *Pneumocystis* pneumonia in immunosuppressed patients cause vomiting (which can be improved by prophylactic anti-emetics), a higher incidence of serious skin reactions, hepatitis and thrombocytopenia.

QUINOLONES

Nalidixic acid was available for many years, but poor tissue distribution and adverse effects limited its use to a second- or third-line treatment for urinary tract infections. Changes to the basic quinolone structure dramatically increased the antibacterial potency of the more modern quinolones, particularly against *Pseudomonas*. Oral bioavailability is good and thus the 4-fluoroquinolones offer an oral alternative to parenteral aminoglycosides and antipseudomonal penicillins for treatment of *Pseudomonas* urinary and chest infections. Although the 4-fluoroquinolones have a very broad spectrum of activity, all of those currently available have very limited activity against streptococci. Most experience has been obtained with **ciprofloxacin**, which has the additional advantage of being available for intravenous use. The quinolones inhibit bacterial DNA gyrase.

Uses

Ciprofloxacin is used for respiratory (but not pneumococcal), urinary, gastro-intestinal and genital infections, septicaemia and meningococcal meningitis contacts. In addition to *Pseudomonas*, it is particularly active against infection with *Salmonella*, *Shigella*, *Campylobacter*, *Neisseria* and *Chlamydia*. It is ineffective in most anaerobic infections. The licensed indications for the other quinolones are more limited. **Ciprofloxacin** is generally well tolerated, but should be avoided by epileptics (it rarely causes convulsions), children (it causes arthritis in growing animals) and individuals with glucose-6-phosphate dehydrogenase deficiency. Anaphylaxis, nephritis, vasculitis, dizziness, hepatic and renal damage have all been reported. An excessively alkaline urine and dehydration can cause urinary crystallization.

Pharmacokinetics

Approximately 80% of an oral dose of **ciprofloxacin** is systemically available. It is widely distributed entering all body compartments including the eye and the CSF. **Ciprofloxacin** is removed primarily by glomerular filtration and tubular secretion. The half-life is four hours.

Drug interactions

Co-administration of **ciprofloxacin** and **theophylline** causes elevated blood **theophylline** concentrations due to inhibition of cytochrome P450. As both drugs are epileptogenic, this interaction is particularly significant.

RECENTLY INTRODUCED ANTIBACTERIAL AGENTS

Increasing antibiotic resistance (especially meticillin-resistant *Staphylococcus aureus* (MRSA) and vancomycin-resistant enterococci) is a matter of deep concern. Although the spread of multi-resistant organisms can be minimized by judicious use of antibiotics and the instigation of tight infection-control measures, there is a continuing need for the development of well-tolerated, easily administered, broad-spectrum antibiotics. Table 43.2 lists some recently introduced antibiotics which fulfil these criteria, together with their main features. At present, their use is restricted and should be administered under close microbiological supervision.

Case history

While on holiday in Spain, a 66-year-old man develops a cough, fever and breathlessness at rest. He is told that his chest x-ray confirms that he has pneumonia. He is started on a seven-day course of oral antibiotics by a local physician and stays in his hotel for the remainder of his ten-day holiday. When he returns home, he is reviewed by his own GP who notices that he looks pale and sallow and is still breathless on exertion, but his chest examination no longer reveals any signs of pneumonia. A full blood count reveals a haemoglobin level of 6.7 g/dL (previously normal), normal white blood count and platelets, and a reticulocyte count of 4.1%.
Question
What other tests should you do and what antibiotics would be most likely to cause this clinical scenario?
Answer
The patient received a course of antibiotics for pneumonia and then developed what appears to be a haemolytic anaemia. This could be further confirmed by raised unconjugated bilirubin levels and low haptoglobin levels, and observation of target cells and poikilocytosis on the blood film. *Mycoplasma* pneumonia should be excluded by performing *Mycoplasma* titres, as this can itself be complicated by a haemolytic anaemia.

However, considering the drugs as the potential cause, it is important to define the patient's glucose-6-phosphate dehydrogenase status, and if he was deficient then to consider such agents as co-trimoxazole (containing sulfamethoxazole, a sulphonamide), the fluoroquinolones (e.g. ciprofloxacin or nitrofurantoin) or chloramphenicol, which can cause haemolytic anaemia in susceptible individuals. Note that chloramphenicol is more commonly prescribed in certain countries on the European mainland. Aplastic anaemia (not the picture in this patient) is a major concern with the use of systemic chloramphenicol. If the patient's glucose-6-phosphate dehydrogenase status is normal, then rarely the β-lactams (penicillins or early (first- and second-) generation cephalosporins) or (less likely) rifampicin may cause an autoimmune haemolytic anaemia due to the production of antibodies to the antibiotic which binds to the red blood cells. This could be further confirmed by performing a direct Coombs' test in which the patient's serum in the presence of red cells and the drug would cause red cell lysis. Management involves stopping the drug, giving folic acid and monitoring recovery of the haemoglobin. It should be noted in the patient's record that certain antibiotics led him to have a haemolytic anaemia.

Table 43.2: New antibacterial agents

	Linezolid	Moxifloxacin	Telithromycin	Ertapenem
Antibiotic class	Oxazolidinone	Fluoroquinolone with an 8-methoxyquinolone structure	Ketolide; a semisynthetic member of the macrolide-lincosamide-streptogramin B family of antibiotics	Carbapenem
Mechanism of action	Inhibits formation of the 70S ribosomal initiation complex, preventing bacterial protein synthesis; primarily bacteriostatic action	Inhibits topoisomerase II and IV with bactericidal activity	Inhibits bacterial protein synthesis by direct binding to the 50S subunit of bacterial ribosomes, preventing translation and ribosome assembly	Attaches to penicillin-binding proteins, inhibiting bacterial cell wall synthesis; bactericidal activity
Spectrum of activity	Gram-positive bacteria and a few Gram-negative anaerobic bacteria; active against staphylococci, pneumococci and enterococci, including those resistant to penicillin and vancomycin	Gram-positives, including staphylococci, enterococci, *Streptococcus pneumoniae*, including penicillin-resistant strains; atypicals, including *Legionella* and *Mycoplasma pneumoniae*; Gram-negatives, including *Haemophilus influenzae*, *Moraxella catarrhalis*, coliforms, *Neisseria gonorrhoeae*; low activity against *Pseudomonas* and some enterobacteriaceae; active against *Mycobacterium tuberculosis*, including multiresistant strains; inhibits 90% of anaerobic bacteria including clostridia, *Bacteroides*, *Fusobacterium*, *Porphyromonas*	Gram-positives, including *Streptococcus pneumoniae* (including erythromycin resistant strains), *Streptococcus pyogenes*, MRSA; some Gram-negative bacteria, including *Haemophilus influenzae*, *Moraxella catarrhalis*; atypicals, including *Mycoplasma pneumoniae*, *Chlamydia pneumoniae* and *Legionella*; not active against erythromycin resistant strains of MRSA	Most enteric bacteria, including those producing beta-lactamase; Gram-negative respiratory pathogens, including *Moraxella catarrhalis* and *Haemophilus influenzae*; Gram-positive bacteria, including *Streptococcus pneumoniae* (including those resistant to penicillin) and MRSA; also effective against many anaerobes, including *Bacteroides*, *Prevotella* and *Porphyromonas*; limited activity against *Pseudomonas aeruginosa* *Acinetobacter*, *Enterococcus*, *Lactobacillus*, MRSA

From Lever A. Recently introduced antibiotics: a guide for the general physician. *Clinical Medicine* 2004; **4**: 494–8.

Case history

A 70-year-old man with a history of chronic obstructive pulmonary disease visits his GP in December during a local flu epidemic. He complains of worsening shortness of breath, productive cough, fever and malaise. On examination, his sputum is viscous and green, his respiratory rate is 20 breaths per minute at rest but, in addition to wheezes, bronchial breathing is audible over the right lower lobe. The GP prescribes amoxicillin which has been effective in previous exacerbations of chronic obstructive pulmonary disease in this patient. Twenty-four hours later, the patient is brought to the local Accident and Emergency Department confused, cyanosed and with a respiratory rate of 30 breaths per minute. His chest x-ray is consistent with lobar pneumonia.

Question

In addition to controlled oxygen and bronchodilators, which three antibacterial drugs would you prescribe and why?

Answer

This patient is seriously ill with community-acquired lobar pneumonia. The previously abnormal chest, the concurrent flu epidemic and the rapid deterioration suggest *Staphylococcus*, but *Streptococcus pneumoniae* and *Legionella* are also possible pathogens. The following antibacterial drugs should be prescribed:

- Flucloxacillin – active against *Staphylococcus* and Gram-positive organisms;
- Cefuroxime – broad spectrum and active against *Staphylococcus*;
- Erythromycin – active against *Legionella* and *Mycoplasma*, and also some *Staphylococcus* and other Gram-positive bacteria.

Case history

A 20-year-old man presented to his GP during a flu epidemic complaining of a throbbing headache which was present when he woke up that morning. He had been studying hard and was anxious about his exams. Physical examination was normal and he was sent home with paracetamol and vitamins. He presented to casualty 12 hours later with a worsening headache. Examination revealed a temperature of 39°C, blood pressure of 110/60 mmHg, neck stiffness and a purpuric rash on his arms and legs which did not blanch when pressure was applied.

Question

Which antibacterial drugs would you use and why?

Answer

This young man has meningococcal meningitis and requires benzylpenicillin i.v. immediately.

REMEMBER: Treatment of bacterial meningitis must never be delayed.

FURTHER READING

British National Formulary, www.bnf.org.

MYCOBACTERIAL INFECTIONS

INTRODUCTION

Tuberculosis ('consumption') was the most common cause of death in Victorian England, but its prevalence fell markedly with the dramatic improvement in living standards during the twentieth century. However, the incidence of *Mycobacterium tuberculosis* infection world-wide (including Europe, UK and USA) is increasing, particularly among immigrants and in human immunodeficiency virus (HIV)-related cases. Infection with *Mycobacterium tuberculosis* usually occurs in the lungs, but may affect any organ, especially the lymph nodes, gut, meninges, bone, adrenal glands or urogenixtal tract. Other atypical (non-tuberculous) mycobacterial infections are less common, but are occurring with increasing frequency in HIV-1-infected individuals. *Mycobacterium tuberculosis* is an intracellular organism, an obligate aerobe in keeping with its predilection for the well-ventilated apical segments of the lungs (Figure 44.1).

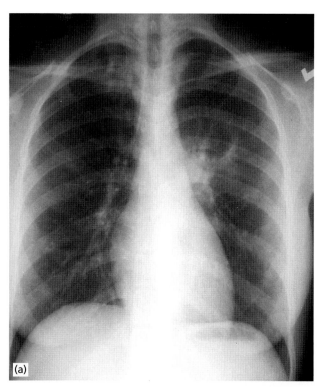
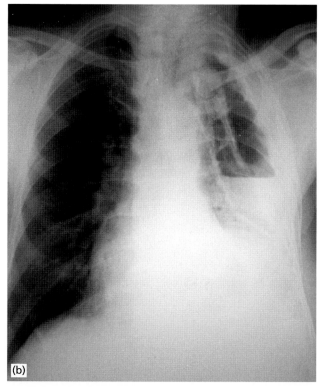

Figure 44.1: Chest x-rays showing pulmonary tuberculosis: (a) cavitating tuberculosis; (b) tuberculous empyema.

PRINCIPLES OF MANAGEMENT OF *MYCOBACTERIUM TUBERCULOSIS* INFECTIONS

The treatment of pulmonary tuberculosis is summarized in Figure 44.2. Successful *M. tuberculosis* therapy requires an initial combination with at least three (and often four) drugs. The use of several drugs reduces the risk of 'missing' the occasional drug-resistant individual which will multiply free of competition from its drug-sensitive companions. The multi-drug strategy is therefore more likely to achieve a cure, with a low relapse rate (0–3%) and reduced drug resistance. The British Thoracic Society now recommends standard therapy for pulmonary tuberculosis for six months. A combination of **isoniazid**, **rifampicin**, **pyrazinamide** and **ethambutol** (or **streptomycin**) is administered for the first two months, followed by **rifampicin** and **isoniazid** for a further four months. **Ethambutol** and/or **streptomycin** may be omitted in patients who are at relatively low risk of carrying multi-drug resistant (MDR) *M. tuberculosis*, which includes 99% of the UK-born population. However, the initial use of four drugs is advisable in HIV patients and in immigrants from countries where MDR *M. tuberculosis* infection is likely. The initial four-drug combination therapy should also be used in all patients with non-tuberculous mycobacterial infection, which often involves organisms that are resistant to both **isoniazid** and **pyrazinamide**. Patients with open active tuberculosis are initially isolated to reduce the risk of spread, but may be considered non-infectious after 14 days of therapy. Those with MDR *M. tuberculosis* are isolated

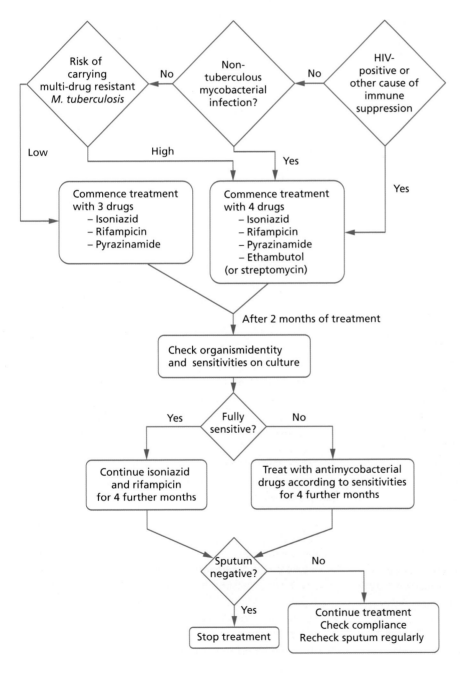

Figure 44.2: Principles of treatment of pulmonary tuberculosis.

and considered non-infectious when they have been treated for at least 14 days and three sputum examinations are negative during a 14-day period. In cases where compliance with a daily regimen is a problem, the initial two months of triple or quadruple chemotherapy can be given on an intermittent supervised basis two or three times a week. At the end of the two-month period, the precise identification and sensitivities of the organism will be available. If they are fully sensitive, treatment will continue with daily **rifampicin** plus **isoniazid** for a further four months. After six months, treatment can usually be discontinued unless the sputum remains positive or the patient is immunocompromised or poorly compliant. If the initial drug sensitivities reveal isoniazid resistance, treatment with **ethambutol** plus **rifampicin** must be continued for a total of 12 months. The duration of chemotherapy will also need to be extended if either **isoniazid**, **rifampicin** or **pyrazinamide** has to be discontinued because of side effects.

The treatment of tuberculosis which is resistant to multiple drugs is more difficult, and regimens have to be individualized according to drug sensitivity.

FIRST-LINE DRUGS IN TUBERCULOSIS THERAPY

ISONIAZID (ISONICOTINIC ACID HYDRAZIDE, INH)

Uses

Isoniazid is bactericidal only to *Mycobacterium tuberculosis*. It is used as a single agent for chemoprophylaxis (a strategy used in some countries, including the USA, that do not use bacillus Calmette–Guérin (BCG)) as a preventive measure – where otherwise healthy people who are Mantoux test positive are assumed to be infected with very small numbers of organisms and are treated for one year with **isoniazid** as a single agent. In countries such as the UK, **isoniazid** is used only in combination with other drugs, usually **rifampicin** plus **pyrazinamide** and/or **ethambutol**. When using high-dose **isoniazid** (e.g. treating tuberculous meningitis) or in patients with special risk factors (e.g. diabetes, alcoholism), **pyridoxine** is given to prevent peripheral neuropathy (see Chapter 35).

Mechanism of action

Isoniazid is a competitive inhibitor of bacterial fatty acid synthase II, an enzyme involved in the synthesis of mycolic acid, a constituent of the *M. tuberculosis* cell wall. **Isoniazid** only acts on growing bacteria.

Adverse effects

Adverse effects include

- restlessness, insomnia and muscle twitching;
- sensory peripheral neuropathy, observed more commonly in slow acetylators, and prevented by supplemental **pyridoxine**;
- biochemical hepatitis, which is clinically significant in 1% of patients, and rarely progresses to hepatic necrosis.

Acetylisoniazid may be responsible for this effect, since enzyme inducers, such as **rifampicin**, result in higher production of this metabolite in the liver and are associated with increased toxicity;

- bone marrow suppression, anaemia and agranulocytosis;
- drug-induced systemic lupus erythematosus.

Pharmacokinetics

Isoniazid is readily absorbed from the gut and is widely distributed to tissues, including the cerebrospinal fluid (CSF), and into macrophages where it kills intracellular tubercle bacilli. It undergoes acetylation in the liver. Between 40 and 45% of people in European populations are rapid acetylators (Chapter 14). The $t_{1/2}$ of **isoniazid** is less than 80 minutes in fast acetylators and more than 140 minutes in slow acetylators. Approximately 50–70% of a dose is excreted in the urine within 24 hours as a metabolite or free drug. Abnormally high and potentially toxic concentrations of **isoniazid** may occur in patients who are both slow acetylators and have renal impairment.

Drug interactions

Isoniazid undergoes hepatic metabolism by CYP450s. It inhibits the metabolism of several anticonvulsants, including **phenytoin** and **carbamazepine**, causing toxic concentrations of these drugs in some patients.

RIFAMPICIN

Uses

Rifampicin is a derivative of rifamycin, which is produced by Amycolatopsis mediterranei (known as *Streptomyces mediterranei*). Because of its high lipophilicity, it diffuses easily through cell membranes to kill intracellular organisms, such as *Mycobacterium tuberculosis*. It is also used to treat nasopharyngeal meningococcal carriers (it enters well into saliva, tears and nasal secretions), Legionnaires' disease and refractory deep-sited staphylococcal infections (e.g. osteomyelitis).

Mechanism of action

Rifampicin acts by binding to the β-subunit of the DNA-directed bacterial RNA polymerase, forming a stable drug–enzyme complex and suppressing initiation of chain formation in RNA synthesis.

Adverse effects

Large doses of **rifampicin** produce toxic effects in about one-third of patients:

- after a few hours influenza-like symptoms, flushing and rashes;
- abdominal pain;
- hepatotoxicity – hepatitis and cholestatic jaundice. It is important to monitor hepatic transaminases, particularly in patients at high risk of liver dysfunction (e.g. alcoholics). Serious liver damage is uncommon.
- thrombocytopenia (rare);
- urine and tears become orangey-pink.

Pharmacokinetics

Absorption from the gut is almost complete, but delayed by food. **Rifampicin** penetrates well into most tissues, cavities and exudates, but little enters the brain and CSF. The $t_{1/2}$ is between one and five hours. It is metabolized by deacetylation and both the metabolite and parent compound are excreted in the bile and undergo enterohepatic circulation. Toxicity is increased by biliary obstruction or impaired liver function. Less than 10% appears unchanged in the urine and thus standard dosing is unaffected by renal failure.

Drug interactions

Rifampicin markedly induces a wide range of hepatic microsomal CYP450 enzymes, thereby accelerating the metabolism of many commonly used drugs (Chapter 13). Clinically important interactions associated with reduced concentration and therapeutic failure are common, and include:

- corticosteroids;
- **warfarin**;
- sex steroids (rendering oral contraception unreliable);
- immunosuppressants (including **ciclosporin**, **tacrolimus**, **sirolimus** leading to graft rejection);
- oral hypoglycaemic drugs (e.g. **glibenclimide**, **gliburide**);
- anticonvulsants (**phenytoin**, **carbamazepine**);
- HIV protease inhibitors.

Clinically important interactions may occur after **rifampicin** is discontinued. The dose of a second drug (e.g. **warfarin**) may be increased during **rifampicin** therapy to compensate for the increased metabolism. If the effect of such a drug is not closely monitored in the weeks following cessation of **rifampicin** treatment and the dose reduced accordingly, serious complications (e.g. bleeding) may ensue.

ETHAMBUTOL

This is the D-isomer of ethylenediiminodibutanol. It inhibits some strains of *Mycobacterium tuberculosis*, but other organisms are completely resistant. Resistance to **ethambutol** develops slowly and the drug often inhibits strains that are resistant to **isoniazid** or **streptomycin**.

Mechanism of action

The mechanism of action of **ethambutol** is unclear. It inhibits bacterial cell wall synthesis and is bacteriostatic.

Adverse effects

These include:

- retrobulbar neuritis with scotomata and loss of visual acuity occurs in 10% of patients on high doses. The first signs are loss of red–green perception. Prompt withdrawal of the drug may be followed by recovery. Testing of colour vision and visual fields should precede initiation of high-dose treatment, and the patient should be regularly assessed for visual disturbances;
- rashes, pruritus and joint pains;
- nausea and abdominal pain;
- confusion and hallucinations;
- peripheral neuropathy.

Pharmacokinetics

Ethambutol is well absorbed (75–80%) from the intestine. The plasma $t_{1/2}$ is five to six hours. Because **ethambutol** is 80% excreted unchanged in the urine, it is contraindicated in renal failure.

PYRAZINAMIDE

Uses

Pyrazinamide is a bactericidal drug which is well tolerated as oral therapy. Because of its ability to kill bacteria in the acid intracellular environment of a macrophage, it exerts its main effects in the first two to three months of therapy. **Pyrazinamide** is most active against slowly or intermittently metabolizing organisms, but is inactive against atypical mycobacteria. Resistance to **pyrazinamide** develops quickly if used as monotherapy. **Pyrazinamide** should be avoided if there is a history of alcohol abuse, because of the occurrence of hepatitis (see below).

Mechanism of action

The enzyme pyrazinamidase in mycobacteria cleaves off the amide portion of the molecule, producing pyrazinoic acid which impairs mycolic acid synthesis by inhibiting the bacterial enzyme fatty acid synthase I.

Adverse effects

These include:

- flushing, rash and photosensitivity;
- nausea, anorexia and vomiting;
- hyperuricaemia and gout;
- biochemical hepatitis (in approximately 5–15% of patients);
- sideroblastic anaemia (rare);
- hypoglycaemia (uncommon).

Pharmacokinetics

Pyrazinamide is converted by an amidase in the liver to pyrazinoic acid. This then undergoes further metabolism by xanthine oxidase to hydroxypyrazinoic acid. **Pyrazinamide** is well absorbed, and has a $t_{1/2}$ of 11–24 hours. **Pyrazinamide** and its metabolites are excreted via the kidney, and renal failure necessitates dose reduction. It crosses the blood–brain barrier to achieve CSF concentrations almost equal to those in the plasma, and is a drug of first choice in tuberculous meningitis.

STREPTOMYCIN

Use

Streptomycin is an aminoglycoside antibiotic. It has a wide spectrum of antibacterial activity, but is primarily used to treat mycobacterial infections. It is only administered parenterally (intramuscularly). Therapeutic drug monitoring of trough plasma concentrations allows dosage optimization.

Mechanism of action

Like other aminoglycosides, it is actively transported across the bacterial cell wall, and its antibacterial activity is due to specific binding to the P12 protein on the 30S subunit of the bacterial ribosome, inhibiting protein synthesis.

Adverse effects

These are the same as for other aminoglycosides (see Chapter 43). The major side effects are eighth nerve toxicity (vestibulotoxicity more than deafness), nephrotoxicity and, less commonly, allergic reactions.

Contraindications

Streptomycin is contraindicated in patients with eighth nerve dysfunction, in those who are pregnant and in those with myasthenia gravis, as it has weak neuromuscular blocking activity.

Pharmacokinetics

Oral absorption is minimal and it is given intramuscularly. **Streptomycin** is mainly excreted via the kidney and renal impairment requires dose adjustment. The $t_{1/2}$ of streptomycin is in the range of two to nine hours. It crosses the blood–brain barrier when the meninges are inflamed.

PREPARATIONS CONTAINING COMBINED ANTI-TUBERCULOUS DRUGS

Several combination preparations of the first-line drugs are available. They are helpful when patients are established on therapy, and the reduced number of tablets should aid compliance and avoid monotherapy. Combined preparations available include **Mynah** (**ethambutol** and **INH**, in varying dosages), **Rifinah** and **Rimactazid** (containing **rifampicin** and **INH**) and **Rifater** (containing **INH**, **rifampicin** and **pyrazinamide**).

TUBERCULOSIS AND THE ACQUIRED IMMUNE DEFICIENCY SYNDROME

It is difficult to eradicate the tubercle bacillus in patients with HIV infection. The absence of a normal immune defence necessitates prolonged courses of therapy. Treatment is continued either for nine months or for six months after the time of documented culture negativity, whichever is longer. Quadruple drug therapy should be used initially, because of increasing multi-drug resistance in this setting. Adverse drug reactions and interactions are more common in HIV-positive patients, who must be carefully monitored.

SECOND-LINE DRUGS AND TREATMENT OF REFRACTORY TUBERCULOSIS

The commonest cause of *M. tuberculosis* treatment failure or relapse is non-compliance with therapy. The previous drug regimen used should be known and the current bacterial

Table 44.1: Second-line antituberculous drugs, used mainly for multi-drug-resistant TB

Drug	Route	Major adverse effects
Ethionamide and prothionamide	Oral	Hepatitis, gastro-intestinal and CNS disturbances, insomnia
PAS	Oral	Gastro-intestinal, rash, hepatitis
Thiacetazone	Oral	Gastro-intestinal, rash, vertigo and conjunctivitis
Capreomycin[a]	i.m.	Similar to streptomycin
Kanamycin[a]	i.m.	Similar to streptomycin
Cycloserine[a]	Oral	Depression, fits and psychosis

PAS, para-aminosalicylic acid.
[a]Adults only.

sensitivity defined. If the organisms are still sensitive to the original drugs, then better supervised and prolonged therapy with these drugs should be prescribed. Alternative drugs are needed if bacterial resistance has arisen. Organisms that are resistant to **INH**, **rifampicin**, **pyrazinamide** and **ethambutol** are now emerging. Second-line antituberculous drugs are listed in Table 44.1.

Key points

Mycobacterium tuberculosis infection

M. tuberculosis:

- is a slow-growing, obligate aerobe;
- pulmonary infections are the most common, in the upper lobes;
- easily and rapidly develops resistance to anti-tuberculous drugs.

Key points

Mycobacterium tuberculosis treatment

- Treatment is with drug combinations to minimize the development of resistance.
- Triple (pyrazinamide plus rifampicin plus INH) or quadruple (pyrazinamide plus rifampicin plus INH and ethambutol or streptomycin) therapy is given for the first two months.
- Two drugs (usually rifampicin and INH, depending on sensitivity) are given for a further four months, or longer if the patient is immunosuppressed.
- Formulations containing two (e.g. rifampicin/isoniazid) or three (e.g. rifampicin/isoniazid/pyrazinamide) drugs may improve compliance.
- Multi-drug-resistant *M. tuberculosis* requires four drugs initially, while awaiting sensitivity results.
- Drug combinations using second-line agents (e.g. ethionamide, cycloserine, capreomycin), based on sensitivities, are required to treat multi-drug-resistant *M. tuberculosis*. These drugs are toxic and should only be used by a clinician experienced in their use.

MYCOBACTERIUM LEPRAE INFECTION

Leprosy manifests in two forms, lepromatoid (the organism being localized to skin or nerve) or lepromatous (a generalized bacteraemic disease that effects many organs, analogous to miliary tuberculosis). The main drugs used to treat leprosy are **dapsone**, **rifampicin** and **clofazimine**. The current World Health Organization (WHO) regimen for multibacillary leprosy is:

1. **rifampicin**, once a month;
2. **dapsone**, daily unsupervised given for 24 months;
3. **clofazimine**, daily unsupervised, plus a larger dose under supervision every four weeks.

Other anti-lepromatous drugs include **ofloxacin**, **minocycline**, **clarithromycin** (see Chapter 43) and **thalidomide**.

DAPSONE

Uses

Dapsone (4,4-diaminodiphenyl sulphone) is a bacteriostatic sulphone. It has been the standard drug for treating all forms of leprosy, but irregular and inadequate duration of treatment as a single agent has produced resistance. **Dapsone** is used to treat dermatitis herpetiformis, as well as leprosy, pneumocystis and, combined with **pyrimethamine**, for malaria prophylaxis.

Mechanism of action

Dapsone is a competitive inhibitor of dihydropteroate (folate) synthase, thereby impairing production of dihydrofolic acid.

Adverse effects

These include:

- anaemia and agranulocytosis;
- gastro-intestinal disturbances and (rarely) hepatitis;
- allergy and rashes, including Stevens–Johnson syndrome;
- peripheral neuropathy;
- methaemoglobinaemia;
- haemolytic anaemia, especially in glucose-6-phosphate dehydrogenase (G6PDH)-deficient patients.

Pharmacokinetics

Dapsone is well absorbed (>90%) from the gastro-intestinal tract. The $t_{1/2}$ is on average 27 hours. It is extensively metabolized in the liver, partly by *N*-acetylation, with only 10–20% of the parent drug being excreted in the urine. There is some enterohepatic circulation.

Drug interactions

The metabolism of **dapsone** is increased by hepatic enzyme inducers (e.g. **rifampicin**) such that its $t_{1/2}$ is reduced to 12–15 hours.

Case history

A 27-year old Asian woman presents to her physician with a history of streaky haemoptysis and weight loss for the past two months. Clinical examination is reported as normal. Her chest x-ray shows patchy right upper lobe consolidation and her sputum is positive for acid-fast bacilli. After having obtained three sputum samples, she is started, while in hospital, on a four-drug regimen, pyrazinamide (800 mg/day), ethambutol (600 mg/day), isoniazid (300 mg/day) and rifampicin (450 mg/day). She is also prescribed pyridoxine 10 mg daily (to reduce the likelihood of developing peripheral neuropathy secondary to INH). She tolerates the therapy well, without evidence of hepatic dysfunction, and her systemic symptoms improve. Three months later, when reviewed in the outpatient clinic, she has been off pyrazinamide and ethambutol for just over one month, and she complains of daily nausea and vomiting, and is found to be eight weeks pregnant. She is taking the low-dose oestrogen contraceptive pill and is adamant that she has been meticulously compliant with all of her anti-TB medications and the contraceptive pill.
Question
What therapeutic problem has occurred here and how can you explain the clinical situation?
How could this outcome have been avoided?
Answer
Ethambutol, isoniazid, rifampicin and pyrazinamide are all inducers of hepatic CYP450 enzymes. Rifampicin is most potent. and affects many CYPs. Over a period of several weeks her drug therapy induced several CYP450 isoenzymes, especially CYP3A4, so that hepatic metabolism of oestrogen and progesterone was markedly enhanced, reducing their systemic concentrations and efficacy as contraceptives. Therefore, drug-induced hepatic CYP450 enzyme induction caused a failure of contraceptive efficacy and so the patient was 'unprotected' and became pregnant. The patient should continue on her anti-TB drug regimen, as there is no evidence that these agents are harmful to the developing fetus, except for streptomycin, which should never be given in pregnancy.

This outcome could have been prevented by advising the patient to double her usual dose of her oral contraceptives while taking anti-TB therapy, and to take additional contraceptive precautions (e.g. barrier methods), or to abandon the pill altogether and use alternative effective contraceptive measures (e.g. an intrauterine contraceptive device) during her anti-TB drug treatment.

FURTHER READING

Joint Tuberculosis Committee of the British Thoracic Society. Control and prevention of tuberculosis in the United Kingdom: code of practice 2000. *Thorax* 2000; **55**: 887–901.

Joint Tuberculosis Committee Guidelines 1999. Management of opportunist mycobacterial infections: Subcommittee of the Joint Tuberculosis Committee of the British Thoracic Society. *Thorax* 2000; **55**: 210–8.

Joint Tuberculosis Committee of the British Thoracic Society. Chemotherapy and management of tuberculosis in the United Kingdom: recommendations 1998. *Thorax* 1998; **53**: 536–48.

CHAPTER 45

FUNGAL AND NON-HIV VIRAL INFECTIONS

ANTIFUNGAL DRUG THERAPY

INTRODUCTION

Fungi, like mammalian cells but unlike bacteria, are eukaryotic and possess nuclei, mitochondria and cell membranes. However, their membranes contain distinctive sterols, ergosterol and lanesterol. The very success of antibacterial therapy has created ecological situations in which opportunistic fungal infections can flourish. In addition, potent immunosuppressive and cytotoxic therapies produce patients with seriously impaired immune defences, in whom fungi that are non-pathogenic to healthy individuals become pathogenic and cause disease. Table 45.1 summarizes an approach to antifungal therapy in immunocompromised patients. Sites of action of antifungal drugs are summarized in Figure 45.1.

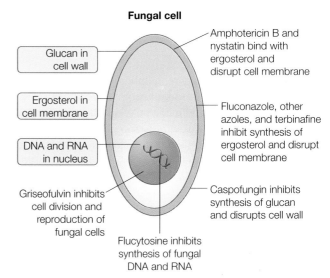

Fungal cell

- Glucan in cell wall
- Ergosterol in cell membrane
- DNA and RNA in nucleus
- Amphotericin B and nystatin bind with ergosterol and disrupt cell membrane
- Fluconazole, other azoles, and terbinafine inhibit synthesis of ergosterol and disrupt cell membrane
- Caspofungin inhibits synthesis of glucan and disrupts cell wall
- Griseofulvin inhibits cell division and reproduction of fungal cells
- Flucytosine inhibits synthesis of fungal DNA and RNA

Figure 45.1: Sites of action of antifungal drugs.

Table 45.1: An approach to antifungal drug therapy in the immunocompromised host

Fungal infection	Drug therapy for superficial infection	Drug therapy for deep-seated infection
Candida	Nystatin – topical	Amphotericin B with or without flucytosine
	Clotrimazole – topical	
	Miconazole – topical	Fluconazole – oral or i.v.
	Fluconazole – oral	Itraconazole or voriconazole oral
		Caspofungin if failing azole therapy
Aspergillus		Amphotericin B i.v. (liposomal)
		Voriconazole or caspofungin if failing azole therapy
Cryptococcus		Amphotericin B plus flucytosine or fluconazole i.v. (oral continuation therapy)
Disseminated histoplasmosis		Itraconazole or amphotericin B i.v. (or fluconazole)
Disseminated coccidiomycosis		Fluconazole or amphotericin B i.v. (plus flucytosine) or itraconazole
Blastomycosis		Amphotericin B i.v. or itraconazole

POLYENES

AMPHOTERICIN B

Uses

Amphotericin is invaluable in treating life-threatening systemic fungal infections, but has considerable toxicity. Its spectrum is broad and includes *Aspergillus* and *Candida* species, *Blastomyces dermatitidis* (which causes North American blastomycosis), *Histoplasma capsulatum* (which causes histoplasmosis), *Cryptococcus neoformans* (which causes cryptococcosis), *Coccidioides immitis* (which causes coccidioidomycosis) and *Sporotrichum schenckii* (which causes sporotrichosis). Resistance is seldom acquired. Amphotericin is insoluble in water, but can be complexed to bile salts to give an unstable colloid which can be administered intravenously. Amphotericin B is normally given as an intravenous infusion given over four to six hours. Several liposomal or lipid/colloidal complex amphotericin preparations have now been formulated, and are less toxic (particularly less nephrotoxic), but more expensive than the standard formulation. **Liposomal amphotericin** is reserved for patients who experience unacceptable adverse effects from regular **amphotericin** or in whom nephrotoxicity needs to be minimized. Topical **amphotericin** lozenges or suspension are used for oral or pharyngeal candidiasis.

Mechanism of action

Amphotericin is a polyene macrolide with a hydroxylated hydrophilic surface on one side of the molecule and an unsaturated conjugated lipophilic surface on the other. The lipophilic surface has a higher affinity for fungal sterols than for cholesterol in mammalian cell membranes and increases membrane permeability by creating a 'membrane pore' with a hydrophilic centre which causes leakage of small molecules, e.g. glucose and potassium ions.

Adverse effects

These include:

- fever, chills, headache, nausea, vomiting, and hypotension during intravenous infusion.
- reversible nephrotoxicity; this is dose dependent and almost invariable. It results from vasoconstriction and tubular damage leading to acute renal impairment and sometimes renal tubular acidosis.
- tubular cationic losses, causing hypokalaemia and hypomagnesaemia;
- normochromic normocytic anaemia due to temporary marrow suppression is common.

Pharmacokinetics

Poor gastro-intestinal absorption necessitates intravenous administration for systemic infections. **Amphotericin** distributes very unevenly throughout the body. Cerebrospinal fluid (CSF) concentrations are 1/40 of the plasma concentration, but it is concentrated in the reticulo-endothelial system. The $t_{1/2}$ is 18–24 hours. **Amphotericin** elimination is unaffected by renal dysfunction.

NYSTATIN

Nystatin works in the same way as **amphotericin B**, but its greater toxicity precludes systemic use. Its indications are limited to cutaneous/mucocutaneous and intestinal infections, especially those caused by *Candida* species. Little or no **nystatin** is absorbed systemically from the oropharynx or gastrointestinal tract, and resistance does not develop during therapy. Preparations of **nystatin** include tablets, pastilles, lozenges or suspension. Patients often prefer topical **amphotericin B** because **nystatin** has a bitter taste. Cutaneous infections are treated with ointment and vaginitis is treated by suppositories.

Adverse effects

Nystatin can cause nausea and diarrhoea when large doses are administered orally.

> ### Key points
>
> Polyene antifungal drugs
>
> - Wide spectrum of antifungal activity, fungicidal; makes 'pores' in fungal membranes.
> - Available for topical (nystatin and amphotericin) treatment of common mucocutaneous fungal infections.
> - Amphotericin is used intravenously for deep-seated and severe fungal infections (e.g. Aspergillus or histoplasmosis).
> - Intravenous amphotericin is toxic, causing fever, chills, hypotension during infusion, nephrotoxicity, electrolyte abnormalities and transient bone marrow suppression.
> - Systemic toxicity (especially nephrotoxicity) of amphotericin is reduced by using the liposomal/lipid/micellar formulations.
> - Amphotericin combined with 5-flucytosine may be used in severe infections and immunosuppressed patients.

AZOLES

IMIDAZOLES

Imidazoles are fungistatic at low concentrations and fungicidal at higher concentrations. They are used topically and are active both against dermatophytes and yeasts (e.g. *Candida*). Some imidazoles are also used systemically, although they have limited efficacy and significant toxicity.

Mechanism of action of azoles (imidazoles and triazoles)

Imidazoles competitively inhibit lanosterol 14-α-demethylase (a fungal cytochrome-haem P450 enzyme), which is a major enzyme in the pathway that synthesizes ergosterol from squalene. This disrupts the acyl chains of fungal membrane phospholipids, increasing membrane fluidity and causing membrane leakage and dysfunction of membrane-bound enzymes. The imidazoles have considerable specificity/affinity for fungal cytochrome-haem P450 enzymes. Azole resistance occurs due to mutations in the gene encoding for lanosterol 14-α-demethylase (ERG11) or less commonly due to increased azole efflux by fungal drug transport proteins.

Ketoconazole was the first imidazole to be used therapeutically but it has been superseded by newer group members because of its hepatotoxicity, its incomplete specificity (it inhibits testosterone and cortisol synthesis) and because it interacts adversely with many drugs. It is still used to treat metastatic prostate cancer and adrenocortical carcinoma (see Chapter 48).

The use and properties of more commonly used imidazoles are listed in Table 45.2.

TRIAZOLES

This group of drugs (e.g. **fluconazole**, **itraconazole** and **voriconazole**) is derived from the imidazoles. Triazole drugs work by the same mechanism as imidazoles but have a wider antifungal spectrum and are more specific for fungal CYP450.

FLUCONAZOLE

Uses

Fluconazole is a potent and broad-spectrum antifungal agent. It is active against many *Candida* species, *Cryptococcus neoformans* and *Histoplasma capsulatum*. However, *Aspergillus* species are resistant and resistant *Candida* species are problematic in immunocompromised patients. **Fluconazole** is used clinically to treat superficial *Candida* infections and oesophageal *Candida*, for the acute therapy of disseminated *Candida*, systemic therapy for blastomycosis and histoplasmosis, for dermatophytic fungal infections and, in low doses, for prophylaxis in neutropenic and immunocompromised patients. It is administered orally or intravenously as a once daily dose.

Adverse effects

Adverse effects include:

- nausea, abdominal distension, diarrhoea and flatulence;
- rashes, including erythema multiforme;
- hepatitis (rarely, hepatic failure).

Contraindications

Fluconazole is contraindicated in pregnancy because of fetal defects in rodents and humans. Breast milk concentrations are similar to those in plasma and **fluconazole** should not be used by nursing mothers.

Pharmacokinetics

Fluconazole is well absorbed after oral administration and is widely distributed throughout the body. CSF concentrations reach 50–80% of those in the plasma. About 80% is excreted by the kidney and dose reduction is required in renal failure. The **fluconazole** mean elimination $t_{1/2}$ is 30 hours in patients with normal renal function. **Fluconazole** is a weaker inhibitor than **ketoconazole** of human CYP3A.

Drug interactions

Fluconazole reduces the metabolism of several drugs by inhibiting CYP3A, including benzodiazepines, calcium channel blockers, **ciclosporin**, **docetaxel** and, importantly, **warfarin**. The plasma concentrations and toxicity of these drugs will increase during concomitant treatment with **fluconazole**. **Rifampicin** enhances the metabolism of **fluconazole**.

ITRACONAZOLE AND VORICONAZOLE

Itraconazole and **voriconazole** are available as oral and parenteral formulations. Oral bioavailability is good for both agents, but intravenous use is indicated for severe fungal infections. The antifungal spectrum is similar to that of **fluconazole** and is broad. They are fungicidal at high concentrations. Both are metabolized by hepatic CYP450s and are inhibitors of hepatic CYP450s. The mean **itraconazole** $t_{1/2}$ is 30–40 hours and that for **voriconazole** is six hours. For **intraconazole**, once daily

Table 45.2: Properties of other commonly used imidazoles

Drug[a]	Use (other specific comments)	Standard formulation	Side effects	Pharmacokinetics
Clotrimazole	Topical therapy for dermatophytes and not used systemically for *Candida* infections	1% cream or powder	Local irritation	Poorly absorbed from gastro-intestinal tract. Induces its own metabolism
Miconazole	Oral *Candida* (topical therapy for ringworm, *Candida* and pityriasis	Oral gel, four times daily 2% cream or powder applied twice daily	Nausea and vomiting, rashes. Local irritation	Systemic absorption is very poor, undergoes extensive hepatic metabolism
Tiaconazole	Topical treatment for nail infections with dermatophytes and yeasts	Apply 28% solution to nails and local skin twice daily for 6 months	Minor local irritation	Systemic absorption is negligible

[a]Other drugs in this group that are used topically include butoconazole, econazole, fenticonazole, isoconazole and sulconazole (see also Chapter 50).

therapy is adequate though more frequent dosing is required for **voriconazole**. Adverse effects include gastro-intestinal upsets, rashes and hepatitis with rare case of hepatic failure. **Voriconazole** causes visual disturbances. CYP450 (especially CYP3A but CYP2C9 > CYP3A in the case of **voriconazole**) inhibition related drug–drug interactions are problematic for both agents. Drugs which decrease gastric acid (e.g. proton-pump inhibitors) reduce the bioavailablity of both agents and drugs that induce hepatic CYP3A decrease systemic drug concentrations. Neither drug should be used in pregnancy and i.v. formulations of both should be avoided in patients with significant renal dysfunction (GFR < 30 mL/min) because of accumulation of the drug diluent (sulphobutylether beta cyclodextrin sodium) which has nephro- and hepatoxic effects in animals.

Posaconazole is a novel agent with considerable potential due to its extended antifungal spectrum.

Key points

Azole antifungal drugs

- Relatively wide spectrum of antifungal activity, fungistatic, but fungicidal with higher concentrations.
- Impair ergosterol biosynthesis by inhibiting lanosterol 14-alpha-demethylase (fungal cytochrome enzyme).
- Available as intravenous, oral and topical formulations.
- Can be used as therapy for superficial (e.g. *Candida*) and serious deep-seated (e.g. *Cryptococcus*) fungal infections.
- Fluconazole, itraconazole and voriconazole are currently much more widely used than ketoconazole.
- Azole-related common toxicities are gastro-intestinal upsets, rashes, hepatitis and CYP3A inhibition-related drug–drug interactions.

ALLYLAMINES

TERBINAFINE

Terbinafine is an allylamine and is fungicidal. It may be administered orally to treat ringworm (*Tinea pedis, T. cruris* or *T. corporis*) or dermatophyte infections of the nails. It is given once daily for two to six weeks (longer in infections of the nailbed, as an alternative to **griseofulvin**, see below). It acts by inhibiting the enzyme squalene epoxidase, which is involved in fungal ergosterol biosynthesis. It interferes with human CYP450, but only to a limited extent (e.g. 10–15% increase in **ciclosporin** concentrations). It is well absorbed, strongly bound to plasma proteins and concentrated in the stratum corneum. It is eliminated by hepatic metabolism with a mean elimination $t_{1/2}$ of 17 hours. Its major side effects are nausea, abdominal discomfort, anorexia, diarrhoea and rashes (including urticaria). Dose reduction is needed in hepatic failure or if co-prescribed with drugs which are potent CYP3A inhibitors (e.g. HIV protease inhibitors). **Rifampicin** increases **terbinafine** metabolism,

requiring a dose increase. **Naftifine**, another allylamine, is available for topical administration.

ECHINOCANDINS

Caspofungin and **micafungin** are novel echinocandins that are fungicidal to susceptible species. Echinocandins are semi-synthetic lipopeptides.

Use

Echinocandins are active against *Candida* and *Aspergillus* species. They are used primarily for fungal infections that are resistant to azoles or where patients are intolerant of azoles and are administered by intravenous infusion, usually once daily.

Mechanism of action

Echinocandins are non-competitive inhibitors of 1,3-β-D glucan synthase, an enzyme necessary for synthesis of a glucose polymer crucial to the structure and integrity of the cell walls of some fungi. Fungal cells unable to synthesize this polysaccharide cannot maintain their shape and lack adequate rigidity to resist osmotic pressure, which results in fungal cell lysis. Glucan also appears essential for fungal cell growth and division. The mechanism of action of echinocandins is unique and drugs of this class are potentially additive or synergistic with polyenes and azoles.

Adverse effects

Adverse effects (usually mild and seldom problematic) include:

- infusion phlebitis and fever, histamine-like infusion reactions, if infused rapidly;
- infrequently nausea, diarrhoea, hyperbilirubinaemia;
- rarely hepatitis, leukopenia.

Pharmacokinetics

Caspofungin and **micafungin** are not absorbed from the gastro-intestinal tract and are administered intravenously. Both agents are eliminated by hydrolysis and *N*-acetylation to inactive metabolites. The mean elimination $t_{1/2}$ for **caspofungin** is 9–11 hours and for **micafungin** is 11–17 hours. Urine excretion of parent drug is insignificant and dose reduction is not indicated in renal failure. The dose of **caspofungin** should, however, be reduced in significant hepatic dysfunction.

Drug interactions

These are minimal compared to the azoles. **Ciclosporin** increases **caspofungin** AUC by 35% and **micafungin** increases the bioavailability of **sirolimus** and **nifedipine**.

Other agents in this expanding class include **anidulafungin**.

OTHER ANTIFUNGAL AGENTS

GRISEOFULVIN

Uses

Griseofulvin is orally active, but its spectrum is limited to dermatophytes. It is concentrated in keratinized cells. It is given orally with meals and treatment is recommended for six weeks for skin infections and up to 12 months for nail infections.

Mechanism of action

Griseofulvin is concentrated in fungi and binds to tubulin, blocking polymerization of the microtubule, disrupting the mitotic spindle.

Adverse effects

These include:

- headaches and mental dullness or inattention;
- diarrhoea or nausea;
- rashes and photosensitivity;

Pharmacokinetics

Griseofulvin is metabolized by the liver to inactive 6-demethylgriseofulvin, which is excreted in the urine. Less than 1% of the parent drug is excreted in the urine. **Griseofulvin** induces hepatic CYP450s and consequently can interact with many drugs.

FLUCYTOSINE (5-FLUOROCYTOSINE)

Flucytosine is used to treat systemic candidiasis and cryptococcosis, provided that the strain is sensitive. Its spectrum is relatively restricted and acquired resistance is a major problem. Consequently, it is only used in combination therapy (e.g. with **amphotericin B**). It is deaminated to 5-fluorouracil in the fungus and converted to an antimetabolite 5-FdUMP. This inhibits thymidylate synthetase, impairing fungal DNA synthesis. Adverse effects include gastro-intestinal upset, leukopenia and hepatitis. **Flucytosine** is well absorbed after oral administration and penetrates the CSF well (thus it is usefully combined with **amphotericin B** to treat cryptococcal meningitis).

It is excreted unchanged by glomerular filtration (<10% of a dose is metabolized). The normal $t_{1/2}$ is six hours and this is prolonged in renal failure.

ANTIVIRAL DRUG THERAPY (EXCLUDING ANTI-HIV DRUGS)

INTRODUCTION

Many viral illnesses are mild and/or self-limiting, but some are deadly (e.g. the now extinct smallpox, some strains of influenza, the global HIV-1 epidemic and various exotic diseases, including Marburg disease, and various encephalitides). Some produce chronic disease (e.g. hepatitis B and C). Even the mild common cold is economically significant, as is its deadly relative SARS (severe acute respiratory syndrome). Patients who are immunocompromised, especially by HIV-1 infection, are at risk of serious illness from viruses that are seldom serious in healthy individuals. Antiviral drug therapy is therefore increasingly important. Antiviral therapy is more difficult than antibacterial therapy because viruses are intimately incorporated in host cells and the therapeutic targets are often similar to the equivalent enzymes/structures in human cells. To summarize these problems:

- Viral replication is intracellular, so drugs must penetrate cells in order to be effective.
- Viral replication usurps the metabolic processes of host cells.
- Although viral replication begins almost immediately after the host cell has been penetrated, the clinical signs and symptoms of infection often appear after peak viral replication is over.

Several events in the viral life cycle may prove susceptible as drug targets:

- when the virus is outside cells it is susceptible to antibody attack; however, finding drugs that are non-toxic but which can destroy viruses in this situation remains a challenge;
- viral coat attachment to the cell surface probably involves interaction between the virus coat and the cell membrane surface;
- penetration of the cell membrane can be prevented (e.g. for influenza A by **amantadine** or neuraminidase inhibitors);
- uncoating of the virus with release of viral nucleic acid intracellularly;
- viral nucleic acid acts as a template for new strands of nucleic acid that in turn direct the production of new viral components utilizing the host cell's synthetic mechanisms. Most non-HIV antiviral drugs act at this stage of viral replication;
- extracellular release of new viral particles.

Figure 45.2 summarizes the sites of action of antiviral drugs.

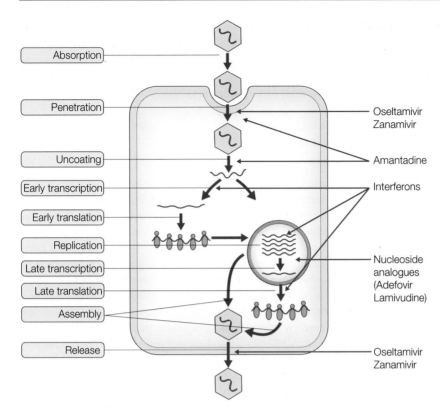

Figure 45.2: Sites of action of antiviral drugs. (Adapted and updated from de Clercq E. *Biochemical Journal* 1982; 205: 1–13.)

NUCLEOSIDE ANALOGUES

ACICLOVIR

Uses

Aciclovir is effective against herpes (simplex and zoster), but is much less active against cytomegalovirus (also a herpes virus). **Aciclovir** and its analogues have replaced **idoxuridine**.

1. **Aciclovir** ointment (3%) accelerates healing in herpetic keratitis. The efficacy of topical **aciclovir** in genital and labial herpes simplex has been unimpressive.

2. **Aciclovir** given orally accelerates healing in genital herpes. It is much less effective in secondary than in primary infection. It does not eliminate vaginal carriage, so Caesarean section is indicated to avoid neonatal herpes.

3. Treatment of shingles (herpes zoster) should be started within 72 hours of the onset and is useful for patients with severe pain, although it shortens the illness only modestly.

4. In generalized herpes simplex or herpetic meningoencephalitis, **aciclovir** is given intravenously.

Mechanism of action

Aciclovir undergoes intracellular metabolic activation to its monophosphate, selectively in infected cells, by a specific thymidine kinase that is coded for by the virus but not by the host genome. **Aciclovir** monophosphate is subsequently converted to the corresponding di- and triphosphate (ACIC-TP).

The viral DNA polymerase is inhibited competitively by ACIC-TP from synthesizing nascent viral DNA.

Adverse effects

These include:

1. a reversible rise in plasma urea and creatinine;
2. neurological disturbance;
3. rash;
4. nausea and vomiting;
5. hepatitis.

Contraindications

Aciclovir is relatively contraindicated in pregnancy as it is an analogue of guanosine and so potentially teratogenic in the first trimester.

Pharmacokinetics

Aciclovir bioavailability is approximately 20% after administration of a standard (200 mg) dose orally, and may be dose dependent. The mean elimination $t_{1/2}$ of **aciclovir** is three hours and it crosses the blood–brain barrier producing a CSF concentration that is approximately 50% of that in plasma. Clearance is largely renal and includes an element of tubular secretion; renal impairment requires dose/schedule adjustment.

Drug interactions

Probenecid prolongs the half-life of **aciclovir** by 20% by inhibiting renal tubular secretion.

Key points

Aciclovir and its analogues

- Aciclovir is an acyclic guanosine analogue that is active against the herpes virus.
- Aciclovir and its analogues are initially phosphorylated by virally coded thymidine kinase and further phosphorylated intracellularly to their triphosphate form, which inhibits the viral DNA polymerase.
- They are used to treat oral herpes simplex (topical), genital herpes simplex (oral therapy) and herpes encephalitis (intravenous therapy).
- Aciclovir has low oral bioavailability.
- Famciclovir (prodrug of penciclovir) and valaciclovir (an aciclovir prodrug) have much greater bioavailability than aciclovir.
- Aciclovir side-effects are mild: increased creatinine levels, rashes, hepatitis and gastro-intestinal disturbances.
- Viral resistance to aciclovir is an increasing problem.

FOSCARNET (TRISODIUM PHOSPHONOFORMATE)

Uses

Foscarnet is active against several important viruses, notably HIV-1 and all human herpes viruses, including **aciclovir**-resistant herpes viruses and cytomegalovirus (CMV). It is used to treat CMV infections (retinitis, pneumonitis, colitis and oesophagitis) and **aciclovir**-resistant herpes simplex virus (HSV) infections in immunocompetent and immunosuppressed hosts. **Foscarnet** is given intravenously as loading dose followed by infusions. Dose reduction is required in patients with renal failure.

Mechanism of action

Foscarnet is a nucleotide analogue that acts as a non-competitive inhibitor of viral DNA polymerase and inhibits the reverse transcriptase from several retroviruses. It is inactive against eukaryotic DNA polymerases at concentrations that inhibit viral DNA replication.

Adverse effects

These include the following:

- nephrotoxicity: minimized by adequate hydration and dose reduction if the serum creatinine rises; monitoring of renal function is mandatory;
- central nervous system effects include irritability, anxiety and fits;
- nausea, vomiting and headache;
- thrombophlebitis;
- hypocalcaemia and hypomagnaesemia;
- hypoglycaemia (rare).

Pharmacokinetics

Foscarnet is poorly absorbed (2–5%) after oral administration. Plasma concentrations decay in a triphasic manner and the terminal $t_{1/2}$ is 18 hours. **Foscarnet** is excreted renally by glomerular filtration and tubular excretion. Approximately 20% remains in the body bound in bone.

Drug interactions

The nephrotoxicity of **foscarnet** is potentiated in the presence of other nephrotoxins, e.g. **pentamidine**, **gentamicin**, **ciclosporin** and **amphotericin B**. Administration with **pentamidine** can cause marked hypocalcaemia.

GANCICLOVIR (DIHYDROXYPROPOXYMETHYL-GUANINE, DHPG)

Uses

Ganciclovir, a guanine analogue, is used to treat sight- or life-threatening CMV infections (e.g. retinitis, pneumonitis, colitis and oesophagitis) in immunocompromised hosts. It also has potent activity against herpes viruses 1 and 2 and is used to treat **aciclovir**-resistant herpes. A loading dose is administered intravenously followed by maintenance infusions. Oral **ganciclovir** is available for therapy despite its poor bioavailability and is only slightly less effective than intravenous therapy in CMV retinitis in AIDS patients. It is easier for the patients and less expensive. Intravitreal **ganciclovir** implants are effective in treating CMV retinitis and are more effective at suppressing progression of disease than systemic **ganciclovir**.

Valganciclovir is the L-valyl ester prodrug of **ganciclovir**. It can be used orally on a twice daily schedule for initial control and suppression of CMV retinitis.

Mechanism of action

Ganciclovir is metabolized intracellularly to its monophosphate in herpes-infected cells by the virally encoded thymidine kinase. It undergoes further phosphorylation by host kinases to its triphosphate anabolite which competitively inhibits the CMV (or HSV) DNA polymerase. If it is incorporated into nascent viral DNA, it causes chain termination. **Ganciclovir** is concentrated ten-fold in infected cells compared to uninfected cells.

Adverse effects

These include:

- neutropenia and bone marrow suppression (thrombocytopenia and less often anaemia); cell counts usually return to normal within two to five days of discontinuing the drug;
- temporary or possibly permanent inhibition of spermatogenesis or oogenesis;
- phlebitis and pain at intravenous infusion site;
- rashes and fever;
- gastro-intestinal upsets;
- transient increases in liver enzymes and serum creatinine in underhydrated patients.

Contraindications

Ganciclovir is contraindicated in pregnancy (it is teratogenic in animals) and in breast-feeding women.

Pharmacokinetics

Only 4–7.5% of an oral dose of **ganciclovir** is absorbed. **Valganciclovir** is well absorbed orally and is converted to

Table 45.3: Summary of available aciclovir-like antiviral agents

Drug[a]	Use	Side effects	Pharmacokinetics	Other specific comments
Famciclovir	Herpes simplex virus (HSV) and recurrent genital HSV varicella zoster (VZV)	See aciclovir	Prodrug of penciclovir. Bioavailability of penciclovir is 77% from famciclovir. $t_{1/2}$ is 2.5 h. Renal excretion	High bioavailability prodrug of penciclovir. Aciclovir-resistant isolates are cross-resistant
Penciclovir	Systemic therapy, for HSV and VZV and hepatitis B. Topical therapy for HSV	See aciclovir. Same as placebo for topical use	Bioavailability is very good. $t_{1/2}$ is 2.5 h. Renal excretion (in renal failure $t_{1/2}$ = 18 h). Intracellular triphosphate is longer lasting (7–20 h) than aciclovir	High bioavailability. Viral DNA polymerase not as sensitive to Pen-Triphosphate. Aciclovir-resistant isolates are cross-resistant.
Valaciclovir	HSV infection but uncertainty about VZV and CMV in future	L-Valyl ester of aciclovir. Haemolytic–uraemic/TTP syndrome in immunosuppressed individuals	Rapid absorption bioavailability is 54%. Converted to aciclovir before phosphorylation	High bioavailability. Aciclovir-resistant isolates are cross-resistant
Cidofovir	Intravenous therapy for HSV and CMV	See ganciclovir, but has been noted to cause renal failure	Plasma $t_{1/2}$ of cidofovir is 2.6 h and of cidofovir diphosphate (active) is 17–30 h. Cidofovir is renally eliminated	CMV isolates resistant to ganciclovir are sensitive. Not to be used in patients with renal failure

[a]Other drugs in the antiviral arena with recent availability or undergoing further clinical development include sorivudine (nucleoside analogue for VZV) n-Docosanol (topical cream for recurrent herpes labialis) and Fomiversen (an antisense phosphorothioate oligonucleotide complementary to human CMV immediate–early mRNA, used in AIDS patients).

ganciclovir, yielding a **ganciclovir** bioavailability of 60%. **Ganciclovir** has a mean elimination $t_{1/2}$ of between two and five hours and is virtually totally excreted by the kidney. Dose reduction is needed in renal failure.

Drug interactions

Probenecid reduces renal clearance of **ganciclovir**. Antineoplastic drugs, **co-trimoxazole** and **amphotericin B** increase its toxic effects on rapidly dividing tissues including bone marrow, skin and gut epithelium. **Zidovudine** (AZT) should not be given concomitantly with **ganciclovir** because of the potentiation of bone marrow suppression.

The pharmacology and therapeutics of other available nucleoside analogue anti-herpes drugs are shown in Table 45.3.

RIBAVIRIN (TRIBAVIRIN)

Uses

Ribavirin is active against a number of RNA and DNA (HSV-1 and HSV-2, influenza) viruses. It is used to treat hepatitis C (combined with **interferon**) or bronchiolitis secondary to respiratory syncytial virus infection in infants and children. Administration for bronchiolitis is via aerosol inhalation.

Mechanism of action

Ribavirin is taken up into cells and phosphorylated to trib-avirin 5′-monophosphate by adenosine kinase and is then phosphorylated to its di- and triphosphates by other cellular kinases. Ribavirin-triphosphate inhibits the guanylation reaction in the formation of the 5′ cap of mRNA and inhibits viral RNA methyltransferase. It has little or no effect on mammalian RNA methyltransferase.

Adverse effects

Systemic administration can cause:

- dose-related haemolytic anaemia and haematopoietic suppression;
- rigors (during infusion);
- rash, pruritus;
- teratogenesis.

No systemic adverse effects of **ribavirin** have been reported following administration by aerosol or nebulizer.
General adverse effects include:

- worsening respiration and bacterial pneumonia (super-infection);
- pneumothorax;
- teratogenesis (a concern even with aerosol exposure of healthcare workers).

Pharmacokinetics

Following nebulized administration, only small amounts of **ribavirin** are absorbed systemically.

ANTI-INFLUENZA AGENTS

AMANTADINE (OR RIMANTADINE)

Amantadine is effective in preventing the spread of influenza A and has an unrelated action in Parkinson's disease (Chapter 21). Its usefulness as an antiviral agent is limited to influenza A. Its mode of action is unknown. Prophylaxis with **amantadine** has an advantage over immunization in that the latter can be ineffective when a new antigenic variant arises in the community and spreads too rapidly for a killed virus vaccine to be prepared and administered. Prophylaxis with **amantadine** during an epidemic should be considered for people at special risk (e.g. patients with severe cardiac or lung disease, or healthcare personnel). **Amantadine** is less effective during periods of antigenic variation than during periods of relative antigenic stability. Treating established influenza with **amantadine** within the first 48 hours may ameliorate symptoms. The mean elimination $t_{1/2}$ is 12 hours and elimination is via renal excretion. Thus, dose reductions are needed when **amantadine** is given to patients with renal failure.

Adverse effects

These include:

- dizziness, nervousness and headaches;
- livedo reticularis.

OSELTAMIVIR PHOSPHATE

Oseltamivir phosphate is an ethyl ester prodrug of **oseltamivir carboxylate**. It is used to prevent and treat influenza A and B infections, when given orally twice a day for five days. **Oseltamivir carboxylate** is an analogue of sialic acid and is a competitive inhibitor of the influenza virus neuraminidase that cleaves the terminal sialic acid residues and destroys the receptors recognized by viral haemagglutinin present on the cell surface of progeny virions and in respiratory secretions. Neuraminidase activity is needed for release of new virions from infected cells. When **oseltamivir carboxylate** binds to the neuraminidase it causes a conformational change at the active site, thereby inhibiting sialic acid cleavage. This leads to viral aggregation at the cell surface and reduced viral spread in the respiratory tract. Adverse effects include headache, nausea, vomiting and abdominal discomfort (noted more frequently in patients with active influenza than if the agent is used for prophylaxis). Adverse effects are reduced by taking the drug with food. Oral **oseltamivir phosphate** is absorbed orally and de-esterified by gastro-intestinal and hepatic esterases to the active carboxylate. The bioavailability of the carboxylate approaches 80% and its mean elimination $t_{1/2}$ is between six and ten hours. Both parent and metabolite are eliminated by renal tubular secretion. No clinically significant drug interactions have been defined, but **probenacid** doubles the half-life of the active carboxylate. Resistant influenza isolates have mutations in the N1 and N2 neuraminidases, but these variants have reduced virulence in animal models. Activity against the dreaded H5N1 avian flu strain is not proven.

ZANAMIVIR

This is another inhibitor of influenza virus neuraminidase enzymes. If given early during influenza A or B infection via intranasal route it is effective in reducing symptoms.

> **Key points**
>
> Antiviral therapy
>
> - Selective toxicity for viruses is more difficult to achieve than for fungi or bacteria.
> - Viruses survive and proliferate inside human cells and often use human cellular enzymes and processes to carry out their replicative process.
> - Certain viruses encode virus-specific enzymes that can be targeted (e.g. herpes virus and aciclovir; CMV virus and its DNA polymerase which is a target for ganciclovir).

INTERFERONS AND ANTIVIRAL HEPATITIS THERAPY

Interferons are cytokines (mediators of cell growth and function). They are glycoproteins secreted by cells infected with viruses or foreign double-stranded DNA. They are non-antigenic and are active against a wide range of viruses, but unfortunately they are relatively species specific. Thus, it is necessary to produce human interferon to act on human cells. Interferon production is triggered not only by viruses but also by tumour cells or previously encountered foreign antigens. Interferons are important in immune regulation.

Four main types of interferon are recognized:

1. **Interferon-α** – known previously as leukocyte or lymphoblastoid interferon. Subspecies of the human α gene produce variants designated by the addition of a number, e.g. interferon-α_2, or in the case of a mixture of proteins, by Nl, N2, etc. Two methods of commercial production have been developed and these are indicated by *rbe* (produced from bacteria – typically *Escherichia coli* – genetically modified by recombinant DNA technology) and *lns* (produced from cultured lymphoblasts stimulated by Sendai virus). Interferon-α_2 may also differ in the amino acids at positions 23 and 24 and these are shown by the addition of a letter. Thus, α-2a has Lys–His at these sites, while α-2b has Arg–His. It is not yet clear whether these different molecules have different therapeutic properties;
2. **interferon-β** from fibroblasts;
3. **interferon-ω** has 60% homology with interferon-α;
4. **interferon-γ** formerly called 'immune' interferon because it is produced by lymphocytes in response to antigens and mitogens.

Commercial production of interferon by cloning of human interferon genes into bacterial and yeast plasmids is now available, facilitating large-scale production.

Uses

Interferon-α when combined with **ribavirin** (see above) provides effective therapy for chronic hepatitis C infection (Chapter 34). Regular **interferon-α** is given three times a week (or **pegylated interferon-α** is given once weekly) by subcutaneous injection, for 6–12 months. **Interferon-β** is of some benefit in patients with relapsing multiple sclerosis. **Interferon-α** is used to treat condylomata acuminata by intralesional injection. All three interferons are used to treat hairy cell leukaemia. **Interferon-α$_{2a}$** and **interferon-α$_{2b}$** are used to treat Kaposi's sarcoma in AIDS patients and **interferon-α$_{2b}$** is effective in recurrent or metastatic renal cell carcinoma (Chapter 48). Recombinant **interferon-γ** has been used for the treatment of chronic granulomatous disease. Interferon therapy is also beneficial in chronic myelogenous leukaemia, multiple myeloma, refractory lymphoma and metastatic melanoma.

Mechanism of action

Interferons bind to a common cell-membrane receptor, except **interferon-γ**, which binds to its own receptor. Following receptor binding, interferons activate the JAK-STAT signal transduction cascade and lead to nuclear translocation of a cellular protein complex that binds to genes containing IFN-specific response elements and stimulating synthesis of enzymes with antiviral activity, namely 2′5-oligoadenylate synthetase (which activates ribonuclease L, which preferentially cuts viral RNA); a protein kinase activity (important in apoptosis) and a phosphodiesterase that cleaves tRNA. The onset of these effects takes several hours, but may then persist for days even after plasma interferon concentrations become undetectable. Interferon also increases the presentation of viral antigens in infected cells and upregulates macrophage activation and T cell and natural killer cell cytotoxicity, thereby increasing viral elimination. The interferon concentrations needed to produce antiviral effects are lower than those required for their antiproliferative effects.

Adverse effects

These include:

* fever, malaise, chills – an influenza-like syndrome, and neuropsychiatric symptoms similar to a postviral syndrome;
* lymphocytopenia and thrombocytopenia are reversible, and tolerance may occur after a week or so;
* anorexia and weight loss;
* alopecia;
* transient loss of higher cognitive functions, confusion, tremor and fits;
* transient hypotension or cardiac dysrhythmias;
* hypothyroidism.

Pharmacokinetics

Most clinical experience has been gained with **interferon-α**, administered subcutaneously. Following subcutaneous administration, peak plasma concentrations occur at between four and eight hours and decline over one to two days. The mean elimination $t_{1/2}$ is three to five hours. Polyethylene glycol (PEG)-conjugated (PEG-ylated) interferons are now used clinically, have protracted half-lives and may be administered weekly. Elimination of interferons is complex. Inactivation occurs in the liver, lung and kidney, but interferons are also excreted in the urine.

ADEFOVIR DIPIVOXIL

Adefovir dipivoxil is a prodrug diester of **adefovir**, an acyclic phosphonate nucleotide analogue of adenosine monophosphate. It is used in the treatment of chronic hepatitis B, especially if **interferon-α** treatment has failed or is not tolerated. It is given orally once a day until seroconversion occurs (or indefinitely in patients with uncompensated liver disease or cirrhosis). **Adefovir dipivoxil** enters cells and is de-esterified to **adefovir**. **Adefovir** is converted by cellular kinases to its diphosphate which is a competitive inhibitor of viral DNA polymerase and reverse transcriptase. Hepatitis B DNA polymerase has a higher affinity for the **adefovir diphosphate** than other cellular enzymes. Adverse effects include dose-related reversible nephrotoxicity and tubular dysfunction, gastro-intestinal upsets and headaches. It is genotoxic, nephrotoxic and hepatotoxic at high doses. The parent compound has low bioavailability, but the prodrug is rapidly absorbed and hydrolysed by blood and gastro-intestinal hydrolases to yield **adefovir** at 30–60% bioavailability. **Adefovir** is eliminated unchanged by the kidney with a mean elimination $t_{1/2}$ of 5–7.5 hours. Dose reduction is needed in patients with renal dysfunction. Drugs that reduce renal function or compete with tubular secretion may increase systemic drug exposure.

LAMIVUDINE (3-THIACYTIDINE)

Lamivudine is a nucleoside analogue reverse transcriptase/DNA polymerase inhibitor. It is used as chronic oral therapy for hepatitis B and HIV. Oral administration twice daily is well tolerated in hepatitis B patients and the most common adverse effects are worsening hepatic transaminases during and after therapy (Chapter 46).

A number of newer oral nucleoside reverse transcriptase/DNA polymerase inhibitors for hepatitis B are in late clinical development.

IMMUNOGLOBULINS

For information related to immunoglobulins, see Chapter 50.

Key points

Non-HIV antiviral drugs

* Specific anti-CMV agents are ganciclovir (valganciclovir) and foscarnet.
* Both are active against aciclovir-resistant herpes viruses.
* Ganciclovir and foscarnet are best given intravenously, poorly or not absorbed orally, both are renally excreted.
* Valganciclovir is a prodrug ester of ganciclovir and yields 60% bioavailable ganciclovir with oral dosing.
* Ganciclovir (bone marrow suppression) and foscarnet (nephrotoxicity) are much more toxic than aciclovir.

Case history

A 35-year-old female with schizophrenia and insulin-dependent diabetes mellitus developed a severe oral *Candida* infection. She was being treated with pimozide for her psychosis and combined glargine insulin with short-acting insulins at meal times. She was started on itraconazole, 100 mg daily, and after a few days her oropharyngeal symptoms were improving. About five days into the treatment, she was brought into a local hospital Accident and Emergency Department with torsades de pointes (polymorphic ventricular tachycardia) that was difficult to treat initially, but which eventually responded to administration of intravenous magnesium and direct current (DC) cardioversion. There was no evidence of an acute myocardial ischaemia/infarction on post-reversion or subsequent ECGs. The patient's cardiac enzymes were not diagnostic of a myocardial infarction. Her electrolyte and magnesium concentrations measured immediately on admission were normal.

Question

What is the likely cause of this patient's life-threatening dysrhythmia and how could this have been avoided?

Answer

In this case, the recent prescription of itraconazole and the serious cardiac event while the patient was on this drug are temporally linked. It is widely known that all azoles can inhibit CYP3A which happens to be the enzyme responsible for metabolizing pimozide. Pimozide has recently been found (like cisapride and terfenadine – now both removed from prescription) to cause prolongation of the QT interval in humans in a concentration-dependent manner. Thus, there is an increased likelihood of a patient developing ventricular tachycardia (VT) if the concentrations of pimozide are increased, as occurs when its metabolism is inhibited by a drug (e.g. itraconazole) that inhibits hepatic CYP3A. This is exactly what happened here. Other common drugs whose concentrations increase (with an attendant increase in their toxicity) if prescribed concurrently with azoles (which should be avoided) are listed in Table 45.4.

Table 45.4: Important interactions with azole antifungals

Drug or drug class	Toxicity caused by azole-mediated reduced hepatic metabolism
Ciclosporin (and Tacrolimus-FK 506)	Nephroxicity and seizures
Warfarin	Haemorrhage
Benzodiazepines – alprazolam, triazolam diazepam, etc.	Increased somnolence
HMG CoA reductase inhibitors (statins, except pravastatin)	Myositis and rhabdomyolysis
Calcium channel blockers	Hypotension
Sildenafil citrate (Viagra)	Protracted hypotension

In this patient, the problem could have been avoided by either changing to an alternative anti-psychotic with least QTc prolonging properties (e.g. clozapine, quetiapine) prior to starting the azole or, if pimozide was such a necessary component of therapy, using a topical polyene, such as amphotericin or nystatin lozenges, to cure her oral *Candida*. Neither of these polyene antifungal agents inhibit CYP3A-mediated hepatic drug metabolism.

Key points

Anti-influenza and antiviral hepatitis agents

- Influenza virus is susceptible to neuraminidase inhibitors, oseltamivir/zanamivir.
- Neuraminidase inhibitors produce viral aggregation at cell surface and reduce respiratory spread of virus.
- Oseltamivir adverse effects mainly involve gastro-intestinal upsets.
- Interferon-alfa plus ribavirin is effective against chronic hepatitis B and C.
- Resistant hepatitis B or C: use lamivudine or adefovir dipiroxil.

FURTHER READING

Albengeres E, Le Leouet H, Tillement JP. Systemic antifungal agents: drug interactions and clinical significance. *Drug Safety* 1998; **18**: 83–97.

Boucher HW, Groll AH, Chiou CC, Walsh TJ. Newer systemic antifungal agents: pharmacokinetics, safety and efficacy. *Drugs* 2004; **64**: 1997–2020.

Como JA, Dismukes WE. Oral azole drugs as systemic antifungal therapy. *New England Journal of Medicine* 1994; **330**: 263–72.

De Clercq E. Antiviral drugs in current clinical use. *Journal of Clinical Virology* 2004; **30**: 115–33.

Francois IE, Aerts AM, Cammue BP, Thevissen K. Currently used antimycotics: spectrum, mode of action and resistance occurrence. *Current Drug Targets* 2005; **6**: 895–907.

McCullers JA. Antiviral therapy of influenza. *Expert Opinion on Investigational Drugs* 2005; **14**: 305–12.

HIV AND AIDS

INTRODUCTION

In June 2006, a cumulative total of approximately 80 000 cases of HIV infection had been reported in the UK and 21 000 of these individuals had acquired immunodeficiency syndrome (AIDS), of whom 80% had died. Approximately 7500 new cases of HIV were reported in the UK in 2005. The most recent World Health Organization (WHO) report estimated that 38.6 million adults and 2.3 million children world-wide were living with HIV at the end of 2005. Globally, heterosexual transmission accounts for 85% of HIV infections. During 2005, an estimated 4.1 million became newly infected with HIV and an estimated 3 million people died from AIDS. World-wide, the HIV incidence rate is believed to have peaked in the late 1990s and to have stabilized subsequently, notwithstanding an increasing incidence in South-East Asia and China.

Key points

HIV-1 epidemiology, life-cycle and dynamics

- By the end of 2005, the number of individuals infected with HIV world-wide was approximately 40 million.
- HIV exposed individuals have CD4/CCR5-expressing cells (mainly lymphoid tissues) invaded; HIV produces its own DNA (from RNA) which is then incorporated into the host DNA, and this is then replicated.
- The production rate of HIV virions is $1–3 \times 10^9$ virions per day.
- HIV genome has 10^4 nucleotides, and all single base DNA mutations are generated daily, three-base mutations are unlikely to be produced before treatment.
- Plasma virions have a half-life of six hours.
- Infected CD4 cells have a half-life of 1.1 days.
- The mean time period needed for HIV generation (time from release of virion into plasma until it infects another cell and causes release of a new generation of viruses) is 2.6 days.
- HIV viral load should be assessed by measurement of the number of copies of HIV RNA/mL of plasma.
- The HIV RNA copy number/mL of plasma is inversely correlated with CD4 count and survival.

IMMUNOPATHOGENESIS OF HIV-1 INFECTION

Following inoculation of a naive host with biological fluid (e.g. blood, blood products or sexual secretions) containing HIV-1, the virus adheres to cells, e.g. lymphocytes, macrophages and dendritic cells in the blood, lymphoid organs or central nervous system, expressing the CD4 receptor and chemokine coreceptors (e.g the CXC chemokine receptor 4 (CXCR4) and the chemokine receptor 5 (CCR5)). During entry, gp120 attaches to the cell membrane by binding to the CD4 receptor. Subsequent interactions between virus and chemokine co-receptors (e.g. CXCR4 and CCR5) trigger irreversible conformational changes. The fusion event takes place within minutes by pore formation and releases the viral core into the cell cytoplasm. The virus then disassembles and the viral reverse transcriptase produces complementary DNA (cDNA) coded by viral RNA. This viral DNA is then integrated into the host genome by the HIV-1 integrase enzyme. Viral cDNA is then transcribed by the host, producing messenger RNA (mRNA) which is translated into viral peptides. These peptides are then cleaved by HIV protease to form the structural viral proteins that, together with viral RNA, assemble to form new infectious HIV virions. These exit the cell by endosomal budding. Figure 46.1 illustrates the HIV-1 life cycle, together with current and potential therapeutic targets.

Newly formed HIV-1 virions infect previously uninfected CD4/CCR5-positive cells and subsequently impair the host immune response by killing or inhibiting CD4/CCR5-positive cells, thus rendering the host immunosuppressed and consequently at high risk of infections by commensal and opportunistic organisms. The diagnosis of HIV-1 infection is based on a combination of the enzyme-linked immunosorbent assay

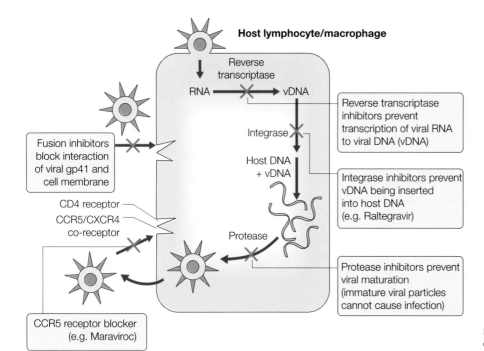

Figure 46.1: Sites of action of anti-HIV drugs.

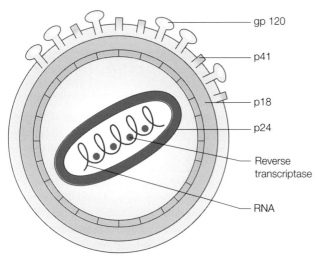

Figure 46.2: HIV structure consisting of membrane glycoprotein gp120 and peptide protein p41 plus an outer membrane of p18 and a nuclear membrane of p24 protein containing viral RNA and the HIV-1 reverse transcriptase and integrase.

(ELISA) techniques that identify HIV-1 antibodies and Western blotting is then used to confirm the presence of HIV-1 structural proteins in blood (see Figure 46.2). Massive viral replication (3×10^9 virions per day) occurs in the four to eight weeks immediately post HIV-1 infection. Viral replication falls in 8–12 weeks, and stabilizes within 6–12 months, initiating a latent period of good health which may last 5–12 years. During this latent period, the viral load falls from an initial peak and remains stable at a plateau of 10^2–10^6 HIV RNA copy number/mL of plasma. The HIV RNA copy number then rises before the development of AIDS. During the latent phase, there is a dynamic equilibrium of HIV replication, T-cell infection and destruction and new T-cell generation with a slow and inexorable decline in CD4$^+$ cell numbers. Only after the CD4 lymphocyte cell count has fallen to <200–500/μL is the

individual predisposed to opportunistic infections (e.g. pneumocystis, tuberculosis) or malignancies (e.g. Kaposi's sarcoma, lymphoma). It is these infections and malignancies that define the later stages of HIV-1 infection, known as AIDS.

GENERAL PRINCIPLES FOR TREATING HIV-SEROPOSITIVE INDIVIDUALS

The accepted standard for HIV treatment is that combination highly active antiretroviral therapy (HAART) should be administered before substantial immunodeficiency intervenes. The primary aim of treating patients with HIV infection is maximal suppression of HIV replication for as long as possible. This improves survival. HAART comprises two nucleoside analogues plus either a boosted protease inhibitor or a non-nucleoside reverse transcriptase inhibitor and reduces viral load to <500 copies of HIV RNA/mL in 80% of patients after 12 months treatment. Not all patients tolerate triple therapy due to toxicity, and alternate double therapy may be used.

Current British HIV Association (BHIVA) recommendations for initiating anti-HIV therapy are as follows. All HIV seropositive patients with symptoms (or AIDS-defining disease) should receive HAART. If the CD4 count is <350 cells per μL or if there is a rapid decline in CD4 count of >300 cells per μL over 12 months, such patients should be treated. Treatment may be deferred and the patient monitored if asymptomatic and CD4 counts are stable in the range 350–500 cells per μL. The recommended regimens for initial therapy are shown in Table 46.1 and are expected to reduce the HIV RNA copy number per mL of plasma by >0.5 log by week 8 of therapy, and ultimately to undetectable levels, and to maintain this state. The plasma HIV RNA copy number is the accepted gold standard for monitoring therapy and is inversely correlated with CD4 count and survival. HIV therapy guidelines are evolving rapidly, requiring

Table 46.1: Examples of combinations to be used as initial anti-HIV drug therapy[a]

Two nucleoside analogues + HIV protease inhibitor	e.g. ZDV + 3-TC or FTC + Lop/rit
Two nucleoside analogues + non-nucleoside reverse transcriptase inhibitor	e.g. ZDV or TDF + 3-TC or FTC + Efav or Nvp
Three nucleoside reverse transcriptase inhibitors	e.g. ABC + ZDV + 3-TC

ABC, abacavir; ZDV, zidovudine; FTC, emtracitabine; 3-TC, 3-thiacytidine (lamivudine); d4T, didehydrothymidine (stavudine); Lop, lopinavir; rit, ritonavir; Efav, efavirenz; Nvp, nevirapine; TDF, tenofovir.
[a]Combinations usually include ZDV or d4T because they have better CSF penetration than other nucleoside analogues and combinations attempt to avoid overlapping toxicities, and to avoid using agents that are phosphorylated by the same enzymes (combinations of ZDV+ d4T and 3-TC + ddC are avoided. ddC = 2'3-dideoxycytidine, also known as zalcitabine).

specialist care. Current principles emphasize combination therapy, regime convenience, tolerability and lifelong therapy. Anti-HIV therapy is a complex therapeutic arena, necessitating specialist supervision.

Key points

General guidelines for anti-HIV-1 therapy

- Treat before significant immunosuppression develops.
- BHIVA treatment criteria are CD4 count (if <350/μL) or symptoms or in USA HIV RNA >100,000 copies/mL plus CD4 <350/μL.
- Standard therapy is highly active antiretroviral therapy (HAART) combination therapy.
- HAART is two nucleoside analogue inhibitors plus one protease inhibitor, e.g. ZDV + 3-TC + amprenavir (or lopinavir/ritonavir).
- If there is drug treatment failure or resistance, change at least two and preferably all three drugs being used.
- The revised regimen may be guided by genotyping of the HIV genome for mutations associated with drug resistance.

ANTI-HIV DRUGS

NUCLEOSIDE ANALOGUE REVERSE TRANSCRIPTASE INHIBITORS (NRTIs)

Of these agents, only **zidovudine** (ZDV) has been proved to reduce mortality in late-stage AIDS. It reduces the incidence of opportunistic infections and possibly also the rate of progression of HIV-1 infection to AIDS. Other members of the class include **lamivudine** (3-TC), **stavudine** (d4T), **didanosine** (ddI), **emtricitabine** (FTC) and **abacavir** (ABC). These drugs are used in combinations and are available as combined products, e.g. 3-TC/ZDV, ABC/3-TC, ZDV/**tenofovir**. They

reduce HIV-1 viral replication as indicated by plasma HIV RNA load.

ZIDOVUDINE (AZIDOTHYMIDINE)

This was originally synthesized in 1964 in the hope that it would be useful in treating malignancies. These hopes were not fulfilled, but it was the first nucleoside analogue effective in treating HIV-1 infection.

Use

Zidovudine (ZDV) is given orally to patients with HIV infection.

Mechanism of action

The parent drug, ZDV, enters virally infected cells by diffusion and undergoes phosphorylation first to its monophosphate (ZDV-MP) then to the diphosphate (ZDV-DP), the rate-limiting step, and finally to the triphosphate (ZDV-TP). The intracellular $t_{1/2}$ of ZDV-TP is two to three hours. ZDV-TP is a competitive inhibitor of the HIV-1 reverse transcriptase and when incorporated into nascent viral DNA causes chain termination. Human cells lack reverse transcriptase and human nuclear DNA polymerases are much less sensitive (by at least 100-fold) to inhibition by ZDV-TP, thus producing a selective effect on viral replication. This mechanism of action is common to all anti-HIV nucleoside analogues.

Adverse effects

These include the following:

- dose-dependent bone marrow suppression causing anaemia with reticulocytopenia and granulocytopenia. This occurred in 15% of patients in the original studies with high-dose ZDV. At currently recommended doses, it occurs in only 1–2% of patients;
- nausea and vomiting;
- fatigue and headache;
- melanonychia (blue-grey nail discoloration);
- lipodystrophy;
- mitochondrial myopathy (uncommon);
- hepatic steatosis with lactic acidosis (rarely);
- it is mutagenic and carcinogenic in animals. However, ZDV is used in HIV-positive pregnant women as it reduces HIV maternal–fetal transmission and thus fetal/neonatal HIV-1 infection and has not been shown to be teratogenic if given to women after the first trimester.

Pharmacokinetics

Zidovudine is almost totally absorbed (>90%) from the gastro-intestinal tract, it achieves cerebrospinal fluid (CSF) concentrations that are 50% of those in plasma. The ZDV plasma elimination $t_{1/2}$ is one to two hours. About 25–40% of a dose undergoes presystemic metabolism in the liver. The major metabolite (80%) is the glucuronide and approximately 20% of a dose appears unchanged in the urine.

Drug interactions

These are numerous and clinically important; the following list is not comprehensive:

1. **probenecid** inhibits the glucuronidation and renal excretion of ZDV;
2. ZDV glucuronidation is reduced by **atovaquone**;
3. rifamycins increase ZDV metabolism;
4. ZDV and antituberculous chemotherapy cause a high incidence of anaemia;
5. **ganciclovir** and ZDV combined therapy produces profound bone marrow suppression;
6. ZDV/ddI or ZDV/3-TC combinations (but not ZDV/D4T) are synergistic.

Table 46.2 shows the properties of other NRTIs used in HIV therapy.

NUCLEOTIDE REVERSE TRANSCRIPTASE INHIBITOR

Tenofovir is the first nucleotide (as distinct from nucleoside) reverse transcriptase inhibitor (NERTI) and is used in combination with NRTIs. It is a derivative of adenosine monophosphate, but lacks the ribose ring. It is phosphorylated sequentially to the diphosphate and then the triphosphate which is a competitive inhibitor of HIV reverse transcriptase. It is adequately absorbed orally and administered once a day (half life 14–17 hours). It is renally eliminated. **Tenofovir** is well tolerated with few adverse effects (mainly flatulence). Occasional cases of renal failure and Fanconi syndrome have been reported, so it should be used with caution in patients with pre-existing renal dysfunction. Although it is not a CYP450 inhibitor or inducer, it increases the AUC of didanosine and reduces the AUC of **atazanavir**. **Ritonavir** and **atazanavir** increase the AUC of **tenofovir**. **Tenofovir** is also active against hepatitis B virus (HBV).

> ### Key points
>
> Anti-HIV drugs – nucleoside analogue reverse transcriptase inhibitors – ZDV
>
> - Used in combinations to increase anti-HIV efficacy and reduce resistance.
> - Zidovudine is phosphorylated intracellularly to ZDV-TP, which inhibits viral reverse transcriptase.
> - Good oral absorption, penetration of CSF, hepatic metabolism and short half-life.
> - Adverse effects include bone marrow suppression and myopathy in the long term.
> - Used in HIV-positive pregnant women, in whom it reduces transmission to the fetus/neonate by approximately 60%.
> - Combination NRTI therapy, e.g. ZDV/3-TC form the 'backbone components' of HAART.
> - Resistance develops slowly to NRTIs.
> - Genotyping of the HIV mutations for drug resistance may guide drug choice.

Table 46.2: Properties of other anti-HIV NRTIs

Anti-HIV nucleoside analogue	Side effects	Pharmacokinetics	Additional comments
Emtricitabine (FTC) – a cytosine analogue, chemically related to lamivudine	One of the least toxic NRTIs. Skin pigmentation, hepatitis, pancreatitis	Well absorbed. Food – no effect on AUC, $t_{1/2}$ is 8–10 h. Renal excretion	FTC-TP long intracellular half-life
Didanosine (ddI; dideoxyinosine)	Peripheral neuropathy, pancreatitis, bone-marrow toxicity is rare. Gastro-intestinal upsets and hyperuricaemia	Acid-labile absorption affected by pH – given as a buffered capsule. Plasma $t_{1/2}$ is 0.5–1.5 h. Renal excretion (50%) and hepatic metabolism	Intracellular triphosphate anabolite ddA-TP has a $t_{1/2}$ of 24–40 h. Didanosine decreases absorption of drugs requiring acid pH (e.g. keto- or itraconazole)
Stavudine (d4T; didehydro-thymidine)	Peripheral neuropathy	Well absorbed (86% bioavailability). T_{max} is 2 h; plasma $t_{1/2}$ is 1 h, rapidly cleared by renal (50%) and non-renal routes	Intracellular triphosphate has $t_{1/2}$ of 3–4 h. In vitro data show antagonism with ZDV against HIV
Lamivudine (3-TC; 2-deoxy-3-thiacytidine)	Well tolerated. Uncommon gastro-intestinal upsets, hair loss, myelosuppression, neuropathy	Well absorbed; $t_{1/2}$ of 3–6 h. Renal excretion (unchanged), requires dose reduction in renal impairment	Intracellular triphosphate has $t_{1/2}$ of 12 h. Synergy in vitro with ZDV against HIV. Co-trimoxazole reduces clearance by 40%

NON-NUCLEOSIDE ANALOGUE REVERSE TRANSCRIPTASE INHIBITORS

The non-nucleoside analogue reverse transcriptase inhibitors (NNRTIs) are used as part of triple-therapy schedules in combination with nucleoside analogue RT inhibitors (e.g. ZDV/3-TC). Agents in this group include **efavirenz, nevirapine** and **delavirdine**. **Efavirenz** is administered orally and causes a marked (>50%) reduction in viral load during eight weeks of therapy. They are synergistic with NRTIs. NNRTIs should only be used in combination therapy due to the rapid development of viral resistance.

Mechanism of action

Non-nucleoside agents inhibit HIV reverse transcriptase by binding to an allosteric site and causing non-competitive enzyme inhibition, reducing viral DNA production.

Adverse effects

These include the following:

* abdominal pain and nausea/vomiting/diarrhoea;
* lipodystrophy;
* arthralgia, myalgia;
* drug–drug interactions: complex effects on other CYP450 metabolized drugs (see below);
* neural tube defects in the fetus.

Pharmacokinetics

Efavirenz is well absorbed. It has a plasma $t_{1/2}$ of 40–60 hours, is highly protein bound and metabolized by hepatic CYP2B6 > CYP3A) to its hydroxylated metabolite, which is glucuronidated and excreted in the urine.

Drug interactions

Efavirenz inhibits CYP3A4, CYP2C9 and CYP2C19 and may reduce the clearance of co-administered drugs metabolized by these isoenzyme systems. **Efavirenz** autoinduces its own metabolism. In contrast, **nevirapine** induces CYP3A and thus increases the clearance of drugs metabolized by this isoenzyme.

Key points

Anti-HIV drugs – Non-nucleoside analogue reverse transcriptase inhibitors (NNRTIs)

* Used in combination, because of synergy with NRTIs, e.g. ZDV.
* Efavirenx, nevirapine and delavirdine are allosteric (non-competitive) inhibitors of the HIV reverse transcriptase.
* Oral absorption is good, hepatic metabolism by CYP3A or 2B6, short–intermediate half-lives.
* Adverse effects include gastro-intestinal disturbances, rashes and drug interactions.
* Resistance develops quickly; not to be used as monotherapy.

HIV PROTEASE INHIBITORS

Uses

Compounds in this class include **amprenavir, ritonavir, indinavir, lopinavir, nelfinavir, saquinavir, atazanavir** and **tipranavir** (Table 46.3). They cause a rapid and marked reduction of HIV-1 replication as measured by a fall of 100- to 1000-fold over 4–12 weeks in the number of HIV RNA copies per mL of plasma. Reductions in viral load are paralleled by increases in CD4 count of approximately 100–150 cells/μL. Resistance is a problem and leads to cross-resistance between protease inhibitors (PIs), so they are used in combination therapy (see Table 46.1).

Mechanism of action

These agents prevent HIV protease from cleaving the gag and gag–pol protein precursors encoded by the HIV genome, arresting maturation and blocking the infectivity of nascent virions. The HIV protease enzyme is a dimer and has aspartyl-protease activity. Anti-HIV protease drugs contain a synthetic analogue structure of the phenylalanine–proline sequence of positions 167–168 of the gag–pol polyprotein. Thus they act as competitive inhibitors of the viral protease and inhibit maturation of viral particles to form an infectious virion.

Adverse effects

These include the following:

* nausea, vomiting and abdominal pain;
* fatigue;
* glucose intolerance (insulin resistance or frank diabetes mellitus) and hypertriglyceridaemia;
* fat redistribution – buffalo hump, increased abdominal girth;
* drug–drug interactions – complex effects on many other drugs that are hepatically metabolized (see Chapter 13).

Key points

Anti-HIV protease inhibitors

* Used in combination, because of synergy with anti-HIV RT inhibitors and reduced resistance.
* They competitively inhibit the HIV protease enzyme, and are the most potent and rapid blockers of HIV replication available.
* Oral absorption is variable, hepatic metabolism is mainly by CYP3A.
* Boosted PI therapy involves combinations such as lopinavir/ritonavir where low-dose ritonavir potentiates the bioavailability of lopinavir by inhibiting gastrointestinal CYP3A and P-glycoprotein (MDR1).
* Side-effects: include gastrointestinal upsets, hyperglycaemia, fat redistribution and drug–drug interactions.
* HIV resistance to one agent usually means cross-resitance to others in this class.

Table 46.3: Properties of commonly available HIV-1 protease inhibitors

Protease inhibitors	Side effects	Pharmacokinetics	Additional comments
Amprenavir (fosamprenavir)	Gastro-intestinal upsets, skin rashes, fat redistribution	Well absorbed T_{max} 1–2 h, $t_{1/2}$ 7–10 h. Hepatic metabolism CYP3A	Inhibits CYP3A
Atazanavir	Hyperbilirubinaemia, gastro-intestinal upsets hyperglycaemia, fat redistribution	Well absorbed with food. T_{max} 2 h, $t_{1/2}$ is 6–8 h, 80–90% protein bound. Hepatic metabolism. No autoinduction of metabolism	Does not induce CYP450, but does inhibit CYP3A drug interactions
Indinavir	Renal stones (5–15%), gastro-intestinal upsets fewer than with other PIs, hepatic dysfunction, hyperglycaemia, fat redistribution	Well absorbed (65% bioavailable). T_{max} is 0.8–1.5 h, $t_{1/2}$ is 2 h. 60–65% protein bound. Hepatic metabolism	Does not induce CYP450, but does inhibit it, especially CYP3A
Saquinavir (soft gel)	Gastro-intestinal upsets, hepatitis hyperglycaemia, fat redistribution	Poorly absorbed (13% bioavailable). Hepatic metabolism	Does not induce CYP450, but inhibits it, at the concentrations achieved clinically (CYP3A)
Nelfinavir	Gastro-intestinal upsets 20%, hyperglycaemia, fat redistribution, transaminitis	Well absorbed (20–80% bioavailable). T_{max} is 2–4 h, $t_{1/2}$ is 3.5–5 h, 98% protein bound. Hepatic metabolism	Does induce CYP450 and inhibits it, especially CYP3A
Tipranavir	Gastro-intestinal disturbances, hyperglycaemia, hepatitis-transaminitis cerebral haemorrhage	Well absorbed (40–60% bioavailable). $t_{1/2}$ is 5–6 h	Induces CYP450, especially CYP3A

Pharmacokinetics

Lopinavir is well absorbed with food and 98–99% protein bound (albumin and alpha-1-acid glycoprotein). It undergoes oxidative metabolism by the CYP3A isozyme, with a half-life of five to six hours. The majority of **lopinavir** is excreted as metabolites in the faeces, with only about 4% appearing in urine. **Ritonavir** is also well absorbed (bioavailability >60%). It is 60% plasma protein bound and metabolized by CYP3A > CYP2D6. It has a half life of between three and five hours. **Ritonavir** inhibits the metabolism of certain CYP3A substrates (and certain drugs metabolized by CYP2D6) and induces its own metabolism. Therefore drug–drug interactions are complex.

Drug interactions

These are numerous and clinically important; the following list is not comprehensive:

1. Most protease inhibitors are inhibitors of hepatic CYP3A. This leads to reduced clearance and increased toxicity of a number of drugs often causing severe adverse effects (e.g. increased sedation with **midazolam, triazolam** and excessive hypotension with calcium channel blockers). Protease inhibitors inhibit the metabolism of **rifabutin** increasing the risk of **rifabutin** toxicity.

2. Enzyme inducers (e.g. rifamycins – **rifampicin/rifabutin** or **nevirapine**) enhance the metabolism of protease inhibitors, making them less effective, producing subtherapeutic plasma concentrations and increasing the likelihood of HIV resistance.

3. Several protease inhibitors reduce gastro-intestinal metabolism (by CYP3A) and luminal transport (via P-gp/MDR1) of co-administered protease inhibitors, thereby increasing plasma concentrations. Combining two agents from this group is called 'boosted protease inhibitor' therapy, e.g. **lopinavir** is available combined with low-dose **ritonavir**; **ritonavir** inhibits CYP3A and P-glycoprotein (MDR1) increasing the bioavailability of **lopinavir**. The same principle applies if **saquinavir**/low-dose **ritonavir** or **amprenavir**/low-dose **ritonavir** are combined.

FUSION INHIBITORS

Uses

Currently, **enfuvirtide** is the only available HIV fusion inhibitor. This agent is reserved for HIV patients who have evidence of progressive HIV replication despite HAART therapy. It is a 36 amino acid peptide analogue of part of the transmembrane region of gp41 that is involved in the fusion of the virus particle with the host cell membranes. It is given subcutaneously on a twice daily basis.

Mechanism of action

The peptide **enfuvirtide** blocks the interaction between the HIV gp41 protein and the host cell membrane by binding to a hydrophobic groove in the N36 region of gp41. Due to this unique mechanism of action, **enfuvirtide** is active against HIV which has developed resistance to HAART. Resistance to **enfuvirtide** can arise by mutations in its gp41 binding site.

Adverse effects

These include:

- injection site reactions – pain, erythema, induration (98% of patients) and nodules; approximately 5% of patients discontinue therapy because of these local skin reactions;
- lymphadenopathy;
- flu-like syndrome;
- eosinophilia;
- biochemical hepatitis.

Pharmacokinetics

Enfuvirtide is well absorbed after subcutaneous administration and is distributed in the plasma volume, with 98% bound to albumin. The plasma $t_{1/2}$ is three to four hours. The major route of clearance is unknown.

Drug interactions

Enfuvirtide is not known to cause drug–drug interactions with other anti-HIV drugs.

CHANGING ANTI-HIV THERAPY FOR TREATMENT FAILURE AND/OR RESISTANCE

A change in anti-HIV therapy may be required because of treatment failure, adverse effects, poor compliance, potential drug–drug interactions or current use of a suboptimal regimen. Viral resistance to NRTIs and NNRTIs and protease inhibitors may cause treatment failure. Reduced susceptibility of HIV-1 isolates to NRTIs/NNRTIs and PIs is developing. Genetic testing of the HIV genome for mutations leading to drug resistance in isolates from individual patients is becoming more widely available and may guide therapy. Resistance to ZDV emerges more quickly and to a greater degree in the later stages of the disease. Progressive stepwise reductions in susceptibility of the HIV reverse transcriptase (RT) correlate with the acquisition of mutations in the gene for the RT protein. In the case of ZDV, the only cross-resistance is to other nucleosides with the 3'-azido side-chain and therefore such isolates are still sensitive to 3-TC, d4T/ddI.

Future prospects include more potent protease inhibitors, novel entry inhibitors e.g. **maraviroc**, HIV-integrase inhibitors e.g. **raltegravir** and effective anti-HIV vaccines.

OPPORTUNISTIC INFECTIONS IN HIV-1-SEROPOSITIVE PATIENTS

PNEUMOCYSTIS CARINII

In moderate to severe *Pneumocystis carinii* pneumonia (PCP) (arterial $PO_2 < 60\,\text{mmHg}$), treatment consists not only of anti-*Pneumocystis* therapy but, in addition, involves the use of glucocorticosteroids. This reduces the number of patients who require mechanical ventilation and improves survival.

CO-TRIMOXAZOLE

High-dose **co-trimoxazole** (Chapter 43) is first-line therapy for PCP in patients with HIV infection. It is given in divided doses for 21 days. Initial treatment is intravenous; if the patient improves after five to seven days, oral therapy may be substituted for the remainder of the course. The major adverse effects of this therapy are nausea and vomiting (which is reduced by the prior intravenous administration of an anti-emetic), rashes, hepatitis, bone marrow suppression and hyperkalaemia. Treatment may have to be discontinued in 20–55% of cases because of side effects and one of the alternative therapies listed below substituted. After recovery, secondary prophylaxis with oral **co-trimoxazole** (one double strength tablet two or three times daily) is preferred to nebulized **pentamidine**, as it reduces the risk of extrapulmonary, as well as pulmonary relapse. **Dapsone** is also effective for secondary prophylaxis.

PENTAMIDINE

Uses

This is an aromatic amidine and is supplied for parenteral use as **pentamidine isetionate**. It has activity against a range of pathogenic protozoa, including *P. carinii*, African trypanosomiasis (*Trypanosoma rhodesiense* and *T. congolese*) and kala-azar (*Leishmania donovani*).

Mechanism of action

Pentamidine has a number of actions on protozoan cells. It damages cellular DNA, especially extranuclear (mitochondrial) DNA and prevents its replication. It also inhibits RNA polymerase and, at high concentrations, it damages mitochondria. Polyamine uptake into protozoa is also inhibited by **pentamidine**. *P. carinii* is killed even in the non-replicating state.

Adverse effects

The adverse effects of the nebulized route include cough and bronchospasm, pre-administration of a nebulized β_2-agonist minimizes these effects.

Intravenous route adverse effects include:

- hypotension and acidosis (due to cardiotoxicity) if given too rapidly;
- dizziness and syncope;
- hypoglycaemia due to toxicity to the pancreatic β-cells, producing hyperinsulinaemia;
- nephrotoxicity (rarely irreversible);
- pancreatitis;
- reversible neutropenia;
- prolongation of the QTc interval.

Pharmacokinetics

Pentamidine is administered parenterally. The $t_{1/2}$ is six hours and it is redistributed from plasma by tissue binding. Renal excretion is low (<5% of dose). Nebulized therapy yields lung concentrations that are as high or higher than those achieved after intravenous infusion.

Drug interactions

Pentamidine inhibits cholinesterase. This suggests potential interactions in enhancing/prolonging the effect of **suxamethonium** and reducing that of competitive muscle relaxants, but it is not known whether this is of clinical importance.

Alternative regimens for treating PCP are summarized in Table 46.4.

Table 46.4: Alternative regimens for treating PCP

Alternative PCP treatment	Additional comments
Trimethoprim, in two divided doses plus dapsone, daily	Oral therapy for 21 days, used in mild to moderate PCP. Check glucose-6-phosphate dehydrogenase
Primaquine, p.o. and clindamycin, i.v. for 11 days and then p.o. for 10 days	Used in mild to moderate PCP. Check glucose-6-phosphate dehydrogenase
Atovaquone (a hydroxynaphthoquinone), for 21 days	Oral therapy used in mild to moderate PCP. Blocks protozoan mitochondrial electron transport chain and de novo pyrimidine synthesis. Side effects include nausea, vomiting, rash and hepatitis

TOXOPLASMA GONDII

PYRIMETHAMINE AND SULFADIAZINE

Use

This combination is the first-line therapy for cerebral and tissue toxoplasmosis. **Pyrimethamine** is given as an oral loading dose followed by a maintenance dose, together with **sulfadiazine**. Treatment is continued for at least four to six weeks after clinical and neurological resolution, and for up to six months thereafter. Folinic acid is given prophylactically to reduce drug-induced bone marrow suppression.

Mechanism of action

Sulfadiazine acts as a competitive inhibitor of dihydropteroate (folate) synthase (competing with p-aminobenzoic acid) in folate synthesis. **Pyrimethamine** is a competitive inhibitor of dihydrofolate reductase, which converts dihydrofolate to tetrahydrofolate. Together they sequentially block the first two major steps in the synthesis of folate in the parasite. Their selective toxicity is due to the fact that humans can utilize exogenous folinic acid and dietary folate, whereas the parasite must synthesize these.

Adverse effects

The major toxic effects of the combination are:

- nausea and vomiting;
- fever and rashes which may be life-threatening (Stevens–Johnson syndrome);
- bone marrow suppression, especially granulocytopenia;
- hepatitis;
- nephrotoxicity, including crystalluria and obstructive nephropathy.

Pharmacokinetics

Oral absorption of **pyrimethamine** is good (>90%). It undergoes extensive hepatic metabolism, but approximately 20% is recovered unchanged in the urine. It has a long plasma $t_{1/2}$ (35–175 hours). Because of its high lipid solubility it has a large volume of distribution, and achieves CSF concentrations that are 10–25% of those in plasma.

Sulfadiazine is rapidly and completely absorbed after oral administration. However, there is substantial first-pass hepatic metabolism. The mean plasma $t_{1/2}$ is ten hours. Cerebrospinal fluid concentrations are 70% of those in plasma. Clearance is a combination of hepatic metabolism and renal excretion, with 50% of a dose being excreted in the urine, so dose reduction is needed in patients with renal failure.

Drug interactions

These are primarily due to **sulfadiazine** (Chapter 43) and the combined bone marrow suppressive effect of **pyrimethamine** with other antifolates.

An alternative anti-toxoplasmosis regimen consists of **pyrimethamine** in combination with **clindamycin** with folinic acid as above. Newer therapies for cerebral toxoplasmosis as salvage therapy include **azithromycin** or **clarithromycin** (Chapter 43) and **atovaquone**.

MYCOBACTERIUM TUBERCULOSIS THERAPY IN HIV PATIENTS

For more information, see also Chapter 44. Bacille Calmette–Guérin (BCG) vaccine should not be given to HIV-1-infected individuals as it is a live, albeit attenuated, strain. Quadruple therapy with **isoniazid** plus **rifampicin** and **pyrazinamide**, plus either **ethambutol** or **streptomycin** is recommended. This quadruple regimen should be given for two months and then **rifampicin** and **isoniazid** continued for nine months or for six months after the sputum converts to negative for bacterial growth, whichever is longer. If there is drug resistance, the regimen is based on the sensitivities of the isolated organism. This may require therapy with second-line anti-TB drugs. Response rates in HIV patients are generally high (around 90%), provided that there is good compliance, with a relatively low recurrence rate (10%). The incidence of adverse effects from anti-tuberculous therapy is high in HIV patients, and may necessitate a change in medication. *M. tuberculosis* strains are becoming multi-drug resistant and are present in this population, so in vitro sensitivity determinations are essential.

MYCOBACTERIUM AVIUM-INTRACELLULARE COMPLEX THERAPY

This infection is a systemic multi-organ system infection in HIV-infected patients. It has not been convincingly shown to be communicable to other individuals as has *M. tuberculosis*. The regimens used for treatment are three- or four-drug combination therapies because of the resistance patterns of the organism. One such successful regimen consists of **rifabutin**, **ethambutol** and **clarithromycin**. If a clinical response is produced (usually within two to eight weeks), secondary prophylaxis (suppressive therapy) should be given for life. Prophylactic treatment is with either **clarithromycin** or **azithromycin**.

ANTIFUNGAL THERAPY

For further information on antifungal therapy, see Chapter 45.

CANDIDA

If the disease is confined locally then initial therapy is with topical **nystatin** or **amphotericin**. If infection is more extensive, treatment should be with **fluconazole**. Alternatives are **itraconazole** or **voriconazole**. Prophylaxis is with **fluconazole**, once weekly. Echinocandins (e.g. **caspofungin**/**mycofungin**) are used for azole-resistant candida.

CRYPTOCOCCUS NEOFORMANS

First-line therapy is with intravenous **amphotericin B**, sometimes in combination with intravenous **flucytosine**. However, **flucytosine** often causes bone marrow suppression in HIV-1-infected patients. Such combination therapy is preferred in severely ill patients. **Fluconazole** and liposomal **amphotericin B** is a less toxic alternative.

HISTOPLASMOSIS

Treatment is with **amphotericin B** or **itraconazole**, daily intravenously for six weeks. Prophylactic maintenance **itraconazole** is recommended.

COCCIDIOMYCOSIS

Treatment is with **amphotericin B** daily intravenously for six weeks, followed by **itraconazole** as maintenance prophylaxis.

ANTI-HERPES VIRUS THERAPY

For more information on anti-herpes therapy, see Chapter 45.

HERPES SIMPLEX VIRUS 1

Aciclovir is used for treatment, and sometimes as maintenance prophylaxis. Unfortunately, this has led to the development of **aciclovir** resistance of herpes virus isolates in many HIV patients. The **aciclovir** prodrugs (e.g. **famciclovir**) achieve higher intracellular concentrations of **aciclovir** and are useful here, as are **foscarnet** or **cidofovir**.

CYTOMEGALOVIRUS INFECTION

Cytomegalovirus (CMV) infection may be multi-system or confined to the eyes, lungs, genito-urinary system or gastro-intestinal tract. Therapeutic regimens are induction with either **ganciclovir** or **foscarnet**, followed by a maintenance regimen (see also Chapter 45). In the treatment of CMV retinitis, studies suggested that **foscarnet** was superior and allowed the continued use of ZDV with an improved survival time. This was perhaps due to its lack of bone marrow suppression, unlike **ganciclovir**, which together with ZDV causes profound marrow suppression. The tolerance of **ganciclovir** in AIDS patients is improved when it is combined with G-CSF to minimize granulocytopenia. Slow-release implants of **ganciclovir** from a reservoir inserted into the vitreous humour are effective in patients with retinal CMV infection.

Case history

A 69-year-old man has had a blood transfusion 12 years ago following surgery for a perforated gastric ulcer. He now complains of a history of fatigue for 18 months and recent weight loss of 5 lb. After thorough clinical assessment and investigation, he was found to be HIV-1-positive. His HIV-1 RNA was 150 000 copies/mL and his CD4 count was 200 cells/μL on two occasions. He was started on ZDV (300 mg twice a day) and lamivudine (150 mg twice a day) given as the combination tablet 'Combivir' one tablet twice a day, and lopinavir 200 mg/ritonavir 50 mg capsules; one capsule twice a day. Two months later, he does not feel significantly better and despite his HIV isolate being sensitive to all agents in the regimen, his plasma HIV RNA is 110 000 copies/mL. He was adamant that he was taking his medication correctly and was tolerating it well and this was confirmed by his wife. His physician increased his lopinavir/ritonavir combination capsules to two capsules twice a day, When reviewed four weeks later, he had put on weight and felt less tired, and his plasma HIV RNA was 45 000 copies/mL.

Question

What is the underlying pharmacological principle of the benefit of combining lopinavir with low-dose ritonavir?

Answer

This patient with late-stage HIV-1 infection was started on a 'triple' combination therapy regimen consisting of two nucleoside analogue reverse transcriptase inhibitors (ZDV and 3-TC) and 'boosted protease' inhibitor regimen. The explanation for the therapeutic benefit of the lopinavir/low-dose ritonavir combination is that ritonavir causes the systemic lopinavir exposure (AUC) to be increased by between 10- and 15-fold, yielding more effective anti-HIV lopinavir concentrations at a lower lopinavir dose. In addition, lopinavir potentially increases the AUC of ritonavir, although the extent and clinical relevance of this interaction is less important as the IC_{50} of HIV-1 for lopinavir is ten times lower than that for ritonavir, thus most of the anti-HIV effect of the lopinavir/ritonavir combination is due to the lopinavir. These effects on the oral bioavailability of lopinavir and 'first-pass' metabolism of each of these protease inhibitors are thought to be primarily due to mutual inhibition of metabolism by the gastro-intestinal and hepatic CYP3A isoenzyme. Data also show that lopinavir is a P-glycoprotein substrate and that inhibition of the gastro-intestinal P-glycoprotein drug efflux transporter by ritonavir increases the bioavailability of lopinavir in this complex drug–drug interaction. Additionally, the bioavailability of lopinavir from the lopinavir/low-dose ritonavir combination shows less variability between individuals, than does the same dose of lopinavir given without ritonavir.

FURTHER READING AND WEB MATERIAL

Dybul M, Fauci AS, Bartlett JG et al. Panel on Clinical Practices for Treatment of HIV. Guidelines for using antiretroviral agents among HIV-infected adults and adolescents. *Annals of Internal Medicine* 2002; **137**: 381–433.

Gazzard B; BHIVA Writing Committee. British HIV Association (BHIVA) guidelines for the treatment of HIV-infected adults with antiretroviral therapy. *HIV Medicine* 2005; **6** (Suppl 2): 1–61.

Lalezari JP, Henry K, O'Hearn M et al. Enfuvirtide, an HIV-1 fusion inhibitor, for drug-resistant HIV infection in North and South America. *New England Journal of Medicine* 2003; **348**: 2175–85.

Martin AM, Nolan D, Gaudieri S et al. Pharmacogenetics of antiretroviral therapy: genetic variation of response and toxicity. *Pharmacogenomics* 2004; **5**: 643–55.

Mofenson LM, Oleske J, Serchuck L et al. Treating opportunistic infections among HIV-exposed and infected children recommendations from CDC, the National Institutes of Health, and the Infectious Diseases Society of America. *Clinical Infectious Diseases* 2005; **40** (Suppl 1): S1–84.

Schols D. HIV co-receptor inhibitors as novel class of anti-HIV drugs. *Antiviral Research* 2006; **71**: 216–26.

Simon V, Ho DD, Abdool Karim Q. HIV/AIDS epidemiology, pathogenesis, prevention, and treatment. *Lancet* 2006; **368**: 489–504.

Recommended websites: www.bhiva.org, www.hopkins-aids.edu, www.aidsinfo.nih.gov

CHAPTER 47

MALARIA AND OTHER PARASITIC INFECTIONS

MALARIA

It estimated that malaria infects 300–500 million humans per year throughout the world, and up to 2 million (mainly children) die annually. Approximately 40% of the world population live in malarious areas, particularly in equatorial regions. Malaria is transmitted to humans in the saliva of the anopheles mosquito and is caused by protozoan organisms of the genus *Plasmodium*. There are four major species, namely *P. falciparum*, *P. vivax*, *P. ovale* and *P. malariae*. *P. falciparum* is the most lethal form. Malaria is one of the most common causes of serious illness in the returning traveller. At least 2000 cases are imported into the UK (10 000 in Europe) per year. Air travel and the incubation period of the disease have raised the awareness of diagnosing and appropriately treating malaria even in areas where it is not endemic (e.g. hospitals near international airports in Western Europe and the USA).

Visitors to endemic areas must be warned of the infection risk and advised that prophylactic drug therapy should be taken, but that it is not 100% effective. They should also be advised to wear long-sleeved clothing to cover extremities (especially in the evenings, when mosquitos feed) to use mosquito-repellent sprays, to sleep in properly screened rooms with mosquito nets (impregnated with pyrethroids) around the bed and/or to burn and vapourize synthetic pyrethroids during the night. In addition to chemoprophylactic drug therapy, travellers to remote areas should be advised to carry standby antimalarial drug treatment with **quinine**. Where there is doubt concerning the suitability of drug therapy for malaria prophylaxis or treatment, the malaria reference laboratory at the London School of Hygiene and Tropical Medicine has advice and guidance (Tel. 020 7636 3924 for health professionals and Tel. 09065 508908 for the general public, regarding malaria prophylaxis: website www.hpa.org.uk/srmd/malaria).

Figure 47.1 illustrates the *Plasmodium* life cycle and the therapeutic targets.

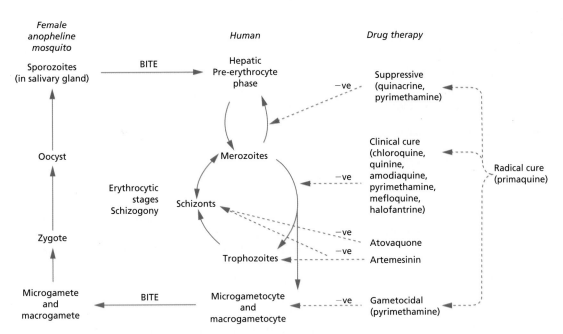

Figure 47.1: Malaria life cycle and type of drug treatment.

MALARIA PROPHYLAXIS

Malaria prophylaxis is relative and the agents are chosen mainly on the basis of the susceptibility patterns of the local *Plasmodium* species. The arylaminoalcohols (e.g. **mefloquine**), 4-aminoquinolines (e.g. **chloroquine**) and the antifolate agents (e.g. **pyrimethamine** and **proguanil**) are the major prophylactic drugs. Prophylaxis must start at least one week (and preferably two weeks) before entering a malaria endemic region, and must continue for four weeks afterwards.

Chloroquine is only used as a prophylactic in regions where falciparum malaria is not **chloroquine** resistant. Drugs for the prophylaxis of **chloroquine**-resistant falciparum malaria are shown below; items 3 and 4 appear to be well tolerated.

1. **mefloquine**, weekly;
2. **chloroquine**, weekly plus **proguanil** daily;
3. **doxycycline** daily;
4. **atovaquone** and **proguanil** daily.

PREVENTION OF MALARIA IN PREGNANCY

Chloroquine or **mefloquine** (in **chloroquine**-resistant areas) are believed to be the most effective and safest antimalarial drugs for chemoprophylaxis in pregnancy.

DRUG TREATMENT OF ACUTE MALARIA

THE 4-AMINOQUINOLINES (E.G. CHLOROQUINE) CHLOROQUINE

Uses

Chloroquine is still one of the most commonly used antimalarial drugs world-wide, but increasing resistance (especially *P. falciparum*) has reduced its efficacy. It is used in:

- acute malaria – chloroquine is effective in terminating an acute attack of benign vivax malaria, but is not radically curative because it does not eradicate the latent hepatic forms of the parasite, and relapses can occur subsequently. If given intravenously, chloroquine can cause encephalopathy. Following a course of **chloroquine**, **primaquine** may be given for 14–21 days to achieve a radical cure (i.e. to eliminate hepatic forms and prevent relapse). Before starting **primaquine**, the possibility of glucose-6-phosphate dehydrogenase (G6PD) deficiency should be considered (Chapter 14).
- malaria prophylaxis (see above);
- rheumatoid arthritis or systemic lupus erythematosis may be treated with **chloroquine** or **hydroxychloroquine** (Chapter 26).

Antimalarial mechanism of action

The erythrocyte stages of *Plasmodium* are sensitive to **chloroquine**. At this stage of its life cycle, the parasite digests haemoglobin in a food vacuole to provide energy for the parasite. The food vacuole is acidic and the weak base **chloroquine** is concentrated within it by diffusion ion-trapping. **Chloroquine** and other 4-aminoquinolines are believed to inhibit the malarial haem polymerase within the food vacuole of the plasmodial parasite, thereby inhibiting the conversion of toxic haemin (ferriprotoporphyrin IX) to haemozoin (a pigment which accumulates in infected cells and is not toxic to the parasite). Ferriprotoporphyrin IX accumulates in the presence of **chloroquine** and is toxic to the parasite, which is killed by the waste product of its own appetite ('hoist with its own petard').

Adverse effects

Short-term therapy These include the following:

1. mild headache and visual disturbances;
2. gastro-intestinal upsets;
3. pruritus.

Prolonged therapy These include the following:

1. retinopathy, characterized by loss of central visual acuity, macular pigmentation ('bull's-eye' macula) and retinal artery constriction. Progressive visual loss is halted by stopping the drug, but is not reversible;
2. lichenoid skin eruption;
3. bleaching of hair;
4. weight loss;
5. ototoxicity (cochleovestibular paresis in fetal life).

Pharmacokinetics

Chloroquine is rapidly and well absorbed from the intestine. It is approximately 50% bound to plasma proteins. About 70% of a dose is excreted unchanged in the urine, and the main metabolite is desethylchloroquine. The mean $t_{1/2}$ is 120 hours. High tissue concentrations (relative to plasma) are found, especially in melanin containing tissues, e.g. the retina.

Drug interactions

Chloroquine and **quinine** are antagonistic and should not used in combination.

ARYLAMINOALCOHOLS (4-AMINOQUINOLINE DERIVATIVES)

This group consists of quinoline methanols (**quinine, quinidine** and **mefloquine**) and the phenanthrene methanol **halofantrine**.

QUININE

Uses

Quinine is the main alkaloid of cinchona bark. The mechanism of its antimalarial activity remains unclear, but may be similar to that of **chloroquine**.

1. **Quinine sulphate** (**quinidine gluconate** in the USA) is the drug of choice in the treatment of an acute attack of falciparum malaria where the parasite is known to be resistant to **chloroquine**. Initially, these drugs may be given intravenously and then orally when the patient improves. The mean $t_{1/2}$ is quite long and in patients with renal or hepatic dysfunction dosing should be reduced to once or twice daily. **Doxycycline** or **clindamycin** may be used as an adjunct to **quinine**.
2. **Quinine** should not be used for nocturnal cramps as its adverse effects outweigh any benefit in this benign condition.

Adverse effects

These include the following:

- large therapeutic doses of **quinine** cause cinchonism (tinnitus, deafness, headaches, nausea and visual disturbances);
- abdominal pain and diarrhoea;
- rashes, fever, delirium, stimulation followed by depression of respiration, renal failure, haemolytic anaemia, thrombocytopenic purpura and hypoprothrombinaemia;
- intravenous **quinine** can produce neurotoxicity such as tremor of the lips and limbs, delirium, fits and coma.

Pharmacokinetics

Quinine is almost completely absorbed in the upper part of the small intestine and peak concentrations occurring 1–3 hours after ingestion are similar following oral or intravenous administration. The mean $t_{1/2}$ is ten hours, but is longer in severe falciparum malaria. Approximately 95% or more of a single dose is metabolized in the liver, principally to inactive hydroxy derivatives, with less than 5% being excreted unaltered in the urine. The uses and properties of other arylaminoalcohols are listed in Table 47.1.

Table 47.1: Uses and properties of other arylaminoalcohols

Drug	Use and pharmacodynamics	Pharmacokinetics	Side effects	Precautions/ comments
Mefloquine	Used for prophylaxis and acute treatment of drug-resistant malaria (especially *P. falciparum*) Schizonticidal in the blood	Acute treatment: oral dosing Hepatic metabolism with enterohepatic circulation $t_{1/2}$ is 14–22 days	Gastro-intestinal disturbances are common (up to 50% of cases) CNS – hallucinations, psychosis, fits	Not used in pregnancy or in patients with neuropsychiatric disorders Do not use in patients with renal or hepatic dysfunction Potentiates bradycardia of beta-blockers and quinine potentiates its toxicity
Halofantrine	Used for only uncomplicated chloroquine-resistant *P. falciparum* Schizonticidal in the blood	Acute treatment: oral dosing Food improves absorption. $t_{1/2}$ is 1–2 days. Hepatic metabolism to an active metabolite	Gastro-intestinal disturbances; less common than with mefloquine Pruritus Prolongs the QTc Hepatitis. CNS – neuromuscular spasm	Embryotoxic in animals – not used in pregnancy Cross-resistance with mefloquine may occur

8-AMINOQUINOLINES (PRIMAQUINE)

Primaquine is used to eradicate the hepatic forms of *P. vivax* or *P. malariae* after standard chloroquine therapy, provided that the risk of re-exposure is low. It may also be used prophylactically with **chloroquine**. It interferes with the organism's mitochondrial electron transport chain. Gastro-intestinal absorption is good and it is rapidly metabolized, with a mean $t_{1/2}$ of six hours. Its major adverse effects are gastro-intestinal upsets, methaemoglobinaemia and haemolytic anaemia in G6PD-deficient individuals.

ARTENUSATE AND ARTEMETHER

Uses

Artemisinin (derived from the weed Quin Hao, *Artemesia annua*) is a sesquiterpene lactone endoperoxide. It has been used in China for at least 2000 years. **Artenusate** and **artemether** are semi-synthetic derivatives of artemisinin and are effective and well-tolerated antimalarials. They should not be used as monotherapy or for prophylaxis because of the risk of resistance developing. In many developed countries, artemisinin derivatives are not yet licensed and can only be used on a named-patient basis. Currently, there is no clinical evidence of resistance to artemesinin derivatives. Treatment can be started i.v. and switched to oral with adjunctive **doxycycline** or **clindamycin** as with **quinine**.

Mechanism of action

Artemesinins undergo haem-mediated decomposition of the endoperoxide bridge to yield carbon-centred free radicals. The involvement of haem explains why they are selectively toxic to malaria parasites. The resulting carbon-centred free radicals alkylate haem and proteins, particularly in the membranes of the parasite's food vacuole and mitochondria, causing rapid death.

Adverse effects

Side effects are mild and include the following:

- nausea, vomiting and anorexia;
- dizziness.

Preclinical toxicology suggested neuro-, hepato- and bone marrow toxicity.

Pharmacokinetics

Oral absorption is fair ($F = 0.3$). **Artenusate** and **artemether** reach peak plasma concentration in minutes and two to six hours, respectively. Both are extensively metabolized to dihydroartemesinin (active metabolite) which has a half-life of one to two hours. They autoinduce their CYP450 catalysed metabolism. Drug–drug interactions are still being elucidated.

ANTI-FOLATES (DAPSONE PROGUANIL, PYRIMETHAMINE)

Combinations of these drugs are taken orally in malaria prophylaxis, but their efficacy in acute malaria treatment is limited due to resistance. These agents inhibit folate biosynthesis at all stages of the malaria parasite's life cycle, acting as competitive inhibitors of the malarial dihydropteroate synthase (**dapsone**) or the malarial dihydrofolate reductase (**proguanil** or **pyrimethamine**). They exhibit typical anti-folate adverse effect profiles (gastro-intestinal upsets, skin rashes, myelosuppression; see Chapters 43 and 46).

TREATMENT OF A MALARIA RELAPSE

Plasmodium falciparum does not cause a relapsing illness after treating the acute attack with schizonticides, because there is no persistent liver stage of the parasite. Infections with *P. malariae* can cause recurrent attacks of fever for up to 30 years, but standard treatment with **chloroquine** eradicates the parasite. Following treatment of an acute attack of vivax malaria with schizonticides, or a period of protection with prophylactic drugs, febrile illness can recur. Such relapsing illness can be prevented (or treated) by eradicating the parasites in the liver with **primaquine**, as described above. **Proguanil hydrochloride** administered continuously for three years, in order to suppress the parasites and allow time for the hepatic stages to die out naturally, is a useful alternative for patients with G6PD deficiency.

Key points

Treatment of acute malaria

- If the infective species is not known or is mixed, initial therapy is with intravenous quinine or mefloquine.
- *P. falciparum* is mainly resistant to chloroquine; treat with quinine, mefloquine or halofantrine.
- Benign malaria (caused by *P. malariae*) is treated with chloroquine alone.
- Benign malaria due to *P. ovale* or *P. vivax* requires chloroquine therapy plus primaquine to achieve a radical cure and prevent relapse.
- Careful attention to hydration and blood glucose is necessary.
- Anticipate complications and monitor the patient frequently.

TRYPANOSOMAL INFECTION

African sleeping sickness is caused by *Trypanosoma gambiense* and *T. rhodesiense*. The insect vector is the *Glossina* (tsetse) fly. Drugs used in antitrypanosomal therapy include:

- those active in blood and peripheral tissues: **melarsoprol, pentamidine, suramin** and **trimelarsan**;
- those active in the central nervous system: **tryparsamide** and **melarsoprol**.

Table 47.2 summarizes the drugs used to treat trypanosomal and other non-malarial protozoan infections.

HELMINTHIC INFECTION

Table 47.3 summarizes the primary drugs used to treat common helminthic infections.

Table 47.2: Drug therapy of non-malarial protozoan infections

Protozoan species	Drug therapy	Additional comments
Trichomonas vaginalis	Metronidazole or tinidazole	The most common protozoan infection. Treat the patient and their sexual partner
T. cruzi (American)	Benznidazole or nifurtimox	Effective in the early acute stages
T. gambiense and *T. rhodesiense* (African)	Pentamidine and suramin are effective in the early stages	Later neurological disease – melarsoprol or eflornithine or nifurtimox
Toxoplasma gondii	Pyrimethamine/sulfadiazine	Add folinic acid to reduce risk of bone marrow suppression
Pneumocystis carinii	Sulfamethoxazole/trimethoprim – high dose	Alternatives: pentamidine, atovaquone, see Chapter 46
Leishmania (visceral)	Sodium stibogluconate or meglumine antimoniate	Resistant cases – add allopurinol plus pentamidine with or without amphotericin B
Leishmania (cutaneous)	Intralesional – antimonials	Lesions usually heal spontaneously
Giardia lamblia	Metronidazole or tinidazole	Treat family and institutional contacts

Table 47.3: Drug therapy for common helminthic infections

Helminthic species	Drug therapy	Comment
Tapeworms		
Taenia saginata	Praziquantel or niclosamide or gastrograffin	A single dose of praziquantel is curative
Cysticercosis		
Taenia solium	Praziquantel or gastrograffin	
Diphyllobothrium latum	Praziquantel or niclosamide or gastrograffin	
Hydatid disease		
Echinococcus granulosus	Albendazole or mebendazole	Surgery for operably treatable cysts
Hookworm		
Ancylostoma duodenale	Mebendazole/albendazole, bephenium or pyrantel pamoate	
Necator americanus		
Strongyloides stercoralis	Albendazole	
Threadworm		
Enterobius vermicularis	Mebendazole/albendazole, bephenium or pyrantel pamoate	
Whipworm		
Trichuris trichiuria	Thiabendazole	
Tissue nematodes		
Ancylostoma braziliensae	Thiabendazole	
Guinea worm		
Dracunculus medinensis	Metronidazole	Symptoms quickly relieved
Visceral larvae/roundworms		
Toxocara canis	Diethylcarbamazine	Progressively increasing dose, allergic reactions to dying larvae, glucocorticosteroids required for ocular disease
Toxocara catis		

(continued)

Table 47.3: Continued

Helminthic species	Drug therapy	Comment
Lymphatic filariasis		
Wuchteria bancrofti	Diethylcarbamazine	
Onchocerciasis		
Onchocerca volvulus	Ivermectin	Single dose is curative
Schistosomiasis/blood flukes		
Schistosoma mansoni	Praziquantel	Oxamiquine (*S. mansoni*)
Schistosoma japonicum		
Schistosoma hematobium		Metriphonate (*S. hematobium*)
Liver flukes/fascioliasis		
Fasciola hepatica, etc.	Praziquantel	
Other gut nematodes		
Ascariasis		
Ascaris lumbricoides	Pyrantel pamoate or levamisole	
Trichinosis		
Trichinella spiralis	Mebendazole, albendazole or pyrantel pamoate	

Case history

A 27-year-old male student goes on elective medical internship at a rural hospital in West Africa. He is taking malaria prophylaxis with chloroquine 250 mg weekly, and proguanil 200 mg daily. Two weeks after arriving at his destination he complains of lethargy, breathlessness on exertion, ankle swelling and paraesthesiae in his hands. He is seen by a physician's assistant who gives him some iron tablets as he looks pale and investigations show a haemoglobin level of 6.8 g/dL with 5% reticulocytes.

Question

What is the underlying problem here that has not been completely defined? How should he be further managed?

Answer

This patient has a significant haemolytic anaemia, which is of recent onset and is thus most likely to be due to his treatment with prophylactic antimalarial drugs. He was tested for glucose-6-phosphate dehydrogenase (G6PD) deficiency and found to have a low activity of this enzyme in his red cells. The lack of this enzyme often only becomes clinically manifest when the red cell is stressed, as in the presence of an oxidant such as chloroquine (other common drugs that precipitate haemolysis include primaquine, dapsone, sulphonamides, the 4-quinolones, nalidixic acid and ciprofloxacin, nitrofurantoin, aspirin and quinidine). The patient's erythrocytes cannot handle the increased oxidation stress and cannot utilize the hexose monophosphate shunt to synthesize NAPDH in order to reduce oxidized glutathione (which is the only way to achieve this in red cells) and are thus damaged by excessive redox stress. The patient should be asked whether anyone in his family has ever experienced a similar condition, as it is inherited as an X-linked defect. Patients whose ethnic origins are from Africa, Asia, southern Europe (Mediterranean) and Oceania are more commonly affected. Stopping the chloroquine and treating with folate and iron should improve the anaemia and symptoms. The patient should be warned about other drugs that can precipitate G6PD deficiency-related haemolysis and advised to inform his physician that he has this condition. He should also carry a card or bracelet that bears this information.

FURTHER READING

Bradley DJ, Bannister B, on behalf of the Health Protection Agency Advisory Committee on Malaria Prevention for UK Travellers. Guidelines for malaria prevention in travellers from the United Kingdom for 2003. *Communicable Diseases and Public Health* 2003; **6**: 180–99.

Liu LX, Weller PF. Antiparasitic drugs. *New England Journal of Medicine* 1996; **334**: 1178–84.

Molyneux M, Fox R. Diagnosis and treatment of malaria in Britain. *British Medical Journal* 1993; **306**: 1175–80.

Pasvol G. The treatment of complicated and severe malaria. *British Medical Bulletin* 2006; **75**: 29–47.

White NJ. The treatment of malaria. *New England Journal of Medicine* 1996; **335**: 800–6.

Zuckerman JN. Preventing malaria in UK travellers. *British Medical Journal* 2004; **329**: 305–6.

CANCER CHEMOTHERAPY

INTRODUCTION

In 2004, there were approximately 153 000 deaths from cancer in the UK. Malignant disease needs a multidisciplinary approach. In addition to surgery, radiotherapy and chemotherapy, attention to psychiatric and social factors is also essential. Accurate staging is important and where disease remains localized cure, using surgery or radiotherapy, may be possible. In some cases, chemotherapy is given following surgery in the knowledge that widespread microscopic dissemination almost certainly has occurred (this is termed 'adjuvant chemotherapy'). If the tumour is widespread at presentation, systemic chemotherapy is more likely to be effective than radiotherapy or surgery, although these may be used to control local disease or reduce the tumour burden before potentially curative chemotherapy.

PATHOPHYSIOLOGY OF NEOPLASTIC CELL GROWTH

Clones of neoplastic cells expand, invade adjacent tissue and metastasize via the bloodstream or lymphatics. Pathogenesis depends on both environmental (e.g. exposure to carcinogens) and genetic factors which derange the molecular mechanisms that control cell proliferation. The hallmarks of a malignant cell are autonomous growth signalling coupled with insensitivity to anti-growth signals, immortalization, invasion and metastasis, evasion of apoptosis, sustained angiogenesis and DNA instability. In approximately 50% of human cancers, genetic mutations contribute to the neoplastic transformation. Some cancer cells overexpress oncogenes (first identified in viruses that caused sarcomas in poultry). Oncogenes encode growth factors and mitogenic factors that regulate cell cycle progression and cell growth. Alternatively, neoplastic cells may overexpress growth factor receptors, or underexpress proteins (e.g. wild-type p53 and the retinoblastoma protein-Rb) coded by tumour suppressor genes that inhibit cellular proliferation. The overall effect of such genetic and environmental factors is to shift the normal balance to dysregulated cell proliferation. Unlike normal adult somatic cells, neoplastic cells are immortal and do not have a programmed finite number of cell divisions before they become senescent. The element of cell replication responsible for this programme is the telomere, located at the end of each chromosome. Telomeres pair and align at mitosis. Telomeres are produced and maintained by telomerase in germ cells and embryonic cells. Telomerase loses its function in the course of normal cell development and differentiation. In healthy somatic cells, a component of the telomere is lost with each cell division, and such telomeric shortening functions as an intrinsic cellular clock. Approximately 95% of cancer cells re-express telomerase, allowing them to proliferate endlessly.

Many drugs used to treat cancer interfere with synthesis of DNA and/or RNA, or the synthesis and/or function of cell cycle regulatory molecules, resulting in cell death (due to direct cytotoxicity or to programmed cell death – apoptosis) or inhibition of cell proliferation. These drug effects are not confined to malignant cells, and many anti-cancer agents are also toxic to normal dividing cells, particularly those in the bone marrow, gastrointestinal tract, gonads, skin and hair follicles. The newest, so-called 'molecularly targeted', anti-cancer agents target ligands or receptors or pivotal molecules in signal transduction pathways involved in cell proliferation, angiogenesis or apoptosis.

Key points
Principal properties of neoplastic cells
<ul><li>Abnormal growth with self-sufficient growth signalling and insensitivity to anti-growth signals</li><li>Immortalization</li><li>Invasion and metastasis</li><li>Evasion of apoptosis</li><li>Sustained angiogenesis</li><li>DNA instability.</li></ul>

CYTOTOXIC THERAPY: GENERAL PRINCIPLES

The number of cytotoxic drugs available has expanded rapidly and their cellular and biochemical effects are now better defined, facilitating rational drug combinations. This has been crucial in

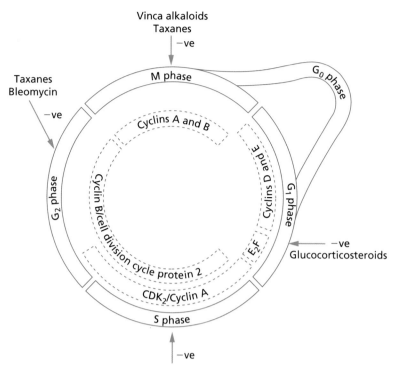

Vinca alkaloids
Taxanes
−ve

Taxanes
Bleomycin
−ve

−ve
Glucocorticosteroids

−ve

Antimetabolites (6-MP, MTX, 5-fluorouracil, etc.)
Topoisomerase inhibitors (I/II) – Anthracyclines, camptothecins, etoposide

Figure 48.1: The cell cycle regulatory systems and sites of drug actions. 6-MP, 6-mercaptopurine; MTX, methotrexate.

several malignancies, especially lymphomas and leukaemias. There are two main groups of cytotoxic drugs, classified by their effects on cell progression through the cell cycle (see Figure 48.1).

CELL CYCLE PHASE-NON-SPECIFIC DRUGS

These drugs act at all stages of proliferation, but not in the G_0-resting phase. Because of this, their dose–cytotoxicity relationships follow first-order kinetics (cells are killed exponentially with increasing dose). The linear relationship between dose and log cytotoxicity (Figure 48.2a) is exploited in the use of high-dose chemotherapy. Cytotoxic drugs are given at very high doses over a short period, thus rendering the bone marrow aplastic, but at the same time achieving a very high tumour cell kill. Clinical efficacy has been established in haematological malignancies (e.g. leukaemias, lymphomas) using such agents. Alkylating agents are examples of cycle-non-specific drugs (e.g. **cyclophosphamide**, **melphalan**) as are nitrosoureas (e.g. **cis-chloroethylnitrosourea (CCNU)**, **lomustine** and **bis-chloroethylnitrosourea (BCNU)**, **carmustine**).

CELL CYCLE PHASE-SPECIFIC DRUGS

These drugs act only at a specific phase in the cell cycle. Therefore, the more rapid the cell turnover, the more effective they are. Their dose–cytotoxicity curve is initially exponential, but at higher doses the response approaches a maximum (see Figure 48.2b). Table 48.1 classifies the commonly used cytotoxic drugs according to their effect on the cell cycle. Until the kinetic behaviour of human tumours can be adequately characterized in individual patients the value of this classification is limited. The distinction between cell cycle phase-non-specific and phase-specific drugs, although clear-cut in animal and in vitro experiments, is also probably an over-simplification.

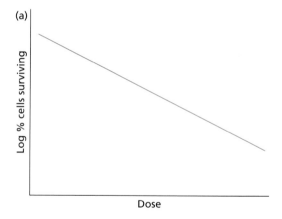

(a)

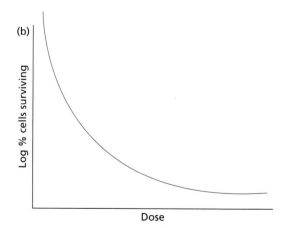

(b)

Figure 48.2: The dose–response relationship (a) for a cell cycle phase-non-specific drug and (b) for a cell cycle phase-specific drug.

Table 48.1: Classification of common traditional cytotoxic drugs according to their effect on the cell cycle

Predominantly cell cycle phase-non-specific	Predominantly cell cycle phase-specific
Actinomycin D	Etoposide
Busulfan	5-Fluorouracil
Carmustine (BCNU)	Camptothecins – irinotecan
Chlorambucil	Capecitabine
Cyclophosphamide	Cytosine arabinoside
Dacarbazine (DTIC)	Gemcitabine
Daunomycin	Methotrexate (MTX)
Doxorubicin	6-Mercaptopurine (6-MP)
Ifosfamide	Taxanes –
Lomustine (CCNU)	paclitaxel/docetaxel
Melphalan	6-tioguanine
Mitomycin C	Vinca alkaloids
Mitoxantrone	
Nitrogen mustard	

CCNU, cis-chloroethylnitrosourea; BCNU, bis-chloroethylnitrosourea.

Cytotoxic cancer chemotherapy is primarily used to induce and maintain a remission or tumour response according to the following general principles. It often entails complex regimens of two to four drugs, including pulsed doses of a cytotoxic agent with daily treatment with agents with different kinds of actions. Knowing the details of such regimens is not expected of undergraduate students and graduate trainees in oncology will refer to advanced texts for this information.

- Drugs are used in combination to increase efficacy, to inhibit the development of resistance and to minimize toxicity.
- Drugs that produce a high fraction cell kill are preferred.
- Drugs are usually given intermittently, but in high doses. This is less immunosuppressive and generally more effective than continuous low-dose regimens.
- Toxicity is considerable and frequent blood counts and intensive clinical support are essential.
- Treatment may be prolonged (for six months or longer) and subsequent cycles of consolidation or for relapsed disease may be needed.

Key points

Principles of cytotoxic chemotherapy

- Cytotoxic drugs kill a constant percentage of cells – not a constant number.
- Cells have discrete periods of the cell cycle during which they are sensitive to cytotoxic drugs.
- Cancer chemotherapy slows progression through the cell cycle.
- Cytotoxic drugs are not totally selective in their toxicity to cancer cells.
- Cell cytotoxicity is proportional to total drug exposure.
- Cytotoxic drugs should be used in combination.

Key points

Combination chemotherapy

- Develop combinations in which the drugs have:
  - individual antineoplastic actions;
  - non-overlapping toxicities;
  - different mechanisms of cytotoxic effects.
- The dose and schedule used must be optimized.
- Combination therapy is better than single drug therapy because:
  - there is improved cell cytotoxicity;
  - heterogeneous tumour cell populations are killed;
  - it reduces the development of resistance.

RESISTANCE TO CYTOTOXIC DRUGS

Drug resistance may be primary (i.e. a non-responsive tumour) or acquired. Acquired tumour drug resistance results from the selection of resistant clones as a result of killing susceptible cells or from an adaptive change in the neoplastic cell. The major mechanisms of human tumour drug resistance are summarized in Table 48.2. The ability to predict the sensitivity of bacterial pathogens to antimicrobial substances in vitro produced a profound change in the efficacy of treatment of infectious diseases. The development of analogous predictive tests has long been a priority in cancer research. Such tests would be desirable because, in contrast to antimicrobial drugs, anticancer agents are administered in doses that produce toxic effects in most patients. Unfortunately, currently, clinically useful predictive drug sensitivity assays against tumours do not exist.

COMMON COMPLICATIONS OF CANCER CHEMOTHERAPY

Chemotherapeutic drugs vary in adverse effects and there is considerable inter-patient variation in susceptibility. The most frequent adverse effects of cytotoxic chemotherapy are summarized in Table 48.3.

NAUSEA AND VOMITING

Cytotoxic drugs cause nausea and vomiting to varying degrees (see Table 48.4). This is usually delayed for one to two hours after drug administration and may last for 24–48 hours or even be delayed for 48–96 hours after therapy. The mechanisms of chemotherapy-induced vomiting include stimulation of the chemoreceptor trigger zone (in the floor of the fourth ventricle) and release of serotonin in the gastrointestinal tract – stimulating 5-HT$_3$ receptors which also stimulate vagal afferents leading to gastric atony and inhibition of peristalsis.

Table 48.2: Multiple mechanisms of acquired tumour drug resistance

Mechanism	Examples
1. Reduced intracellular drug concentration	
(i) increased drug efflux (MDR-1, Pgp and related proteins)	Anthracyclines (e.g. doxorubicin), vinca alkaloids (e.g. vincristine), taxanes (paclitaxel), podophyllotoxins (etoposide)
(ii) decreased inward transport	Antimetabolites – methotrexate, nitrogen mustards
2. Deletion of enzyme to activate drug	Cytosine arabinoside; 5-fluorouracil
3. Increased detoxification of drug	6-Mercaptopurine, alkylating agents
4. Increased concentration of target enzyme	Methotrexate, hydroxyurea
5. Decreased requirement for specific metabolic product	L-Asparaginase
6. Increased utilization of alternative pathway	Antimetabolites (e.g. 5-fluorouracil)
7. Rapid repair of drug-induced lesion	Alkylating agents (e.g. mustine, cyclophosphamide and cisplatin)
8. Decreased number of receptors for drug	Hormones, glucocorticosteroids

Table 48.3: Common adverse effects of cytotoxic chemotherapy

Immediate	Delayed
1. Nausea and vomiting	1. Bone-marrow suppression predisposing to infection, bleeding and anaemia
2. Extravasation with tissue necrosis	2. Alopecia
3. Hypersensitivity reactions	3. Agent-specific organ toxicity (e.g. nervous system – peripheral neuropathy with vinca alkaloids, taxanes)
	4. Psychiatric morbidity and cognitive impairment
	5. Infertility/teratogenicity
	6. Second malignancy

Sometimes vomiting may be anticipatory and this may be minimized by treatment with benzodiazepines. It is often routine to use two- or three-drug combinations as prophylactic anti-emetic therapy (e.g. glucocorticosteroids + 5HT₃

Table 48.4: Emetogenic potential of commonly used cytotoxic drugs

Severe	Moderate	Low
Doxorubicin	Lomustine, carmustine	Bleomycin
Cyclophosphamide (high dose)	Mitomycin C	Cytarabine
Dacarbazine	Procarbazine	Vinca alkaloids
Mustine	Etoposide	Methotrexate
Cisplatin	Ifosfamide	5-Fluorouracil
	Taxanes	Chlorambucil
	Camptothecins	Mitozantrone

antagonists + NK1 antagonist; see Chapter 34) which are tailored to the emetogenic potential of the chemotherapy to be administered. It may also be necessary to give the patient a supply of as-needed medication for the days after chemotherapy. No prophylactic anti-emetic treatment is 100% effective, especially for **cisplatin**-induced vomiting.

EXTRAVASATION WITH TISSUE NECROSIS

Tissue necrosis, which may be severe enough to require skin grafting, occurs with extravasation of the following drugs: **doxorubicin**, **BCNU**, **mustine**, vinca alkaloids and **paclitaxel**. Careful attention to the correct intraluminal location of vascular catheters for intravenous cytotoxic drug administration is mandatory.

BONE MARROW SUPPRESSION

There are two patterns of bone marrow recovery after suppression (see Figure 48.3), namely rapid and delayed. The usual pattern is of rapid recovery, but **chlorambucil**, **BCNU**, **CCNU**, **melphalan** and **mitomycin** can cause prolonged myelosuppression (for six to eight weeks). Support with blood products (red cells and platelet concentrates) and early antibiotic treatment (see below) is crucial to chemotherapy, since aplasia is an anticipated effect of many effective regimens. The availability and use of recombinant haematopoietic growth factors (erythropoietin (Epo), granulocyte colony-stimulating factor (G-CSF), granulocyte macrophage colony-stimulating factor (GM-CSF)), to minimize the bone marrow suppression caused by various chemotherapeutic regimens is a clear-cut advance in supportive care for patients undergoing cancer chemotherapy. In the future, the availability of additional haematopoietic growth factors, e.g. **interleukin-3** (IL-3), **thrombopoietin** (Tpo) and **interleukin-11**, may further enhance the ability to minimize cytotoxic induced bone marrow suppression. **Vincristine**, **bleomycin**, glucocorticosteroids and several of the recently developed molecularly

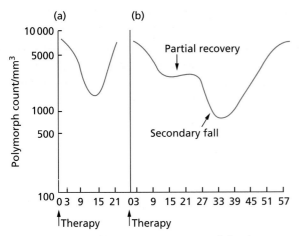

Figure 48.3: Patterns of bone marrow recovery following cytotoxic therapy: (a) rapid (17–21 days) and (b) delayed (initial fall 8–10 days, secondary nadir at 27–32 days, recovery 42–50 days) (after DE Bergasagel).

targeted (e.g. **sunitinib**, **trastuzumab**) therapies seldom cause myelosuppression.

INFECTION

Infection is a common and life-threatening complication of chemotherapy. It is often acquired from the patient's own gastro-intestinal tract flora. Effective isolation is achieved in purpose-built laminar-airflow units, but this does not solve the problem of the patient's own bacterial flora. Classical signs of infection – other than pyrexia – are often absent in neutropenic patients, and constant vigilance is required to detect and treat septicaemia early. Broad-spectrum antibiotic treatment must be started empirically in febrile neutropenic patients before the results of blood and other cultures are available. Combination therapy with an aminoglycoside active against *Pseudomonas* and other Gram-negative organisms (e.g. **tobramycin**, **netilmicin** or **amikacin**) plus a broad-spectrum ureidopenicillin (e.g. **piperacillin**) may be used. Alternatively, monotherapy with a third- or fourth-generation cephalosporin active against β-lactamase-producing organisms (e.g. **ceftazidime**, **cefotaxime** or **cefipime**) can provide suitable empiric coverage. Therapeutic decisions need to be guided by knowledge of local organisms, the patient's previous antimicrobial therapy and culture results (see Chapter 43). Opportunistic infections with fungi or protozoa (e.g. *Pneumocystis carinii*) can occur; details of the treatment for such infections are to be found in Chapters 43, 45 and 46.

ALOPECIA

Doxorubicin, **ifosfamide**, parenteral **etoposide**, camptothecins, anti-metabolites, vinca alkaloids and taxanes all commonly cause alopecia. This may be ameliorated in the case of **doxorubicin** by cooling the scalp with, for example, ice-cooled water caps. Some hair loss occurs with many cytotoxic agents.

INFERTILITY AND TERATOGENESIS

Cytotoxic drugs predictably impair fertility and cause fetal abnormalities. Most women develop amenorrhoea if treated with cytotoxic drugs. However, many resume normal menstruation when treatment is stopped and pregnancy is then possible, especially in younger women who are treated with lower total doses of cytotoxic drugs. In men, a full course of cytotoxic drugs usually produces azoospermia. Alkylating agents are particularly harmful. Recovery can occur after several years. Sperm storage before chemotherapy can be considered for males who wish to have children in the future. Reproductively active men and women must be advised to use appropriate contraceptive measures during chemotherapy, as a reduction in fertility with these drugs is not universal and fetal malformations could ensue. It is best to avoid conception for at least six months after completion of cytotoxic chemotherapy.

SECOND MALIGNANCY

Up to 3–10% of patients treated for Hodgkin's disease (particularly those who received both chemotherapy and radiation therapy) develop a second malignancy, usually acute non-lymphocytic leukaemia. This malignancy is also approximately 20 times more likely to develop in patients with ovarian carcinoma treated with alkylating agents with or without radiotherapy. This delayed treatment complication is likely to increase in prevalence as the number of patients who survive after successful cancer chemotherapy increases.

Key points

Adverse effects of cytotoxic chemotherapy

- *Immediate effects*:
  - nausea and vomiting (e.g. cisplatin, cyclophosphamide);
  - drug extravasation (e.g. vinca alkaloids, anthracyclines, e.g. doxorubicin).
- *Delayed effects*:
  - bone marrow suppression – all drugs;
  - infection;
  - alopecia;
  - drug-specific organ toxicities (e.g. skin and pulmonary – bleomycin; cardiotoxicity – doxorubicin);
  - psychiatric-cognitive morbidity;
  - teratogenesis.
- *Late effects*:
  - gonadal failure/dysfunction;
  - leukaemogenesis/myelodysplasia;
  - development of secondary cancer.

DRUGS USED IN CANCER CHEMOTHERAPY

These include the following:

1. alkylating agents;
2. antimetabolites;

3. DNA-binding agents;
4. topoisomerase inhibitors;
5. microtubular inhibitors (vinca alkaloids and taxanes);
6. molecularly targeted agents; small molecules and monoclonal antibodies;
7. hormones;
8. biological response modifiers.

ALKYLATING AGENTS

Alkylating agents are particularly effective when cells are dividing rapidly, but are not phase-specific. They combine with DNA and thus damage malignant and dividing normal cells (see Table 48.5). If a tumour is sensitive to one alkylating agent, it is usually sensitive to another, but cross-resistance does not necessarily occur. The pharmacokinetic properties of the different drugs are probably important in this respect. For example, although most alkylating agents diffuse passively into cells, **mustine** is actively transported by some cells.

MUSTINE (MECHLORETHAMINE)

Uses

Mustine is used in combination cytotoxic regimes (e.g. in refractory Hodgkin's disease).

Mechanism of action

Mustine forms highly reactive ethyleneimine ions that alkylate and cross-link guanine bases in DNA (Figure 48.4) and alkylate other macromolecules, including proteins.

Adverse effects

Adverse effects are listed in Table 48.5.

Pharmacokinetics

Mustine is given intravenously. The reactive ethyleneimine ion forms spontaneously due to cyclization in solution. The plasma $t_{1/2}$ is approximately 30 minutes.

Other oral agents in this class of nitrogen mustards include **carmustine** (BCNU) and **lomustine** (CCNU).

CYCLOPHOSPHAMIDE

Uses

Cyclophosphamide is an oxazaphosphorine alkylating agent (**ifosfamide** is another). It is an inactive prodrug given orally or intravenously. Several combination cytotoxic regimens include **cyclophosphamide**. Very high marrow ablative

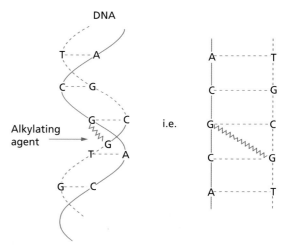

Figure 48.4: Mechanism of intramolecular bridging of DNA by alkylating agents. A, adenine; C, cytosine; G, guanine; T, thymidine.

Table 48.5: Comparative pharmacology of classical alkylating agents

Drug	Route of administration	Nausea and vomiting	Granulocytopenia	Thrombocytopenia	Special toxicity
Mustine	i.v.	+++	+++	+++	Tissue necrosis if extravasated
Cyclophosphamide	Oral/i.v.	++	+++	+	Alopecia (10–20%)
					Chemical cystitis (reduced by mesna)
					Mucosal ulceration
					Impaired water excretion
					Interstitial pulmonary fibrosis
Ifosfamide	i.v.	++	++	+	Chemical cystitis (reduced by mesna)
					Alopecia
Chlorambucil	Oral	+	++	++++	Bone marrow suppression
Melphalan	Oral	0	+++	+++	Chemical cystitis (very rare)
Busulfan	Oral	0	++++	+++	Skin pigmentation
					Interstitial pulmonary fibrosis
					Amenorrhoea
					Gynaecomastia (rare)

doses are used to prepare patients with acute leukaemia or aplastic anaemia for allogeneic bone marrow transplantation. **Cyclophosphamide** is highly effective in treating various lymphomas, leukaemias and myeloma, but also has some use in other solid tumours. It is an effective immunosuppressant (Chapter 50).

Adverse effects

Adverse effects are listed in Table 48.5.

Pharmacokinetics

Cyclophosphamide undergoes metabolic activation in the liver via CYP2B6 and chronic use autoinduces the metabolic activation to cytotoxic alkylating metabolites, the most potent of which is the short-lived phosphoramide mustard. Absorption from the gastro-intestinal tract is excellent (essentially 100% bioavailabilty). **Cyclophosphamide** and its metabolites are excreted in the urine. Renal excretion of one of its metabolites, acrolein, causes the haemorrhagic cystitis that accompanies high-dose therapy.

MESNA (UROPROTECTION AGENT)

Use

Mesna (2-mercaptoethane sulphonate) is solely used to protect the urinary tract against the urotoxic metabolites of **cyclophosphamide** and **ifosfamide**. **Mesna** is given by intravenous injection or by mouth. Because **mesna** is excreted more rapidly ($t_{1/2}$ is 30 minutes) than **cyclophosphamide** and **ifosfamide**, it is important that it is given at the initiation of treatment, and that the dosing interval is no more than four hours. The **mesna** dose and schedule vary with the dose of **cyclophosphamide** or **ifosfamide**. Urine is monitored for volume, proteinuria and haematuria. The side effects of **mesna** include headache, somnolence and rarely rashes.

Mechanism of action

Mesna protects the uro-epithelium by reacting with acrolein in the renal tubule to form a stable, non-toxic thioether.

OTHER ALKYLATING AGENTS

PROCARBAZINE

Uses

Procarbazine, a hydrazine, is a component of combination therapy for Hodgkin's disease and brain tumours. **Procarbazine** is given daily by mouth. The other agent in this class is **dacarbazine**.

Mechanism of action

Procarbazine is activated in the liver by CYP450 enzymes to reactive azoxy compounds that alkylate DNA. In addition, it methylates DNA and inhibits DNA and protein synthesis.

Adverse effects

These include the following:

- dose-related haematopoietic suppression, leukopenia and thrombocytopenia at 10–14 days after treatment;
- nausea and vomiting.

Pharmacokinetics

Procarbazine is well absorbed. The plasma $t_{1/2}$ is approximately ten minutes. **Procarbazine** and its metabolites penetrate the blood–brain barrier. It is converted to active metabolites in the liver (see above); these are excreted by the kidneys.

Drug interactions

Procarbazine blocks aldehyde dehydrogenase (for comparison see **disulfiram**, Chapter 53) and consequently causes flushing and tachycardia if **ethanol** is taken concomitantly. It is also a weak monoamine oxidase inhibitor and may precipitate a hypertensive crisis with tyramine-containing foods (Chapter 20).

PLATINUM COMPOUNDS

CISPLATIN

Uses

Cisplatin is an inorganic platinum (II) co-ordination complex in which two amine (NH_3) and two chlorine ligands occupy *cis* positions (the *trans* compound is inactive). **Cisplatin** is markedly effective for testicular malignancies and several other solid tumours, including carcinoma of the ovary, lung, head and neck, and bladder may also respond well. **Cisplatin** is given intravenously in combination with other cytotoxic agents. Because of the efficacy of platinum compounds and the toxicity of **cisplatin**, there has been a search for less toxic analogues, yielding **carboplatin** and **oxaliplatin**. The comparative pharmacology of **carboplatin** and **oxaliplatin** is summarized in Table 48.6.

Mechanism of action

Platinum compound cytotoxicity results from selective inhibition of tumour DNA synthesis by the formation of intra- and inter-strand cross-links at guanine residues in the nucleic acid backbone. This unwinds and shortens the DNA helix.

Adverse effects

These include the following:

- severe nausea and vomiting;
- nephrotoxicity (especially **cisplatin**) which is dose-related and dose-limiting. Prehydration and fluid diuresis reduce the immediate effects, but cumulative and permanent damage still occurs;
- hypomagnesaemia and hypokalaemia;
- ototoxicity develops in up to 30% of patients: audiometry should be carried out before, during and after treatment;

Table 48.6: Comparative pharmacology of some platinum compounds

Drug	Standard dosing regimen	Side effects	Pharmacokinetics	Additional comments
Carboplatin (CBP)	i.v. dose is calculated based on the desired AUC by the Calvert formula	Like cisplatin, but less vomiting and nephrotoxicity. Low potential for ototoxicity and neuropathy	Activation slower than cisplatin $t_{1/2}$ 2–3 h, 60–70% excreted in the urine in first 24 h	Anti-tumour spectrum similar to that of cisplatin
Oxaliplatin	i.v. administration. Bulky DACH carrier ligand. Unlike cisplatin or carboplatin	Mild bone marrow suppression. Little nephro- or ototoxicity, cf. cisplatin but cold-induced neurosensory toxicity	Biotransformed in blood. Renal and tissue elimination. Good tissue distribution due to DACH	Third generation platinum analogue. Activity profile differs from cisplatin. Ovarian, colorectal, pancreatic cancer, and mesothelioma

CDDP, cisplatin; DACH, diaminocyclohexane.

- myelosuppression – usually thrombocytopenia;
- nervous system effects – cerebellar syndrome, peripheral neuropathy.

Pharmacokinetics

Cisplatin requires the replacement of the two chloride atoms with water ('aquation') to become active. This process takes approximately 2.5 hours. Plasma disappearance of **cisplatin** is multiphasic and traces of platinum are detectable in urine months after treatment.

Drug interactions

Additive nephrotoxicity and ototoxicity occurs with aminoglycosides or **amphotericin**.

ANTIMETABOLITES

Antimetabolites are structural analogues of, and compete with, endogenous nucleic acid precursors. Unfortunately, the pathways blocked by antimetabolites are not specific to neoplastic cells. Thus, their selectivity for malignant cells is only partial. They act in the S-phase of the cell cycle.

ANTIFOLATE ANALOGUES
METHOTREXATE
Uses

Methotrexate is curative for choriocarcinoma, also induces remission in acute lymphocytic leukaemia and is often active in breast cancer, osteogenic sarcoma and head and neck tumours. **Methotrexate** is also an immunosuppressant (Chapters 26 and 50) and is used to inhibit cellular proliferation in severe psoriasis (Chapter 51). There are several different dosage schedules, several of which require co-administration of folinic acid (see Figure 48.5).

Mechanism of action

Folic acid is required in the synthesis of thymidylate (a pyrimidine) and of purine nucleotides and thus for DNA synthesis (Figure 48.5). **Methotrexate** is a very slowly reversible competitive inhibitor of dihydrofolate reductase (DHFR). The affinity of DHFR for **methotrexate** is 100 000 times greater than that for dihydrofolate. Thus, **methotrexate** prevents nucleic acid synthesis and causes cell death. Folinic acid circumvents this biosynthetic block and thus non-competitively antagonizes the effect of **methotrexate**.

Determinants of methotrexate toxicity

These consist of:

- a critical extracellular concentration for each target organ;
- a critical duration of exposure that varies for each organ.

For bone marrow and gut, the critical plasma concentration is 2×10^{-8} M and the time factor is approximately 42 hours. Both factors must be exceeded for toxicity to occur in these organs. The severity of toxicity is proportional to the length of time for which the critical concentration is exceeded and is independent of the amount by which it is exceeded.

Folinic acid rescue bypasses the dihydrofolate reductase blockade and minimizes **methotrexate** toxicity. Some malignant cells are less able to take up folinic acid than normal cells, thus introducing a degree of selectivity. Rescue is commenced 24 hours after **methotrexate** administration and continued until the plasma **methotrexate** concentration falls below 5×10^{-8} M. Monitoring of the plasma **methotrexate** concentrations has improved the safe use of this drug and allows identification of patients at high risk of toxicity. If a patient develops severe toxicity with protracted elevation of **methotrexate** concentrations, **methotrexate** metabolism can be rapidly increased by administering an inactivating enzyme, namely **carboxypeptidase-G2** (not routinely available in the UK), when **methotrexate** concentrations exceed 1×10^{-7} M.

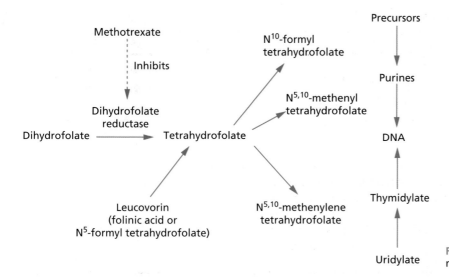

Figure 48.5: Folate metabolism: effects of methotrexate and leucovorin (folinic acid).

Adverse effects

These include the following:

- myelosuppression;
- nausea and vomiting;
- stomatitis;
- diarrhoea;
- cirrhosis – chronic low-dose administration (as for psoriasis) can cause chronic active hepatitis and cirrhosis, interstitial pneumonitis and osteoporosis;
- renal dysfunction and acute vasculitis (after high-dose treatment);
- intrathecal administration also causes special problems, including convulsions, and chemical arachnoiditis leading to paraplegia, cerebellar dysfunction and cranial nerve palsies and a chronic demyelinating encephalitis.

Renal insufficiency reduces **methotrexate** elimination and monitoring plasma **methotrexate** concentration is essential under these circumstances. Acute renal failure can be caused by tubular obstruction with crystals of **methotrexate**. Diuresis (>3 L/day) with alkalinization (pH >7) of the urine using intravenous sodium bicarbonate reduces nephrotoxicity. Renal damage is caused by the precipitation of **methotrexate** and 7-hydroxymethotrexate in the tubules, and these weak acids are more water soluble at an alkaline pH, which favours their charged form (Chapter 6).

Pharmacokinetics

Methotrexate absorption from the gut occurs via a saturable transport process, large doses being incompletely absorbed. It is also administered intravenously or intrathecally. After intravenous injection, **methotrexate** plasma concentrations decline in a triphasic manner, with prolonged terminal elimination due to enterohepatic circulation. This terminal phase is important because toxicity is related to the plasma concentrations during this phase, as well as to the peak **methotrexate** concentration. Alterations in albumin binding affect the pharmacokinetics of the drug. **Methotrexate** penetrates transcellular

water (e.g. the plasma: CSF ratio is approximately 30:1) slowly by passive diffusion. About 80–95% of a dose of **methotrexate** is renally excreted (by filtration and active tubular secretion) as unchanged drug or metabolites. It is partly metabolized by the gut flora during enterohepatic circulation. 7-Hydroxymethotrexate is produced in the liver and is pharmacologically inactive but much less soluble than **methotrexate**, and so contributes to renal toxicity by precipitation and crystalluria.

Drug interactions

- **Probenecid**, sulphonamides, salicylates and other NSAIDs increase **methotrexate** toxicity by competing for renal tubular secretion, while simultaneously displacing it from plasma albumin. Other weak acids including **furosemide** and high-dose vitamin C compete for renal secretion.
- **Gentamicin** and **cisplatin** increase the toxicity of **methotrexate** by compromising renal excretion.

PYRIMIDINE ANTIMETABOLITES

5-FLUOROURACIL

Uses

5-Fluorouracil (5-FU) is used to treat solid tumours of the breast, ovary, oesophagus, colon and skin. **5-Fluorouracil** is administered by intravenous injection. Dose reduction is required for hepatic dysfunction or in patients with a genetic deficiency of dihydropyridine dehydrogenase.

Mechanism of action

5-Fluorouracil is a prodrug that is activated by anabolic phosphorylation (Figure 48.6) to form:

- 5-fluorouridine monophosphate, which is incorporated into RNA, inhibiting its function and its polyadenylation;
- 5-fluorodeoxyuridylate, which binds strongly to thymidylate synthetase and inhibits DNA synthesis.

Incorporation of **5-fluorouracil** itself into DNA causes mismatching and faulty mRNA transcripts.

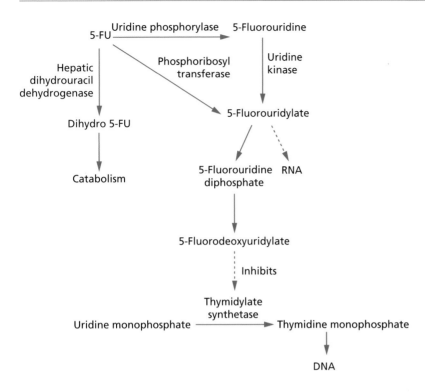

Figure 48.6: Metabolism and activation of 5-fluorouracil (5-FU).

Adverse effects

- Oral ulceration and diarrhoea is an adverse event in approximately 20% of patients.
- Bone marrow suppression – megaloblastic anaemia usually occurs about 14 days after starting treatment.
- Cerebellar ataxia (2% incidence) is attributed to **fluorocitrate**, a neurotoxic metabolite that inhibits the Krebs cycle by lethal synthesis.
- Patients with dihydropyridine dehydrogenase deficiency (enzyme activity <5% of normal) have an increased risk of severe mucositis/haematologic suppression.

Pharmacokinetics

5-Fluorouracil is given intravenously because it is variably absorbed from the gut due to high hepatic first-pass metabolism. Deactivation occurs primarily in the liver, where it is reduced to inactive products that are excreted in the urine. Only 20% is excreted unchanged in the urine.

Capecitabine, an oral prodrug, is de-esterified and deaminated to yield high concentrations of 5-deoxy fluorodeoxyuridine (5-dFdU). 5-dFdU is then converted in the liver, peripheral tissues and tumour to produce 5-FU concentrations that are about 10% of the 5-dFdU concentrations. **Capecitabine** is used to treat breast, lung and colorectal cancer and has the same toxicity profile as 5-FU.

PURINE ANTIMETABOLITES

6-MERCAPTOPURINE

Uses

6-Mercaptopurine (6-MP) is a purine antimetabolite. It is effective as part of combination therapy for acute leukaemias. It is also an immunosuppressant (Chapter 50). Other purine antimetabolites that are used clinically include **tioguanine**, **fludarabine** and **2-chlorodeoxyadenosine** [cladrabine] (see Table 48.7).

Mechanism of action

6-MP requires transformation by intracellular enzymes to 6-thioguanine which inhibits purine synthesis.

Adverse effects

These include the following:

- bone marrow suppression (macrocytosis, leukopenia and thrombocytopenia);
- mucositis;
- nausea, vomiting and diarrhoea with high doses;
- reversible cholestatic jaundice.

Pharma.cokinetics

Only approximately 15% of **6-MP** is absorbed when given orally. Thiopurine-*S*-methyltransferase (TPMT) catalyses the *S*-methylation and deactivation of thiopurines (**6-MP**, **azathioprine** and **6-thioguanine**). TPMT is deficient in one in 300 white Europeans. TPMT-deficient individuals are at very high risk of haematopoietic suppression with standard doses of **6-MP** because of the accumulation of thiopurines. Pretreatment assessment is currently the only pharmacogenetic test in routine use (Chapter 14). Xanthine oxidase also contributes appreciably to inactivation of thiopurine drugs. Approximately 20% of an intravenous dose of **6-MP** is excreted in the urine within six hours, thus renal dysfunction enhances toxicity.

Drug interactions

Allopurinol inhibits xanthine oxidase (Chapter 26). The usual dose of **6-MP** should be reduced by 75% to avoid toxicity in

Table 48.7: Summary of clinical pharmacology properties of common antimetabolites

Drug	Use	Mechanism	Side effects	Additional comments
Cytosine arabinoside (cytarabine)	Acute leukaemia (AML)	Inhibits pyrimidine synthesis and in its triphosphate form inhibits DNA polymerase	Nausea and vomiting, bone marrow suppression, mucositis, cerebellar syndrome	Short half-life, continuous infusions or daily doses intravenously or subcutaneously, dose reduced in renal dysfunction
Fludarabine	Chronic lymphocytic leukaemia (CLL)	Inhibits purine synthesis	Myelosuppression, pulmonary toxicity, CNS toxicity	Daily i.v. dosing, reduce dose in renal failure
2-Chlorodeoxy 2-chlorodeoxy adenosine (cladribine)	CLL and acute leukaemia (ANLL)	Converted to triphosphate and inhibits purine synthesis	Severe neutropenia	i.v. infusion
Gemcitabine	Pancreatic and lung cancer	Cytidine analogue – triphosphate form incorporated into DNA, blocks DNA synthesis	Haematopoietic suppression, mucositis, rashes	i.v. infusion, inactivated by cytidine deaminase, active throughout the cell cycle, dose reduced in renal dysfunction
Hydroxyurea	CML and myelo-proliferative disorders	Inhibits ribonucleotide reductase, affecting DNA and RNA synthesis	Neutropenia, nausea, skin reactions	Oral dosing, short half-life, rapidly reversible toxicity

patients who are concurrently taking **allopurinol**. This is important because **allopurinol** pretreatment is used to reduce the risk of acute uric acid nephropathy due to rapid tumour lysis syndrome in patients with leukaemia.

ANTIBIOTICS

Several antibiotics (e.g. anthracyclines, anthracenediones – **mitoxantrone**) are clinically useful antineoplastic agents (see Table 48.8).

ANTHRACYCLINES

Doxorubicin and **daunorubicin** are the most widely used drugs in this group, but newer analogues (e.g. **epirubicin**, **idarubicin**) have reduced hepatic and cardiac toxicity, and **idarubicin** may be administered orally.

DOXORUBICIN

Uses

Doxorubicin is a red antibiotic produced by *Streptomyces peucetius*. It is the most widely used drug of the anthracycline group, with proven activity in acute leukaemia, lymphomas, sarcomas and a wide range of carcinomas. Liposomal formulations of **doxorubicin** are available.

Mechanism of action

Cytotoxic actions of anthracyclines lead to apoptosis, and include:

- intercalation between adjacent base pairs in DNA, leading to fragmentation of DNA and inhibition of DNA repair, enhanced by DNA topoisomerase II inhibition;
- membrane binding alters membrane function and contributes to cardiotoxicity;
- free-radical formation also causes cardiotoxicity.

Adverse effects

These include the following:

- cardiotoxicity – acute and chronic (see below);
- bone marrow suppression with neutropenia and thrombocytopenia;
- alopecia – may be mitigated by scalp cooling;
- nausea and vomiting;
- 'radiation recall' – anthracyclines exacerbate or reactivate radiation dermatitis or pneumonitis;
- extravasation causes severe tissue necrosis.

Anthracycline cardiotoxicity

- *Acute*: this occurs shortly after administration, with the development of various dysrhythmias that are occasionally life-threatening (e.g. ventricular tachycardia, heart block). These acute effects do not predict chronic toxicity.

Table 48.8: Clinical pharmacology of antitumour antibiotics

Drug	Indications and route of administration	Side effects	Pharmacokinetics	Additional comments
Mitoxantrone	Advanced breast cancer; leukaemia and lymphoma, i.v. dosing	Nausea and vomiting, stomatitis, low incidence of cardiotoxicity (<3%)	Hepatic metabolism, extensively bound to tissues, $t_{1/2} = 20–40$ h	Intercalates into DNA and inhibits DNA topoisomerase II
Mitomycin C	Gastro-intestinal tumours, advanced breast cancer, head and neck tumours. Intravenous infusions	Vesicant cumulative toxicity, myelosuppression, interstitial alveolitis, haemolytic-uraemic syndrome	Pharmacokinetics not affected by renal or hepatic function	It is a prodrug – transformed to an alkylating intermediate; alkylates guanine residues (10% of its adducts form inter-strand breaks); synergistic with 5-FU and radiotherapy
Bleomycin	Lymphomas, testicular carcinoma and squamous cell tumours, i.v. dosing	Fever, shivering, mouth ulcers, skin erythema – pigmentation, interstitial lung disease if dose >300 units	50–70% of a dose is excreted in the urine, $t_{1/2} = 9$ h; prolonged in renal dysfunction. Also metabolized by peptidases; skin and lung have high drug concentrations as they lack peptidases	It causes single- and double-strand breaks in DNA. Arrests cells in G_2/M phase

- *Chronic*: cardiomyopathy, leading to death in up to 60% of those who develop signs of congestive cardiac failure. It is determined by the cumulative dose. Risk factors for cardiomyopathy include prior mediastinal irradiation, age over 70 years and pre-existing cardiovascular disease. Agents to protect against **anthracycline** cardiomyopathy and allow dose intensification are under investigation.

Pharmacokinetics

Doxorubicin is given intravenously. The plasma concentration–time profile shows a triphasic decline. **Doxorubicin** does not enter the central nervous system (CNS). Hepatic extraction is high, with 40% appearing in the bile (as unchanged drug and metabolites, e.g **doxorubicinol**, which has antitumour activity). Renal excretion accounts for less than 15% of a dose. Dose reduction is recommended in patients with liver disease, particularly if accompanied by hyperbilirubinaemia.

TOPOISOMERASE INHIBITORS

DNA TOPOISOMERASE I INHIBITORS

CAMPTOTHECINS

Camptothecins are alkaloids derived from a Chinese tree *Camptotheca acuminata*. **Irinotecan (CPT-11)** and **topotecan** are available for clinical use.

Uses

The camptothecins are active against a broad range of tumours, including carcinomas of the colon, lung and cervix. They are given intravenously.

Mechanism of action

Camptothecins act during the S-phase of the cell cycle. DNA topoisomerase I is necessary for unwinding DNA for replication and RNA transcription. Camptothecins stabilize the DNA topoisomerase I–DNA complex. Cell killing is most likely via induction of apoptosis (programmed cell death).

Pharmacokinetics

Irinotecan is converted to a more potent cytotoxic metabolite SN38, which is inactivated by hepatic glucuronidation (via UGT1A1, see Chapters 5 and 14). **Topotecan** is hydrolysed by the blood carboxylesterase and is excreted in the urine, requiring dose reduction in renal impairment.

Adverse effects

The principal adverse effects are myelosuppression, acute and delayed diarrhoea (particularly **irinotecan**), which can be dose limiting and require prophylactic therapy with anticholinergics (for acute diarrhoea) and **loperamide**, or treatment with **octreotide**. Other less severe side effects include alopecia and fatigue.

Table 48.9: Summary of the clinical pharmacology of the vinca alkaloids

Drug	Route	Side effects	Pharmacokinetics	Additional comments
Vincristine	i.v.	Vesicant if extravasated, reversible peripheral neuropathy, alopecia, SIADH	Hepatic metabolism (CYP3A4). $t_{1/2} = 85$ h, non-linear kinetics	
Vinblastine	i.v.	Less neurotoxic, but more myelo-suppressive than vincristine, SIADH	Hepatic metabolism (CYP3A4) – active metabolite, $t_{1/2} = 24$ h	
Vinorelbine	i.v. injection or infusion, weekly	Bone marrow suppression, SIADH	Hepatic metabolism (CYP3A4), $t_{1/2} = 30$–40 h	Refractory breast and advanced lung cancer

SIADH, syndrome of inappropriate antidiuretic hormone.

DNA TOPOISOMERASE II INHIBITORS

A component of the cytotoxic action of anthracyclines (e.g. **doxorubicin**, see above) is due to inhibition of DNA topoisomerase II. **Etoposide** and **teniposide,** synthetic derivatives of podophyllotoxin (which is extracted from the American mandrake or May apple, and is topically effective against warts), are also reversible inhibitors of topoisomerase II.

ETOPOSIDE

Uses

Etoposide is one of the most active drugs against small-cell lung cancer and is used in combination therapy. It is also used to treat lymphomas, testicular and trophoblastic tumours.

Mechanism of action

DNA topoisomerase II is a nuclear enzyme that binds to and cleaves both strands of DNA. It is necessary for DNA replication and RNA transcription. **Etoposide** stabilizes the topoisomerase II–DNA complex, leading to apoptosis, as for camptothecins.

Adverse effects

These include the following:

- nausea and vomiting;
- alopecia;
- bone marrow suppression (dose-dependent and reversible).

Pharmacokinetics

Etoposide is given by intravenous injection or orally (50% bioavailability). It undergoes hepatic metabolism (CYP3A) to inactive metabolites and a small amount is eliminated in the urine.

MICROTUBULAR INHIBITORS (VINCA ALKALOIDS AND TAXANES)

VINCA ALKALOIDS

The Madagascar periwinkle plant was the source of **vincristine** and **vinblastine**, the first agents in this class. Newer synthetic

analogues include **vinorelbine**. Despite their close structural relationship, these drugs differ in their clinical spectrum of activity and toxicity. **Vincristine** is used in breast cancer, lymphomas and the initial treatment of acute lymphoblastic leukaemia. **Vinblastine** is a component of the cytotoxic combinations used to treat testicular cancer and Hodgkin's disease. **Vinorelbine** has activity against advanced breast cancer and non-small-cell lung cancer, where it is often combined with platinum compounds.

Mechanism of action

Vinca alkaloids bind to β-tubulin, a protein that forms the microtubules which are essential for the formation of the mitotic spindle. They prevent β-tubulin polymerizing with α-tubulin and thus inhibit mitosis. Blockade of microtubular function involved in neuronal growth and axonal transport probably accounts for their neurotoxicity. Further important clinical pharmacology of vinca alkaloids is summarized in Table 48.9.

Key points

Practical 'do's and don'ts' of cytotoxic therapy

- Patients should have recovered fully from the toxic effects of the previous cycles of cytotoxic therapy before starting the next treatment cycle.
- Ensure that the dose and schedule of certain drugs is adjusted for concurrent renal and hepatic impairment.
- Avoid the concomitant use of platelet-inhibiting drugs.
- Haematopoietic growth factors (for myelosuppression) reduce the duration of the nadir neutropenia, but should not be prescribed routinely.

TAXANES

PACLITAXEL AND DOCETAXEL

Uses

Paclitaxel (Figure 48.7) was derived from the bark of the Pacific yew tree and is used as single agent or in combination therapy for the treatment of a broad range of solid tumours, including carcinoma of the lung, breast, ovary and cervix and head and neck tumours, and for lymphomas. **Paclitaxel** is given intravenously.

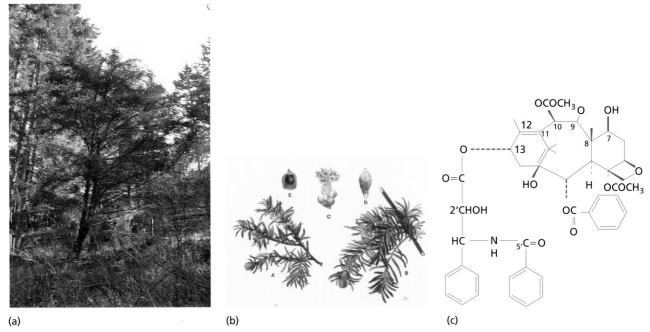

Figure 48.7: *Taxus brevifolia* (a, b), the source of paclitaxel. The chemical structure is shown in panel (c). ((a) Source: Pacific Yew (Taxus brevifolia) O'Daniel Tigner, Canadian Forest Tree Essences, provided courtesy of Tree Canada Foundation. (b) © Natural History Museum, London. Reproduced with permission.)

Mechanism of action

Paclitaxel binds to the β-subunit of tubulin and antagonizes the depolymerization of microtubules, halting mitosis. Cells are blocked in the G_2/M phase of the cell cycle and undergo apoptosis.

Adverse effects

These include the following:

- hypersensitivity reactions;
- bone marrow suppression (dose-dependent and reversible);
- myalgias and arthralgias;
- sensory peripheral neuropathy;
- cardiac dysrhythmias;
- nausea and vomiting;
- alopecia.

Pharmacokinetics

Paclitaxel is poorly absorbed orally and requires intravenous administration. It is inactivated by hepatic CYP450 and <5% of the parent drug is excreted in the urine. The dose should be reduced in hepatic dysfunction.

Docetaxel is a semi-synthetic taxane derivative with a similar anti-tumour spectrum as **paclitaxel**. It causes myelosuppression and peripheral fluid retention, but less cardio- and neurotoxicity than **paclitaxel**.

MOLECULARLY TARGETED AGENTS

This recently developed family of compounds is grouped together because they were developed to target specific molecules or cellular processes on or within the malignant cell. It is likely this heterogeneous group of compounds will grow considerably, as much research is being undertaken in tumour biology and defining targets. The agents discussed here include tyrosine kinase inhibitors (TKIs) (e.g. **imatinib**, **gefitinib** and **erlotinib**), multi-targeted TKIs (**sorafenib, sunitinib**), proteasome inhibitors (**bortezomib**) and histone deacetylase inhibitors (**vorinostat**). Several of these drugs have yet to be licensed in the UK or Europe, but it is important to be aware of them as they are important advances in what had, until recently, been a rather static area of therapeutics.

TYROSINE KINASE INHIBITORS (TKIS)

Tyrosine kinases are critical components of many signal transduction pathways. They signal from the cell membrane or cytoplasm to the nucleus-modulating DNA synthesis and gene transcription. There are approximately 500 protein tyrosine kinases coded in the human genome. They are classified into tyrosine kinases, serine-threonine kinases and tyrosine-serine-threonine kinases. The tyrosine kinases are further subdivided into non-receptor tyrosine kinases and receptor tyrosine kinases. Abnormal activity of tyrosine kinases was found in many cancers and this has proven a useful drug target (Figure 48.8).

NON-RECEPTOR TYROSINE KINASE INHIBITORS (CYTOPLASMIC TKIS)

IMATINIB

Uses

Imatinib mesylate is primarily used to treat Philadelphia-positive chronic myeloid leukaemia (CML) and gastro-intestinal stromal tumours (GIST). It is administered orally on a daily basis. Initial response rates are high, but after 12 months of therapy about 90% of CML patients develop drug-resistant clones.

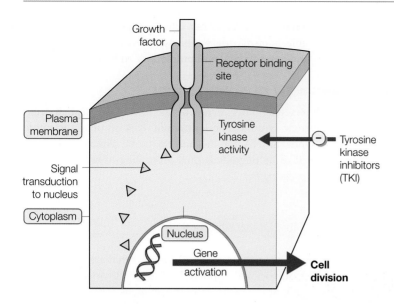

Figure 48.8: Inhibitory effect of tyrosine kinase inhibitors on cell proliferation. (Redrawn with permission from Gardiner-Caldwell communications Ltd.(©1999).)

Mechanism of action

Imatinib is an ATP mimetic. It competitively inhibits several tyrosine kinases, most potently BCR-ABL and platelet-derived growth factor receptor tyrosine kinases (IC_{50}s, 100–300 nM) and a mutated c-KIT. In CML, the BCR-ABL fusion protein is pivotal in driving cellular replication and proliferation pathways. In GIST, it is c-KIT that is overactive and drives proliferation. Inhibition of these tyrosine kinases causes the cell to undergo apoptosis.

Adverse effects

These include the following:

- nausea and vomiting;
- peripheral oedema and effusions (rare);
- leukopenia;
- skin rashes;
- hepatitis.

Pharmacokinetics

Oral absorption is very good with almost 100% bioavailabilty. **Imatinib** and its active *N*-desmethyl metabolite have a half-life of 18 and 40 hours, respectively. It is inactivated by hepatic CYP3A. The kinetics do not change with chronic dosing and little drug appears unchanged in the urine.

Drug interactions

Concurrent use of drugs that induce CYP3A (e.g. anticonvulsants, St John's wort, rifamycins) will lead to reduced drug exposure. In contrast, potent inhibitors of CYP3A (e.g. **ketoconazole**) can increase the **imatinib** AUC by 40%.

    Dasatinib (available in the USA) is another TKI. It is active against most **imatinib**-resistant BCR-ABL kinases and may be useful after **imatinib** resistance has developed. It also inhibits the Rous sarcoma virus (v-Src) kinase.

RECEPTOR TYROSINE KINASE INHIBITORS (RTKIs)

EPIDERMAL GROWTH FACTOR RECEPTOR (EGFR) TKIs

Uses

Erlotinib and **gefitinib** are used as single agents (by mouth once daily) to treat tumours (e.g. non-small cell lung cancers) which overexpress EGFR. **Erlotinib** has the best evidence of survival benefit for advanced lung cancer patients. Tumours that bear a mutation in the EGFR receptor which makes it constitutively activated may be more susceptible, but how to select patients who will benefit from treatment is still under investigation.

Mechanism of action

The EGFR receptor belongs to a family of four receptors expressed/overexpressed on certain tumours. In the non-ligand-binding domain of these receptors, there is a tyrosine kinase which phosphorylates the receptor. **Erlotinib** and **gefitinib** are ATP mimetics and are competitive inhibitors of the EGFR-1 tyrosine kinases. Inhibition of this tyrosine kinase blocks EGFR signal transduction and causes the cell to undergo apoptosis.

Adverse effects

These include the following:

- diarrhoea;
- acneiform skin rash;
- nausea and anorexia;
- hepatitis;
- pneumonitis;
- decreased cardiac contractility (EF).

Pharmacokinetics

Oral absorption is very good for **erlotinib** and **gefitinib**. Their mean elimination half-lives are 36 and 41 hours, respectively. Both **erlotinib** and **gefitinib** are metabolized by hepatic CYP3A to metabolites with little or no tyrosine kinase inhibiting activity.

Drug interactions

Concurrent use of drugs that induce CYP3A (e.g. anticonvulsants, St John's wort, rifamycins) reduces exposure to **erlotinib** and **gefitinib**, whereas use of inhibitors of CYP3A have the opposite effect.

    Multi-EGFR TKIs and irreversible EGFR TKIs are in late phase clinical development, so new agents in this group are anticipated.

MULTI-TARGETED TKIs

Sorafenib and **sunitinib** are used in the USA as single oral agents to treat advanced renal cell carcinoma.

Sorafenib increases median survival by approximately 12 months in patients with advanced refractory renal cell cancer. It is a small molecule ATP mimetic and competitive inhibitor of Raf kinase, the VEGF receptor tyrosine kinase and the platelet-derived growth factor receptor (PDGFR) tyrosine kinase. It undergoes hepatic oxidation mediated by CYP3A and glucuronidation (UGT1A1). Adverse effects include skin rash, hand–foot skin reactions, diarrhoea, hypertension and bleeding.

Sunitinib doubled the survival time of **imatinib**-resistant GIST tumours and improved survival in advanced renal cell cancer. It is a small molecule ATP mimetic and competitive inhibitor of signalling through multiple tyrosine receptor kinases, including platelet-derived growth factor receptor and vascular endothelial growth factor receptor. These kinases are important in angiogenesis. It is metabolized by CYP3A. Adverse effects include diarrhoea, hypertension, skin discoloration, mucositis, fatigue and hypothyroidism. Less frequently, neutropenia, thrombocytopenia and decreases in left ventricular ejection fraction have been noted.

PROTEASOME INHIBITORS

Bortezomib is the first member of this class. It is effective in treating refractory multiple myeloma. It is a reversible competitive inhibitor of the proteolytic function of the chymotrypsin-like activity of the 20S core subunit of the proteasome. The proteasome can be considered the cellular 'garbage can' for proteins. Proteins once ubiquitinated are destined to be degraded by the proteasome and exit the proteasome as small peptides. Proteasome inhibition affects a number of cellular functions, but a major effect is to disable IκB degradation. IκB binds to NF-κB and prevents this transcription factor moving to the nucleus, silencing NF-κB-mediated gene transcription. Additonally, proteasome inhibition disrupts the homeostasis of key regulatory proteins (p21, p27 and p53) involved in cell cycle progression and proliferation. **Bortezomib** is administered intravenously. It undergoes hepatic metabolism via CYP3A and CYP2D6. Adverse effects include thrombocytopenia, fatigue, peripheral neuropathy, neutropenia, gastrointestinal disturbances.

HISTONE DEACETYLASE INHIBITORS

Vorinostat (suberoylanilide hydroxamic acid, SAHA) is effective against refractory cutaneous T-cell lymphoma, producing a 30% response rate with a median response of 168 days. Many tumour cells overexpress histone deacetylase enzymes which deacetylate histones. **Vorinostat** inhibits these enzymes, blocking the transcription of genes involved in cell cycle progression. **Vorinostat** is administered orally. It undergoes hepatic glucuronidation and oxidation. Adverse effects include gastro-intestinal disturbances, fatigue, hyperglycaemia, hyperlipidaemia, bone marrow suppression (anaemia, thrombocytopenia and neutropenia) and pulmonary embolism.

ANTI-BCL-2 OLIGONUCLEOTIDE

Oblimersen is under review by the FDA as an 'orphan drug' for chronic lymphocytic leukaemia. It is an oligonucleotide that binds mRNA for the anti-apoptotic protein Bcl-2 and causes it to be degraded, thus promoting apoptosis in cells overexpressing Bcl-2.

MONOCLONAL ANTIBODIES

Cancer cells express a range of proteins that are suitable targets for monoclonal antibodies. The development of monoclonal antibodies against specific antigens (targets) has been facilitated by advances in hybridoma technology (i.e. immunizing mice with human tumour cells and screening the hybridomas for antibodies of interest). Because murine anti-mouse antibodies have a short half-life and induce human anti-mouse antibody immune response, they are usually chimerized or humanized for therapeutic use (Chapter 16). The nomenclature for therapeutic monoclonal antibodies is to have the suffix '-ximab' for chimeric antibodies and '-umab' for humanized antibodies. **Trastuzumab**, one of the first agents demonstrated to have clinical benefit in cancer therapy, is discussed below. Other monoclonal antibodies that are used therapeutically in cancer are detailed in Table 48.10. All are administered intravenously.

Figure 48.9 shows an example of the 3D structure of a monoclonal antibody.

TRASTUZUMAB

Uses

Trastuzumab is a humanized monoclonal antibody (molecular weight approximately 100 kDa) that is used as a single agent or in combinations (e.g. with **paclitaxel**) to treat metastatic breast cancer that over-expresses the target-HER2/neu (Erb-2, i.e. EGFR-1) – about 30% of such cancers do this.

Mechanism of action

This monoclonal antibody binds tightly to the Her-2/Neu (Erb-B2) glycoprotein, a member of the epidermal growth factor family of cellular receptors (EGFR). EGFR encodes its own tyrosine kinase which, upon receptor–ligand binding, normally autophosphorylates the receptor causing downstream signalling which increases proliferation, metastatic potential and evasion of apoptosis. **Trastuzumab** binding inhibits such downstream signalling of the EGFR receptor.

Adverse effects

These include the following:

- infusion reactions involving fever, chills, nausea, dyspnoea, rashes;

Table 48.10: Monoclonal antibodies used to treat cancer

Drug[a]	Therapeutic use	Pharmacodynamics/pharmacokinetics	Side effects	Additional comments
Alemtuzumab	B-cell lymphoma	Binds to CD52 on neutrophils and lymphs, Causes apoptosis via ADCC. Plasma $t_{1/2} = 12$ days, dose-dependent kinetics	Infusion reactions, opportunistic infections, pancytopenia	Early efficacy in mycosis fungoides and T-cell lymphoma
Bevacizumab	Colorectal and ? lung cancer	Binds to circulating VEGF, inhibits angiogenesis neovascularization, plasma $t_{1/2} =$ mean 20 days (range 11–50)	Hypertension, pulmonary and gastro-intestinal bleeds, proteinuria, cardiac failure	Used as single agent or in combinations in colorectal cancer. It improves median survival by 5 months
Cetuximab	Colorectal and pancreatic and NSCL and ? breast cancer	Targets EGFR (Erb-1), inhibits EGFR-mediated signal transduction. Plasma $t_{1/2} = 3–8$ days	Infusion reactions, skin rashes – 75%, electrolyte losses	Prolongs survival in colon cancer
Gemtuzumab	Acute myeloid leukaemia	Targets CD33 on T cells, plasma $t_{1/2} = 10–20$ days	Infusion reactions, bone marrow suppression, VOD and skin rash	
Rituximab[b]	B-cell lymphoma and CLL (also used for ITP)	Binds to CD20 on B-cells and activates TK, c-myc and MHC class II molecules, plasma $t_{1/2} = 10–14$ days	Infusion reactions: fever, rash, dyspnoea, delayed neutropenia	

[a]Dosing of all monoclonal antibodies is intravenous. Usually a loading dose is followed by weekly or biweekly treatments.
[b]Radioisotope labelled versions of other antibodies to the same target are available.
ADCC, antibody-directed cellular cytotoxicity; EGFR, epidermal growth factor receptor; CLL, chronic lymphatic leukaemia; ITP, idiopathic thrombocytopenia; NSCL, non-small cell lung; TK, tyrosine kinase; VEGF, vascular endothelial growth factor; VOD, vascular occlusive disease.

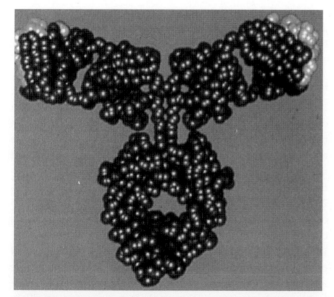

Figure 48.9: Three-dimensional structure of a monoclonal antibody.

- acute hypersensitivity reactions;
- heart failure, especially in patients who have received prior anthracyclines or **cyclophosphamide**.

HORMONES

Hormones can cause remission of sensitive tumours (e.g. lymphomas), but do not eradicate the disease. They often alleviate symptoms over a long period and they do not cause bone marrow suppression. Sex hormones or their antagonists (Chapter 41) are effective in tumours arising from cells that are normally hormone dependent (breast, prostate).

There are several ways in which hormones can affect malignant cells:

- A hormone may stimulate growth of a malignant cell. For example, if a breast carcinoma is oestrogen receptor-positive, oestrogen antagonists can inhibit these cells.
- A hormone may suppress the production of other hormones by a feedback mechanism. This will change the hormonal milieu surrounding the malignant cells and may suppress their proliferation. In breast cancer, patients who respond to one form of endocrine therapy are more likely to respond to subsequent hormone treatment than those who fail to respond initially.

OESTROGENS

Oestrogens are little used in the current management of prostatic carcinoma, because of the availability of gonadotrophin-releasing hormone (GnRH) analogues to suppress testosterone.

ANTI-OESTROGENS

Therapy for hormone receptor-positive breast cancers includes the use of selective oestrogen receptor modulators (SERM), selective oestrogen receptor downregulators (SERD) and aromatase inhibitors.

Selective oestrogen receptor modulators (SERMs) and selective oestrogen receptor downregulators (SERDs)

Tamoxifen (Chapter 41) is the lead compound in the SERM class (others include **raloxifene**). It is used to treat oestrogen receptor-positive breast cancer and may be used as prophylaxis against breast cancer in high-risk patients. It is given orally once or twice a day and metabolized by CYP2D6 and 3A to active metabolites (e.g. **endoxifen**). **Tamoxifen** and its metabolites are competitive inhibitors of oestrogen binding to its receptor. Adverse effects include hot flushes, hair loss, nausea and vomiting, menstrual irregularities, an increased incidence of thrombo-embolic events, and a two- to three-fold increased incidence of endometrial cancer in post-menopausal women.

Fulvestrant is one example of the SERD class. It purportedly has an improved safety profile, faster onset and longer duration of action than SERMs. It is given as a monthly injection. Common adverse effects are nausea, fatigue, injection reactions and hot flushes.

Aromatase inhibitors

This class of agents, for example **anastrazole** (**letrozole**), is used to treat early and advanced-stage oestrogen receptor-positive breast cancer. Original members of this class were **aminoglutethimide** and **formestane**. **Anastrazole** is given orally and metabolized by CYP3A and glucuronidation to inactive metabolites. **Anastrazole** acts by reversibly binding to the haem moiety of the CYP19 gene product. This is the aromatase enzyme responsible in many tissues (including breast tissue) for converting androstenedione and testosterone to oestrogen. Adverse effects are less frequent than with **tamoxifen**, but include hot flushes, menstrual irregularities, thrombo-embolic events and endometrial cancer.

PROGESTOGENS

Endometrial cells normally mature under the influence of progestogens and some malignant cells that arise from the endometrium respond in the same way. About 30% of patients with disseminated adenocarcinoma of the body of the uterus respond to a progestogen, such as **megestrol**. Progestogen bound to its receptor impairs the regeneration of oestrogen receptors and also stimulates 17-β-oestradiol dehydrogenase, the enzyme that metabolizes intracellular oestrogen. These actions may deprive cancer cells of the stimulatory effects of oestrogen. There is also probably a direct cytotoxic effect at high concentrations. Other progestogens that are used include **norethisterone** and **hydroxyprogesterone**. There are no important toxic effects of progestogens that are relevant to cancer chemotherapy (Chapter 41).

GLUCOCORTICOSTEROIDS

Glucocorticosteroids (see Chapters, 33, 40 and 50) are cytotoxic to lymphoid cells and are combined with other cytotoxic agents to treat lymphomas and myeloma, and to induce remission in acute lymphoblastic leukaemia.

HORMONAL MANIPULATION THERAPY IN ADVANCED PROSTATE CANCER

In advanced prostate cancer, manipulation of the androgen environment of the tumour cells can control the disease. Gonadotrophin-releasing hormone (GnRH) analogues (long-acting preparations of drugs, such as **leuprolide/goserelin** (Chapter 42) initially stimulate and then reduce pituitary FSH/LH release. These desensitize and suppress testosterone production and have superseded the use of oestrogens to antagonize the androgen dependency of prostate cancer cells. They are given with an androgen receptor antagonist (e.g. **flutamide**, **bicalutamide**, **cyproterone**) to block the intracellular receptors for dihydrotestosterone and prevent flare of the disease.

Aminoglutethimide (an aromatase inhibitor) and high-dose **ketoconazole** (Chapter 45) block the synthesis of testicular testosterone, adrenal androgens and other steroids. They are given orally to patients with refractory prostate cancer.

BIOLOGICAL RESPONSE MODIFIERS

These agents influence the biological response to the tumour. They may act indirectly to mediate anti-tumour effects, e.g stimulate the immune response against the transformed neoplastic cells or directly on the tumour (e.g. by modulating tumour differentiation). Drugs with proven anti-cancer clinical efficacy in this class are **interleukin-2** and **interferon-alfa 2b**.

INTERLEUKIN-2 (ALDESLEUKIN)

Interleukin-2 (**IL-2**, **aldesleukin**) is a human recombinant form of the native IL-2 produced by T helper cells. It differs from native **IL-2** in that it is not glycosylated, has no terminal alanine and a serine substituted at amino acid 125. It is used to treat metastatic malignant melanoma and renal cell carcinoma. In these patients with advanced cancer, response rates of as high as 20–30%, with durable complete responses in 5–10% have been observed. **IL-2** is not a direct cytotoxic, but it induces/expands cytolytic T cells against tumours. It is administered intravenously. Toxicity is the major determinant of the duration of treatment. Common toxicities are often dose-limiting due to the activation of T cells and release of other cytokines (TNF, interleukins and interferon). They include hypotension, capillary leak syndrome with pulmonary oedema, cardiac dysrhythmias, prerenal uraemia, abnormal transaminases, anaemia-thrombocytopenia, nausea, vomiting, diarrhoea, confusion, rashes and fever.

INTERFERON-ALFA 2B

Interferon-alfa 2b is a glycoprotein (molecular weight 15–27.6 kDa) produced by recombinant expression in *E. coli*. It is used in the treatment of hairy cell leukaemia, refractory chronic myeloid leukaemia, advanced malignant melanoma and follicular lymphoma. Interferons bind to specific cell surface receptors which initiate intracellular events relating to effects on RNA and protein synthesis. Such processes include enzyme induction, inhibition of cell proliferation enhancement of immune effector cells, such as macrophage phagocytic activity and cytotoxic T lymphocytes. Interferons are administered subcutaneously. Pegylated formulations allow once weekly administration. Common adverse effects include flu-like illnesses, fatigue, myalgias and arthralgias, injection site reactions, rashes. Less frequent side effects are hypotension, cardiac failure and CNS effects (memory loss and depression). Chronic interferon therapy may downregulate CYP450s involved in drug metabolism and lead to drug toxicity, e.g to **theophylline**.

Other immunostimulatory drugs that have been used with some success include **thalidomide**, which has anti-angiogenesis properties and decreases TNF production (effective in refractory malignant myeloma), and **levamisole** (as an adjuvant for colon cancer). The optimal use of tumour vaccines is still being actively researched.

Case history

A 19-year-old white male presented with palpable lumps on both sides of his neck and profuse sweating at night. Lymph node biopsy and computed tomography (CT) scanning yielded a diagnosis of stage IVb Hodgkin's disease. He was started on combination chemotherapy with doxorubicin 60 mg/m^2, bleomycin 10 units/m^2, vinblastine 5 mg/m^2 and dacarbazine 100 mg (ABVD). After four cycles of chemotherapy, he developed abdominal pain that was found to be due to acute appendicitis and he underwent emergency appendicectomy and made a good recovery. Four days after completing his fifth cycle of ABVD treatment he noted increased dyspnoea on exertion. This progressed over 48 hours to dyspnoea at rest. Physical examination revealed cyanosis. There was no palpable cervical lymphadenopathy, but he had a sinus tachycardia and bilateral basal and mid-zone late inspiratory crackles. Further investigations revealed normal haemoglobin, white blood count and platelets, normal coagulation screen, PO_2 on air 50 mmHg and fluffy interstitial infiltrates in both lower- and mid-lung fields on chest x-ray. Pulmonary function tests showed an FEV$_1$/FVC ratio of 80%, reduced FVC and a DL$_{CO}$ of 25% of the predicted value. Bronchoalveolar lavage fluid was negative for bacterial, viral and fungal pathogens, including *Pneumocystis jiroveci*.

Question
What was the cause of this patient's respiratory problems? How should he be treated?
Answer
In this patient, the possible causes of such pulmonary symptoms and radiographic findings include opportunistic infection, pulmonary oedema (secondary to fluid overload), pulmonary haemorrhage, progression of disease or drug-induced interstitial alveolitis. Here, with the exclusion of a haemorrhagic diathesis and pulmonary infection, no fluid overload and apparent regression of his cervical lymphadenopathy, the probable diagnosis is bleomycin-induced interstitial pneumonitis. Although the patient had not received more than 300 units of bleomycin, it is likely that during his operation he received high inspired oxygen concentrations, and this could have put him at higher risk of developing 'bleomycin lung'. Currently, he should receive the lowest inspired oxygen concentration that will yield a PO_2 of >60 mmHg. Glucocorticosteroid therapy may be of benefit, but the syndrome may not be fully reversible. Bleomycin, and other cytotoxic agents which cause a pneumonitis (e.g. cyclophosphamide, busulfan, carmustine, methotrexate and mitomycin) and radiation therapy (which can exacerbate bleomycin pulmonary toxicity), should not be used for this patient's future therapy.

FURTHER READING AND WEB MATERIAL

Baker SD, Grochow LB. Pharmacology of cancer chemotherapy in the older person. *Clinics in Geriatric Medicine* 1997; **13**: 169–83.

Chabner BA, Longo DL. *Cancer chemotherapy and biotherapy*, 2nd edn. Philadelphia: Lippincott-Raven, 1996.

Douglas JT. Cancer gene therapy. *Technology in Cancer Research and Treatment* 2003; **2**: 51–64.

Frei E. Curative cancer chemotherapy. *Cancer Research* 1985; **45**: 6523–37.

Kim R, Emi M, Tanabe K et al. The role of apoptotic or nonapoptotic cell death in determining cellular response to anticancer treatment. *European Journal of Surgical Oncology* 2006; **32**: 269–77.

Krause DS, Van Etten RA. Tyrosine kinases as targets for cancer therapy. *New England Journal of Medicine* 2005; **353**: 172–87.

Mooi WJ, Peeper DS. Oncogene-induced cell senescence – halting on the road to cancer. *New England Journal of Medicine* 2006; **355**: 1037–46.

O'Driscoll L, Clynes M. Biomarkers and multiple drug resistance in breast cancer. *Current Cancer Drug Targets* 2006; **6**: 365–84.

Yong WP, Innocenti F, Ratain MJ. The role of pharmacogenetics in cancer therapeutics. *British Journal of Clinical Pharmacology* 2006; **62**: 35–46.

Useful websites: American Society of Clinical Oncology, www.asco.org; National Cancer Institute of America, www.cancer.gov.

PART X

HAEMATOLOGY

CHAPTER 49

ANAEMIA AND OTHER HAEMATOLOGICAL DISORDERS

HAEMATINICS – IRON, VITAMIN B$_{12}$ AND FOLATE

IRON

Biochemistry and physiology

Iron plays a vital role in the body in many proteins including transport proteins (e.g. haemoglobin, myoglobin) and enzymes (e.g. CYP450s, catalase, peroxidase, metalloflavoproteins). It is stored in the reticulo-endothelial system and bone marrow. The total body iron content is 3.5–4.5 g in an adult, of which about 70% is incorporated in haemoglobin, 5% in myoglobin and 0.2% in enzymes. Most of the remaining iron (approximately 25%) is stored as ferritin or haemosiderin. About 2% (80 mg) comprises the 'labile iron pool' and about 0.08% (3 mg) is bound to transferrin (a specific iron-binding protein).

Pharmacokinetics

Gastro-intestinal (GI) absorption is the primary mechanism controlling total body iron. This remains remarkably constant (1–1.4 mg/day) in healthy individuals despite variations in diet, erythropoiesis and iron stores. Iron absorption occurs in the small intestine and is influenced by several factors:

1. The physico-chemical form of the iron:
   (a) Inorganic ferrous iron is better absorbed than ferric iron.
   (b) Absorption of iron from the diet depends on the source of the iron. Most dietary iron exists as non-haem iron (e.g. iron salts) and is relatively poorly absorbed (approximately 5–10%), mainly because it is combined with phosphates and phytates (in cereals). Haem iron is well absorbed (20–40%).
2. Factors increasing absorption:
   (a) Acid: e.g. gastric acid and ascorbic acid facilitate iron absorption.
   (b) Ethanol increases ferric but not ferrous iron absorption.

3. Factors reducing iron absorption:
   (a) Partial gastrectomy reduces gastric acid and iron deficiency is more common than vitamin B$_{12}$ deficiency following partial gastrectomy.
   (b) Malabsorption states, e.g. coeliac disease.
   (c) Drug–iron binding interactions in the GI tract; tetracyclines chelate iron, causing malabsorption of both agents; oral bisphosphonates and magnesium trisilicate reduce iron absorption.

Disposition of iron

Iron in the lumen of the gut is transported across the intestinal membrane either directly into plasma or is bound by mucosal ferritin. A negative regulator of gastro-intestinal mucosal absorption of iron (hepcidin) synthesized by the liver may contribute to the anaemia of chronic disease. Iron is transported in plasma by transferrin, one molecule of which binds two atoms of iron. The iron is transferred to cells (e.g. red-cell precursors in the bone marrow) by transferrin binding to transferrin receptors followed by endocytosis. The iron dissociates from transferrin in the acidic intracellular environment. When red cells reach the end of their life-span, macrophages bind the iron atoms released, which are taken up again by transferrin. About 80% of total body iron exchange normally takes place via this cycle (Figure 49.1). Ferritin is the main storage form of iron. It is a spherical protein with deeply located iron-binding sites, and is found principally in the liver and the reticulo-endothelial system. Aggregates of ferritin form haemosiderin, which accumulates when levels of hepatic iron stores are high.

Iron deficiency

Iron deficiency is the most common cause of anaemia and although it is most common and most severe in Third World countries, it is also prevalent in developed countries. Serum iron concentration in iron-deficient patients falls only when stores are considerably depleted. The total amount of transferrin determines the total iron-binding capacity (TIBC) of plasma,

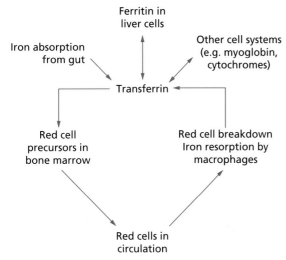

Figure 49.1: Iron metabolism.

and is normally 54–80 µmol/L. Transferrin saturation (i.e. plasma iron divided by TIBC) is normally 20–50% and provides a useful index of iron status. In iron-deficiency states, TIBC rises in addition to the fall in plasma iron, and when transferrin saturation falls to less than 16%, erythropoiesis starts to decline. The cause of iron deficiency is most often multifactorial, e.g. poor diet combined with excessive demands on stores (pregnancy, chronic blood loss, lactation), reduced stores (premature birth) or defective absorption (achlorhydria, surgery to the gastro-intestinal tract). Although treatment of iron deficiency is straightforward, its cause should be determined so that the underlying condition can be treated. Iron-deficiency anaemia in men or post-menopausal women is seldom due solely to dietary deficiency, and a thorough search for other causes (notably colon cancer) should be undertaken.

IRON PREPARATIONS

ORAL IRON

Most patients with iron deficiency respond to simple oral iron preparations. Treatment is continued for 3–6 months after

haemoglobin concentrations enter the normal range, in order to replace iron stores. Failure to respond may be due to:

- wrong diagnosis;
- non-compliance with therapy;
- continued blood loss;
- malabsorption (e.g. coeliac disease, post-gastrectomy).

There are too many iron-containing preparations available, many containing vitamins as well as iron. None of these combinations carries an advantage over iron salts alone, except for those containing folic acid, which are used prophylactically in pregnancy. Treatment should start with a simple preparation such as ferrous sulphate, ferrous fumarate or ferrous gluconate. Examples of commonly available iron preparations are listed in Table 49.1.

Adverse effects

Gastro-intestinal side effects, including nausea, heartburn, constipation or diarrhoea, are common. Patients with ulcerative colitis and those with colostomies suffer particularly severely from these side effects. No one preparation is universally better tolerated than any other, but individual patients often find that one salt suits them better than another. Ferrous sulphate is least expensive, but if it is not tolerated it is worth trying an organic salt, e.g. fumarate. Although iron is best absorbed in the fasting state, gastric irritation is reduced if it is taken after food. Accidental overdose with iron is not uncommon in young children and can be extremely serious, with gastro-intestinal haemorrage, cardiovascular collapse, hepatic and neurotoxicity. Desferrioxamine (an iron-chelating agent) is administered to treat it (Chapter 54).

IRON PREPARATIONS FOR CHILDREN

Sugar-free liquid preparations that do not stain the teeth should be used in paediatrics (e.g. sodium iron edetate). The dose is calculated in terms of the amount of elemental iron.

PARENTERAL IRON

Oral iron is effective, easily administered and cheap. Parenteral iron (formulated with sorbitol and citric acid) is also effective, but can cause anaphylactoid reactions and is expensive. The rate of rise in haemoglobin concentration is no faster than after oral iron, because the rate-limiting factor is the capacity of the

Table 49.1: Ferrous iron content and relative cost of available iron formulations

Iron formulation	Ferrous iron content in one unit dose	Approximate ratio of cost for one unit dose
Ferrous sulphate	60 mg	1
Ferrous fumarate	65 mg	2
Ferrous gluconate	35 mg	2.6
Ferrous succinate	35 mg	3
Sodium ironedetate	27.5–55 mg	6
Polysaccharide iron complex	50–100 mg	11

bone marrow to produce red cells. The only advantages of parenteral iron are the following:

- Iron stores are rapidly and completely replenished.
- There is no doubt about compliance.
- It is effective in patients with malabsorption.

Parenteral iron should therefore only be considered in the following situations:

- malabsorption;
- genuine intolerance of oral iron preparations;
- when continued blood loss is not preventable and large doses of iron cannot be readily given by mouth;
- failure of patient compliance;
- when great demands are to be made on a patient's iron stores (e.g. in an anaemic pregnant woman just before term).

IRON DEXTRAN AND IRON SUCROSE INJECTIONS

Use

These can be administered by deep intramuscular injection (to minimize staining of the skin) or intravenously (anaphylactoid reactions can occur (up 3% of patients) and a small test dose should be given initially). Oral iron should be stopped 24 hours before starting parenteral iron therapy and not restarted until five days after the last injection.

> ### Key points
>
> Iron replacement therapy
>
> - In health, normal iron losses require the absorption of 0.5–1 mg (in males) and 0.7–2 mg (in menstruating females) of iron.
> - Ferrous iron is best absorbed from the small intestine.
> - Iron deficiency is the most common cause of anaemia (e.g. malabsorption, menstrual, occult or gastro-intestinal blood loss – always determine the cause).
> - For iron deficiency, 100–200 mg of elemental iron are given orally per day and continued until iron stores are replete, usually within three to six months.
> - Parenteral iron use is restricted to cases of non-compliance or non-tolerance of oral preparations, or malabsorption states.
> - During erythropoietin therapy, supplemental iron is given to support increased haem synthesis.

VITAMIN B₁₂

Vitamin B₁₂ is an organic molecule with an attached cobalt atom. Linked to the cobalt atom may be a cyanide (cyanocobalamin), hydroxyl (hydroxocobalamin) or methyl (methylcobalamin) group. These forms are interconvertible. Sources of vitamin B₁₂ include liver, kidney heart, fish and eggs.

Use

Replacement therapy is required in vitamin B₁₂ deficiency which may be due to:

- malabsorption secondary to gastric pathology (Addisonian pernicious anaemia, where parietal cells are destroyed by an autoimmune reaction, so intrinsic factor is not produced, resulting in vitamin B₁₂ deficiency; gastrectomy);
- intestinal malabsorption (e.g. Crohn's disease or surgical resection of the terminal ileum);
- competition for vitamin B₁₂ absorption by gut organisms (e.g. blind loop syndrome due to a jejunal diverticulum or other cause of bacterial overgrowth, infestation with the fish tapeworm *Diphyllobothrium latum*);
- nutritional deficiency – this is rare and is limited to strict vegans. The few such individuals who do develop megaloblastic anaemia often have some co-existing deficiency of intrinsic factor.

Vitamin B₁₂ replacement therapy is given by intramuscular injection. **Hydroxocobalamin** is preferred, given as an initial loading dose followed by three monthly maintenance treatment for life.

Cellular mechanism of action

Vitamin B₁₂ is needed for normal erythropoiesis and for neuronal integrity. It is a cofactor needed for the isomerization of methylmalonyl coenzyme A to succinyl coenzyme A, and for the conversion of homocysteine into methionine (which also utilizes 5-methyltetrahydrofolate, see Figure 49.2). Vitamin B₁₂ is also involved in the control of folate metabolism, and B₁₂ and folate are required for intracellular nucleoside synthesis. Deficiency of vitamin B₁₂ 'traps' folate as methylene tetrahydrofolate, yielding a macrocytic anaemia with megaloblastic erythropoiesis in the bone marrow, and possible neurological dysfunction, i.e. peripheral neuropathy, subacute combined degeneration of the spinal cord, dementia and optic neuritis.

Pharmacokinetics

Humans depend on exogenous vitamin B₁₂. Following total gastrectomy liver stores (1–10 mg) are adequate for 3–5 years, following which there is an increasing incidence of vitamin B₁₂ deficiency. The daily vitamin B₁₂ loss is 0.5–3 μg, which results mainly from metabolic breakdown, and 2–3 μg is absorbed daily from the diet. Vitamin B₁₂ is complexed with intrinsic factor (secreted from the gastric parietal cells). Intrinsic factor is a

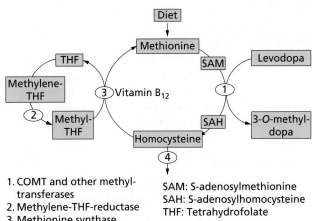

1. COMT and other methyltransferases
2. Methylene-THF-reductase
3. Methionine synthase
4. Cystathionine ß-synthase

SAM: S-adenosylmethionine
SAH: S-adenosylhomocysteine
THF: Tetrahydrofolate

Figure 49.2: Role of vitamin B₁₂ and folate in homocysteine – methionine cycling.

glycoprotein of molecular weight approximately 55 kDa which forms a stable complex with vitamin B_{12}. The complex passes down the small intestine and binds to specific receptors on the mucosa of the terminal ileum (at neutral pH and in the presence of calcium) and is actively absorbed. Once in the circulation, vitamin B_{12} is transported by the beta globulin transcobalamin II (TC II) to tissues, with its primary storage site being the liver (90% body stores). Vitamin B_{12} complexed with other transcobalamins (TCI and III, which are alpha-globulins) probably represent the major intracellular storage form. The normal range of plasma vitamin B_{12} concentration is 170–900 ng/L (150–660 pmol/L). Vitamin B_{12} is secreted into the bile, but enterohepatic circulation results in most of this being reabsorbed via the intrinsic factor mechanism.

FOLIC ACID

Uses

Folic acid is given to correct or prevent deficiency states and prophylactically during pregnancy. It consists of a pteridine ring linked to glutamic acid via p-aminobenzoic acid (PABA). The richest dietary sources are liver, yeast and green vegetables.

Folate deficiency may be due to:

- poor nutrition – in children, the elderly or those with alcoholism;
- malabsorption – caused by coeliac disease, sprue or diseases of the small intestine;
- excessive utilization – in pregnancy, chronic haemolytic anaemias (e.g. sickle cell disease) and leukaemias;
- anti-epileptic drugs (e.g. **phenytoin**).

The normal requirement for folic acid is about 200 μg daily. In established folate deficiency, large doses (5–15 mg orally per day) are given. If the patient is unable to take folate by mouth, it may be given intravenously. Patients with severe malabsorption may be deficient in both folic acid and vitamin B_{12}, and administration of folic acid alone may precipitate acute vitamin B_{12} deficiency. Such patients require replacement of both vitamins concurrently. Many patients on chronic anticonvulsant therapy develop macrocytosis without frank folate deficiency. Treatment is by the addition of folic acid to the anticonvulsant regimen.

Cellular mechanism of action

Folic acid is required for normal erythropoiesis. Deficiency of folic acid results in a megaloblastic anaemia and abnormalities in other cell types. Folate acts as a methyl donor in biochemical reactions, including the methylation of deoxyuridylic acid to form thymidylic acid, as well as other reactions in purine and pyrimidine synthesis.

Pharmacokinetics

Folate is present in food as reduced polyglutamates. These are hydrolysed to monoglutamate, reduced and methylated to methyltetrahydrofolate by the combined action of pteroyl-glutamyl carboxypeptidase and tetrahydrofolate reductase. This occurs in the proximal small intestine, the site of folate absorption into the portal blood. About one-third of total body folate (70 mg) is stored in the liver, representing only about four months supply. The normal range for serum folate concentration is 4–20 μg/L.

IRON AND FOLIC ACID THERAPY IN PREGNANCY

Pregnancy imposes a substantial increase in demand on maternal stores of iron and folic acid. A pregnant woman during the last trimester therefore requires approximately 5 mg of iron daily. Most women are iron depleted by the end of the pregnancy if they do not receive supplements. Requirements for folic acid also increase by two- to three-fold during pregnancy. Folate deficiency is associated with prematurity, low birth weight for gestational age and neural-tube defects (Chapter 9). In the UK, the usual practice is to give iron and folic acid supplements throughout pregnancy. Folate supplementation should be also be given before conception to women who are attempting to become pregnant, in order to reduce the incidence of neural-tube defects. High-dose prophylaxis (folate, 5 mg daily) is advised for women who have previously given birth to a child with a neural-tube defect.

> **Key points**
>
> Vitamin B_{12} and folate therapy
>
> - Healthy subjects require 3–5 μg of vitamin B_{12} and 200 μg of folate daily.
> - Body stores of vitamin B_{12} are 3 mg; folate stores are approximately 200 mg.
> - Vitamin B_{12} and folate are absorbed from the small intestine, and vitamin B_{12} is specifically absorbed from the terminal ileum.
> - The most common cause of B_{12} or folate deficiency is dietary or malabsorption, or due to gastric surgery.
> - Vitamin B_{12} deficiency must not be inappropriately treated with folate alone, as any associated neurological damage may be irreversible.
> - Drugs may cause vitamin B_{12} (e.g. metformin) or folate (e.g. phenytoin, other anti-epileptic drugs) deficiency.

PYRIDOXINE, RIBOFLAVIN

Sideroblastic anaemia with failure of incorporation of iron into haem in the mitochondria, may respond to long-term pyridoxine supplementation. Infrequently, red cell aplasia is due to riboflavin deficiency and will respond to supplementation with this vitamin (Chapter 35).

HAEMATOPOIETIC GROWTH FACTORS

Recombinant DNA technology has been used to synthesize several human haematopoietic growth factors (Figure 49.3 shows an outline of haematopoiesis). Haematopoietic growth factors now have a clear role in the treatment of many forms of bone marrow dysfunction.

RECOMBINANT HUMAN ERYTHROPOIETIN (ERYTHROPOIETIN AND DARBEPOETIN)

Erythropoietin is secreted as a glycosylated protein with a mass of 34 kDa. About 90% of endogenous erythropoietin is

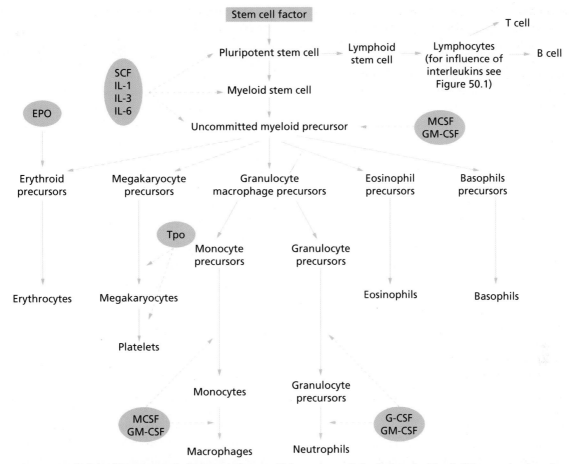

Figure 49.3: Haematopoiesis and haematopoietic growth factors. EPO, erythropoietin; IL, interleukin; G-CSF, granulocyte colony-stimulating factor; MCSF, macrophage colony-stimulating factor; GM-CSF, granulocyte macrophage colony-stimulating factor; SCF, stem-cell factor; Tpo, thrombopoietin.

produced by interstitial cells of the renal cortex adjacent to the proximal tubules and 10% by the liver. Biosynthesis is stimulated by anaemia/tissue hypoxia which increases levels of the active form of a transcription factor called 'hypoxia-inducible factor-1' (HIF), which enhances transcription of the erythropoietin gene. Endogenous erythropoietin homeostasis is further controlled by a negative feedback loop that maintains red-cell mass at an optimal level for oxygen transport.

Uses

Epoetin, the recombinant form of **erythropoietin** and **darbepoetin** (an analogue with a longer plasma half-life) are used to stimulate red cell growth. These agents are given by subcutaneous injection. Haemoglobin is monitored to titrate dosing. Iron supplementation should be used routinely. Recent studies in cancer patients showed that when compared to placebo, erythropoietic agents used to treat patients with weaknesss, malaise and fatigue, but whose Hb was not <12 g/dL and who were not currently receiving cytotoxic chemotherapy, reduced patient survival. This suggests the need to more critically evaluate and use erythropoietic agents in such patients and in cancer patients generally, as many tumours express **erythropoietin** receptors.

Erythropoietin is used in:

- anaemia of chronic renal failure;
- anaemia of drug-induced bone marrow suppression (e.g. cancer chemotherapy or ZDV therapy);
- anaemia with myeloma;
- anaemia of rheumatoid arthritis;
- autologous blood harvesting for transfusion during elective surgery;
- prevention of anaemia in premature babies of low birth weight.

Mechanism of action

Erythropoietin binds to a membrane receptor on erythroid cell precursors. Signal transduction is through a tyrosine kinase, that increases transcription of the genes for key haem biosynthetic enzymes. Thus, **erythropoietin** increases haem biosynthesis and causes differentiation of erythroid precursors into mature erythroid cells.

Pharmacokinetics

Elimination occurs by catabolism in the erythroid cells in the marrow following internalization, by hepatic metabolism and to a lesser extent urinary excretion.

Adverse effects

These include the following:

- hypertension which can be severe;
- thrombosis, for example of shunts, or causing a cardiovascular/cerebrovascular accident;
- influenza-like symptoms;
- iron deficiency may be unmasked;
- pure red cell aplasia associated with antibodies to erythropoietin has been reported during treatment with **epoetin alfa**.

HUMAN GRANULOCYTE COLONY-STIMULATING FACTOR (FILGRASTIM, LENOGRASTIM, PEG-FILGRASTIM).

Granulocyte colony-stimulating factor (G-CSF) is a 174 amino acid glycoprotein. **Filgrastim** is unglycosylated rhG-CSF and **lenograstim** is glycosylated rhG-CSF. Pegylated G-CSF (**PEG-filgrastim**) has a protracted half-life and can be given much less frequently.

Uses

Indications for G-CSF include:

- to prevent and treat the neutropenia induced by cytotoxic cancer chemotherapy (main use);
- congenital neutropenia;
- human immunodeficiency virus (HIV)-related AZT-induced neutropenia (chronic therapy);
- aplastic anaemia;
- mobilization of peripheral blood-cell progenitors and subsequent harvesting for transplant;
- following bone marrow transplantation.

G-CSF is usually administered by subcutaneous injection. Therapy is monitored by regular neutrophil counts. After stopping treatment, neutrophil counts return to baseline after four to seven days.

Mechanism of action

G-CSF stimulates the proliferation and differentiation of progenitor cells of the myelogranulocyte lineage. It binds to the G-CSF receptor on myelogranulocyte precursors, enhancing cell replication and differentation. Once bound to its receptor, G-CSF is internalized and signal transduction involves a number of tyrosine kinase proteins which induce the synthesis of proteins that upregulate cell-cycle and differentiation processes.

Adverse effects

These include the following:

- bone pain;
- injection site reactions;
- myalgia and fevers;
- splenomegaly;
- thrombocytopenia;
- abnormal liver enzymes.

Contraindications

G-CSF should not be given to patients with myeloid or myelomonocytic leukaemia, because it increases proliferation of the malignant clone.

Pharmacokinetics

The bioavailability of subcutaneously administered G-CSF is 54%. The G-CSF plasma $t_{1/2}$ ranges from two to six hours. Clearance of G-CSF is complex and it increases as the granulocyte count rises. In addition, G-CSF is metabolized in the kidney and liver to its component amino acids, with little or no G-CSF found in the urine.

INTERLEUKIN-11 AND THROMBOPOIETIN

Interleukin-11 is a recombinant protein which enhances megakaryocyte maturation and is used to prevent thrombocytopenia in patients who developed platelet counts $<20\,000/\mu L$ with prior cycles of cytotoxic chemotherapy. Interleukin-11 (**oprelvekin**, not yet available in the UK) is given daily via subcutaneous injection until the platelet count $>10\,000/\mu L$. Major side effects include fluid retention and associated cardiac symptoms, injection site reactions, paraesthesias and blurred vision.

Thrombopoietin is a recombinant protein which binds to the mpl-proto-oncogene, stimulates megakaryocyte proliferation and differentiation in humans. It synergizes with stem cell factor and G-CSF in promoting bone marrow production of granulocytes. **Thrombopoietin** may be useful in drug-induced thrombocytopenia and in bone marrow transplantation.

> **Key points**
>
> Haematopoietic growth factors
>
> - The clinically used haematopoietic growth factors are recombinant DNA products of the endogenous glycoprotein.
> - Erythropoietin (Epo)/darbepoetin:
>   - stimulate proliferation of erythroid (red cell) precursors;
>   - are used in the treatment of the anaemia of renal failure (myelodysplasia);
>   - are given parenterally; its toxicities include hypertension and thrombotic episodes.
> - Granulocyte colony-stimulating factor (G-CSF):
>   - stimulates proliferation of myeloid precursors;
>   - is used to treat neutropenia of chemotherapy, aplastic anaemia and bone marrow transplant;
>   - is given parenterally and its toxicities include myalgias, bone pain, fever, thrombocytopenia and hepatitis.

COAGULATION FACTORS AND HAEMOPHILIAS A AND B

Pathophysiology

In haemophilia A there is a deficiency of factor VIII. In haemophilia B there is a deficiency of factor IX. Both types present with excessive bleeding in response to trauma, e.g. muscle haematoma, haemarthrosis, haemorrhage after minor (e.g. dental) or major surgery, and intracranial bleeding following minor head injury.

Therapeutic principles

The extent of haemorrhage depends on the severity of the factor VIII or IX deficiency and the severity of the trauma. Therapy consists of temporarily raising the concentration of the deficient factor, appropriate supportive measures, analgesia and graded physiotherapy. In minor trauma in mild haemophilia A, infusions of a synthetic vasopressin analogue (desmopressin, DDAVP; Chapter 36), produce a short-term two- to four-fold increase in factor VIII. Fluid overload due to the antidiuretic hormone action of DDAVP must be prevented by limiting water intake. DDAVP is usually given with an inhibitor of fibrinolysis, such as tranexamic acid. If the haemophilia and/or trauma is severe, then infusions of factor VIII or IX are required. Patients and their parents or other carers are taught to administer these factors at home in order to minimize delay in therapy.

FACTOR VIII

Factor VIII used to be obtained from purified pooled plasma of blood donors, but recombinant preparations are free of potential viral pathogens, including hepatitis B, hepatitis C, HIV and cytomegalovirus (CMV). It is given as an intravenous infusion. It is highly bound to von Willebrand factor (>95%) and is degraded by reticuloendothelial cells in the liver. The dose of factor VIII is calculated on the basis of the severity of the injury and the required increase in plasma factor VIII concentration. Transient reactions to infusions (e.g. urticaria, flushing and headache) occur, but respond to antihistamines. Anaphylactic reactions are rare.

FACTOR IX

Factor IX is used in patients with factor IX deficiency. It acts as a cofactor for factor VIII and as recombinant factor IX is available for patients with haemophilia B the recombinant form does not contain other factors or potential pathogens. Factor IX is given as an intravenous infusion. The use and adverse effects of factor IX are similar to those described for factor VIII.

FACTOR VIIA

Recombinant activated factor VII (rFVIIa) is a haemostatic protein. It was originally developed to treat bleeding episodes in haemophilic patients with inhibitors against coagulation factors VIII and IX. It is used by specialists to achieve haemostasis in several severe congenital and acquired haemorrhagic states.

> **Key points**
>
> Coagulation factor therapy
>
> - Factor VIII is used to treat haemophilia A (factor IX is used for haemophilia B) when patients present with severe bleeding.
> - These factors are given intravenously and the dose is based on the level of factor deficiency and blood loss.
> - Recombinant coagulation factors are free from the risk of contamination with infectious agents, such as HIV and hepatitis C, and cause less antibody production.

APLASTIC ANAEMIA

Aplastic anaemia is characterized by pancytopenia associated with absence of haematological precurors in the marrow. Some cases are congenital (e.g. Fanconi's anaemia), but many are acquired, and in 50% of these an aetiological agent (a virus, chemical or drug) can be implicated. Certain drugs predictably cause aplastic anaemia if given in sufficient dose (e.g. alkylating agents, such as **cyclophosphamide**), others (e.g. **chloramphenicol**) may cause aplastic anaemia as an idiosyncratic type B adverse reaction (Chapter 12).

TREATMENT

Support is provided with transfusions (of red cells and platelets) and appropriate antibiotics. Successful bone marrow transplantation is curative and is the therapy of choice for young patients. For those who are unsuitable for this treatment, or in cases where there is no available histocompatible donor, anabolic steroids, e.g. **oxymetholone** or **stanozolol** and **epoetin** and G-CSF (see above) may reduce the requirement for transfusions.

IDIOPATHIC THROMBOCYTOPENIC PURPURA

It is important to exclude other causes of thrombocytopenia, including drugs (e.g. **quinine**). Platelet transfusions are required to control active bleeding or to cover operations. Other treatment options include:

- glucocorticosteroids – e.g. **prednisolone**: an increase in platelet count may take one to two weeks. If steroids fail or the disease relapses, splenectomy should be considered. The patient should be immunized against pneumococcal infection several weeks preoperatively. Glucocorticosteroids should be continued after splenectomy until the platelet count rises.

- immunosuppressive drugs (Chapters 48 and 50), especially **vincristine**, are used in refractory cases.

- intravenous immunoglobulin (IVIG), **rituximab**, anti-CD20 antibody (Chapter 50) and **ciclosporin** are alternatives.

> **Key points**
>
> Drug-related haematological toxicity
>
> - Cytotoxic cancer chemotherapy can suppress all haematopoietic lineages.
> - Drugs that cause aplastic anaemia include ticlopidine, indometacin, carbimazole and zidovudine.
> - Drugs that cause agranulocytosis include, for example, carbamazepine, propylthiouracil, NSAIDs, H_2 antagonists and antipsychotics (e.g. chlorpromazine, clozapine).
> - Drugs that cause thrombocytopenia include, for example, heparin, azathioprine, quinidine and thiazides.
> - Drugs that cause haemolytic anaemia include, for example, methyldopa, β-lactams (penicillins and cephalosporins).

A 65-year-old woman presents to the medical out-patient department with a history of fatigue. She has in the last few months been undergoing adjuvant cytotoxic chemotherapy for a node-positive resected breast cancer. The patient is pale, but no other abnormalities are noted. Her full blood count shows a haemoglobin level of 9.8 g/dL with a mean corpuscular volume of 86 fL; other haematological indices and serum transferrin are normal. Her faecal occult blood is negative. She is started on oral iron sulphate and given weekly injections of erythropoietin 40 000 U subcutaneously. Three months later, her haemoglobin level has risen to 13.5 g/dL, but she presents to the Accident and Emergency Department with acute-onset dysphasia and weakness of her right arm. Her supine blood pressure is 198/122 mmHg. Her neurological deficit resolves over 24 hours and her blood pressure settles to 170/96 mmHg. She has no evidence of cardiac dyshythmias or of carotid disease on ultrasonic duplex angiography, and her serum cholesterol concentration was 4.2 mmol/L.

Question

What led to this patient's acute neurological episode? Does she require further therapy?

Answer

Her mild normochromic-normocytic anaemia was most likely related to her cytotoxic cancer therapy. Treatment with iron and erythropoietin was indicated. She was not iron deficient, and using iron and erythropoietin in combination for a haemoglobin <10 g/dL is well justified. The most common dose-limiting side effects of erythropoietic drug administration are hypertension and thrombosis, which are implicated in the left middle cerebral transient ischaemic attack (TIA) she has suffered.

Treatment with erythropoietin and iron should be stopped, and her blood pressure monitored over 8–12 weeks. If hypertension is solely related to the erythropoietin therapy, her blood pressure should normalize and no further treatment will be required. In retrospect it may have been prudent to have more closely monitored her erythropoietic therapy and once her Hb >12 g/dL stopped it as this may have avoided her neurological event.

FURTHER READING

Akkerman JW. Thrombopoietin and platelet function. *Seminars in Thrombosis and Hemostasis* 2006; **32**: 295–304.

Chong BH, Ho SJ. Autoimmune thrombocytopenia. *Journal of Thrombosis and Haemostasis* 2005; **3**: 1763–72.

Franchini M. Recombinant factor VIIa: a review on its clinical use. *International Journal of Hematology* 2006; **83**: 126–38.

Kaushansky K. Lineage-specific hematopoietic growth factors. *New England Journal of Medicine* 2006; **354**: 2034–45.

Limentani SA, Roth DA, Furie BC, Furie B. Recombinant blood clotting proteins for haemophilia therapy. *Seminars in Thrombosis and Hemostasis* 1993; **19**: 62–7.

McGrath K. Treatment of anaemia caused by iron, vitamin B$_{12}$ or folate deficiency. *Medical Journal of Australia* 1989; **157**: 693–7.

Scott J, Weir D. Folate/vitamin B$_{12}$ inter-relationships. *Essays in Biochemistry* 1994; **28**: 63–72.

Umbreit J. Iron deficiency: a concise review. *American Journal of Hematology* 2005; **78**: 225–31.

PART XI

IMMUNOPHARMACOLOGY

CHAPTER 50

CLINICAL IMMUNOPHARMACOLOGY

INTRODUCTION

The introduction of a foreign antigen into the body may provoke an immune reaction. Antigens (usually proteins, glycoproteins or high-molecular-weight carbohydrates) usually have a molecular weight >5000 Da. They are typically processed by macrophages before presentation to T lymphocytes. The effector limb of the immune response is initiated by interaction of the presented antigen with receptors on the surface of the lymphocytes. Immune responses are of two types, namely humoral (via B lymphocytes, plasma cells and antibody) or cellular (via T lymphocytes).

The immune response is an essential defence mechanism. However, it may be defective, disorganized or overactive. The body has the potential to stimulate its own immune system so that antibodies are produced against itself. Normally this situation is prevented, for example, by tolerance, but if this fails then autoimmune disease results. Deficiencies in the immune system may be congenital or result from disease (notably AIDS from HIV-1 infection) or the use of immunosuppressant drugs, particularly cytotoxic agents (e.g. **cyclophosphamide**, **6-mercaptopurine**), glucocorticosteroids and immunophilins (e.g. **ciclosporin** and its analogues). By the same token, these are the very drugs that are used clinically as immunosuppressants when it is necessary to damp down an inappropriate immune response.

IMMUNITY AND HYPERSENSITIVITY

HUMORAL IMMUNITY

The humoral response occurs in two stages:

1. *primary reactions* – these occur with the first exposure to the antigen. There is a small and short-lived rise in antibody titre which consists largely of IgM;

2. *secondary reactions* – these occur with subsequent exposure to the antigen. The rise in antibody titre is greater and persists for a long period. The antibody consists mainly of IgG. This reaction requires the interaction of helper T cells and B lymphocytes.

CELLULAR IMMUNITY

This is mediated by sensitized T lymphocytes which recognize and bind the antigen and subsequently release a cascade of lymphokines which control and amplify both humoral and cellular immune responses. The effector arm of cellular immunity consists of cytotoxic T cells.

ACTIVE IMMUNITY

This consists of immunity that is developed either in response to infection or following inoculation with an attenuated strain of organism, or with a structural protein or toxic protein to which the host produces protective antibodies.

PASSIVE IMMUNITY

This is immunity that is transferred by the administration of preformed antibodies (e.g. immune globulin/serum) either from another host or from recombinant techniques in vitro.

HYPERSENSITIVITY

Sometimes the immune response to an antigen results in damage to the tissue; this is known as hypersensitivity. There are four types of hypersensitivity.

TYPE-I HYPERSENSITIVITY

This results from the combination of antigen with high-affinity IgE (reaginic) antibody on the surface of tissue mast cells and/or blood basophils, releasing potently vasoactive and pro-inflammatory mediators. These mediators include histamine, leukotrienes C_4, D_4 and E_4, eosinophil chemotactic factor (ECF), serotonin, tachykinins and prostaglandins. This can cause anaphylaxis, bronchospasm, hay fever or urticaria.

TYPE-II HYPERSENSITIVITY

These reactions occur when antibody combines with antigenic components on a cell or tissue surface. This leads to cell lysis or tissue damage as a result of antibody-directed cell-mediated cytoxicity (ADCC) by macrophages and natural killer (NK) cells through Fc receptors or by activation of complement. This reaction may form the basis of a drug reaction (e.g. **penicillin**- or **quinidine**-induced haemolytic anaemia or thrombocytopenia). This is because although most drugs are low molecular weight, they can bind to a protein to form an immunologically active entity ('hapten'). Another example of this type of reaction is haemolytic disease of the newborn, when antibodies produced by a rhesus-negative mother against the rhesus factor on the red cells of the fetus cross the placental barrier and cause haemolysis. Such reactions may be mediated by IgM or IgG antibodies.

TYPE-III HYPERSENSITIVITY (ARTHUS REACTION – IMMUNE COMPLEX MEDIATED)

This is the result of the deposition of soluble antigen–antibody complexes in small blood vessels (e.g. in the renal glomeruli) or other tissues. Immune complex deposition activates complement and initiates a sequence which results in chemotaxis of polymorphs, tissue injury and vasculitis. This reaction is slower in onset than the immediate type I reaction. Serum sickness is an example of this type of response.

TYPE-IV (DELAYED OR CELL-MEDIATED HYPERSENSITIVITY)

This is mediated by sensitized CD41 circulating T lymphocytes reacting with antigen. Circulating antibodies are not involved. Activation of primed CD41 T cells causes their proliferation and the release of cytokines which produce local inflammation, attracting and activating NK cells, macrophages and granulocytes. This type of reaction takes place after one to two days and is exemplified by contact dermatitis, the Mantoux reaction and organ transplant rejection.

IMMUNOSUPPRESSIVE AGENTS

For therapeutic purposes, immunosuppression should ideally be specific and not impair immune responses indiscriminately.

The sites of action of immunosuppressive agents are shown in Figure 50.1. Immunosuppressive agents are inevitably a two-edged sword and before considering individual agents it is worth considering some of their general adverse effects.

GENERAL ADVERSE EFFECTS OF IMMUNOSUPPRESSION

Increased susceptibility to infection Bacterial infections are common and require prompt treatment with appropriate antibiotics. Tuberculosis may also occur and sometimes takes unusual forms. Viral infections may be more severe than usual and include the common herpes infection, but occasionally also such rarities as progressive multifocal leukoencephalopathy. Fungal infections are also common, including *Candida albicans* (which may be local or systemic). Protozoal infections (e.g. *Pneumocystis carinii*) also occur with increased frequency.

Sterility Azoospermia in men is common, especially with alkylating agents (Chapter 48). In women, hormone failure leading to amenorrhoea is common.

Teratogenicity This is less common than might be anticipated. However, it is prudent to avoid conception while on these drugs. Men should wait 12 weeks (the time required to clear abnormal sperm) after stopping treatment.

Carcinogenicity Immunosuppression is associated with an increased incidence of malignant disease. Large-cell diffuse lymphoma can present early in treatment, but with prolonged treatment other types of malignancy may arise. The incidence in transplant patients is about 1%.

GLUCOCORTICOSTEROIDS

For more information, see Chapter 40.

Uses

Glucocorticosteroids are used in each of the four kinds of hypersensitivity disease:

1. Glucocorticosteroids are used in the treatment of allergic rhinitis, atopic dermatitis, acute severe asthma, chronic asthma and anaphylaxis. In allergic rhinitis and atopic dermatitis (type-I reactions), the principal benefit probably arises from their non-specific anti-inflammatory effects, including vasoconstriction and decreased vascular permeability.
2. Glucocorticosteroids are often effective in type-II autoimmune diseases. They are the drugs of choice for pemphigus vulgaris and autoimmune haemolytic anaemia, and are often effective in idiopathic thrombocytopenic purpura (ITP).
3. Immune complex disease (type-III hypersensitivity) may also be treated with glucocorticosteroids, although they often produce symptomatic relief without altering the underlying disease process.
4. Glucocorticosteroids are potent inhibitors of the cell-mediated hypersensitivity (type IV) reactions. Clinically they are used to prevent acute graft rejection and improve severe contact dermatitis.

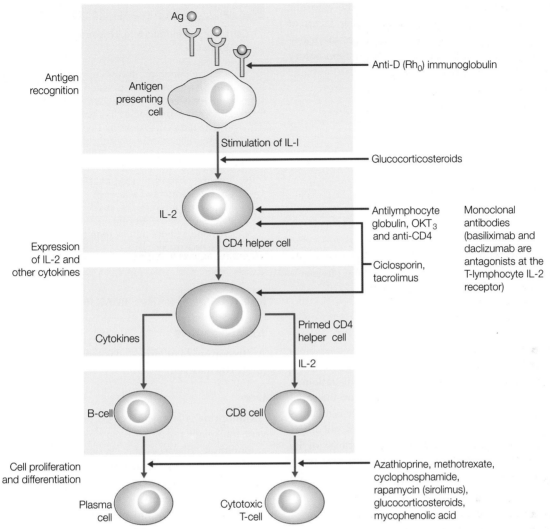

Figure 50.1: Sites of action of certain immunosuppressive agents.

Glucocorticosteroids as immunosuppressants

- Topical (e.g. beclometasone) or systemic (e.g. prednisolone) glucocorticosteroids are very effective immunosuppressants.
- Appropriate dosing schedules of glucocorticoids are effective in diseases due to all types of hypersensitivity.
- Cellular pharmacodynamics:
  - inhibits expression of pro-inflammatory cytokines IL-2, 3 and 6, TNF, GM-CSF and IFN-γ;
  - inhibits production of adhesion molecules – ICAM-1, E-selectin and vascortin – leading to reduced vascular permeability;
  - reduces synthesis of arachidonic acid metabolites (prostaglandins, leukotrienes) and reduces histamine release;
  - reduces synthesis of Fc and C3 receptors.
- Hepatic metabolism (CYP3A), dosed to minimize HPA suppression – lowest dose, once a day.
- Adverse effects include:
  - acute effects – metabolic disturbances (glucose/hypokalaemia), CNS (mood disorders, insomnia);
  - chronic-effects – features of Cushing's syndrome;
  - immunosuppression, risk of infection and HPA axis suppression.

CALCINEURIN INHIBITORS: CICLOSPORIN (AND ITS CONGENERS)

Ciclosporin is a cyclic hydrophobic decapeptide that was originally extracted from fungal cultures.

Uses

The main use of **ciclosporin** is in immunosuppression for solid-organ transplantation, but it is also effective in refractory psoriasis and bone marrow transplantation and graft-versus-host disease. A high dose of **ciclosporin** is given 4–12 hours before transplantation and then various oral maintenance dose regimens are used. Therapeutic drug monitoring is used to optimize therapy.

Mechanism of action

Ciclosporin is a specific T-lymphocyte suppressor, primarily acting on the T-helper (Th1) cells, with a unique effect on the primary immune response. It inhibits the production of interleukin-2 (IL-2) and other cytokines by activated lymphocytes. **Ciclosporin** binds to a cytosolic protein cyclophilin. This conjugate subsequently interacts with a Ca^{2+}–calmodulin-dependent calcineurin complex and inhibits its phosphorylase activity. This impairs access to the nucleus of the cytosolic component of the transcription promoter nuclear factor of activated T cells (NF-ATc), which in turn reduces the transcription of messenger RNA for IL-2, other pro-inflammatory lymphokines and IL-2 receptors.

Adverse effects

These include the following:

- nephrotoxicity, which may be minimized by concomitant use of calcium channel blockers;
- hyperkalaemia;
- nausea and gastro-intestinal disturbances;
- hypertension;
- hirsutism;
- gingival hypertrophy;
- tremor (which can be an early sign of increasing plasma concentrations), paraesthesia and fits;
- hepatotoxicity;
- anaphylaxis with intravenous administration.

Pharmacokinetics

Ciclosporin is variably absorbed after oral administration. It undergoes variable presystemic metabolism by gastro-intestinal cytochrome P450 3A4. The major route of clearance is metabolism via hepatic CYP3A. Renal dysfunction does not affect **ciclosporin** clearance, but caution is needed because of its nephrotoxicity. Dose reduction is required in patients with hepatic impairment.

Therapeutic drug monitoring

Ciclosporin is assayed by radioimmunoassay (RIA) or high-performance liquid chromatography (HPLC). Effective immunosuppression occurs at trough concentrations of 100–300 μg/L.

Drug interactions

These include **allopurinol**, **cimetidine**, **ketoconazole** (and other azoles), **erythromycin**, **diltiazem** (and other calcium-channel blockers), anabolic steroids, **norethisterone** and other inhibitors of cytochrome P450 3A4, which reduce the hepatic clearance of **ciclosporin** leading to increased toxicity. **Phenytoin** and **rifampicin** increase hepatic clearance, thus reducing plasma concentrations. Concomitant use of nephrotoxic agents such as aminoglycosides, **vancomycin** and **amphotericin** increases nephrotoxicity. ACE inhibitors increase the risk of hyperkalaemia.

Tacrolimus (**FK506**) is another calcineurin inhibitor. It is more potent than **ciclosporin** and often used in patients who are refractory to **ciclosporin**. It can be given intravenously or orally, and has variable absorption, and is metabolized by hepatic CYP3A4. Therapeutic drug monitoring of trough concentrations is useful. The side effect and drug–drug interaction profile of **tacrolimus** is similar to that of **ciclosporin**, but it may cause more neurotoxicity and nephrotoxicity.

Key points

Calcineurin inhibitors (e.g. ciclosporin) as immuno-suppressants

- First-line immunosuppressive agent in solid-organ transplant immunosuppression.
- Used in severe refractory psoriasis.
- Inhibits transcription of IL-2 and other pro-inflammatory cytokines by T lymphocytes.
- Given orally or intravenously, shows variable absorption and hepatic metabolism (CYP3A) to many inactive metabolites.
- Toxicity – nephrotoxicity, nausea, hypertension, CNS effects (tremor and seizures).
- Many drug interactions – toxicity potentiated by azoles, macrolides and diltiazem.
- Tacrolimus (more potent than ciclosporin, but possibly more neurotoxicity).

ANTI-PROLIFERATIVE IMMUNOSUPPRESSANTS

AZATHIOPRINE

Azathioprine is a prodrug and is converted to **6-mercaptopurine (6-MP)** by the liver.

Uses

Azathioprine is less widely used now than previously to prevent transplant rejection. It may also be used to treat certain autoimmune diseases (e.g. systemic lupus erythematosus, rheumatoid arthritis, inflammatory bowel disease, chronic active hepatitis and some cases of glomerulonephritis). Owing to its potential toxicity, it is usually reserved for patients in whom glucocorticosteroids alone are inadequate. The **azathioprine** mechanism of action, adverse reactions, pharmacokinetics and drug interactions are those of **6-MP** and are detailed in Chapter 48.

Key points

Anti-proliferative agents as immunosuppressants

- These include azathioprine (prodrug of 6-MP), methotrexate, cyclophosphamide and mycophenolate mofetil.
- They are used as components of combination therapy with ciclosporin and/or steroids.
- Azathioprine's haematopoietic suppression is a major limitation of its use.
- Sirolimus, which also synergizes with calcineurin inhibitors, is an alternative.

CYCLOPHOSPHAMIDE AND METHOTREXATE

For more information on **cyclophosphamide** and **methotrexate**, see Chapter 48.

MYCOPHENOLATE MOFETIL
Uses

Mycophenolate mofetil is an ester of a product of the *Penicillium* mould. It is used in combination with immunophilins (e.g **ciclosporin**) and glucocorticosteroids in solid-organ (e.g. renal,

Table 50.1: Novel anti-proliferative immunosuppressants

Drug	Comments on use	Side effects	Pharmacokinetics
Sirolimus (rapamycin)	Used with ciclosporin to prevent graft rejection	Mild gastro-intestinal disturbances. Thrombocytopenia leukopenia, anaemia, increased cholesterol and triglycerides. Not nephrotoxic	Well absorbed. Elimination $t_{1/2}$ is 57 h. Hepatic metabolism by CYP3A. Linear kinetics
	Molecular target/mechanism: binds and inhibits mTOR, a protein kinase involved in cell cycle progression	Drug interactions similar to ciclosporin. Sirolimus AUC increased if given with ciclosporin	Therapeutic drug monitoring advised
Everolimus	Analogue of sirolimus		Shorter $t_{1/2}$ than sirolimus

mTOR, mammalian target of rapamycin.

cardiac) transplantation and is a more effective alternative than **azathioprine**. **Mycophenolate mofetil** may also be effective in the treatment of other autoimmune disorders, such as rheumatoid arthritis and psoriasis.

Mechanism of action

In vivo the active entity, mycophenolic acid, inhibits inosine monophosphate dehydrogenase (a pivotal enzyme in purine synthesis). It suppresses proliferation both of T and B lymphocytes. In addition, **mycophenolic acid** inhibits the production of pro-inflammatory cytokines.

Adverse effects

These include the following:

- gastro-intestinal disturbances – diarrhoea and haemorrhage;
- bone marrow suppression, especially leukopenia and anaemia;
- CMV infection;
- lymphomas.

Pharmacokinetics

Mycophenolate mofetil is a prodrug ester of **mycophenolic acid**, with improved absorption. After oral administration in humans, the ester is rapidly and completely cleaved to **mycophenolic acid**. **Mycophenolic acid** undergoes hepatic elimination to its inactive glucuronide metabolite.

Drug interactions

Antacids decrease **mycophenolate** absorption.

For novel anti-proliferative agents, such as **sirolimus** and **everolimus** – see Table 50.1.

BIOLOGIC IMMUNOSUPPRESSANTS

POLYCLONAL ANTIBODIES

ANTILYMPHOCYTE GLOBULIN

Antilymphocyte globulin (ALG, also known as **antithymocyte globulin**) is prepared by injecting human T lymphocytes into animals (e.g. rabbits or horses) to raise antibodies. The active immunoglobulin is largely in the IgG fraction and ALG is a polyclonal antilymphocyte antibody with inherent variability from batch to batch. The major effect is probably to prevent antigen from accessing the antigen-recognition site on the T-helper cells. It is given intravenously for acute organ transplant rejection. Adverse effects include anaphylaxis and serum sickness.

MONOCLONAL ANTIBODIES

ANTI-CD3 ANTIBODY (MUROMONAB-CD3)

Uses

These monoclonal antibodies are used as adjuvant (often as second-line) immunosuppressive therapy in patients with acute transplant rejection. They are IgG2a antibodies produced from murine hybridoma cells and are given intravenously. After a 10- to 14-day course, some patients develop neutralizing antibodies.

Mechanism of action

Anti-CD3 antibodies bind CD3 protein, blocking antigen binding to the T-cell antigen–recognition complex, and decreasing the number of circulating CD3-positive lymphocytes. In addition, binding of anti-CD3 to its receptor causes cytokine release (see Adverse effects below). The overall effect is to reduce T-cell activation in acute solid-organ graft rejection.

Adverse effects

These include the following:

- cytokine release syndrome, with chest pain, wheezing and dyspnoea (pulmonary oedema occurs after the first dose in 1% of patients);
- hypersensitivity reactions ranging from anaphylaxis to an acute influenza-like syndrome;
- CNS effects – seizures, reversible meningo-encephalitis and cerebral oedema.

Other humanized monoclonal antibodies used as immuno-suppressants include:

- **Daclizumab** and **basilixumab** (organ transplant rejection) which are anti-IL-2 receptor antibodies, inhibiting IL-2-mediated T-cell activation. They have similar toxicities as the anti-CD-3 monoclonal antibody, but do not cause cytokine release syndrome on first dose.
- **Infliximab** and **etanercept** (which bind to TNF-alpha) are used in the treatment of refractory rheumatoid arthritis and inflammatory bowel disease (Chapter 34).
- **Natalizumab** (an anti-alpha-4 beta-3 integrin monoclonal antibody) used in patients with progressive multiple sclerosis.

Other drugs that attenuate the immune response include **penicillamine**, **gold** and **chloroquine**. These drugs are used in an attempt to modify disease progression in patients with severe rheumatoid arthritis (Chapter 26).

CHEMICAL MEDIATORS OF THE IMMUNE RESPONSE AND DRUGS THAT BLOCK THEIR ACTIONS

Several important therapeutic drugs block the release or action of mediators of immune reactions.

HISTAMINE

Histamine is widely distributed in the body and is derived from the decarboxylation of histidine. It is concentrated in mast-cell and basophil granules. The highest concentrations are found in the lung, nasal mucous membrane, skin, stomach and duodenum (i.e. at interfaces between the body and the outside environment). Histamine is liberated by several basic drugs (usually when these are given in large quantities intra-venously), including **tubocurarine**, **morphine**, **codeine**, **vancomycin** and **suramin**. Histamine controls some local vascular responses, is a neurotransmitter in the brain, releases gastric acid (Chapter 34) and contributes to allergic responses. There are two main types of histamine receptors, H_1 and H_2.

H_1-RECEPTORS

In humans, stimulation of H_1-receptors causes dilatation of small arteries and capillaries, together with increased permeability, which leads to formation of oedema. Histamine induces vascular endothelium to release nitric oxide, which causes vasodilatation and lowers systemic blood pressure. Inhaled histamine induces bronchospasm. In fetal vessels (e.g. the umbilical artery), histamine causes vasoconstriction. Histamine contributes to the triple response to mechanical stimulation of the skin which consists of localized pallor, which gives way to a wheal (localized oedema caused by increased vessel permeability and attributable to histamine) surrounded by a more distant and slowly developing flare (due to arteriolar dilatation via an axon-reflex mechanism and involving tachykinins such as substance P, rather than histamine). Local injection of histamine causes itching and sometimes pain due to stimulation of peripheral nerves. Inhaled histamine is used as a challenge to determine bronchial hyperreactivity and assist in the diagnosis of asthma.

H_2- AND H_3-RECEPTORS

H_2-receptors are principally concerned with the stimulation of gastric acid release (Chapter 34). Their contribution to most vascular responses is minor, but some (e.g. in the pulmonary vasculature) are H_2-receptor mediated. H_3-receptors are involved in neurotransmission.

HYPERSENSITIVITY REACTIONS INVOLVING HISTAMINE RELEASE

Anaphylactic shock (acute anaphylaxis)

In certain circumstances, injection of an antigen is followed by the production of reaginic IgE antibodies. These coat mast cells and basophils, and further exposure to the antigen results in rapid degranulation with release of histamine and other mediators, including tachykinins, prostaglandin D_2 and leukotrienes. Clinically, the patient presents a picture of shock and collapse with hypotension, bronchospasm and oropharyngeal-laryngeal oedema, often accompanied by urticaria and flushing. A similar so-called 'anaphylactoid reaction' may occur after the non-IgE-mediated release of mediators by x-ray contrast media.

> **Key points**
>
> Anaphylaxis and anaphylactoid reactions
>
> - Anaphylaxis:
>   - is IgE-mediated hypersensitivity (type-1) that occurs in a previously sensitized individual;
>   - its pathophysiology is major cardiovascular and respiratory dysfunction due to vasoactive mediator release from mast cells;
>   - common causes are penicillins, cephalosporins and many other drugs, insect stings and food allergies (e.g. strawberries, fish, peanuts).
> - Anaphylactoid reactions:
>   - are due to drug dose-related pharmacologically induced mediator release from mast cells and basophils;
>   - common causes include aspirin, NSAIDs and radiographic contrast media.

Atopy

Some individuals with a hereditary atopic diathesis have a propensity to develop local allergic reactions if exposed to appropriate antigens, causing hay fever, allergic asthma or urticaria. This is due to antigen combining with mast-cell-associated IgE in the mucosa of the respiratory tract or the skin.

Treatment of anaphylactic shock

Anaphylactic shock is a medical emergency and its treatment is as follows:

- Stop the offending drug or blood/blood product infusion.
- Check the patient's blood pressure (lie them flat) and check for the presence of stridor/bronchospasm.
- Administer oxygen (FiO_2 40–60%).
- Administer adrenaline (epinephrine) 0.5–1 mg intramuscularly, and repeat after ten minutes if necessary.
- Give intravenous colloids (0.9% NaCl) for refractory hypotension.
- Administer hydrocortisone, 100–200 mg i.v.
- Administer chlorpheniramine, 12.5 mg i.v.
- Give nebulized salbutamol, 2.5–5 mg for refractory bronchospasm.

DRUGS THAT BLOCK THE EFFECTS OF MEDIATORS OF ALLERGY

Therapeutic approaches to the management of allergic disease produced by mediators include the following:

- inhibition of their biosynthesis;
- blockade of their release;
- antagonism of their effects.

INHIBITION OF BIOSYNTHESIS OF PRO-INFLAMMATORY MEDIATORS

INTRANASAL AND TOPICAL GLUCOCORTICOSTEROIDS

These are covered in Chapters 33 and 40.

Uses

These preparations are used in the therapy of allergic rhinitis and they are very effective in reducing the symptoms of nasal itching, sneezing, rhinorrhoea and nasal obstruction (they are more effective than **cromoglicate**). Common agents used to treat hay fever include **beclometasone**, **budesonide** and **fluticasone**.

Adverse effects

The adverse effects of all these preparations are similar, namely sneezing, and dryness and irritation of the nose and throat. Occasionally, epistaxis is a problem.

BLOCKADE OF RELEASE OF PRO-INFLAMMATORY MEDIATORS

SODIUM CROMOGLICATE AND NEDOCROMIL

See also Chapter 33.

Uses

Sodium cromoglicate and **nedocromil** are effective in preventing exercise-induced and allergic asthma (but less effective than inhaled glucocorticosteroids for the latter). They are also effective in preventing hay fever and its symptoms. **Cromoglicate** is used as nasal or eye drops for allergic rhinitis and conjunctivitis. Local adverse effects include occasional nasal irritation or transient stinging in the eye.

ANTAGONISM OF THE EFFECTS OF PRO-INFLAMMATORY MEDIATORS

ANTIHISTAMINES

There are a large number of antihistamines (H_1-receptor antagonists) available, several of which are available without prescription. Some of those in common use are listed in Table 50.2. Their

Table 50.2: Properties of commonly used H_1-antagonists

Drug	Duration of effect (h)	Degree of sedation	Anti-emetic action	Risk of ventricular tachycardia when prescribed with other drugs inhibiting their metabolism
First generation				
Promethazine	20	Marked	Some	?
Diphenhydramine	6	Some	Little	?
Chlorphenamine	4–6	Moderate	Little	?
Cyclizine	6	Some	Marked	?
Triprolidine (slow release)	24	Moderate	Little	?
Second generation				
Acrivastine	6–8	Nil	Little	None
Fexofenadine	12	Nil	Little	None
Cetirizine	24	Nil	Little	None
Loratadine	24	Nil	Little	None

antihistaminic actions are similar when used in clinically appropriate dosage, but their major differences are in duration of effect, degree of sedation and anti-emetic potential.

Uses

These include the following:

- hypersensitivity reactions;
- urticaria and hay fever;
- bee and wasp stings;
- anti-emetic (e.g. **cyclizine**).

Mechanism of action

Antihistamines are competitive antagonists of histamine at H_1-receptors.

Pharmacokinetics

Antihistamines are rapidly absorbed from the intestine and are effective within about 30 minutes. They generally undergo hepatic metabolism. Newer agents, such as **fexofenadine, cetirizine** and **loratadine** have half-lives that permit once or twice daily dosing. They do not penetrate the blood–brain barrier and cause less psychomotor impairment than first-generation antihistamines.

Adverse effects

These include the following:

- sedation and psychomotor impairment, especially with older (first-generation) agents;
- photosensitivity rashes;
- antimuscarinic effects: dry mouth, blurred vision, etc. (first-generation agents);
- prolongation of the QTc and torsades de pointes.

Key points

Antihistamines and therapy of allergic disorders

- Antagonists at H_1-receptors; widely available agents, often without prescription (e.g. chlorpheniramine).
- Used to treat hay fever and urticaria, and also used as therapy for motion sickness.
- Should not be applied topically for skin irritation, as they may cause dermatitis.
- Hepatically metabolized (CYP3A – long- and shorter-acting drugs.
- Duration of effects often outlasts their presence in the blood.
- First-generation agents are shorter acting (e.g. chlorpheniramine), sedating and anticholinergic, better anti-emetics, and have some 5HT and α-adrenoceptor antagonist activity.
- Second-generation agents have few or no sedative or ancilliary properties, and are longer acting (e.g. cetirizine).
- Second generation agents (e.g. cetirizine, loratadine) are safe (i.e. ventricular tachycardia is not a risk) if co-prescribed with macrolides or azoles.

Contraindications

Antihistamines should be avoided in porphyria and in the Ward–Romano syndrome (congenital long-QT syndrome).

ADRENALINE (EPINEPHRINE)

Adrenaline (epinephrine) is uniquely valuable therapeutically in anaphylactic shock. Its rapid action may be life-saving in general anaphylaxis due to insect venom allergy and reaction to drugs. The usual dose is 0.5–1.0 mg, repeated after ten minutes if necessary, given intramuscularly or if necessary intravenously. It is effective by virtue of its α-agonist activity which reverses vascular dilatation and oedema, and its β_2-agonist activity which produces cardiac stimulation and bronchodilatation. It also reduces the release of pro-inflammatory mediators and cytokines.

TREATMENT OF ANAPHYLACTIC SHOCK

1. Stop any drug or blood/blood product that is being administered intravenously.
2. Adrenaline 0.5–1 mg i.m. or 0.25–0.5 mg i.v.
3. Intravenous fluid (e.g. 0.9% NaCl, normal saline).
4. Oxygen (high concentration FiO_2 28–40%).
5. Hydrocortisone 100–200 mg intravenously.
6. Antihistamine intravenously (e.g. **chlorpheniramine**, 12.5 mg).
7. Consider nebulized **salbutamol** (2.5–5 mg) for residual bronchospasm.

THERAPY OF ALLERGIC RHINITIS (HAY FEVER)

The patient who presents with symptoms of allergic rhinitis should be assessed to ensure that infection is not the primary problem. If infection is the cause, the presence of a foreign body should be excluded and appropriate antibacterial therapy prescribed. If the symptoms are due to allergy, the first step in therapy is allergen avoidance and minimization of exposure (e.g. to ragweed pollen). However, complete avoidance is difficult to achieve. For patients with mild intermittent symptoms, either intranasal antihistamine (e.g. **olopatadine** or **azelastine**) or intranasal **cromoglicate** or a shorter-acting non-sedating systemic antihistamine (e.g. **acrivastine** or **fexofenadine**) is effective. Short-term use of a nasal decongestant such as **pseudoephedrine** is effective, but if used for longer periods causes rebound vasomotor rhinitis. **Ipratropium bromide** administered intra-nasally may be added if rhinorrhoea is the predominant symptom. If symptoms are more chronic, the first-line therapy is intranasal glucocorticosteroids because these are effective against all symptoms, and are more effective than antihistamines or **cromoglicate**. In children, topical **cromoglicate** given by insufflator or nasal spray is useful. If rhinorrhoea is the main problem, **ipratropium bromide** may be added with or without a long-acting antihistamine (e.g. **cetirizine**). If these measures are ineffective, consider low-dose intranasal steroids, or immunotherapy or surgery if there is evidence of sinusitis.

DRUGS THAT ENHANCE IMMUNE SYSTEM FUNCTION

ADJUVANTS

Adjuvants non-specifically augment the immune response when mixed with antigen or injected into the same site. This is achieved in the following ways:

- release of the antigen is slowed and exposure to it is prolonged;
- various immune cells are attracted to the site of injection and the interaction between such cells is important in antibody formation.

There are a number of such substances, usually given as mixtures and often containing lipids, extracts of inactivated tubercle bacilli and various mineral salts.

IMMUNOSTIMULANTS

Immunostimulants non-specifically enhance immune responses, examples include bacille Calmette-Guérin (BCG) or killed *Corynebacterium parvum*.

INTERLEUKIN-2 (IL-2)

Interleukin-2 is effective treatment for metastatic melanoma and renal cell carcinoma (Chapter 48).

VACCINES

IMMUNOLOGY AND GENERAL USE

Vaccines stimulate an immune response. They may consist of:

- an attenuated form of the infectious agent, such as the live vaccines used to prevent rubella, measles or polio, or BCG to prevent tuberculosis;
- inactivated preparations of virus (e.g. influenza virus) or bacteria (e.g. typhoid vaccine);
- detoxified exotoxins ('toxoids'), e.g. tetanus vaccine.

Live vaccine immunization is generally achieved with a single dose, but three doses are required for oral polio (to cover different strains). Live vaccine replicates while in the body and produces protracted immunity, albeit not as long as that acquired after natural infection. When two live vaccines are required (and are not in a combined preparation) they may be given at different sites simultaneously or at an interval of at least three weeks. Inactivated vaccines usually require sequential doses of vaccine to produce an adequate antibody response. Booster injections are required at intervals. The duration of immunity acquired with the use of inactivated vaccines ranges from months to years. The vaccination programmes recommended by the Department of Health (DH) in the UK are described in detail in a memorandum entitled 'Immunization against infectious disease', available to doctors from the Department of Health. The British National Formulary summarizes the recommended schedule of vaccinations.

Contraindications

Postpone vaccination if the patient is suffering from acute illness. Ensure that the patient is not sensitive to antibiotics used in the preparation of the vaccine (e.g. **neomycin** and **polymyxin**). Egg sensitivity excludes the administration of several vaccines (e.g. influenza). Live vaccines should not be given to pregnant women, nor should they be given to patients who are immunosuppressed. Live vaccines should be postponed until at least three months after stopping glucocorticosteroids and six months after chemotherapy. Live vaccines should not be administered to HIV-1-positive individuals.

Key points

Vaccine therapy

- Vaccines generally stimulate the production of protective antibodies or activated T cells.
- Vaccines consist of:
  - attenuated infectious agents – antiviral vaccines (e.g. mumps, rubella, etc.).
  - inactivated viral/bacterial preparations (e.g. influenza virus or typhoid vaccine).
  - extracts of detoxified toxins (e.g. tetanus toxin).
- Live vaccines produce protracted immunity and some (e.g. measles and mumps vaccines) have a low risk of causing a mild form of the disease.
- Different countries have different vaccination schedules based on the prevalence of the disease in the population and the level of herd ('population') immunity.

IMMUNOGLOBULINS AS THERAPY

Immunoglobulin injection gives immediate passive protection for four to six weeks. Recombinant technology will yield antibodies of consistent quality in the future, but it is a challenge to replicate the diversity present in polyclonal human normal immunoglobulin. Currently, there are two types of immunoglobulin, namely normal and specific.

HUMAN NORMAL IMMUNOGLOBULIN

Human normal immunoglobulin (HNIG) is prepared from pooled donations of human plasma. It contains antibodies to measles, mumps, varicella, hepatitis A and other viruses.

Uses

HNIG is used to protect susceptible subjects from infection with hepatitis A and measles and, to a lesser extent, to protect the fetus against rubella in pregnancy when termination is not an option. Special formulations for intravenous administration are available for replacement therapy in agammaglobulinaemia, hypogammaglobulinaemia and IgG subclass deficiency (e.g. Bruton's agammaglobulinaemia, Wiskott–Aldrich syndrome), idiopathic thrombocytopenic purpura and for prophylaxis of infection in bone marrow transplant patients.

Adverse effects

The most common adverse effects occur during the first infusion and are dependent on the antigenic load (dose) given. They include the following:

- fever, chills and rarely anaphylaxis – most commonly seen with the first dose, and reduced by slow administration and premedication with antihistamines and glucocorticosteroids;
- increased plasma viscosity – caution is needed in patients with ischaemic heart disease;
- aseptic meningitis (high dose).

Contraindications

Normal immunoglobulin is contraindicated in patients with known class-specific antibody to IgA.

Interactions

Live virus vaccinations may be rendered less effective.

SPECIFIC IMMUNOGLOBULINS

These antibodies are prepared by pooling the plasma of selected donors with high levels of the specific antibody required. The following are currently available and effective: rabies immunoglobulin, tetanus immunoglobulin (human origin-HTIG), varicella zoster immunoglobulin (VZIG) (limited supply); anti-CMV immunoglobulin (on a named patient basis).

ANTI-D (RHO) IMMUNOGLOBULIN

This immunoglobulin is used to prevent a rhesus-negative mother from forming antibodies to fetal rhesus-positive cells that enter the maternal circulation during childbirth or abortion. An intramuscular injection is given to rhesus-negative mothers up to 72 hours after the birth/abortion. This prevents a subsequent child from developing haemolytic disease of the newborn.

Case history

A 35-year-old woman had a cadaveric renal transplant for polycystic kidneys two years previously and was stable on her immunosuppressive regimen of ciclosporin, 300 mg twice a day, and mycophenolate mofetil, 1 g twice a day. Her usual trough ciclosporin concentrations were 200–250 µg/L and her hepatic and liver function was normal. She went on holiday to southern California for ten days, where she was well, but drank plenty of fluids (but no alcohol) as she was warned about the dangers of dehydration. By the end of her visit, she noted some nausea and a mild tremor. Following a long return flight, she went to her local hospital and sustained a brief spontaneously remitting epileptic fit in the outpatient department where she was having her blood ciclosporin concentration checked. The fit lasted about one minute and she was taken to the Accident and Emergency Department.

Examination revealed no abnormalities apart from slight tremor which she said she had noted for the last 48 hours. Her ciclosporin concentration was 650 µg/L. All other medical biochemistry tests were normal. She was not taking any other prescribed medications or over-the-counter drugs.
Questions
What caused this patient's seizures?
How can you explain the markedly elevated trough ciclosporin concentration?

Answer
In this patient, the development of an acute epileptic seizure in the context of a very high ciclosporin trough concentration indicates ciclosporin toxicity; epilepsy is a well-recognized toxic effect of high ciclosporin concentrations. The difficult issue in the case is why she developed high ciclosporin blood concentrations (in the face of normal renal and hepatic function) when she was adamant that there had been no alteration in the daily dose of ciclosporin she was taking, nor had she started any other drugs (prescribed or over-the-counter agents). Further questioning defined that she was drinking about 1 L/day of grapefruit juice – a taste she had acquired while on holiday in California. Grapefruit juice contains psoralens and flavonoids which inhibit CYP3A (gastrointestinal and hepatic) and flavonoids which inhibit P-gp in the gut wall, increasing the bioavailability of ciclosporin by 19–60%, the combined effect leading to higher concentrations without a change in dose. The patient had her ciclosporin dosing stopped until the concentration was <300 µg/L. She had no further fits, her nausea and tremor subsided, and she was then restarted on her normal dose with clear instructions not to drink grapefruit juice.

Examples of other drugs whose oral bioavailability is increased in humans with co-ingestion of grapefruit juice include midazolam, oestrogens, atorvastatin (and most statins except pravastatin), testosterone, felodipine, nifedipine (but not diltiazem), some anti-HIV protease inhibitors, other calcinerin inhibitors. Patients who are taking these agents or other drugs metabolized by CYP3A/P-gp should be warned not to ingest even single cupfuls of grapefruit juice, as this may precipitate toxic drug concentrations.

FURTHER READING

Golightly LK, Greos LS. Second-generation antihistamines: actions and efficacy in the management of allergic disorders. *Drugs* 2005; **65**: 341–84.

Lindenfeld J, Miller GG, Shakar SF et al. Drug therapy in the heart transplant recipient: part II: immunosuppressive drugs. *Circulation* 2004; **110**: 3858–65.

Lipsky JJ. Drug profile. Mycophenolate mofetil. *Lancet* 1996; **348**: 1357–9.

Plaut M, Valentine MD. Clinical practice. Allergic rhinitis. *New England Journal of Medicine* 2005; **353**: 1934–44.

Simons ERF, Simons KJ. Drug therapy:the pharmacology and use of H$_1$-receptor antagonist drugs. *New England Journal of Medicine* 1994; **330**: 1663–70.

Waldman TA. Immunotherapy: past, present and future. *Nature Medicine* 2003; **9**: 269–77.

PART XII

THE SKIN

DRUGS AND THE SKIN

INTRODUCTION

Skin conditions account for up to 2% of consultations in general practice. The ability of the practitioner to make a correct diagnosis is paramount, and is aided by the ease of biopsy of the abnormal tissue. The non-specific use of drugs which can modify the appearance of skin lesions (e.g. potent topical glucocorticosteroids) should be avoided in the absence of a diagnosis. Adverse reactions to topical or systemic drugs produce a wide variety of skin lesions. Drugs applied topically to the skin may act locally and/or enter the systemic circulation and produce either a harmful or beneficial systemic pharmacological effect. Further details of transdermal drug absorption/delivery are discussed in Chapter 4.

ACNE

Incidence and pathophysiology

Acne vulgaris is one of the most common skin disorders, occurring in 80–90% of adolescents. It is associated with *Propionibacterium acnes* infection of the sebaceous glands and causes inflammatory papules, pustules, nodules, cysts and scarring, mainly on the face, chest, back and arms.

PRINCIPLES OF TREATMENT

An algorithm for treatment of acne is outlined in Figure 51.1. The topical use of keratolytic (peeling) agents, such as **benzoyl peroxide** or **retinoic acid** (**tretinoin**) on a regular basis in conjunction with systemic antibiotic therapy is successful in most cases. The main side effect of keratolytic agents is skin irritation. **Azelaic acid** is a natural product of *Pityrosporum ovale*, and has both antibacterial and anti-keratinizing activity. It is less irritant than **benzoyl peroxide** and preferred by some patients for this

reason, especially for facial lesions. Because of the powerful teratogenic effects of oral vitamin A analogues, there has been concern about the safety of topical retinoic acid derivatives in the first trimester of pregnancy. However, a large study from the USA has shown that topical **retinoic acid** is not associated with an increased risk of major congenital abnormalities. Suitable antibiotic treatment includes low-dose **doxycycline** or **erythromycin** given until improvement occurs, which may take several months. Tetracyclines should not be used until the secondary dentition is established (i.e. after the age of 12 years). *Pseudomembranous colitis* has occurred in patients on long-term tetracyclines for acne, as has the development of microbial resistance. Topical antibiotic preparations (e.g. **tetracycline** or **clindamycin**) are less effective than systemic therapy.

For patients with disease that is refractory to these therapies, the use of either low-dose anti-androgens or **isotretinoin** (see below) should be considered, but only under the supervision of a consultant dermatologist.

HORMONAL THERAPY OF ACNE

Acne depends on the actions of androgens on the sebaceous glands. Hormone manipulation is often successful in women with acne that is refractory to antibiotics and is useful in patients who require contraception, which is essential because of the potential for feminizing a male fetus. **Cyproterone acetate** is an anti-androgen with central and peripheral activity, and is combined with low-dose oestrogen, **ethinylestradiol**. Some women with hirsutism may also benefit because hair growth is also androgen-dependent. Contraindications include pregnancy and a predisposition to thrombosis.

RETINOID THERAPY IN ACNE

The management of severe acne has changed dramatically with the advent of the synthetic vitamin A analogues.

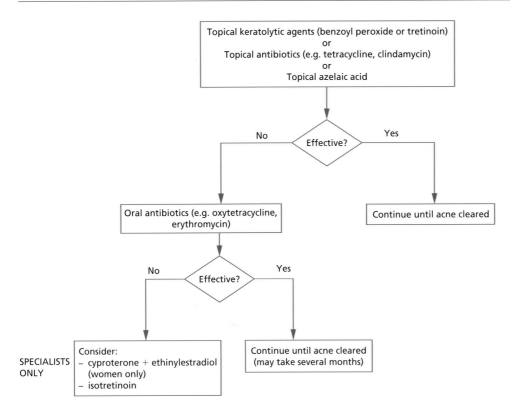

Figure 51.1: Pathway for treatment of acne.

ISOTRETINOIN

Uses

Isotretinoin is the D-isomer of **tretinoin**, another vitamin A analogue. It is given orally for severe acne or rosacea and should only be prescribed under hospital supervision. The usual course is four months, with 80% improvement. Clinical benefit continues after discontinuation of therapy.

Mechanism of action

The primary action of retinoids is inhibition of sebum production, reducing the size of the sebaceous glands by 90% in the first month. These drugs also inhibit keratinization of the hair follicle, resulting in reduced comedones.

Adverse effects

These include the following:

- teratogenic effects;
- mucocutaneous effects – cheilitis, dry mouth, epistaxis, dermatitis, desquamation, hair and nail loss;
- central nervous system (CNS) effects – ocular (papilloedema, night blindness), raised intracranial pressure;
- musculoskeletal effects – arthralgia, muscle stiffness, skeletal hyperostosis, premature fusion of epiphyses;
- hepatotoxic effects;
- hypertriglyceridaemia.

Contraindications

Systemic use of any vitamin A analogue is contraindicated in pregnant or breast-feeding women.

Pharmacokinetics

Isotretinoin is well absorbed (>90%). Tissue binding is high and it is eliminated over a period of at least one month after treatment has been discontinued. This explains the ongoing clinical benefit after stopping drug therapy and also the persistent risk of teratogenicity after a course of treatment. **Isotretinoin** is almost totally cleared from the body by hepatic metabolism.

Drug interactions

There is an increased incidence of raised intracranial pressure if **isotretinoin** is prescribed with tetracyclines.

ALOPECIA AND HIRSUTISM

In androgenic baldness, it is possible to promote hair growth by topical application of **minoxidil sulphate** (the active metabolite of **minoxidil**). This is believed to have a mitogenic effect on the hair follicles. Adverse effects include local itching and dermatitis. Approximately 30% of subjects respond within 4–12 months, but hair loss recurs once therapy is discontinued. In women, **cyproterone acetate** combined with **ethinylestradiol** prevents the progression of androgenic alopecia.

The anti-androgen activity (both central and peripheral) of **cyproterone acetate** makes it the systemic drug of choice for female hirsutism, if topical depilation has failed or the hirsutism is too general. It is given with **ethinylestradiol** to prevent pregnancy (feminization of the fetus). Clinical improvement may take 6–12 months.

Eflornithine, an irreversible inhibitor of ornithine decarboxylase, is a topical cream licensed for female facial hirsutism.

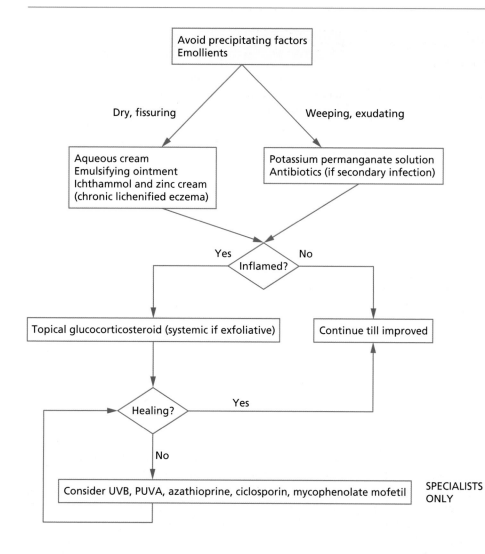

Figure 51.2: Pathway for treatment of dermatitis.

DERMATITIS (ECZEMA)

PRINCIPLES OF TREATMENT

The most common forms of dermatitis that present to physicians are atopic dermatitis, synonymous with atopic eczema, seborrhoeic dermatitis and contact dermatitis. An algorithm for treatment of dermatitis is shown in Figure 51.2.

Management of atopic eczema should include avoidance of trigger factors and the use of emollients. Dry skin is a major factor and emollients should be used when bathing and applied as often as necessary. A simple emollient (an aqueous cream, e.g. E45 or Alpha Keri) is usually all that is necessary for dry, fissured scaly lesions. Inflammation should be treated with short courses of mild to moderate topical glucocorticosteroids. A more potent glucocorticosteroid may be required for particularly severely affected areas or for a more general flare up. Oral antihistamines are often effective in reducing pruritus. **Ichthammol** and **zinc cream** may be used in chronic lichenified forms of eczema. **Potassium permanganate** solution can be used in exudating eczema for its antiseptic and astringent effect; treatment should be stopped when weeping stops.

Weeping eczema may require topical glucocorticosteroids and often antibiotics to treat secondary infection. Immunosuppressant therapy, such as **ciclosporin**, is sometimes effective in severe, resistant eczema. Ultraviolet B or psoralen + ultraviolet A (PUVA), or an immunosuppressive agent (e.g. **azathioprine**, **ciclosporin** or **mycophenolate mofetil**, Chapter 50) are also used.

Seborrhoeic dermatitis may respond to a mild topical glucocorticosteroid. Scalp seborrhoeic dermatitis is often improved by coal tar, salicylic acid and sulphur preparations. (Fungal infection should be ruled out if there is no response.)

Contact dermatitis is caused by external agents (e.g. nickel), but often complicates a pre-existing dermatitis. Avoidance of precipitating factors, emollients and topical glucocorticosteroids are used.

GLUCOCORTICOSTEROIDS

Topical glucocorticosteroids act as anti-inflammatory vasoconstrictors and reduce keratinocyte proliferation. They include **hydrocortisone** and its fluorinated semi-synthetic derivatives, which have increased anti-inflammatory potency compared to hydrocortisone (Chapter 40).

Table 51.1: Topical glucocorticosteroids and their anti-inflammatory potency

Potency	Drug and strength
Extremely potent	Clobetasol (0.05%)
	Halcinonide (0.1%)
	Diflucortolone (0.3%)
Potent	Beclometasone (0.025%)
	Budesonide (0.025%)
	Fluocinolone (0.025%)
	Fluocinonide (0.05%)
Moderately potent	Clobetasone (0.05%)
	Flurandrenolone (0.0125%)
Mild	Hydrocortisone (0.5–2.5%)
	Alclometasone (0.05%)
	Methylprednisolone (0.25%)

Uses

The use of systemic glucocorticosteroids (e.g. oral **prednisolone**) is limited to serious disorders such as pemphigus or refractory exfoliative dermatitis (e.g. Stevens Johnson syndrome). Topical glucocorticosteroids are widely used and effective in treating eczema, lichen planus, discoid lupus erythematosus, lichen simplex chronicus and palmar plantar pustulosis, but rarely in psoriasis. The symptoms of eczema are rapidly suppressed, but these drugs do not treat the cause. In the presence of infection, they are combined with an antimicrobial agent. The lowest potency glucocorticosteroid preparation that will control the disease is preferred. Occlusive dressings should be used only in the short term (two to three days) and increase potency considerably. Potent fluorinated glucocorticosteroids should not be used on the face because they cause dermatitis medicamentosa.

Many preparations are available, some of which are listed in descending order of anti-inflammatory potency in Table 51.1.

Adverse effeccts of cutaneoulsly applied glucocorticosteroids

These include the following:

- hypothalamic–pituitary–adrenal suppression where very potent drugs are used long term on large areas of skin or when systemic absorption is increased under occlusive dressing;
- spread of local infection – bacterial or fungal;
- atrophic striae;
- depigmentation and vellus hair formation;
- perioral dermatitis when applied to the face;
- rebound exacerbation of disease (e.g. pustular psoriasis) when treatment is stopped;
- exacerbation of glaucoma if applied to the eyelids;
- contact dermatitis (rare);
- hirsutism and acne if systemic absorption is very high.

PSORIASIS

Psoriasis occurs in approximately 2% of the population. Its cause is unknown and no treatment is curative. The skin lesions are characterized by epidermal thickening and scaling due to increased epidermal undifferentiated cell proliferation with abnormal keratin. Figure 51.3 shows an algorithm for treatment.

Therapy in mild cases consists of reassurance and a simple emollient cream. More resistant cases are treated with a keratolytic, e.g. **salicylic acid**, **coal tar** or **dithranol** applied accurately to the lesions. Topical and systemic steroids are reserved for cases that do not respond to these simple remedies and their use should be monitored by a specialist, as they can worsen the disease in some patients (e.g. pustular psoriasis on stopping treatment). **Calcitriol** (a vitamin D analogue) is effective topically. In some cases, therapy with PUVA (see below) is effective. Refractory cases are treated with oral retinoids (e.g. **acetretin**).

Occasionally refractory cases justify immunosuppression with **methotrexate** (Chapters 48 and 50), but chronic use can cause cirrhosis. Potential recipients need to be warned about this and their liver function must be monitored meticulously. **Ciclosporin** is an alternative (Chapter 50), but causes hypertension and nephrotoxicity. Regular monitoring of blood pressure and plasma **ciclosporin** concentration is essential. Recently, the use of biological agents (**alefacept**, **etanercept**, **efalizumab**, **infliximab**) has been found to produce good remissions in otherwise refractory psoriasis (see Table 51.2); these agents are discussed more fully in Chapter 50. Second-line therapies (phototherapy or systemic drugs) should only be used under the supervision of a dermatologist.

CALCIPOTRIOL (1-α, 24-DIHYDROXYVITAMIN D$_3$)

This analogue of vitamin D$_3$ is used as a cream applied to mild to moderate psoriasis. Vitamin D receptors are present in keratinocytes, T and B lymphocytes and dermal fibroblasts of psoriatics, and the stimulation of vitamin D receptors on keratinocytes inhibits proliferation and differentiation. Adverse effects include local irritation, facial and perioral dermatitis, and possible hypercalcaemia and hypertriglyceridaemia if used too extensively. It should not be used in pregnancy.

PSORALEN WITH ULTRAVIOLET A LIGHT

Psoralen with ultraviolet A light (PUVA) is a well-established but somewhat inconvenient therapy for chronic plaque psoriasis. Psoralens intercalate DNA bases and, when activated by light, produce highly reactive oxygen species which sensitize the skin to the cytotoxic effects of long-wave UVA (320–400 nm wavelength) radiation. **Psoralen** is taken orally two hours before phototherapy, or applied topically immediately before phototherapy; the usual course lasts for four to six weeks. Skin burning and ageing, cataracts and skin cancer are potential complications, especially with the higher total doses of UVA. Sunglasses are worn during UVA exposure in order to reduce the risk of cataract formation, if the **psoralen** has been administered orally. Technological advances in psoralens and

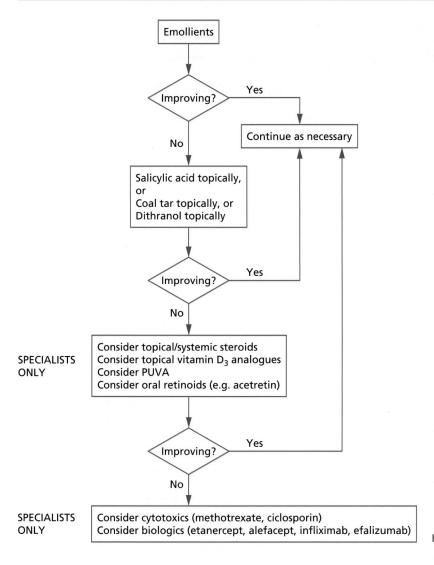

Figure 51.3: Pathway for treatment of psoriasis.

Table 51.2: Novel biological treatments used in psoriasis

	Alefacept	Efalizumab	Etanercept	Infliximab
Mechanism of action	T cell targeting	T cell targeting	TNF-α inhibition	TNF-α inhibition
Licensed for psoriasis in the UK	No	Yes	Yes	Yes
Method of administration	15 mg i.m. (7.5 mg i.v.) weekly for 12 weeks	Initial dose 0.7 mg/kg, then 1 mg/kg s.c. weekly	25–50 mg s.c. twice weekly	5 mg/kg i.v. at 0, 2 and 6 weeks, then 8-weekly
Onset of action	6–8 weeks	2–3 weeks	2–3 weeks	1 week
Percentage of patients with PASI 75	20% after 12 weeks	25% after 12 weeks	34% with 25 mg, 49% with 50 mg at 12 weeks	>80% at 10 weeks
Effects on psoriatic arthritis	In phase II trials	Modest	Yes	Yes
Efficacy as monotherapy	Yes	Yes	Yes	Yes
Monitoring investigations	Peripheral CD4 T cell count	Monthly FBC for first 3 months, then 3-monthly	FBC, renal and LFTs at 3 months, then 6-monthly	FBC, renal and LFTs at 3 months, then 6-monthly
Safety and efficacy data for long-term use	Up to 12, 12-week cycles	Up to 3 years	Up to 24 weeks	Up to 50 weeks

From Ghaffar SA, Clements SE, Griffiths CEM. Modern management of psoriasis. *Clinical Medicine* 2005; **5**: 564–68.
FBC, full blood count; i.m., intramuscular; i.v., intravenous; LFT, liver function test; PASI, Psoriasis Area Severity Index; s.c., subcutaneous; TNF, tumour necrosis factor.

UVA light, notably optimization of the dose regimen, have reduced the risk of carcinogenicity. Phototherapy combined with coal tar, **dithranol**, vitamin D or vitamin D analogues allows reduction of the cumulative dose of phototherapy required to treat psoriasis.

ACITRETIN

Acitretin is the active carboxylated metabolite of **etretinate**. It is given orally for the treatment of severe resistant or complicated psoriasis and other disorders of keratinization. It should only be given under hospital supervision. A therapeutic effect occurs after two to four weeks, with maximal benefit after six weeks. Because it is highly teratogenic, women must take adequate contraceptive precautions for one month prior to and during therapy and for two years after stopping the drug.

Retinoids bind to specific retinoic acid receptors (RARs) in the nucleus. RARs have many actions, one of which is to inhibit AP-1 (transcription factor) activity.

Acitretin is well absorbed. Unlike its parent compound, **etretinate**, **acetretin** is not highly bound to adipose tissue. Its elimination $t_{1/2}$ is shorter than that of the parent drug, but even so pregnancy must be avoided for two years after stopping treatment. Hepatic metabolism is the major route of elimination.

Acitretin is contraindicated in the presence of hepatic and renal impairment. Other contraindications and adverse effects are as for **isotretinoin** (see above).

Drug interactions

Drug interactions include the following:

- Concomitant therapy with **tetracycline** increases the risk of raised intracranial pressure.

- Hypertriglyceridaemia: other drugs (e.g. vitamin D analogues) can have additive effects.
- It increases **methotrexate** plasma concentrations and the risk of heptotoxicity.
- It possibly antagonizes the action of **warfarin**.

URICARIA

Acute urticaria is usually due to a type-1 allergic reaction: treatment is discussed in Chapter 50.

SUPERFICIAL BACTERIAL SKIN INFECTIONS

Skin infections are commonly due to staphylococci or streptococci. Impetigo or infected eczema is treated topically for no more than two weeks with antimicrobial agents, e.g. **mupirocin**.

FUNGAL SKIN AND NAIL INFECTIONS

For a summary of the drug therapy of fungal skin and nail infections see Table 51.3. Chapter 45 gives a more detailed account of the clinical pharmacology of antifungal drugs.

VIRAL SKIN INFECTIONS

For a detailed account of the pharmacology of anti-viral drugs see Chapter 45. Table 51.4 gives a summary of the drug therapy of viral skin infections.

Table 51.3: Drug therapy of fungal skin and nail infections

Fungal skin infection	Drug therapy	Comment
Candida infection of the skin, vulvovaginitis or balanitis	Topical antifungal therapy with nystatin cream (100 000 units/g) or ketoconazole 2%, clotrimazole 1% or miconazole 2% cream	Alternative topical agents are terbinafine 1% or amorolfine 0.25% creams. Systemic therapy may be necessary in refractory cases. Consider underlying diabetes mellitus
Fungal nail infections, onychomycosis dermatophytes	Griseofulvin, 10 mg/kg daily for 6–12 months, or alternatively fluconazole, 200 mg daily for 6–12 months	If systemic therapy is not tolerated, tioconazole 28% is applied daily for 6 months. Topical amorolfine 5% is an alternative
Pityriasis capitis, seborrhoeic dermatitis (dandruff)	Topical steroids – clobetasol propionate 0.05%, or betamethasone valerate 0.1%, with cetrimide shampoo	Severe cases may require additional topical ketoconazole 2% or clotrimazole 1%
Tinea capitis	Systemic therapy with fluconazole, itraconazole, miconazole or clotrimazole	–
Tinea corporis	Topical therapy with, for example, ketoconazole 2% or clotrimazole 1% applied for 2–3 weeks	Systemic therapy is only necessary in refractory cases
Tinea pedis	As for tinea corporis	As for tinea corporis

TREATMENT OF OTHER SKIN INFECTIONS (LICE, SCABIES)

The treatment of lice and scabies is covered in Table 51.5.

ADVERSE DRUG REACTIONS INVOLVING THE SKIN

Cutaneous adverse drug reactions can arise from topically or systemically administered drugs. The clinical presentation of an adverse cutaneous drug reaction is seldom pathognomonic and may vary from an erythematous, macular or morbilliform rash to erythema multiforme. Such reactions generally occur within the first one or two weeks of therapy. However, immunologically mediated reactions may take months to become clinically manifest. Contact dermatitis is usually eczematous and is most commonly seen with antimicrobial drugs or antihistamines. Sometimes the vehicle is the culprit.

The diagnosis of a drug-induced cutaneous reaction requires an accurate drug history from the patient, especially defining the temporal relationship of the skin disorder to concomitant drug therapy. In milder cases and fixed drug eruptions, re-administration (rechallenge) with the suspect agent may be justified. Patch testing is useful for contact dermatitis. The treatment of drug-induced skin disorders involves removing the cause, applying cooling creams and antipruritics, and reserving topical steroids only for severe cases.

Table 51.6 lists some of the most common drug-related cutaneous reactions.

PHOTOSENSITIVITY

The term 'photosensitivity' combines both phototoxicity and photoallergy. Phototoxicity (like drug toxicity) is a predictable

Table 51.4: Summary of drug therapy of viral skin infections

Viral skin infection	Drug therapy	Comment
Initial or recurrent genital labial or herpes simplex	Topical 5% aciclovir cream, 4-hourly for 5 days is used, but is of questionable benefit. Systemic aciclovir therapy is required for buccal and vaginal herpes simplex	Topical penciclovir (2% cream) is an alternative for recurrent orolabial herpes. Systemic valaciclovir or famciclovir are new alternatives to aciclovir
Skin warts, papilloma virus infections	All treatments are destructive. Cryotherapy (solid carbon dioxide, liquid nitrogen). Daily keratolytics, such as 12% salicylic acid	For plantar warts use 1.5% formaldehyde or 10% glutaraldehyde. For anal warts use podophyllin resin 15% or podophyllotoxin 0.5% solution applied precisely on the lesions once or twice weekly

Table 51.5: Summary of the treatments for other common dermatological infections

Disease	Causal agent	Treatment	Toxicity of therapy	Additional comments
Lice	Caused by *Pediculus humanus capitis*	0.5% malathion or carbamyl are recommended – leave in contact for 12 h	Use aqueous rather than alcohol preparations in asthmatics and small children	Apply to affected area and repeat in 7 days to kill lice that have just emerged from eggs
Scabies	Caused by transmission of *Sarcoptes scabei*	Lindane 1% (apply topically and leave for 24 h, then repeat after 7 days if needed) or malathion 0.5% applied to hair and left for 12 h (if on whole body leave for 24 h)	Major toxicity is skin irritation	Do not use lindane or malathion during pregnancy or in children. Permethrin is an effective alternative pyrethroid

Table 51.6: Adverse effects of drugs on the skin

Cutaneous eruption	Drugs commonly associated	Comment
Acne	Glucocorticosteroids, androgens, anabolic steroids, phenytoin	
Alopecia	Cytotoxic chemotherapy, retinoids, gold, long-term heparin, oral contraceptives, sodium valproate	
Eczema	β-Lactams, phenothiazines	
Erythema multiforme	Sulphonamides, penicillins (β-lactams), barbiturates, allopurinol, rifampicin, all NSAIDs, phenytoin, carbamazepine and lamotrigine	Inclusive of Stevens Johnson syndrome
Erythema nodosum	Sulphonamides, antimicrobials (especially β-lactams), oral contraceptives	
Exfoliative dermatitis and erythroderma	Allopurinol, carbamazepine, gold, penicillins, phenothiazines	
Fixed eruptions	Barbiturates, laxatives, phenolphthalein, naproxen, nifedipine, penicillins, sulphonamides, tetracyclines, quinidine	These eruptions recur at the same site (often circumorally) with each administration of the drug and may be purpuric or bullous
Lichenoid eruptions	Captopril, chloroquine, furosemide, gold, phenothiazines, thiazides	
Lupus erythematosus with butterfly rash	Hydralazine, isoniazid, phenytoin, procainamide	
Photosensitivity		
Systemic drugs	Amiodarone, chlorodiazepoxide, furosemide, griseofulvin, nalidixic acid, thiazides, tetracyclines, piroxicam	
Topical drugs	Coal tar, hexachlorophane, p-aminobenzoic acid and its esters	
Pigmentation	Amiodarone, chloroquine, oral contraceptives, phenothiazines	AZT causes grey nails; chloroquine causes hair and skin depigmentation
Pruritus	Oral contraceptives, phenothiazines, rifampicin	Without any rashes – rifampicin causes biliary stasis
Purpura	Thiazides, phenylbutazone, sulphonamides, sulphonylureas, quinine	May be thrombocytopenic or vasculitic
Toxic epidermal necrolysis	NSAIDs, penicillins (β-lactams), phenytoin, sulphonamides	
Toxic erythema	Ampicillin, sulphonamides, sulphonylureas, furosemide, thiazides	Usually occurs after 7–9 days of therapy or after 2–3 days in those previously exposed
Urticaria		
Acute	Radiocontrast media	
Acute/chronic	Aspirin (NSAIDs), ACE inhibitors, gold, penicillins	
Vasculitis – allergic	NSAIDs, phenytoin, sulphonamides, thiazides, penicillins and retinoids	

NSAIDs, non-steroidal anti-inflammatory drugs; ACE, angiotensin-converting enzyme; AZT, azidothymidine.

effect of too high a dose of UVB in a subject who has been exposed to a drug. The reaction is like severe sunburn and the threshold returns to normal when the drug is discontinued. Photoallergy (like drug allergy) is a cell-mediated immune reaction that only occurs in certain individuals, is not dose related and may be severe. It is due to a photochemical reaction caused by UVA where the drug combines with a tissue protein to form an antigen. These reactions are usually eczematous, and may persist for months or years after withdrawal of the drug. Some agents that commonly cause photosensitivity are shown in Table 51.6.

Key points

- Treatment of skin disorders depends on accurate diagnosis; steroids are not useful for all rashes and indeed may cause harm if used inappropriately.
- Acne is treated first line with keratolytics; if systemic antibiotics are indicated, use oral oxytetracycline or erythromycin (but do not use tetracyclines in children under 12 years). Vitamin A analogues should only used in refractory cases.
- In eczema, it is important to identify the causal agent and minimize/eradicate exposure if possible.
- For dry, scaly eczema, use emollients plus a keratolytic; for wet eczema use drying lotions or zinc-medicated bandages.
- Topical glucocorticosteroids are often required, but do not use high-potency glucocorticosteroids on the face. Use the lowest potency steroid for the shortest time possible required to produce clinical benefit.
- In psoriasis, simple emollients should be used to treat mild cases. Keratolytics may be used in moderate cases.
- Additional therapies for more severe cases of psoriasis include topical vitamin D analogues, PUVA, oral acitretin and cytotoxic drugs. Although glucocorticosteroids are effective, tachyphylaxis occurs, and on withdrawal pustular psoriasis may appear.

Case history

A 45-year-old white woman with a previous history of one culture-positive urinary tract infection (UTI) presents with a three-day history of dysuria and frequency of micturition. Her urinalysis shows moderate blood and protein and is positive for nitrates. She is started on a seven-day course of co-trimoxazole, two tablets twice a day, as she has a history of penicillin allergy with urticaria and wheezing. In the early morning of the last day of therapy, she develops a generalized rash on her body, which is itchy and worsens, despite the fact that she has not taken the last two doses of her antibiotic, her UTI symptoms having resolved. By the following morning she feels much worse, with itchy eyes, has had fevers overnight and is complaining of arthralgia and buccal soreness, and is seen by her community physician. He notes conjunctivitis, with swollen eyelids, soreness and ulceration on her lips and buccal and vaginal mucosa. She has a generalized maculo-papular rash which involves her face and has become confluent in areas on her abdomen and chest, and there is evidence of skin blistering and desquamation on her chest.

Question
What is the most likely diagnosis here? What is the probable cause, and how should this patient be managed?

Answer
The most likely diagnosis of a rapidly progressive generalized body rash involving the eyes, mouth and genitalia with systemic fever and early desquamation is erythema multiforme-major (Stevens Johnson syndrome, see Chapter 12, Figures 12.2 and 12.3). The most common causes of this syndrome are viral infections, especially herpes virus, drugs and (less frequently) systemic bacterial infections, such as meningitis, nephritis and streptococcal infection. Many drugs can cause this adverse reaction, but the most commonly incriminated classes of drugs are antibacterial agents such as sulphonamides, β-lactams (especially penicillins), vancomycin and rifampicin, anticonvulsants, salicylates and other NSAIDs, and allopurinol. In this patient the most likely aetiology is that she is taking co-trimoxazole, which contains 400 mg of sulphamethoxazole and 80 mg of trimethoprim per tablet. Stopping the offending agent is the most important part of her initial management. Her further management should include admission to hospital for intravenous fluids to maintain hydration, supportive care for the skin in order to minimize further desquamation and secondary infection with sterile wet dressings and an aseptic environment, analgesia if necessary, and maintenance and monitoring of her hepatic and renal function. If her condition is very severe, the patient may need to be transferred to a burns unit. Short courses of high-dose glucocorticosteroids early in the disease have been recommended, but controlled clinical studies have not demonstrated the benefit of glucocorticosteroids in this condition. The disease may progress for up to four or five days and recovery may take from one to several weeks. The mortality rate for Stevens Johnson syndrome is <5%, but increases to about 30% if the diagnosis is toxic epidermal necrolysis with more extensive desquamation.

FURTHER READING

Series of articles relating to current treatment of dermatological conditions. *Clinical Medicine* 2005; **5**: 551–75.

PART XIII

THE EYE

CHAPTER 52

DRUGS AND THE EYE

INTRODUCTION: OCULAR ANATOMY, PHYSIOLOGY AND BIOCHEMISTRY

The eye is protected by a series of barriers, namely the blood–retinal, blood–aqueous and blood–vitreous barriers, and so represents both an opportunity for localized drug administration and also a challenge to drug delivery. See Figure 52.1 for a cross-sectional view of the anatomy of the eye.

The structures of the eye itself are divided into the anterior and posterior segments. The anterior segment includes the cornea, limbus, anterior and posterior chambers, trabecular meshwork, Schlemm's canal, the iris, lens and the ciliary body. The posterior segment consists of the sclera, choroid, retina, vitreous and optic nerve. The anterior surface of the eye is covered by the conjunctiva. The ocular secretory system is composed of the main lacrimal gland located in the upper outer orbit, and accessory glands located in the conjunctiva. The lacrimal gland has both sympathetic and parasympathetic innervation. Parasympathetic innervation is relevant in that many drugs with anticholinergic side effects cause the symptom of dry eyes (see Table 52.1). Tear drainage starts through small puncta located in the medial aspects of the eyelids. Blinking causes tears to enter the puncta and drain through the canaliculi, lacrimal sac and nasolacrimal duct into the nose. The nose is lined with highly vascular epithelium which permits direct access of absorbed drugs to the systemic circulation. Consequently, even though the dose administered as eye drops is much smaller than the usual dose of the same drug (e.g. **timolol**) administered by mouth, the lack of first-pass metabolism may nonetheless lead to unwanted systemic effects.

THE IRIS AND CILIARY BODY

In the iris, dilator smooth muscle is orientated radially and innervated by the sympathetic system, which produces dilatation (mydriasis). At the pupillary margin, the sphincter smooth muscle is organized in a circular orientation with parasympathetic innervation which, when stimulated, leads to pupillary constriction (miosis) (see Table 52.1 for a summary of the autonomic pharmacology of the eye).

The ciliary body serves two specialized functions, namely secretion of the aqueous humour and accommodation. Parasympathetic stimulation contracts the ciliary muscle and allows the lens to become more convex, focusing on near objects. Contraction of this muscle also widens the spaces in the trabecular meshwork and this also explains, in part, the effect of parasympathomimetics in lowering intra-ocular pressure.

GENERAL PHARMACOKINETICS OF INTRA-OCULAR DRUG ADMINISTRATION

The bioavailability of intra-ocularly administered drugs depends on pH and other pharmaceutical properties of the vehicle. Most ophthalmic drugs in general use are delivered as drops, usually in aqueous solution. Formulations which prolong the time for which a drug remains in contact with the eye surface include gels, ointments, solid inserts, soft contact lenses and collagen shields. Drug penetration into the eye itself is approximately linearly related to the concentration of drug applied.

Nasolachrymal drainage plays a key role in the systemic absorption of drugs administered to the eye, and drugs absorbed via this route circumvent hepatic first-pass metabolism. Thus ocular drugs such as β-adrenergic antagonists can cause wheezing in asthmatic patients. Figure 52.2 shows potential pathways for drug absorption in the eye.

DRUGS USED TO DILATE THE PUPIL

Mydriasis (pupillary dilatation) is often required for detailed examination of the retina. Two major groups of drugs are used

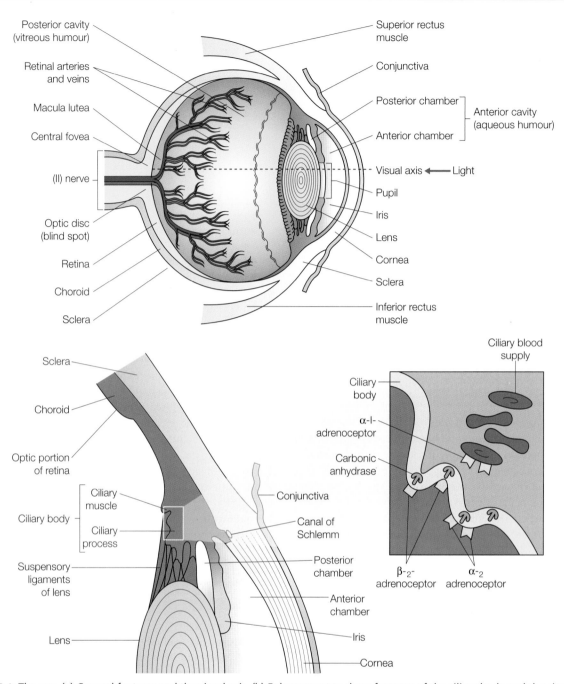

Figure 52.1: The eye. (a) General features and the visual axis. (b) Enlargement to show features of the ciliary body and the circulation of aqueous humour, and high magnification area detailing the distribution of adrenergic receptors and carbonic anhydrase location. (Redrawn with permission from Clancy J, McVicar AJ. *Physiology and anatomy*. London: Edward Arnold, 1995).

Table 52.1: Autonomic pharmacology/physiology of the eye and associated structures

Tissue	Adrenergic receptor and subtype	Response	Cholinergic receptor and subtype	Response
Iris radial muscle	α_1	Mydriasis		
Iris sphincter muscle	–	–	M_3	Miosis
Ciliary epithelium	α_2/β_2	Aqueous humour production		
Ciliary muscle	β_2	Relaxation	M_3	Accommodation
Lacrimal gland	α_1	Secretion	M_2/M_3	Secretion

to cause pupillary dilatation, namely muscarinic antagonists (anticholinergics) and sympathomimetics. Short-acting relatively weak mydriatics, such as **tropicamide**, facilitate retinal examination. **Cyclopentolate** and **atropine** are preferred for producing cycloplegia (paralysis of the ciliary muscle) for refraction in young children. **Atropine** is also used for the treatment of iridocyclitis mainly to prevent posterior synechiae, when it is often combined with **phenylephrine**.

Table 52.2 shows some commonly used agents, their receptor effects, dose schedule and toxicity. Agents that dilate the pupil may abruptly increase the intra-ocular pressure in closed-angle glaucoma by causing obstruction to the outflow tract, and are contraindicated in this condition. Patients should be asked whether they are driving before having their pupils dilated and should be warned not to drive afterwards until their vision has returned to normal.

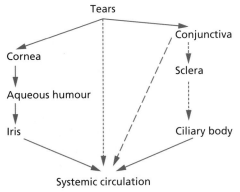

Figure 52.2: Potential absorption pathways for drugs applied to the eye.

DRUGS USED TO CONSTRICT THE PUPIL AND TO TREAT GLAUCOMA

PHYSIOLOGY OF AQUEOUS HUMOUR DYNAMICS AND REGULATION OF INTRA-OCULAR PRESSURE

Aqueous humour is produced at a rate of 2–2.5 mL per minute and flows from the posterior chamber through the pupil into the anterior chamber. Around 80–95% of it exits via the trabecular meshwork and into the canal of Schlemm and subsequently into the episcleral venous plexus and eventually into the systemic circulation. Fluid can also flow via the ciliary muscles into the suprachoroidal space. The geometry of the anterior chamber differentiates the two forms of glaucoma, namely open-angle glaucoma (the more common form) and angle-closure glaucoma (closed-angle glaucoma). Open-angle glaucoma is usually treated medically in the first instance, by reducing aqueous humour flow and/or production. Closed-angle glaucoma is treated by iridectomy following urgent medical treatment to reduce the intra-ocular pressure in preparation for surgery.

PRINCIPLES OF THERAPY FOR GLAUCOMA

Acute glaucoma is a medical emergency. **Mannitol** can reduce the intra-ocular pressure acutely by its osmotic effect. In addition, therapy with a carbonic anhydrase inhibitor (intravenous **acetazolamide** or topical **dorzolamide**) may be required. This is then supplemented with either a topical β-adrenergic antagonist (e.g. **timolol**) or a cholinergic agonist (e.g. **pilocarpine**), or both.

Table 52.2: Drugs commonly used to dilate the pupil

Drug	Receptor	Dose, onset of mydriasis and schedule	Toxicity and other comments
Anticholinergics			
Tropicamide		Single drop of 0.5% solution, maximum onset of effect is in 20–40 min and lasts 3–6 h	Photosensitivity, blurred vision and systemic absorption can occur
Cyclopentolate	All anticholinergics are antagonists at the M$_3$ receptor on the ciliary muscle	Single drops of 0.5 or 1.0% solution, maximum onset of effect is in 30–60 min and lasts 24 h	As for tropicamide
Atropine		Single drop of 0.5 or 1.0% solution, maximum onset of effect is 30–40 min and lasts 7–10 days	As for tropicamide
Sympathomimetics			
Phenylephrine		One of two drops of 10% solution, lasts up to 12 h	Systemic absorption can occur (avoid in patients with coronary artery disease or hypertension)

Chronic simple glaucoma is due to a limitation of flow through the trabecular meshwork. Initial treatment is with a topical β-blocker. Other drugs (e.g. **dipivefrine**, a prodrug of **adrenaline (epinephrine)** designed to penetrate the cornea readily, or **pilocarpine**) are added as necessary. Disappointingly, visual impairment may progress despite adequate control of intra-ocular pressure and surgery has a place in this, as well as in the acute form of glaucoma.

DRUGS USED TO TREAT GLAUCOMA

MANNITOL

Mannitol (Chapter 36) is an osmotic diuretic. It is used in an emergency or before surgery, and is given as an intravenous infusion (e.g. 100–200 mL of a 20% solution) over 30–60 minutes. It shifts water from intracellular and transcellular compartments (including the eye) into the plasma, and promotes loss of fluid by its diuretic action on the kidney. Its major adverse effect is dehydration.

CARBONIC ANHYDRASE INHIBITORS

Acetazolamide is used in acute and chronic glaucoma, and it also has highly specialized uses in certain seizure disorders in infants, and in adapting to altitude. It was previously used as a diuretic (see Chapter 36). It is a sulphonamide. It is a competitive inhibitor of carbonic anhydrase, the enzyme that converts CO_2 and H_2O into H_2CO_3. Inhibition of this enzyme in the eye reduces aqueous humour production by the ciliary body.

Adverse effects

Adverse effects include the following:

- paraesthesiae and tingling;
- nausea, vomiting and loss of taste;
- metabolic acidosis;
- polyuria due to its mild diuretic properties;
- hypersensitivity reactions – particularly of the skin;
- bone marrow suppression (rare).

Acetazolamide is poorly tolerated orally, although a slow-release preparation exists which can be given twice daily and has reduced incidence of side effects. **Dorzolamide** is a topically applied carbonic anhydrase inhibitor, whose use may reduce the need for systemic **acetazolamide** therapy (see below). **Acetazolamide** should not be used in patients with renal failure, renal stones or known hypersensitivity to sulphonamides, or in pregnant women.

TOPICAL AGENTS FOR GLAUCOMA

DORZOLAMIDE

Dorzolamide is a topically applied carbonic anhydrase inhibitor, which may be used either alone or as an adjunct to a β-blocker. Systemic absorption does occur and systemic side effects (e.g. rashes, urolithiasis) may require drug withdrawal. Typical adverse effects include local irritation of the eye and eyelid with burning, stinging and visual blurring, and a bitter taste.

PROSTAGLANDIN ANALOGUES

Latanoprost is a prostaglandin $F_{2\alpha}$ analogue. It can be used in patients who are intolerant of β-blockers or as add-on therapy when the response to the first drug has been inadequate. **Latanoprost** is an inactive prodrug which readily penetrates the cornea and is hydrolysed to the free acid. The free acid diffuses out of the cornea into the aqueous humour and lowers the intra-ocular pressure by increasing uveoscleral outflow. Systemic absorption does occur via conjunctival and mucous membranes. **Latanoprost** is cleared by hepatic metabolism. The main side effects are local irritation with stinging, burning and blurred vision. Punctate keratopathy has occurred, and it increases the amount of brown pigment in the iris in patients with mixed-coloured eyes, which may be a cosmetic problem, especially if treatment is only needed for one eye. **Travoprost** and **bimatoprost** are related prostaglandin analogues.

α₂-AGONISTS

Brimonidine is a selective α₂-agonist, used for chronic open-angle glaucoma when other drugs are unsatisfactory. It is used alone or as an adjunct to β-blocker therapy in chronic glaucoma. It decreases aqueous humour production and increases uveoscleral flow. Trace amounts do get into the circulation and undergo hepatic metabolism. The major toxicities include local ocular irritation and occasional corneal staining, and systemic adverse effects include dry mouth (25% of cases), headache, fatigue, drowsiness and allergic reactions. It is contraindicated in patients taking monoamine oxidase inhibitors (MAOIs) and should be used with caution in those with severe coronary artery disease (CAD) or taking tricyclic antidepressants.

Apraclonidine is another selective α₂-agonist which is formulated for ophthalmic use.

Key points

Drugs and the pupil

- Miosis (pupillary constriction)
  - Parasympathetic stimulation: muscarinic agonists (e.g. carbachol, pilocarpine); cholinesterase inhibitors (e.g. neostigmine, physostigmine).
  - Sympathetic blockade: α₁-antagonists (e.g. phentolamine).
- Mydriasis (pupillary dilatation)
  - Parasympathetic blockade: muscarinic antagonists (e.g. atropine, tropicamide).
  - Sympathetic stimulation: α₁-agonists (e.g. phenylephrine).

Table 52.3: Antibacterial agents used to treat conjunctivitis and blepharitis

Drug class or drug	Indication and use	Toxicity
Chloramphenicol Fluoroquinolones (e.g. norfloxacin, ofloxacin, ciprofloxacin) Framycetin sulphate Aminoglycosides (e.g. gentamicin sulphate, neomycin sulphate)	Broad-spectrum antibacterials	Local irritation and hypersensitivity reactions
Ciprofloxacin hydrochloride	Corneal ulceration	Causes local burning and itching; best avoided in children
Chlortetracycline	Chlamydial infections	Local irritation and hypersensitivity reactions
Gentamicin sulphate Tobramycin	*Pseudomonas aeruginosa* infections	Local irritation and hypersensitivity reactions
Sodium fusidate	Staphylococcal infections	Hypersensitivity reactions

Table 52.4: Antiviral agents for eye infections

Drug	Route	Indication for use	Toxicity
Idoxuridine	Topical	Herpes simplex keratitis	Punctate keratopathy and hypersensitivity
Aciclovir	Topical (3%) Oral/intravenous	Herpes simplex keratitis Herpes zoster ophthalmicus	
Foscarnet	Intravenous/intravitreal	Cytomegalovirus retinitis	
Ganciclovir	Intravenous/intravitreal	Cytomegalovirus retinitis	

DRUGS USED TO TREAT EYE INFECTIONS

Several antimicrobial agents are formulated for ophthalmic use (see Tables 52.3 and 52.4). Appropriate selection of an antibacterial agent and the route of administration depend on the clinical findings and culture and sensitivity results. Acute bacterial conjunctivitis is usually due to *Staphylococcus aureus* or *Streptococcus*. **Chloramphenicol**, **gentamicin**, **fusidic acid** or one of the fluoroquinolones (e.g. **ciprofloxacin**, **ofloxacin**), all of which are available as eye drops, may be appropriate.

DRUGS USED TO TREAT INFLAMMATORY DISORDERS IN THE EYE

POST SURGERY

Non-steroidal anti-inflammatory drugs (NSAIDs) are used to reduce post-operative inflammation. Several such ophthalmic preparations are available, including **diclofenac**, **flurbiprofen** and **ketorolac**.

OTHER ANTI-INFLAMMATORY OCULAR DRUG THERAPIES

GLUCOCORTICOSTEROIDS

Topical ocular glucocorticosteroids should only be used under specialist supervision to treat uveitis and scleritis, and sometimes in the post-operative setting. They should never be used to treat the undiagnosed 'red-eye' which could be due to a herpes infection, which is aggravated by glucocorticosteroids and may progress to loss of the eye. Furthermore, topical steroids produce or exacerbate glaucoma in genetically predisposed individuals (Chapter 14). Thinning of the cornea or perforation of the sclera may occur in susceptible patients. A number of preparations are available (e.g. **hydrocortisone** or **betametasone** – both available as drops or ointment).

ANTIHISTAMINES AND MAST CELL STABILIZERS

These agents are used to treat allergic or seasonal conjunctivitis. Topical antihistamines for ophthalmic use include **antazoline** and **azelastine**. Ocular irritation, oedema of the eyelids or blurred vision can occur, as can systemic effects (e.g. drowsiness).

Table 52.5: Adverse ocular effects of drugs

Drug class or drug	Ocular structure affected	Adverse ocular effects
Anticholinergic drugs (anti-spasmodics; tricyclic anti-depressants, phenothiazines, first-generation antihistamines)	Lacrimal apparatus	Dry secretions, ocular irritation and burning
Cholinergic agents (methacholine, neostigmine)	Lacrimal apparatus	Increased tear secretions
Amiodarone Amodiaquone Phenothiazine Gold	Corneal – microdeposits	Few symptoms, but reduced vision and ocular discomfort
Glucocorticosteroids and antimitotics (e.g. busulfan, nitrogen mustards)	Lens	Cataract formation
Anticholinergics	Lens	Impaired accommodation – blurred vision
Oral contraceptives, sulphonamides, tetracyclines	Lens	Lens hydration increased – blurred vision
Anticholinergics in people with glaucoma; systemic and topical glucocorticosteroids	Intra-ocular pressure is increased	Reduced visual acuity
Chloroquine Ethambutol Chloramphenicol	Optic nerve	Retrobulbar neuritis, optic atrophy; permanent visual loss may occur
Digoxin	Retina	Impaired yellow–green vision
Sildenafil	Retina	Blue vision

Sodium cromoglicate or **nedocromil** drops are widely used in the longer-term treatment of allergic conjunctivitis. **Sodium cromoglicate** in particular is very safe and only causes local stinging as its main side effect.

DRUGS FOR AGE-RELATED MACULAR DEGENERATION

Pegaptanib and **ranibizumab** are two newly licensed agents for the treatment of age-related macular degeneration. They work by inhibiting the new blood vessel formation that is characteristic of this disease, by blocking the action of vascular endothelial growth factor (VEGF), and are given by periodic intravitreal injection. **Bevacizumab** is another VEGF inhibitor that has been used in this condition because of its considerably lower cost, but its use in this situation is presently unlicensed because of lack of robust evidence of efficacy and safety; currently, its licensed indications are metastatic colorectal or breast carcinoma (see Chapter 48).

LOCAL ANAESTHETICS AND THE EYE

Oxybuprocaine and **tetracaine** are widely used in the eye as topical local anaesthetics. **Proxymetacaine** causes less initial stinging and is useful in paediatric patients. **Tetracaine** causes more profound anaesthesia and is suitable for minor surgical procedures. **Oxybuprocaine** or a combination of **lidocaine** and **fluorescein** is used for tonometry. **Lidocaine** with or without **adrenaline** is often injected into the eyelids for minor surgery. **Lidocaine** is also often injected for surgical procedures on the globe of the eye.

ADVERSE EFFECTS ON THE EYE OF SYSTEMIC DRUG THERAPY

One of the most devastating ocular complications of systemic drug therapy is the Stevens Johnson syndrome (erythema multiforme major). Ocular involvement occurs in up to two-thirds of patients, of whom approximately one-third suffer permanent visual sequelae. Table 52.5 illustrates the diversity of adverse ocular effects of drugs.

Table 52.6: Common drug-induced problems in patients with contact lenses

Drug	Adverse effects	Comment
Oral contraceptives (high oestrogen)	Swelling of the corneal surface – poorly fitting lenses	Visual acuity deterioration
Anxiolytics, hypnotics, first-generation antihistamines (e.g. diphenhydramine, etc.)	Reduced rate of blinking	Dry eyes and higher risk of infections
Antihistamines, anticholinergics, phenothazines, diuretics and tricyclic antidepressants	Reduced lacrimation	Dry eyes – irritation and burning
Hydralazine and ephedrine	Increased lacrimation	
Isotretinoin, aspirin	Conjunctival inflammation and irritation	
Rifampicin and sulfasalazine	Discolour lenses	

CONTACT LENS WEARERS

As the number of patients who wear contact lenses increases, an awareness has developed that these patients represent a special subgroup in whom particular care is needed when prescribing, as they may develop specific additional problems related to commonly prescribed drugs. A summary of such agents is given in Table 52.6.

Case history

A 68-year-old man has hypertension and ischaemic heart disease. His angina and blood pressure are well controlled while taking oral therapy with bendroflumethiazide, 2.5 mg daily, and slow-release diltiazem 120 mg daily. His visual acuity gradually declines and he is diagnosed as having simple open-angle glaucoma. His ophthalmologist starts therapy with pilocarpine 2% eye drops, one drop four times a day, and carteolol drops, two drops twice a day. A week after starting to see his ophthalmologist he attends his GP's surgery complaining of shortness of breath on exertion, paroxysmal nocturnal dyspnoea and othopnoea. Clinical examination reveals a regular pulse of 35 beats per minute, blood pressure of 158/74 mmHg and signs of mild left ventricular failure. His ECG shows sinus bradycardia with no evidence of acute myocardial infarction.
Question
How can you explain this problem and what should your management be?
Answer
Carteolol is a non-selective β-adrenergic antagonist that can gain access to the systemic circulation via the nasolachrymal apparatus thus avoiding heptic first-pass metabolism. It can thus act (especially in conjunction with a calcium antagonist – diltiazem in this case) on the cardiac conducting system and on the working myocardium. Discontinuing the ocular carteolol should resolve the problem.

Key points

Drugs used to lower intra-ocular pressure
- Systemic administration of:
  - osmotic agents (e.g. mannitol);
  - acetazolamide (carbonic anhydrase inhibitor).
- Topical administration of:
  - pilocarpine (muscarinic agonist);
  - timolol (β-adrenoceptor antagonist);
  - dorzolamide (carbonic anhydrase inhibitor);
  - latanoprost ($PGF_{2\alpha}$ analogue);
  - brimonidine (α_2-agonist).

FURTHER READING

Ghate D, Edelhauser HF. Ocular drug delivery. *Expert Opinion on Drug Delivery* 2006; **3**: 275–87.

Marquis RE, Whitson JT. Management of glaucoma: focus on pharmacological therapy. *Drugs and Aging* 2005; **22**: 1–21.

PART XIV

CLINICAL TOXICOLOGY

DRUGS AND ALCOHOL ABUSE

INTRODUCTION

The World Health Organization's (WHO) definition of drug dependence is 'a state, psychic and sometimes physical, resulting from the interaction between a living organism and a drug characterized by behavioural and other responses that always include a compulsion to take the drug on a continuous or periodic basis in order to experience its psychic effects and sometimes to avoid the discomfort of its absence'. More recent definitions include the WHO's ICD-10 and the American Psychiatric Association's DSM-IV diagnostic criteria for Substance-Related Disorders, which emphasize the importance of loss of control over drug use and its consequences in limiting other, non-drug-related activities, in addition to tolerance and physical dependence.

In the above definitions, a distinction is made between physical and psychological dependence. Although psychological dependence has not been shown to produce gross structural changes, it must be assumed that changes have occurred in the brain at a molecular or receptor level. Central to the definition of psychological dependence is the compulsion or craving to take a drug repeatedly. In contrast, physical dependence occurs in the absence of a drug, when a range of symptoms – a withdrawal state – is present. The ease and degree to which withdrawal symptoms develop defines the liability of a particular drug to produce physical dependence. As a generalization, the withdrawal syndrome seen after cessation of a drug tends to be the opposite of the symptoms produced by acute administration of that drug (e.g. anxiety, insomnia and arousal seen after withdrawal of alcohol or benzodiazepines, or depression and lethargy seen after withdrawal of stimulants). Physical and psychological dependence may be distinguished clinically. For instance, abrupt cessation of tricyclic antidepressants leads to sympathetic nervous system activation, without psychological dependence, whereas **nicotine** withdrawal produces predominantly psychological changes, with minimal physical symptoms. The major difference between drug abuse and drug dependence is quantitative.

Tolerance, when repeated exposure to a drug produces progressively diminished effects, is another important concept. It may be caused by changes in the rate at which the drug is distributed or metabolized in the body, or by adaptive processes occurring in the brain. A distinct feature is cross-tolerance, where tolerance to one type of drug is associated with tolerance to other drugs. Cross-tolerance, which can encompass chemically distinct drugs, has been clearly demonstrated for alcohol, benzodiazepines and other sedative drugs. It forms the basis for substitution treatment of dependency.

Key points

Features of drug dependence

- A subjective awareness or compulsion to use a drug, often related to unsuccessful efforts to reduce drug intake.
- Continued drug use despite awareness of its harmful effects on physical health, social functioning, etc.
- Priority of drug-taking or obtaining drugs over other activities, limiting normal social or work roles.
- The development of tolerance and withdrawal symptoms.
- After abstinence, dependence may recur rapidly with reuse of the drug.

PATHOPHYSIOLOGY OF DRUG DEPENDENCE

Most people who are exposed to drugs do not become dependent on them. Factors that increase the likelihood of addiction include:

- *Genetic factors*: Genetic factors can predispose to dependency, but can also protect against alcoholism (e.g. defective aldehyde dehydrogenase genes – common in East Asians – produce unpleasant flushing/headache after drinking alcohol).
- *Personality/environment*: Drinking or drug-taking behaviour is influenced by the example set by family or peer group, or by cultural norms.

- *Drug availability and economic factors*: Rates of dependence are increased if a drug is easily available. This may explain why dependence on **nicotine** and **alcohol** is a much greater public health problem than dependence on illegal drugs, because of their greater availability. Drug use is sensitive to price (e.g. rates of alcoholism are reduced by increasing alcohol prices).
- *Biochemical reinforcement*: Drugs of abuse and dependence have a common biochemical pathway: they all increase dopamine in the nucleus accumbens, associated with mood elevation and euphoria. Behaviourally, this is linked with reinforcement of drug-taking. Dependence-potential of different drugs is related to potency in releasing dopamine (**cocaine** is most potent). The rate of dopamine release is also important, e.g. smoked and intravenous drugs give a more rapid effect than oral drugs.

GENERAL PRINCIPLES OF TREATING ADDICTIONS

By the time an addict presents for assessment and treatment, he or she is likely to have diverse and major problems. There may be physical or mental illness, and emotional or attitudinal problems, which may have contributed to the addiction and/or resulted from it. Their financial and living circumstances may have been adversely affected by their drug habit and they may have legal problems relating to drug possession, intoxication (e.g. drink–driving offences), or criminal activities carried out to finance drug purchases. Attitudes to drug use may be unrealistic (e.g. denial). The best chance of a successful outcome requires that all of these factors are considered, and the use of a wide range of treatment options is likely to be more successful than a narrow repertoire.

Treatment objectives vary depending on the drug. Complete abstinence is emphasized for **nicotine**, **alcohol** or **cocaine** addiction, whereas for **heroin** addiction many patients benefit from **methadone** maintenance. Other objectives are to improve the health and social functioning of addicted patients. Treatment success can only be determined over a long time, based on reduction in drug use and improvements in health and social functioning. A treatment programme should include medical and psychiatric assessment and psychological and social support. Addicts should be referred to specialist services if these are available. Other services based in the voluntary sector (e.g. Alcoholics Anonymous) are also valuable and complementary resources. Medical and psychiatric assessment may need to be repeated once the patient is abstinent, as it is often difficult to diagnose accurately certain disorders in the presence of withdrawal symptoms (e.g. anxiety, depression and hypertension are features of alcohol withdrawal, but are also common in abstinent alcoholics).

The pharmacological treatment of addictions, which includes treatment of intoxication, detoxification (removal of the drug from the body, including management of withdrawal symptoms) and treatment to prevent relapse, is discussed below.

Table 53.1: Opioid drugs that are commonly abused

Drugs	Comment
Diamorphine[a]	Mainly obtained on the black market. It is of variable purity and cut with quinine, talc, lactose, etc. It is usually mixed with water, heated until dissolved, and sometimes strained through cotton. It may be used intravenously (mainlining), subcutaneously (skin popping) or inhaled ('snorted'/'chasing the dragon', by heating up on foil and inhaling the smoke) ($t_{1/2}$ = 60–90 min)
Methadone	This is the mainstay of drug addiction clinics, and is usually given as an elixir (long $t_{1/2}$ of 15–55 h). It is very difficult to use elixir for injection
Dipipanone (+ cyclizine = Diconal®)[a]	Previously much used by non-clinic doctors treating addicts. It is easily crushed up and dissolved for intravenous use
Other opoids	All opioids, including mixed agonists/antagonists (e.g. buprenorphine) have the potential to cause dependence

[a]Diamorphine, dipipanone and cocaine (not an opioid) can only be prescribed to addicts for treatment of their addiction by doctors with a special licence.

OPIOID/NARCOTIC ANALGESICS

Diamorphine ('heroin') is preferred by most opioid addicts. It is often adulterated with other white powders, such as **quinine** (which is bitter, like opiates), caffeine, lactose and even chalks, starch and talc. Due to the variable purity, the dose of black-market **heroin** is always uncertain. The drug is taken intravenously, subcutaneously, orally or by inhalation of smoked **heroin**. In addition to the illegal supply of **heroin** from Afghanistan and elsewhere, opioids are obtained from pharmacy thefts and the legal prescription of drugs for treatment of the addiction. Some of the drugs used are listed in Table 53.1.

The pharmacological actions of opioids are described in Chapter 25 and their effects on the central nervous system (CNS) are summarized in Table 53.2.

MEDICAL COMPLICATIONS

Medical complications of opioid addiction are common and some of them are listed in Table 53.3. The majority of these relate to use of infected needles, the effects of contaminating substances used to cut supplies or the life-style of opioid addicts. These are the principal reasons for the development of **methadone** clinics and needle-exchange programmes

Table 53.2: Central nervous system effects of opioids

Analgesia

Euphoria

Drowsiness → sleep → coma

Decrease in sensitivity of respiratory centre to CO_2

Depression of cough centre

Stimulation of chemoreceptor trigger zone (vomiting in 15% of cases)

Release of antidiuretic hormone

Table 53.3: Medical complications of opioid addiction

Infection	Endocarditis – bacterial, often tricuspid valve, staphyloccocal, fungal (e.g. *Candida*)
	HIV/hepatitis B virus (HBV)/hepatitis C virus (HCV)
	Abscesses
	Tetanus
	Septicaemia
	Hepatitis
Pulmonary	Pneumonia – bacterial, fungal, aspiration
	Pulmonary oedema – 'heroin lung'
	Embolism
	Atelectasis
	Fibrosis/granulomas
Skin	Injection scars
	Abscesses
	Cellulitis
	Lymphangitis
	Phlebitis
	Gangrene
Neurological	Cerebral oedema
	Transverse myelitis
	Horner's syndrome
	Polyneuritis
	Crush injury
	Myopathy
Hepatic	Cirrhosis
Renal	Nephrotic syndrome with proliferative glomerulonephritis
Musculoskeletal	Osteomyelitis (usually lumbar vertebrae, Pseudomonas, *Staphylococcus*, *Candida*), crush injury, myoglobinuria, rhabdomyolysis

as a way of minimizing medical complications of opioid dependence.

INTOXICATION AND OVERDOSE

For several seconds following intravenous injection, **heroin** produces an intense euphoria (rush) which may be accompanied by nausea and vomiting, but is nevertheless pleasurable. Over the next few hours the user may describe a warm sensation in the abdomen and chest. However, chronic users often state that the only effect they obtain is remission from abstinence symptoms. On examination, the patient may appear to be alternately dozing and waking. The patient may be hypotensive with a slow respiratory rate, pin-point pupils and infrequent and slurred speech. These signs can be reversed with **naloxone**. Opioids predispose to hypothermia.

Overdose is commonly accidental due to unexpectedly potent **heroin** or waning tolerance (e.g. after release from prison). Severe overdose may cause immediate apnoea, circulatory collapse, convulsions and cardiopulmonary arrest. Alternatively, death may occur over a longer period of time, usually due to hypoxia from direct respiratory centre depression with mechanical asphyxia (tongue and/or vomit blocking the airway).

A common complication of opioid poisoning is non-cardiogenic pulmonary oedema. This is usually rapid in onset, but may be delayed. Therefore, any patient who is admitted following **heroin** overdose should usually be hospitalized for approximately 24 hours. **Naloxone** reverses opioid poisoning with a rapid increase in pupil diameter, respiratory rate and depth of respiration. It may precipitate an acute abstinence syndrome in addicts and (very rarely) convulsions. This does not contraindicate its use in opioid overdoses in addicts. Severe hypoxia causes mydriasis and some opioids (notably **pethidine**) have an anti-muscarinic **atropine**-like mydriatic effect, so absence of small pupils should not preclude a trial of **naloxone** when the clinical situation suggests the possibility of opioid overdose. **Naloxone** is eliminated more rapidly than **morphine** and may need to be administered repeatedly (Chapter 25).

TOLERANCE AND WITHDRAWAL

Increasing doses of opioid must be administered in order to obtain the effect of the original dose. Such tolerance affects the euphoric and analgesic effects, so the addict requires more and more opioid for his or her 'buzz'. Changes in tolerance are much less apparent in the therapeutic use of opioids for the treatment of pain.

Withdrawal symptoms usually start at the time when the next dose would normally be given, and their intensity is related to the usual dose. For **heroin**, symptoms usually reach a maximum at 36–72 hours and gradually subside over the next five to ten days. Table 53.4 lists features of the opioid abstinence syndrome.

Table 53.4: Symptoms of the opioid abstinence syndrome

Early	Intermediate	Late
Yawning	Mydriasis	Involuntary muscle spasm
Lacrimation	Piloerection	Fever
Rhinorrhoea	Flushing	Nausea and vomiting
Perspiration	Tachycardia	Abdominal cramps
	Twitching	Diarrhoea
	Tremor	
	Restlessness	

Withdrawal symptoms can be treated acutely by substitution with a longer-acting opioid agonist (e.g. **methadone** by mouth) or a partial agonist (e.g. **buprenorphine**, administered sublingually). The dose can be tapered over one to two weeks. Alternatively, withdrawal symptoms are alleviated by **lofexidine** (an α_2-antagonist with less marked hypotensive effects than **clonidine**) and an antidiarrhoeal agent, such as **loperamide**, administered over 48–72 hours.

MANAGEMENT OF OPIOID ADDICTS

Opioid addicts should be managed by specialized addiction clinics when possible. A highly simplified outline of management is summarized in the Key points below. Morbidity of opioid dependence is related more to the use of infected needles, injection of unsterile material, adulterants and cost (e.g. theft, prostitution) than to the acute toxicity of opioids per se.

Key points

Management of opioid addicts in hospital

- Attempt to confirm addiction by telephoning prescriber. Confirm dosing regimen.
- Obtain urine screen for a full drug misuse screen.
- Look for evidence of needle marks.
- Look for signs of opioid withdrawal.
- Contact psychiatric liaison team.
- In the Accident and Emergency Department, it is rarely appropriate to prescribe methadone. If clear withdrawal signs are evident, treat symptomatcially (e.g. with antidiarrhoeal agent); discuss with psychiatric liaison team regarding dose titration.
- For in-patients, methadone may be appropriate – consult with psychiatric liaison regarding dose titration.
- Analgesia – address needs as for other patients, but note the effects of tolerance.
- On discharge, contact the patient's usual prescriber, or if this is a new presentation make arrangements through psychiatric team.

An orally available long-acting opioid antagonist, such as **naltrexone**, is sometimes used as an adjunct to maintain abstinence once opioid-free. (If given prematurely **naltrexone** precipitates withdrawal.) Few opioid addicts choose to remain on long-term antagonist therapy, in contrast to long-term **methadone**.

Opioid addicts rarely present to hospital asking for treatment of their addiction, but more commonly present to physicians during routine medical or surgical treatment for a condition which may or may not be related to their addiction. Some patients will deny drug abuse and clinical examination should always include a search for signs of needle-tracking and withdrawal. Acute abstinence in a casualty/general hospital setting is uncomfortable for the patient, but most unlikely to be dangerous. Physicians are not allowed to prescribe **diamorphine** or **cocaine** to addicts for treatment of their addiction or abstinence unless they hold a special licence. It is reasonable to treat a genuine opioid withdrawal syndrome with a low dose of opioid (e.g. sublingual **buprenorphine**). If a patient says that they are being treated for addiction it is always wise to confirm this by telephoning their usual prescriber and/or the supplying pharmacist. If the patient is admitted to hospital, expert advice must be obtained. Knowledge of local policies towards drug addicts is essential for anyone working in the Accident and Emergency Department or who comes into contact with drug addicts. Newborn children of addicted mothers may be born with an abstinence syndrome or, less commonly, with features of drug overdose. Assisted ventilation is preferred to **naloxone** if apnoeic at birth in this situation.

Key points

Management of opioid dependence

- Refer to specialized addiction clinic.
- Conduct assessment (to include two urine samples positive for opioids).
- Give maintenance treatment (e.g. full agonists such as methadone, or partial agonists such as buprenorphine).
- Give antagonist treatment (e.g. naltrexone).
- Provide detoxification regimens (e.g. lofexidine plus loperamide).
- Give counselling/social support.
- Repeat urine testing to confirm use of methadone and not other drugs.
- Contract system.
- Avoid prescriptions of other opioids/sedatives.
- Special 'drug-free' centres – concentrate on psychological and social support through the acute and chronic abstinence phases, and are successful in some patients.

There are legal requirements for the prescription of controlled drugs (Misuse of Drugs Regulations, 1985) distinguished in the British National Formulary by the symbol CD (e.g. **diamorphine**, **morphine**, injectable **dihydrocodeine**, **dipipanone**, **fentanyl**, **buprenorphine**, dexamfetamine, **methylphenidate**, **Ritalin**®, barbiturates, **temazepam**). Among the requirements are that the prescription must be written by hand by the prescriber, in ink, with the dose and quantity of dose units stated in both figures and words (see British National Formulary). **Diamorphine**, **dipipanone** and **cocaine** may only be prescribed to an addict for their addiction by doctors with a special licence. Doctors are expected to continue to report the treatment demands of all drug misusers by returning the local drug misuse database reporting forms, which provide anonymized data to the appropriate national or regional Drug Misuse Database (DMD).

Key points

Prescription of controlled drugs

Preparations which are subject to the prescription requirements of the Misuse of Drugs Regulations 2001 are labelled CD. The principal legal requirements are as follows:

Prescriptions ordering Controlled Drugs subject to prescription requirements must be signed and dated by the prescriber and specify the prescriber's address. The prescription must always state in the prescriber's own handwriting in ink or otherwise so as to be indelible:

* the name and address of the patient;
* in the case of a preparation, the form and, where appropriate, the strength of the preparation;
* the total quantity of the preparation, or the number of dose units, in both words and figures;
* the dose.

Prescriptions ordering 'repeats' on the same form are not permitted.
It is an offence for a doctor to issue an incomplete prescription (see the British National Formulary for full details).

DRUGS THAT ALTER PERCEPTION

Cannabis (marijuana) is the most widely used illicit drug in the UK. The most active constituent is Δ-9-tetrahydrocannabinol, which produces its effects through actions on cannabinoid CB1 receptors. It is most commonly mixed with tobacco and smoked, but it may be brewed into a drink or added to food. The pleasurable effects of **cannabis** include a sensation of relaxation, heightened perception of all the senses and euphoria. The nature and intensity of the effects varies between individuals, and is related to dose, and to the mood of the subject. The effects usually occur within minutes and last for one to two hours. Conjunctival suffusion is common. **Tetrahydrocannabinol** and other cannabinoids are extremely lipid soluble and are only slowly released from body fat. Although the acute effects wear off within hours of inhalation, cannabinoids are eliminated in the urine for weeks following ingestion. It is claimed that **cannabis** may be of value in the symptomatic management of multiple sclerosis, particularly if nausea is a prominent symptom. It has no approved medicinal use in the UK.

Acute adverse effects include dysphoric reactions, such as anxiety or panic attacks, the impairment of performance of skilled tasks, and sedation. This may lead to road traffic accidents. Chronic use has been associated with personality changes, including 'amotivational syndrome' which is characterized by extreme lethargy. The association of chronic **cannabis** use with onset of schizophrenia is unproven. A physical dependence syndrome has been reported for **cannabis**, but only after extremely heavy and frequent intake. Dependence on **cannabis** as a primary problem is rare and there are no specific treatments for **cannabis** dependence. Similarly, there are no treatments for **cannabis** intoxication, although dysphoric reactions may require brief symptomatic treatment (e.g. with benzodiazepines).

LYSERGIC ACID DIETHYLAMIDE AND OTHER PSYCHEDELICS

Psychedelics produce hallucinations (e.g. visual, somatic, olfactory) and other changes in perception, e.g. feelings of dissociation and altered perception of time. Psychedelics can be divided into serotonin- or indoleamine-like psychedelics (e.g. **lysergic acid diethylamide** (**LSD**) and **psilocybin**) and phenylethylamines (e.g. **mescaline**, **phencyclidine** – angel dust – and **methylenedioxymethylamphetamine** – MDMA or 'ecstasy, XTC'). These are agonists at the serotonin 5-HT_2-receptor and their potency as hallucinogens is closely correlated with their affinity for this receptor. Some phenethylamine psychedelics stimulant properties and can produce feelings of increased energy and euphoria and heightened perception.

MDMA is the most commonly abused recreational hallucinogenic central stimulant in the UK. The most common users are adolescents.

In high-dose hyperpyrexia, trismus, dehydration, hyponatraemia, rhabdomyolysis, seizures, coma, hepatic damage and death have been reported. Interactions with antidepressants are life-threatening. Impulsivity and impaired memory are serious long-term effects. Chronic MDMA usage produces degeneration of serotonergic neurones. MDMA is metabolized via the CYP 2D6 system and is a potent CYP 2D6 inhibitor. The elimination kinetics are saturable.

Psychedelics were used historically as adjunctive treatment in psychotherapy, but were subsequently found to be of no benefit. Most are taken orally and perceptual changes occur approximately one hour later. The duration depends on dose and clearance, and is often several hours to one day. Tolerance to behavioural effects can occur, but no withdrawal syndrome has been demonstrated.

In addition to the uncommon life-threatening adverse effects caused by MDMA, physicians come into contact with psychedelic drug abusers when they contact emergency services, e.g. as a result of dysphoric reactions or 'bad trips'. These symptoms can respond to reassurance and quiet surroundings, although **chlorpromazine** (which has 5-HT_2-antagonist effects) or **diazepam** may be of benefit.

Phencyclidine ('PCP', 'angel dust') was originally developed as an injectable anaesthetic. It binds to the glutamate ion channel. Its therapeutic use in humans was stopped after early clinical studies showed that it produced confusion, delirium and hallucinations. It is used for anaesthetic purposes by veterinarians. Patients may show extreme changes in behaviour and mood (e.g. rage and aggression, lethargy and negativism, euphoria), hallucinations, autonomic arousal (hypertension, hyperthermia) and, in extreme cases, coma and seizures. Symptoms of PCP intoxication should be treated symptomatically. PCP abuse is rare in the UK.

CENTRAL STIMULANTS

Amphetamines are abused for their stimulant properties, which are related acutely to the release of **dopamine** and **noradrenaline**. Their therapeutic use is limited to specialist treatment of narcolepsy and hyperactivity in children. They should not be prescribed in the management of depression or obesity. Acutely they may alleviate tiredness and induce a feeling of cheerfulness and confidence, and because of their sympathomimetic effects they raise blood pressure and heart rate. With high doses, particularly after intravenous use, a sensation of intense exhilaration may occur. Users tend to become hyperactive at high doses, especially if these are repeated over several days. Repeated use of amphetamines can produce 'amphetamine psychosis', which is characterized by delirium, panic, hallucinations and feelings of persecution, and can be difficult to distinguish from acute schizophrenia. Anxiety, irritability and restlessness are also common. Prolonged use leads to psychological dependence, tolerance and hostility, as well as irritation due to lack of sleep and food. The most commonly used amphetamine is **amphetamine sulphate** in oral or injectable forms, which are only available illegally. More recently, free-base amphetamine has become available ('ice'), which can be smoked, and this has pharmacokinetic and subjective effects similar to those of injected **amphetamine sulphate**. There are no specific drug treatments for amphetamine dependence, and the mainstay of therapy involves counselling and social management. MDMA is described under drugs that alter perception.

Cocaine is derived from the Andean coca shrub. It has powerful stimulant properties which are related to its action in blocking synaptic re-uptake of dopamine, and to a lesser extent noradrenaline and serotonin. As the salt it is most commonly sniffed up the nose, although it can also be injected. In the USA, the free base of cocaine ('crack') is widely available. The pharmacokinetics of smoked crack **cocaine** are almost identical to those of intravenous **cocaine**.

Acutely **cocaine** causes arousal, hypertension, exhilaration, euphoria, indifference to pain and fatigue, and the sensation of having great physical strength and mental capacity. Repeated large doses commonly precipitate an extreme surge of agitation and anxiety. Myocardial infarction or arterial dissection can occur acutely. In contrast to alcohol and opioids, which addicts tend to use on a regular basis, **cocaine** is used in binges, where doses may be taken several times an hour over a day or several days until exhaustion or lack of money prevents this. Tolerance of the euphoric effects occurs. However, upon stopping a **cocaine** binge, withdrawal symptoms including excessive sleep, fatigue and mild depression, may occur. Repeated **cocaine** use may produce adverse effects including anorexia, confusion, exhaustion, palpitations, damage to the membranes lining the nostrils and, if injected, blood-borne infections. Use of **cocaine** in pregnancy is associated with damage to the central nervous system of the fetus. 'Crack babies' can usually be cured of their 'addiction' by abstinence over a few weeks. Currently, there are no specific drug treatments for **cocaine** dependence. Counselling and social management of patients have been shown to be of only modest benefit in maintaining abstinence.

Nicotine is an alkaloid present in the leaves of the tobacco plant. The only medical use of **nicotine** is as an aid in smoking cessation. Its importance relates to its addictive properties and its presence in tobacco. The smoke of a completely burned cigarette usually contains 1–6 mg and that of a cigar contains 15–40 mg of nicotine. Acute administration of 60 mg of **nicotine** orally may be fatal. **Nicotine** first stimulates the nicotinic receptors of autonomic ganglia and then blocks them. Thus smoking can accelerate the heart via sympathetic stimulation, or slow it by sympathetic block or parasympathetic stimulation. Adrenaline and noradrenaline are secreted from the adrenal medulla. The motor end-plate acetylcholine receptors are initially stimulated and then blocked, producing a paralysis of voluntary muscle. The results of extensive central stimulation include wakefulness, tremor, fits, anorexia, nausea, vomiting, tachypnoea and secretion of antidiuretic hormone (ADH).

Adverse effects of smoking

Smoking is a potent risk factor for malignant and cardiovascular disease. Some of the specific causes of death which are related to smoking are listed in Table 53.5.

Chronic obstructive pulmonary disease including chronic bronchitis and emphysema are also associated with smoking as is peptic ulcer disease. Smoking during pregnancy is associated with spontaneous abortion, premature delivery, small babies, increased perinatal mortality and an increased incidence of sudden infant death syndrome (cot death). In households where the parents smoke, there is an increased risk of pneumonia and bronchitis in preschool and school-age children, which is most marked during the first year of life.

Pharmacokinetics

About 90% of **nicotine** from inhaled smoke is absorbed, while smoke taken into the mouth results in only 25–50% absorption. As well as being absorbed via the gastro-intestinal (GI), buccal and respiratory epithelium, **nicotine** is absorbed through the skin. A high concentration of **nicotine** may be present in the breast milk of smokers. Around 80–90% of circulating **nicotine** is metabolized in the liver, kidneys and lungs. The plasma elimination $t_{1/2}$ is 25–40 minutes. **Nicotine** and its metabolites are excreted in the urine. The metabolite cotinine can be used to quatitate exposure.

Table 53.5: Principal causes of death associated with smoking

Ischaemic heart disease (strongest correlation)

Cancers of the lung, other respiratory sites and the oesophagus, lip and tongue

Chronic bronchitis and emphysema, respiratory tuberculosis

Pulmonary heart disease

Aortic aneurysm

Peak plasma levels after smoking cigarettes can be matched by **nicotine** gum or patches but the rate of increase is much slower after chewing gum or applying transdermal patches.

Effect of smoking on drug disposition and effects

The most common effect of tobacco smoking on drug disposition is an increase in elimination consistent with induction of drug-metabolizing enzymes. **Nicotine** itself is metabolized more extensively by smokers than by non-smokers. Substrates for cytochrome P450 1A2 (e.g. **theophylline**, **caffeine**, **imipramine**) are metabolized more rapidly in smokers than in non-smokers.

Drug treatment for nicotine dependence

Nicotine is a potent drug of dependence. Withdrawal can lead to an abstinence syndrome consisting of craving, irritability and sometimes physical features (e.g. alimentary disturbances).

Substitution of **nicotine** via skin patches or **nicotine** gum as part of a smoking cessation programme significantly increases success rates. The antidepressant **bupropion** appears to reduce the desire to smoke and is licensed as an adjunct to motivational support in smoking cessation. It is contraindicated in patients with a history of seizures or of eating disorders, or who are experiencing acute alcohol or benzodiazepine withdrawal.

Varenicline, a selective nicotinic receptor partial agonist, is an oral adjunct to smoking cessation. It is started 1–2 weeks before stopping smoking. It is contraindicated in pregnancy. Side effects include gastro-intestinal disturbances, headache, dizziness and sleep disorders.

XANTHINES

This group of compounds includes **caffeine** (present in tea and colas, as well as coffee), **theobromine** (present in chocolate) and **theophylline** (Chapter 33). **Caffeine** is included in a number of proprietary and prescription medicines, particularly in analgesic combinations. The major effects of these compounds are mediated by inhibition of phosphodiesterase, resulting in a raised intracellular cyclic adenosine monophosphate (AMP) concentration.

Adverse effects

In large doses, **caffeine** exerts an excitatory effect on the CNS that is manifested by tremor, anxiety, irritability and restlessness, and interference with sleep. Its use does not lead to improved intellectual performance except perhaps when normal performance has been impaired by fatigue.

Circulatory effects include direct myocardial stimulation producing tachycardia, increased cardiac output, ectopic beats and palpitations. **Caffeine** use should be curtailed in patients who suffer paroxysmal dysrhythmias. Its effect on blood pressure is unpredictable. Cerebral vasoconstriction provides some rationale for use of **caffeine** in migraine. Bronchial smooth muscle relaxes and respiration is stimulated centrally. Mild diuresis occurs due to an increased glomerular filtration rate subsequent to dilatation of the afferent arterioles. **Caffeine** increases gastric acid secretion via its action on cyclic AMP.

Pharmacokinetics

Caffeine is rapidly and completely absorbed after oral administration and undergoes hepatic metabolism. The plasma $t_{1/2}$ of caffeine is 2.5–12 hours.

Caffeine dependence

Tolerance is low grade and dependence is not clinically important.

CENTRAL DEPRESSANTS

ALCOHOL

Ethyl alcohol (alcohol) has few clinical uses when given systemically, but is of great medical importance because of its pathological and psychological effects when used as a beverage. **Alcohol** is the most important drug of dependence, and in Western Europe and North America the incidence of alcoholism is about 5% among the adult population.

Pharmacokinetics

Ethyl alcohol is absorbed from the buccal, oesophageal, gastric and intestinal mucosae – approximately 80% is absorbed from the small intestine. **Alcohol** delays gastric emptying and in high doses delays its own absorption. Following oral administration, **alcohol** can usually be detected in the blood within five minutes. Peak concentrations occur between 30 minutes and two hours. Fats and carbohydrates delay absorption.

Alcohol is distributed throughout the body water. About 95% is metabolized (mainly in the liver) and the remainder is excreted unchanged in the breath, urine and sweat. Hepatic oxidation to acetaldehyde is catalysed by three parallel processes. The major pathway (Figure 53.1) is rate limited by cytoplasmic alcohol dehydrogenase using nicotinamide adenine dinucleotide (NAD) as coenzyme.

Alcohol elimination follows Michaelis–Menten kinetics, with saturation occurring in the concentration range encountered during social drinking. A small additional 'dose' can thus have a disproportionate effect on the concentration of **alcohol** in the plasma.

Effects of alcohol

Nervous system: **Alcohol** decreases concentration, judgement, discrimination, and reasoning and increases self-confidence. Progressively increasing plasma concentrations are associated with sensations of relaxation followed by mild euphoria, incoordination, ataxia and loss of consciousness. At high blood concentrations, the gag reflex is impaired, vomiting may occur and death may result from aspiration of gastric contents. The importance of **alcohol** as a factor in road traffic accidents is well known (see Figure 53.2). The central depressant actions of **alcohol** greatly enhance the effects of other central depressant drugs. In patients with organic brain damage, **alcohol** may induce unusual aggression and destructiveness, known as pathological intoxication. Death may also result from direct

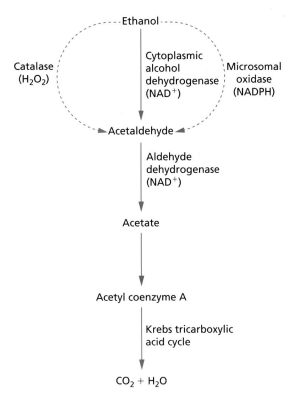

Figure 53.1: Pathways of ethanol oxidation. →, major pathway. – – –, minor pathways; NAD, nicotinamide adenine dinucleotide; NADP, nicotinamide adenine dinucleotide phosphate.

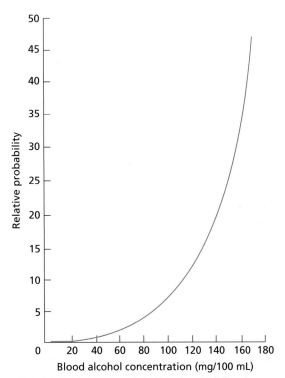

Figure 53.2: Relative probability of causing a road accident at various blood alcohol concentrations. (Redrawn with permission from Harvard JDJ. *Hospital Update* 1975; **1**: 253).

respiratory depression. Chronic neurological accompaniments of persistent **alcohol** abuse include various forms of central and peripheral neurodegeneration, most commonly involving the vermis of the cerebellum, and a peripheral neuropathy. Nutritional deficiencies may contribute to the pathogensesis of neurodegeneration. Wernicke's encephalopathy (difficulty in concentrating, confusion, coma, nystagmus and ophthalmoplegia) and Korsakov's psychosis (gross memory defects with confabulation and disorientation in space and time) are mainly due to the nutritional deficiency of thiamine associated with alcoholism. Any evidence of Wernicke's encephalopathy should be immediately treated with intravenous thiamine followed by oral thiamine for several months. Psychiatric disorder is common and devastating, with social and family breakdown.

Circulatory: Cutaneous vasodilatation causes the familiar drunkard's flush. Atrial fibrillation (± embolization) is important. Chronic abuse is an important cause of cardiomyopathy. Withdrawal (see below) causes acute hypertension and heavy intermittent **alcohol** consumption can cause variable hypertension by this mechanism which can exacerbate or be mistaken for essential hypertension (Chapter 28).

Gastrointestinal: Gastritis, peptic ulceration, haematemesis (including the Mallory–Weiss syndrome, which is haematemesis due to oesophageal tearing during forceful vomiting, as well as from peptic ulcer or varices). Liver pathology includes fatty infiltration, alcoholic hepatitis and cirrhosis. **Alcohol** can cause pancreatitis (acute, subacute and chronic).

Metabolic: Alcohol suppresses ADH secretion and this is one of the reasons why polyuria occurs following its ingestion. Reduced gluconeogenesis leading to hypoglycaemia may cause fits. The accumulation of lactate and/or keto acids produces metabolic acidosis. Hyperuricaemia occurs (particularly, it is said, in beer drinkers) and can cause acute gout.

Haematological effects: Bone marrow suppression occurs. Folate deficiency with macrocytosis is common and chronic GI blood loss causes iron deficiency. Sideroblastic anaemia is less common but can occur. Mild thrombocytopenia is common and can exacerbate haemorrhage. Neutrophil dysfunction is common even when the neutrophil count is normal, predisposing to bacterial infections (e.g. pneumococcal pneumonia), which are more frequent and serious in alcoholics.

In pregnancy: Infants of alcoholic mothers may exhibit features of intra-uterine growth retardation and mental deficiency, sometimes associated with motor deficits and failure to thrive. There are characteristic facial features which include microcephaly, micrognathia and a short upturned nose. This so-called fetal alcohol syndrome is unlike that reported in severely undernourished women. Some obstetricians now recommend total abstinence during pregnancy.

Key points

Acute effects of alcohol

- Central effects include disinhibition, impaired judgement, inco-ordination, trauma (falls, road traffic accidents), violence and crime.
- Coma and impaired gag reflex; asphyxiation on vomit.
- Convulsions, enhancement of sedative drugs.
- Atrial fibrillation, vasodilation.
- Gastritis, nausea, vomiting, Mallory – Weiss syndrome.
- Hepatitis.
- Hypoglcycaemia, metabolic acidosis, etc.

Key points

Chronic effects of alcohol

- Dependence
- Behavioural changes
- Encephalopathy (sometimes thiamine deficient), dementia, convulsions
- Cardiomyopathy
- Gastritis, nausea and vomiting; peptic ulceration
- Pancreatitis
- Cirrhosis
- Myopathy
- Bone marrow suppression
- Gout
- Hypertension
- Fetal alcohol syndrome.

Medical uses of alcohol

Alcohol is used topically as an antiseptic. Systemic **alcohol** is used in poisoning by methanol or ethylene glycol, since it competes with these for oxidation by alcohol dehydrogenase, slowing the production of toxic metabolites (e.g. formaldehyde, oxalic acid).

Management of alcohol withdrawal

A withdrawal syndrome develops when **alcohol** consumption is stopped or severely reduced after prolonged heavy alcohol intake. Several features of acute withdrawal are due to autonomic overactivity, including hypertension, sweating, tachycardia, tremor, anxiety, agitation, mydriasis, anorexia and insomnia. These are most severe 12–48 hours after stopping drinking, and they then subside over one to two weeks. Some patients have seizures ('rum fits' generally 12–48 hours post abstinence). A third set of symptoms consists of alcohol withdrawal delirium or 'delirium tremens' (acute disorientation, severe autonomic hyperactivity, and hallucinations – which are usually visual). Delirium tremens often follows after withdrawal seizures and is a medical emergency. If untreated, death may occur as a result of respiratory or cardiovascular collapse. Management includes thiamine and other vitamin replacement, and a long-acting oral benzodiazepines (e.g. **chlordiazepoxide** or **diazepam**), given by mouth if possible. The initial dose requirement is determined empirically and is followed by a regimen of step-wise dose reduction over the

next two to three days. The patient should be nursed in a quiet environment with careful attention to fluid and electrolyte balance. Benzodiazepines (intravenous if necessary, Chapters 18 and 22) are usually effective in terminating prolonged withdrawal seizures – if they are ineffective the diagnosis should be reconsidered (e.g. is there evidence of intracranial haemorrhage or infection). Psychiatric assessment and social support are indicated once the withdrawal syndrome has receded.

Key points

Delirium tremens

- Mortality is 5–10%.
- There is a state of acute confusion and disorientation associated with frightening hallucinations and sympathetic overactivity. Delirium tremens occurs in less than 10% of alcoholic patients withdrawing from alcohol.
- Management includes:
  - nursing in a quiet, evenly illuminated room;
  - sedation (either clomethiazole or diazepam);
  - vitamin replacement with adequate thiamine;
  - correction of fluid and electrolyte balance;
  - psychiatric referral.

Long-term management of the alcoholic

Psychological and social management: Some form of psychological and social management is important to help the patient to remain abstinent. Whatever approach is used, the focus has to be on abstinence from alcohol. A very small minority of patients may be able to take up controlled drinking subsequently, but it is impossible to identify this group prospectively, and this should not be a goal of treatment. Voluntary agencies such as Alcoholics Anonymous are useful resources and patients should be encouraged to attend them.

Alcohol-sensitizing drugs: These produce an unpleasant reaction when taken with **alcohol**. The only drug of this type used to treat alcoholics is **disulfiram**, which inhibits aldehyde dehydrogenase, leading to acetaldehyde accumulation if **alcohol** is taken, causing flushing, sweating, nausea, headache, tachycardia and hypotension. Cardiac dysrhythmias may occur if large amounts of **alcohol** are consumed. The small amounts of **alcohol** included in many medicines may be sufficient to produce a reaction and it is advisable for the patient to carry a card warning of the danger of **alcohol** administration. **Disulfiram** also inhibits **phenytoin** metabolism and can lead to **phenytoin** intoxication. Unfortunately, there is only weak evidence that **disulfiram** has any benefit in the treatment of alcoholism. Its use should be limited to highly selected individuals in specialist clinics.

Acamprosate: The structure of **acamprosate** resembles that of GABA and glutamate. It appears to reduce the effects of excitatory amino acids and, combined with counselling, it may help to maintain abstinence after **alcohol** withdrawal.

Interactions of alcohol with other drugs

Alcohol potentiates the effects of other CNS depressants (e.g. benzodiazepines). Increased metabolism of **warfarin** and **phenytoin** have been reported in alcoholics. **Alcohol** enhances the gastric irritation caused by **aspirin**, **indometacin** and other gastric irritants. **Disulfiram**-type reactions (flushing of the face, tachycardia, sweating, breathlessness, vomiting and hypotension) have been reported with **metronidazole, chlorpropamide** and **trichloroethylene** (industrial exposure). Enhanced hypoglycaemia may occur following coadministration of **alcohol** with **insulin** and oral hypoglycaemic agents.

BARBITURATES

Thiopental is currently used i.v. to induce general anaesthesia and to treat refractory status epilepticus. Earlier therapeutic uses of barbiturates as hypnotics and anxiolytics are obsolete. Tolerance with physical and psychological dependence occurred after chronic administration. Central effects are similar to **alcohol**. During withdrawal, convulsions are more often seen in barbiturate-dependent patients than in those dependent on alcohol. Barbiturate overdoses were commonly fatal due to respiratory depression and/or asphyxia. **Chloral hydrate** and **clomethiazole** have similar potential for dependence, and their use is difficult to justify.

BENZODIAZEPINES

For more information on benzodiazepines, see Chapter 18.

SOLVENTS

Solvent abuse is common in adolescents. It is often part of more widespread antisocial behaviour. A dependence syndrome has not been identified. Solvents such as glues or paints are sniffed, often with the aid of a plastic bag to increase the concentration of vapour. The effect may be enhanced by reduced oxygen and occur almost instantly (because of the rapid absorption of volatile hydrocarbons from the lungs) and usually resolve within 30 minutes. Disinhibition can lead to excessively gregarious, aggressive or emotional behaviour. Some sniffers just vomit. Accidents are common; coma and asphyxiation occur. Cardiac dysrhythmia can occur (as with hydrocarbon anaesthetics, Chapter 24). Most deaths are associated with asphyxia as a result of aerosol inhalations or bags placed over the head. Excessive chronic use is rare, but may lead to major organ failure, as well as permanent brain damage. There are no specific drug therapies for solvent abusers and psychological and/or social management is required.

MISCELLANEOUS

ANABOLIC STEROIDS

Anabolic steroids are abused by athletes in order to build up muscle tissue. Most synthetic anabolic steroids are derived from **testosterone** and are popular among body builders. The prevalence of anabolic steroid abuse among athletes is uncertain. It is likely that chronic use is associated with hypertension, unusual hepatic and renal tumours, psychotic reactions and

depression on withdrawal, and possibly sudden death from cardiac dysrhythmias. Other 'performance-enhancing' drugs, usually of doubtful benefit but with side effects, include **human chorionic gonadotrophin**, **growth hormone**, **caffeine**, amphetamines, β-blockers and **erythropoietin**.

AMYL NITRATE AND BUTYL NITRATE

These inhaled drugs cause almost instant vasodilatation, hypotension, tachycardia and a subjective 'rush'. They are claimed to enhance sexual pleasure and dilate the anus. The hypotension can cause coma and frequent use of these drugs is associated with methaemoglobinaemia. They work via cGMP, so combination with **sildenafil** (Chapter 41) results predictably in dangerously enhanced vasodilatation and hypotension.

GAMMA-HYDROXYBUTYRIC ACID (GHB)

GHB is a 'popular' drug of abuse whose effects may include euphoria, sedation, amnesia (implicated as 'date rape' drug), aggression, vomiting, coma, respiratory depression and seizure. Management is supportive. **Atropine** may be required to treat bradycardia.

Case history

A 70-year-old man is admitted with confusion, nystagmus and ophthalmoplegia. His breath does not smell of alcohol. Laboratory tests reveal a raised mean corpuscular volume (MCV) and gamma-glutamyl transferase (GT), but are otherwise unremarkable.
Question 1
What is the likely diagnosis?
Question 2
What does the initial treatment involve?
Answer 1
Wernicke's encephalopathy.
Answer 2
Intravenous thiamine.

Case history

A 20-year-old man is brought by the police to the Accident and Emergency Department unconscious. The police believe that he ingested condoms full of diamorphine prior to his arrest following a drugs raid. He had been in police custody for approximately one hour. On examination he is centrally cyanosed, breathing irregularly, with pinpoint pupils and no response to painful stimuli. There is bruising over many venepuncture sites.
Question 1
What is the immediate management?
Question 2
Abdominal radiography reveals six unbroken condoms in the patient's intestine. Is surgery indicated?
Answer 1
Give oxygen, maintain an airway and give intravenous naloxone.
Answer 2
Since naloxone is an effective antidote to diamorphine poisoning, close observation with repeated injections or infusion of naloxone, inhaled oxygen and bulk laxatives should be sufficient.

FURTHER READING

Goldman D, Oroszi G, Ducci F. The genetics of addictions: Uncovering the genes. *Nature Reviews. Genetics* 2005; **7**: 521–32.

Green AR, Mechan AO, Elliott JM et al. The pharmacology and clinical pharmacology of 3, 4-methylenedioxymethamphetamine. *Pharmacological Reviews* 2003; **55**: 463–508.

Hall AP, Henry JA. Acute toxic effects of ecstasy (MDMA) and related compounds. *British Journal of Anaesthesia* 2006; **6**: 675–85.

Mottram DR (ed.). *Drugs in sport*, 4th edn. London: Routledge, 2005.

Winger G, Woods JH, Hofmann FG. *A handbook of drug and alcohol abuse*, 4th edn. Oxford: Oxford University Press, 2004.

CHAPTER 54

DRUG OVERDOSE AND POISONING

INTENTIONAL SELF-POISONING

Self-poisoning creates 10% of the workload of Accident and Emergency departments in the UK. Opioids (diamorphine (heroin), morphine and methadone), compound analgesics (e.g. **codeine** plus paracetamol), paracetamol alone and antidepressants are the most common drugs used in fatal overdose. **Temazepam**, **cocaine**, **MDMA/ecstasy**, lithium, **paraquat**, salicylates, **digoxin** and **aminophylline** continue to cause fatalities. This list of agents that cause death from overdose does not reflect the drugs on which individuals most commonly overdose. Self-poisoning often involves multiple drugs and alcohol. Benzodiazepines (often taken with alcohol) are commonly taken in an overdose, but are seldom fatal if taken in isolation. Around 75% of deaths from overdose occur outside hospital, with the mortality of those treated in hospital being less than 1%. The majority of cases of self-poisoning fall into the psychological classification of suicidal gestures (or a cry for help). However, the prescription of potent drugs with a low therapeutic ratio can cause death from an apparently trivial overdose.

DIAGNOSIS

HISTORY

Self-poisoning may present as an unconscious patient being delivered to the Accident and Emergency Department with or without a full history available from the patient or their companions. Following an immediate assessment of vital functions, as full a history as possible should be obtained from the patient, relatives, companions and ambulance drivers, as appropriate. A knowledge of the drugs or chemicals that were available to the patient is invaluable. Some patients in this situation give an unreliable history. A psychiatric history, particularly of depressive illness, previous suicide attempts or drug dependency, is relevant.

EXAMINATION

A meticulous, rapid but thorough clinical examination is essential not only to rule out other causes of coma or abnormal behaviour (e.g. head injury, epilepsy, diabetes, hepatic encephalopathy), but also because the symptoms and signs may be characteristic of certain poisons. The clinical manifestations of some common poisons are summarized in Table 54.1. The effects may be delayed.

LABORATORY TESTS

Routine investigation of the comatose overdose patient should include blood glucose (rapidly determined by stick testing) and biochemical determination of plasma electrolytes,

Table 54.1: Clinical manifestations of some common poisons

Symptoms/signs of acute overdose	Common poisons
Coma, hypotension, flaccidity	Benzodiazepines and other hypnosedatives, alcohol
Coma, pinpoint pupils, hypoventilation	Opioids
Coma, dilated pupils, hyper-reflexia, tachycardia	Tricyclic antidepressants, phenothiazines; other drugs with anticholinergic properties
Restlessness, hypertonia, hyper-reflexia, pyrexia	Amphetamines, MDMA, anticholinergic agents
Convulsions	Tricyclic antidepressants, phenothiazines, carbon monoxide, monoamine oxidase inhibitors, mefenamic acid, theophylline, hypoglycaemic agents, lithium, cyanide
Tinnitus, overbreathing, pyrexia, sweating, flushing, usually alert	Salicylates
Burns in mouth, dysphagia, abdominal pain	Corrosives, caustics, paraquat

MDMA, methylenedioxymethylamphetamine.

Table 54.2: Common indications for emergency measurement of drug concentration.

Suspected overdose	Effect on management
Paracetamol	Administration of antidotes – acetylcysteine or methionine
Iron	Administration of antidote – desferrioxamine
Methanol/ethylene glycol	Administration of antidote – ethanol or fomepizole with or without dialysis
Lithium	Dialysis
Salicylates	Simple rehydration or alkaline diuresis or dialysis
Theophylline	Necessity for intensive care unit (ITU) admission

Table 54.3: Gastric aspiration and lavage

1. If the patient is unconscious, protect airway with cuffed endotracheal tube. If semiconscious with effective gag reflex, place the patient in the head-down, left-lateral position. An anaesthetist with effective suction must be present
2. Place the patient's head over the end/side of the bed, so that their mouth is below their larynx
3. Use a wide-bore lubricated orogastric tube
4. Confirm that the tube is in the stomach (not the trachea) by auscultation of blowing air into the stomach; save the first sample of aspirate for possible future toxicological analysis (and possible direct identification of tablets/capsules)
5. Use 300 –600 mL of tap water for each wash and repeat three to four times. Continue if ingested tablets/capsules are still present in the final aspirate
6. Unless an oral antidote is to be administered, leave 50 g of activated charcoal in the stomach

urea, creatinine, oxygen saturation and arterial blood gases. Drug screens are often requested, although they are rarely indicated as an emergency.

Table 54.2 lists those drugs where the clinical state of a patient may be unhelpful in determining the severity of the overdose in the acute stages. In these, emergency measurement of the plasma concentration can lead to life-saving treatment. For example, in the early stages, patients with **paracetamol** overdoses are often asymptomatic, and although it only rarely causes coma acutely, patients may have combined **paracetamol** with alcohol, a hypnosedative or an opioid. As such, an effective antidote (**acetylcysteine**) is available, it is recommended that the **paracetamol** concentration should be measured in all unconscious patients who present as cases of drug overdose.

When there is doubt about the diagnosis, especially in coma, samples of blood, urine and (when available) gastric aspirate should be collected. Subsequent toxicological screening may be necessary if the cause of the coma does not become apparent or recovery does not occur. Avoidable morbidity is more commonly due to a missed diagnosis, such as head injury, than to failure to diagnose drug-induced coma.

PREVENTION OF FURTHER ABSORPTION

Syrup of ipecacuanha is no longer recommended in the management of poisoning.

Gastric aspiration and lavage should only be performed if the patient presents within one hour of ingestion of a potentially fatal overdose. If there is any suppression of the gag reflex, a cuffed endotracheal tube is mandatory. Gastric lavage is unpleasant and is potentially hazardous. It should only be performed by experienced personnel with efficient suction apparatus close at hand (see Table 54.3).

If the patient is uncooperative and refuses to give consent, this procedure cannot be performed. Gastric lavage is usually contraindicated following ingestion of corrosives and acids, due to the risk of oesophageal perforation and following ingestion of hydrocarbons, such as white spirit and petrol, due to the risk of aspiration pneumonia.

An increasingly popular method of reducing drug/toxin absorption is by means of oral activated charcoal, which adsorbs drug in the gut. To be effective, large amounts of charcoal are required, typically ten times the amount of poison ingested, and again timing is critical, with maximum effectiveness being obtained soon after ingestion. Its effectiveness is due to its large surface area ($>1000 \, m^2/g$). Binding of charcoal to the drug is by non-specific adsorption. Aspiration is a potential risk in a patient who subsequently loses consciousness or fits and vomits. Oral charcoal may also inactivate any oral antidote (e.g. **methionine**).

The use of repeated doses of activated charcoal may be indicated after ingestion of sustained-release medications or drugs with a relatively small volume of distribution, and prolonged elimination half-life (e.g. salicylates, **quinine, dapsone, carbamazepine**, barbiturates or **theophylline**). The rationale is that these drugs will diffuse passively from the bloodstream if charcoal is present in sufficient amounts in the gut or to trap drug that has been eliminated in bile from being re-absorbed (see below). Metal salts, alcohols and solvents are not adsorbed by activated charcoal.

Whole bowel irrigation using non-absorbable polyethylene glycol solution may be useful when large amounts of sustained-release preparations, iron or lithium tablets or packets of smuggled narcotics have been taken. Paralytic ileus is a contraindication.

SUPPORTIVE THERAPY

Patients are generally managed with intensive supportive therapy whilst the drug is eliminated naturally by the body. After an initial assessment of vital signs and instigation of appropriate resuscitation, repeated observations are necessary, as drugs may continue to be absorbed with a subsequent increase in plasma concentration. In the unconscious patient, repeated measurements of cardiovascular function, including blood pressure, urine output and (if possible) continuous electrocardiographic (ECG) monitoring should be performed. Plasma electrolytes and acid-base balance should be measured. Hypotension is the most common cardiovascular complication of poisoning. This is usually due to peripheral vasodilatation, but may be secondary to myocardial depression following, for example, α-blocker, tricyclic antidepressant or dextropropoxyphine poisoning. Hypotension can usually be managed with intravenous colloid. If this is inadequate, positive inotropic agents (e.g. **dobutamine**) may be considered. If dysrhythmias occur any hypoxia or hypokalaemia should be corrected, but anti-dysrhythmic drugs should only be administered in life-threatening situations. Since the underlying cardiac tissue is usually healthy (unlike cardiac arrests following myocardial infarction), prolonged external cardiopulmonary resuscitation whilst the toxic drug is excreted is indicated. Respiratory function is best monitored using blood gas analysis – a $PaCO_2$ of >6.5 kPa is usually an indication for assisted ventilation. Serial minute volume measurements or continuous measurement of oxygen saturation using a pulse oximeter are also helpful for monitoring deterioration or improvement in self-ventilation. Oxygen is not a substitute for inadequate ventilation. Respiratory stimulants increase mortality.

ENHANCEMENT OF ELIMINATION

Methods of increasing poison elimination are appropriate in less than 5% of overdose cases. Repeated oral doses of activated charcoal may enhance the elimination of a drug by 'gastro-intestinal dialysis'. Several drugs are eliminated in the bile and then reabsorbed in the small intestine. Activated charcoal can interrupt this enterohepatic circulation by adsorbing drug in the gut lumen, thereby preventing reabsorption and enhancing faecal elimination. Cathartics, such as **magnesium sulphate**, can accelerate the intestinal transit time, which facilitates the process. Orally administered activated charcoal adsorbs drug in the gut lumen and effectively leaches drug from the intestinal circulation into the gut lumen down a diffusion gradient. Although studies in volunteers have shown that this method enhances the elimination of certain drugs, its effectiveness in reducing morbidity in overdose is generally unproven. However, it is extremely safe unless aspiration occurs. Forced diuresis is hazardous, especially in the elderly, and is no longer recommended. Adjustment of urinary pH is much more effective than causing massive urine output. Alkaline diuresis (urinary alkalinization) should be considered in cases of **salicylate**, **chlorpropramide**, phenoxyacetate herbicides and **phenobarbital** poisoning, and may be combined with repeated doses of oral activated charcoal. Acid diuresis may theoretically accelerate drug elimination in **phencyclidine** and **amfetamine**/ 'ecstasy' poisoning. However, it is not usually necessary, may be harmful and is almost never recommended.

Table 54.4: Methods and indications for enhancement of poison elimination

Method	Poison
Alkaline diuresis	Salicylates, phenobarbital
Haemodialysis	Salicylates, methanol, ethylene glycol, lithium, phenobarbital
Charcoal haemoperfusion	Barbiturates, theophylline, disopyramide
'Gastro-intestinal dialysis' via multiple-dose activated charcoal	Salicylates, theophylline, quinine, most anticonvulsants, digoxin

Haemodialysis and, much less commonly, charcoal haemoperfusion are sometimes used to enhance drug elimination. Table 54.4 summarizes the most important indications and methods for such elimination techniques. In addition, exchange transfusion has been successfully used in the treatment of poisoning in young children and infants. The risk of an elimination technique must be balanced against the possible benefit of enhanced elimination.

SPECIFIC ANTIDOTES

Antidotes are available for a small number of poisons and the most important of these, including chelating agents, are summarized in Table 54.5.

NALOXONE

Naloxone is a pure opioid antagonist with no intrinsic agonist activity (Chapter 25). It rapidly reverses the effects of opioid drugs, including **morphine**, **diamorphine**, **pethidine**, **dextropropoxyphene** and **codeine**. When injected intravenously, **naloxone** acts within two minutes and its elimination half-life is approximately one hour. The plasma half-life of most opioid drugs is longer (e.g. 12–24 hours) and repeated doses or infusions of **naloxone** may be required. The usual dose is 0.8–1.2 mg, although much higher doses may be needed after massive opioid overdoses, which are common in addicts and especially after a partial agonist (e.g. **buprenorphine**) overdose, because partial agonists must occupy a relatively large fraction of the receptors compared to full agonists in order to produce even modest effects. **Naloxone** can precipitate withdrawal reactions in narcotic addicts. This is not a contraindication, but it is wise to ensure that patients are appropriately restrained if this is a risk.

MANAGEMENT OF SPECIFIC OVERDOSES

PARACETAMOL

This over-the-counter mild analgesic is commonly taken in overdose. Although remarkably safe in therapeutic doses,

Table 54.5: Antidotes and other specific measures.

Overdose drug	Antidote/other specific measures
Paracetamol	Acetylcysteine i.v.
	Methionine p. o.
Iron	Desferrioxamine
Cyanide	Oxygen, dicobalt edetate i.v. or sodium nitrite i.v. followed by sodium thiosulphate i.v.
Benzodiazepines	Flumazenil i.v.
Beta-blockers	Atropine
	Glucagon
	Isoprenaline
Carbon monoxide	Oxygen
	Hyperbaric oxygen
Methanol/ethylene glycol	Ethanol, Fomepizole
Lead (inorganic)	Sodium EDTA i.v.
	Penicillamine p.o.
	Dimercaptosuccinic acid (DMSA) i.v. or p.o.
Mercury	Dimercaptopropane sulphonate (DMPS)
	Dimercaptosuccinic acid (DMSA)
	Dimercaprol
	Penicillamine
Opioids	Naloxone
Organophosphorus insecticides	Atropine, pralidoxime
Digoxin	Digoxin-specific fab antibody fragments
Calcium-channel blockers	Calcium chloride or gluconate i.v.
Insulin	20% dextrose i.v.
	Glucagon i.v. or i.m.

Note: DMSA, DMPS and 4-methyl-pyrazole are not licensed in the UK.

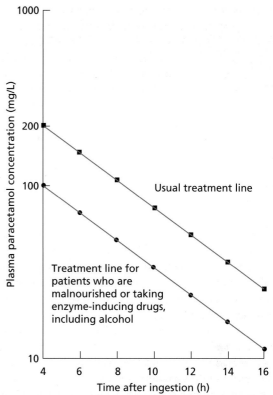

Figure 54.1: Treatment graph for paracetamol overdose. The graph provides guidance on the need for acetylcysteine treatment. The time (in hours) after ingestion is often uncertain. If in doubt – treat.

overdoses of 7.5 g or more may cause hepatic failure, less commonly renal failure, and death (for discussion of the mechanism involved see Chapter 5). The patient is usually asymptomatic at the time of presentation, but may complain of nausea and sweating. Right hypochondrial pain and anorexia may precede the development of hepatic failure. Coma is rare unless a sedative or opioid has been taken as well.

If a potentially toxic overdose is suspected, the stomach should be emptied if within one hour of ingestion. The antidote should be administered and blood taken for determination of **paracetamol** concentration, prothrombin time (INR), creatinine and liver enzymes. The decision to stop or continue the antidote can be made at a later time. The plasma **paracetamol**

concentration should be obtained urgently and related to the graph shown in Figure 54.1, which plots time from ingestion against plasma **paracetamol** concentration and probability of liver damage. A more precise treatment graph is printed in the British National Formulary (it is unreliable for staggered overdoses). If doubt exists concerning the time of ingestion it is better to err on the side of caution and give the antidote.

Intravenous **acetylcysteine** and/or oral **methionine** are potentially life-saving antidotes and are most effective if given within eight hours of ingestion; benefit is obtained up to 24 hours after ingestion. For serious **paracetamol** overdoses seen greater than 24 hours after ingestion, advice should be sought from poisons or liver specialists. **Acetylcysteine** is administered as an intravenous infusion. In approximately 5% of patients, pseudoallergic reactions occur, which are usually mild. If hypotension or wheezing occurs, it is recommended that the infusion be stopped and an antihistamine administered parenterally. If the reaction has completely resolved, **acetylcysteine** may be restarted at a lower infusion rate. Alternatively, **methionine** may be used (see below).

Patients who are taking enzyme-inducing drugs (e.g. **phenytoin**, **carbamazepine**) and chronic alcoholics are at a higher risk of hepatic necrosis following **paracetamol** overdose. The INR is the first indicator of hepatic damage. If the INR and serum creatinine are normal when repeated at least 24 hours after the overdose, significant hepatic or renal damage is unlikely.

Table 54.6: Urinary alkalinization regimen for aspirin

Indicated in adults with a salicylate level in the range 600–800 mg/L and in elderly adults and children with levels in the range 450–750 mg/L

Adults: 1 L of 1.26% sodium bicarbonate (isotonic) + 40 mmol KCl IV over 4 h, and/or 50-mL i.v. boluses of 8.5% sodium bicarbonate (*note*: additional KCl will be required)

Children: 1 mL/kg of 8.4% sodium bicarbonate (= 1 mmol/kg) + 20 mmol KCl diluted in 0.5 L of dextrose saline infused at 2–3 mL/kg/h

Source: National Poisons Information Service, Guy's and St Thomas' Trust London Centre.
Poisons information Services: UK National Poisons Information Services, Tel. 0844 892 0111, directs caller to relevant local centre.

Methionine is an effective oral antidote in **paracetamol** poisoning. It may be useful in remote areas where there will be a delay in reaching hospital or when **acetylcysteine** is contraindicated.

SALICYLATE

Patients poisoned with **salicylate** typically remain conscious, but in contrast to **paracetamol** overdose usually look and feel ill, The typical presentation includes nausea, tinnitus and hyperventilation and the patient is hot and sweating. Immediate management includes estimation of arterial blood gases, electrolytes, renal function, blood glucose (hypoglycaemia is particularly common in children) and plasma **salicylate** concentration. The patient is usually dehydrated and requires intravenous fluids. A stomach washout is performed, if within one hour of ingestion. Activated charcoal should be administered. Multiple dose activated charcoal is advised until the **salicylate** level has peaked. Blood gases and arterial pH normally reveal a mixed metabolic acidosis and respiratory alkalosis. Respiratory alkalosis frequently predominates and is due to direct stimulation of the respiratory centre. The metabolic acidosis is due to uncoupling of oxidative phosphorylation and consequent lactic acidosis. If acidosis predominates, the prognosis is poor. Absorption may be delayed and the plasma **salicylate** concentration can increase over many hours after ingestion. Depending on the **salicylate** concentration (see Table 54.6) and the patient's clinical condition, an alkaline diuresis should be commenced using intravenous sodium bicarbonate. However, this is potentially hazardous, especially in the elderly. Children metabolize **aspirin** less effectively than adults and are more likely to develop a metabolic acidosis and consequently are at higher risk of death. Plasma electrolytes, **salicylate** and arterial blood gases and pH must be measured regularly. **Sodium bicarbonate** acutely lowers plasma potassium, by shifting potassium ions into cells. Supplemental intravenous potassium may cause dangerous hyperkalaemia if renal function is impaired, so frequent monitoring of serum electrolytes is essential. If the **salicylate** concentration reaches 800–1000 mg/L, haemodialysis is likely to be necessary. Haemodialysis may also be life-saving at lower **salicylate** concentrations if the patient's metabolic and clinical condition deteriorates.

TRICYCLIC ANTIDEPRESSANTS

Tricyclic antidepressants cause death by dysrhythmias, myocardial depression, convulsions or asphyxia. If the patient reaches hospital alive they may be conscious, confused, aggressive or in deep coma. Clinical signs include dilated pupils, hyperreflexia and tachycardia. Following immediate assessment, resuscitation and ECG monitoring as necessary, blood should be taken for determination of arterial blood gases and electrolytes. Gastric lavage may be performed up to one hour after ingestion if the patient is fully conscious. ECG monitoring should be continued during this procedure and for at least 12 hours after clinical recovery.

The most common dysrhythmia is sinus tachycardia, predominantly due to anticholinergic effects and does not require any intervention. Broadening of the QRS complex can result from a **quinidine**-like (sodium ion blocking) effect and is associated with a poor prognosis. Anti-dysrhythmic prophylaxis should be limited to correction of any metabolic abnormalities, especially hypokalaemia, hypoxia and acidosis. Intravenous sodium bicarbonate (1–2 mmol/kg body weight) is the most effective treatment for the severely ill patient and its mode action may involve a redistribution of the drug within the tissues. Some centres recommend prophylactic bicarbonate and potassium to keep the pH in the range of 7.45–7.55 and the potassium concentration at the upper end of the normal range if the QRS duration is >100 ms or the patient is hypotensive despite intravenous colloid. If resistant ventricular tachycardia occurs, intravenous magnesium or overdrive pacing have been advocated. If ventricular tachycardia results in hypotension, DC shock is indicated. Convulsions should be treated with intravenous benzodiazepines. Oral benzodiazepines may be used to control agitation.

Occasionally, assisted ventilation is necessary.

SELECTIVE SEROTONIN REUPTAKE INHIBITORS

Substitution of selective serotonin reuptake inhibitors (SSRIs) in place of tricyclic antidepressants has reduced the mortality from antidepressant overdose. SSRIs do not have anticholinergic actions and are much less cardiotoxic. Nausea and diarrhoea are common. Seizures may occur and are associated with **venlafaxine** (which blocks noradrenaline, as well as serotonin reuptake, Chapter 20) overdose in particular.

Supportive and symptomatic measures are usually sufficient. Oral activated charcoal is recommended following the ingestion of more than ten tablets within one hour.

PARACETAMOL/DEXTROPROPOXYPHENE (CO-PROXAMOL) – *NOW DISCONTINUED*

It is usually the **dextropropoxyphene** that causes death from overdose with this mixture of **dextropropoxyphene** and **paracetamol**. The patient may present with coma, hypoventilation and pinpoint pupils. The cardiac toxicity includes a negative inotropic effect and dysrhythmias. Immediate cardiopulmonary resuscitation and intravenous **naloxone** are indicated. The plasma **paracetamol** concentration should be measured and **acetylcysteine** administered as shown in Figure 54.1. The

Commission on Human Medicines (CHM) has advised that **co-proxamol** should no longer be prescribed. Whilst overdose from other paracetamol–opioid compounds (e.g. **co-codamol**) may also present with coma, pinpoint pupils and hypoventilation, the cardiac toxicity should be markedly reduced.

CARBON MONOXIDE

This is a common cause of fatal poisoning. Carbon monoxide suicides are usually men under 65 years of age, who die from carbon monoxide generated from car exhaust fumes (catalytic converters reduce the carbon monoxide emission and this may have reduced the number of deaths). Accidental carbon monoxide poisoning is also common and should be considered in the differential diagnosis of confusional states, headache and vomiting, particularly in winter as a result of inefficient heaters and inadequate ventilation. Measurement of the carboxyhaemoglobin level in blood may be helpful. Carbon monoxide toxicity may also be present in survivors of fires. The immediate management consists of removal from exposure and administration of oxygen. There is evidence that hyperbaric oxygen speeds recovery and reduces neuropsychiatric complications.

> **Key points**
>
> Symptoms of accidental carbon monoxide poisoning
>
> - Headache, 90%
> - Nausea and vomiting, 50%
> - Vertigo, 50%
> - Alteration in consciousness, 30%
> - Subjective weakness, 20%
>
> *Source*: the Chief Medical Officer.

NON-DRUG POISONS

A vast array of plants, garden preparations, pesticides, household products, cosmetics and industrial chemicals may be ingested. Some substances, such as paraquat and cyanides, are extremely toxic, whilst many substances are non-toxic unless enormous quantities are consumed. It is beyond the scope of this book to catalogue and summarize the treatment of all poisons and the reader is strongly advised to contact one of the poisons information services (see Table 54.6 for telephone number) whenever any doubt exists as to toxicity management.

PSYCHIATRIC ASSESSMENT

It is important to assess the mental state of overdose patients following recovery. Although most patients take overdoses as a reaction to social or life events, some overdose patients are pathologically depressed or otherwise psychiatrically unwell and should be reviewed by a psychiatrist. In treating depression decisions regarding drug treatment involve a balance between the efficacy of the drug and the risk of further overdose. Selective serotonin reuptake inhibitors are safer alternatives to tricyclics.

> **Key points**
>
> Diagnosis of acute self-poisoning in comatose patients
>
> - History:
>   from companions, ambulance staff, available drugs/poisons, suicide note.
> - Examination:
>   immediate vital signs;
>   signs of non-poison causes of coma (e.g. intracerebral haemorrhage);
>   signs consistent with drug overdose (e.g. meiosis and depressed respiration due to opioid).
> - Investigation:
>   determine severity (e.g. blood gases, ECG);
>   determine paracetamol level to determine whether acetylcysteine is appropriate;
>   exclude metabolic causes of coma (e.g. hypoglycaemia);
>   diagnose specific drug/poison levels if this will affect management.
>
> *Note*: Acute overdose may mimic signs of brainstem death, yet the patient may recover if adequate supportive care is provided. Always measure the blood glucose concentration in an undiagnosed comatose patient.

ACCIDENTAL POISONING

Accidental poisoning with drugs causes between 10 and 15 deaths per annum in children. Most commonly, tablets were prescribed to the parents and left insecure in the household or handbag. Unfortunately, many drugs resemble sweets. Antidepressants are commonly implicated. The use of child-proof containers and patient education should reduce the incidence of these unnecessary deaths. Non-drug substances that cause significant poisoning in children include antifreeze, cleaning liquids and pesticides.

In adults, accidental poisoning most commonly occurs at work and usually involves inhalation of noxious fumes. Factory and farm workers are at particular risk. Carbon monoxide is associated with approximately 50 accidental deaths and seriously injures at least 200 individuals in the UK per year. The onset of symptoms is often insidious. There is particular concern in the UK about the effect of organophosphate pesticides, not only as a cause of acute poisoning, but also because it is possible that repeated exposure to relatively low doses may result in chronic neurological effects. Those working with sheep dip appear to be most at risk.

CRIMINAL POISONING

This is one mode of non-accidental injury of children. Homicidal poisoning is rare, but possibly underdiagnosed. There is increasing concern that terrorists may use poisons such as nerve agents. Cross-contamination is an issue. 'NAAS pods' are available for emergencies. Specialist advice should be sought from the National Poisons Information Service (0844 892 0111). Suspicion is the key to diagnosis and toxicological screens are invaluable.

Case history

A 21-year-old student is brought into your Accident and Emergency Department having been at a party with his girlfriend. She reports that he drank two non-alcoholic drinks, but had also taken 'some tablets' that he had been given by a stranger at the party. Within about one hour he started to act oddly, becoming uncoordinated, belligerent and incoherent. When you examine him, he is semi-conscious, responding to verbal commands intermittently. During the period when you are interviewing/examining him, he suddenly sustains a non-remitting grand-mal seizure.

Question 1
What are the agents he is most likely to have taken?
Question 2
How would you treat him?
Answer 1
The most likely agents that could have caused an altered mental status and then led to seizures are:

- sympathomimetics (e.g. amphetamines, cocaine, MDMA);
- hallucinogens: LSD, phencyclidine (PCP) – (latter unusual in the UK).
- tricyclic antidepressants;
- selective serotonin reuptake inhibitors.

Much less likely causes are:

- antihistamines (especially first-generation antihistamines in high dose; these are available over the counter);
- theophylline;
- ethanol and ethylene glycol can also do this, but are unlikely in this case, because of the patient's girlfriend's account of events.

Answer 2
This patient should be treated as follows:

1. Ensure a clear airway with adequate oxygenation – avoid aspiration.
2. Ensure that other vital functions are adequate.
3. Prevent him from injuring himself (e.g. by falls (off a trolley) or flailing limbs).
4. Give therapy to stop the epileptic fit:
   diazepam, 10 mg i.v. and repeat if necessary;
   if the patient is refractory to this, consider thiopental anaesthesia and ventilation.
5. Monitor the patient closely, including ECG, and observe for respiratory depression and further seizures. Attempt to define more clearly which agent he ingested to allow further appropriate toxicological management.

Case history

A 20-year-old known heroin addict who is HIV-, hepatitis C- and hepatitis B-positive is brought to the Accident and Emergency Department. It is winter and there is a major flu epidemic in the area. He is certified dead on arrival. Many old venepuncture sites and one recent one are visible on his arms. He does not appear cyanosed.

The history from his girlfriend, also a heroin addict, is that he was released from prison one week earlier and they moved into an old Victorian flat. They had tried to stay off heroin for one week (he had obtained a limited supply while in prison), but both had experienced headaches, nausea, vomiting, stomach cramps, tremor and diarrhoea.
The patient had told his girlfriend that he had to have some heroin. She left the flat for six hours to pick up her unemployment benefit, and returned home to find him prostrate on the floor with a syringe and needle beside him. She called an ambulance and attempted to resuscitate him with CPR and an amphetamine.
Question
Name two possible causes of death.
Answer
Carbon monoxide poisoning and heroin overdose.
Comment
Some of this patient's symptoms are not typical of heroin withdrawal, but are characteristics of carbon monoxide poisoning. His flatmate should be examined neurologically, a sample taken for carboxyhaemoglobin and the flat inspected. Oxygen is the antidote to carbon monoxide poisoning, and naloxone is the antidote to heroin poisoning.

FURTHER READING

Afshari R, Good AM, Maxwell SRJ. Co-proxamol overdose is associated with a 10-fold excess mortality compared with other paracetamol combination analgesics. *British Journal of Clinical Pharmacology* 2005; **60**: 444–7.

Bateman DN, Gorman DR, Bain M. Legislation restricting paracetamol sales and patterns of self-harm and death from paracetamol-containing preparations in Scotland. *British Journal of Clinical Pharmacology* 2006; **62**: 573–81.

Friberg LE, Isbister GK, Duffull SB. Pharmacokinetic-pharmacodynamic modelling of QT interval prolongation following citalopram overdoses *British Journal of Clinical Pharmacology* 2006; **61**: 177–90.

Hawton K, Simkin S, Gunnell D. A multicentre study of coproxamol poisoning suicides based on coroners' records in England. *British Journal of Clinical Pharmacology* 2005; **59**: 207–12.

Jones AL, Dargan PI. *Churchill's pocket book of toxicology*. London: Churchill Livingstone, 2001.

Jones AL, Volans G. Management of self-poisoning. *British Medical Journal* 1999; **319**: 1414–7.

Pakravan N, Mitchell AJ, Goddard J. Effect of acute paracetamol overdose on changes in serum electrolytes. *British Journal of Clinical Pharmacology* 2005; **59**: 650.

Stass H, Kubitza D, Moller JG. Influence of activated charcoal on the pharmacokinetics of moxifloxacin following intravenous and oral administration of a 400 mg single dose to healthy males. *British Journal of Clinical Pharmacology* 2005; **59**: 536–41.

INDEX

Note: Page numbers in *italics* refer to figures and tables.